COMPARATIVE ASPECTS OF TUMOR DEVELOPMENT

Cancer Growth and Progression

SERIES EDITOR: HANS E. KAISER

Department of Pathology, University of Maryland, Baltimore, Md, U.S.A.

Scientific Advisors:

Kenneth W. Brunson / Harvey A. Gilbert / Ronald H. Goldfarb / Alfred L. Goldson / Elizier Gorelik / Anton Gregl / Ronald B. Herberman / James F. Holland / Ernst H. Krokowski [†] / Arthur S. Levine / Annabel G. Liebelt / Lance A. Liotta / Seoras D. Morrison / Takao Ohnuma / Richard L. Schilsky / Harold L. Stewart / Jerome A. Urban / Elizabeth K. Weisburger / Paul V. Woolley

Comparative Aspects of Tumor Development

Edited by

HANS E. KAISER

Department of Pathology, University of Maryland
Baltimore, Md., U.S.A.

Kluwer Academic Publishers

DORDRECHT / BOSTON / LONDON

Library of Congress Cataloging in Publication Data
Comparative aspects of tumor development.

    (Cancer growth and progression ; v. 5)
    Includes index.
    1. Tumors--Growth. 2. Metastasis. 3. Carcinogenesis.
4. Pathology, Comparative. I. Kaiser, Hans E. (Hans
Elmar), 1928-   . II. Series. [DNLM: 1. Cell
Transformation, Neoplastic. 2. Histology, Comparative.
3. Neoplasm Invasiveness. 4. Neoplasm Metastasis.
QZ 200 C2151518 v.5]
RC269.C64 1988   616.99'2071   87-28252

ISBN-13:978-94-010-6981-6   e-ISBN-13:978-94-009-1091-1
DOI: 10.1007/978-3-94-009-1091-1

Published by Kluwer Academic Publishers,
P.O. Box 17, 3300 AA Dordrecht, The Netherlands.

Kluwer Academic Publishers incorporates
the publishing programmes of
Martinus Nijhoff, Dr W. Junk, D. Reidel, and MTP Press.

Sold and distributed in the U.S.A. and Canada
by Kluwer Academic Publishers,
101 Philip Drive, Norwell, MA 02061, U.S.A.

In all other countries, sold and distributed
by Kluwer Academic Publishers Group,
P.O. Box 322, 3300 AH Dordrecht, The Netherlands.

Cover design by Jos Vrolijk.

TABLE OF CONTENTS

B. ENVIRONMENTAL ONCOLOGY OR SPECIES-SPECIFIC ASPECTS OF ENVIRONMENTAL CHAIN REACTIONS

INTRODUCTION

In this volume, aspects of neoplastic spread, already elucidated in Volumes I–IV of this series, are considered against a broad biological background. The mammalian orders constituting the logical framework for man as focal point of a comparative oncology are reviewed. Selected examples of neoplastic progression in various taxonomic units are provided, beginning with the opposite pole of taxonomic development, the vascular plants, where no metastatis of malignant neoplasms occur. Among invertebrates, vertebrates, and vascular plants, lining membranes (epithelia) exhibit the highest degree of comparability. Metastases also occur, but more rarely, in invertebrates; and are discussed as they are found in the nonmammalian vertebrates: in fish, amphibians, reptiles, and birds. Diseases of the leukemia (leucosis)-lymphoma complex are present in invertebrates and particularly well-known in birds (Marek's disease) and, of course, in mammals, to name only some of the most important representatives. Taxonomic examples of the leukemia-lymphoma group are set forth in the separate chapters on aspects of progression in these tumor groups. The lymphatic system, very important in neoplastic distribution in man, is most highly developed in mammals, the only class of animals where the lymph nodes appear to be assigned an active role in tumor spread. The mammary gland, restricted to the mammals, exhibits high tumor regenerative potential in certain human population groups. Comparison of the interaction and relationship of both systems is challenging indeed.

The volume also reviews environmental oncology and species-specific aspects of environmental chain reactions. It is apparent that the environment plays a significant role in the development of neoplasms. Neoplasms among the species have become much more common as a result of man's impact on the environment. The latter chapters present a brief review of geologic and technologic and cultural changes, and the implications of species-specific cancer progression. The remainder of this section outlines a number of selected chain reactions leading to neoplastic development in certain members of these chains. A discussion of the storage of chemical carcinogens in plants and their interaction with other causes of neoplastic growth is also included. Activation and detoxification by gamefish can cause or stimulate the development of neoplasms if the contaminated fish are used as food. Moreover, terrestrial mammals also exhibit signs of chemical carcinogenesis. This volume therefore underscores the realities of water and oil pollution in man, the consumption of contaminated organisms by man and the impact of this phenomenon on cancer progression in various species.

Series/Volume Editor
Hans E. Kaiser

ACKNOWLEDGEMENT

Inspiration and encouragement for this wide ranging project on cancer distribution and dissemination from a comparative biological and clinical point of view, was given by my late friend E. H. Krokowski.

Those engaged on the project included 252 scientists, listed as contributors, volume editors and scientific advisors, and a dedicated staff. Special assistance was furnished by J. P. Dickson, J. A. Feulner, and I. Theloe.

I. Bauer, D. L. Fischer, S. Fleishman, K. Joshi, A. M. Lewis, J. Taylor and K. E. Ÿinug have provided additional assistance.

The firm support of the publisher, especially B. F. Commandeur, is deeply appreciated. The support of the University of Maryland throughout the preparation of the series is acknowledged.

To the completion of this undertaking my wife, Charlotte Kaiser, has devoted her unslagging energy and invaluable support.

CONTRIBUTORS

Miriam R. ANVER, Ph.D.
Clement Associates Inc.
1515 Wilson Boulevard
Arlington, Virginia 22209, USA

Thomas W. BEDNAR, Ph.D.
formerly Michigan Cancer Foundation
110 E Warren Ave.
Detroit, Michigan 48201, USA
mailing address:
P.O. Box 353
Western Springs, Illinois 60558, USA

Michael E. BENDER, Ph.D.
Virginia Institute of Marine Science
School of Marine Science
College of William and Mary
Gloucester Point, Virginia 23062, USA

Keith R. COOPER, Ph.D.
College of Pharmacy
Rutgers Medical School
College of Medicine & Dentistry
Piscataway, New Jersey 08854, USA

C. Austin FARLEY, Ph.D.
National Oceanographic and Aeronautical Administration
Biological Laboratory
National Marine Fishery Service
Oxford, Maryland 21654, USA

Torgeny N. FREDRICKSON, Ph.D.
U-89 Department of Pathology
University of Connecticut
Storrs, Connecticut 06268, USA

Howard M. HAYES, Jr. DVM
Environmental Epidemiology Branch
National Cancer Institute/National Institutes of Health
Landow Building, Bethesda, Maryland 20892, USA

Cornelia HOCH-LIGETI, M.D.[†]
Registry of Experimental Tumors
National Cancer Institute/National Institutes of Health
Bethesda, Maryland 20205, USA

Robert J. HUGGETT, Ph.D.
Virginia Institute of Marine Science
School of Marine Science
College of William and Mary
Gloucester Point, Virginia 23062, USA

Harold E.B. HUMPHREY
Michigan Department of Public Health
3500 N. Logan
P.O. Box 30035
Lansing, Michigan 48909, USA

Elliott R. JACOBSON, DVM Ph.D.
College of Veterinary Medicine
J. Hillis Miller Health Center
University of Florida
Gainesville, Florida 32610, USA

Hans E. KAISER, D.Sc.
Department of Pathology
Sch of Medicine
University of Maryland
10 S. Pine Street
Baltimore, Maryland 21201, USA

Elfriede M. LINSMAIER-BEDNAR, Ph.D.
formerly Michigan Cancer Foundation
110 E Warren Avenue
Detroit, Michigan 48201, USA
mailing address:
P.O. Box 353
Western Springs, Illinois 60558, USA

Samuel V. MACHOTKA, II, DVM
Hazleton Laboratories America, Inc.
9200 Leesburg Turnpike
Vienna, Virginia 22180, USA

Bruce B. McCAIN, Ph.D.
Northwest and Alaska Fisheries Center
Environmental Conservation Division and National
Oceanographic and Aeronautical Administration
2725 Montlake Boulevard
East Seattle, Washington 98112, USA

Wim MISDORP, M.D.
Antoni van Leeuwenhoek Hospital of the Netherlands
  Cancer Institute
Plesmanlaan 121
Amsterdam, The Netherlands

Takao MORI, Ph.D.
Zoological Institute
Faculty of Science
University of Tokyo Bunkyo-Tokyo, 113, Japan

Ryozo MORIGUCHI, DVM
Hokkaido University
Faculty of Veterinary Medicine
Sapporo 060, Japan

[†] deceased May 17th 1986

Mark S. MYERS, Ph.D.
Northwest and Alaska Fisheries Center
Environmental Conservation Division
National Oceanographic and Aeronautical Administration
2725 Montlake Boulevard
East Seattle, Washington 98112, USA

Hiroshi NAGASAWA, Ph.D., M.D.
Experimental Animal Research Laboratory
Meiji University 5158 Ikuta
Tama-ku Kawasaki
Kanagawa 214, Japan

William L. PENGELLY, Ph.D.
Department of Chemical
Biological and Environmental Sciences
Oregon Graduate Center
19600 Von Neumann Drive
Beaverton, Oregon 97006, USA

H. Graham PURCHASE, Ph.D.
MPS, 207005 USDA BARC
West Beltsville, Maryland 20705, USA

Bernard SASS, DVM
Registry of Experimental Cancers/WHO Collaborating
Center for Reference on Tumours of Laboratory Animals
National Cancer Institute/National Institutes of Health
Bethesda, Maryland 20892, USA

Jagden M. SHARMA, Ph.D.
Regional Poultry Research Laboratory
Agricultural Research Service
USDA, 3606 E. Mount Hope Road
East Lansing, Michigan 48823, USA

Theodora STEINECK, DVM
Forschungsinstitut für Wildtierkunde,
der Veterinärmedizinischen Universität Wien
(Research institute about free ranging animals
Veterinary University of Vienna)
Savoyenstrasse 1, A-1160 Vienna, Austria

Harold L. STEWART, M.D.
Registry of Experimental Cancers/WHO Collaborating
Center for Reference on Tumours of Laboratory Animals
National Cancer Institute/National Institutes of Health
Bethesda, Maryland 20892, USA

E. Tom THORNE, DVM
Wyoming State Veterinary Laboratory
University of Wyoming
P.O. Box 250
Laramie, Wyoming 82070, USA

Elizabeth S. WILLIAMS, DVM, Ph.D.
Wyoming State Veterinary Laboratory
University of Wyoming
P.O. Box 950
Laramie, Wyoming 82979, USA

NEOPLASTIC DISSEMINATION AND SPREADING FROM THE VIEWPOINT OF COMPARATIVE PATHOLOGY: DIFFERENCES AND SIMILARITIES BETWEEN ANIMALS AND PLANTS

H.E. KAISER

Neoplastic growth is bound to certain requirements of the particular host species in which it develops; this, especially, is the case for the progression and spread of secondary tumors, caused either by direct spread or local recurrence of the primary tumor or by metastasis. Neoplastic cells with anarchistic autonomous character are derived from normal host cells, which are now attacked by the anarchistic cells. Because the cells of the host transmit certain characteristics to the neoplastic daughter cells, it is the host of the tumor that provides the basis for each neoplastic development.

Since man is the species of which we know the most with regards to the progression of neoplastic diseases, we shall examine this phenomenon briefly in man first before we consider basic aspects of variations as they occur in other organisms, like animals and plants.

Neoplastic growth is bound to cells which have been transformed from normal body cells in any given species. It is not surprising, therefore, that differences, such as condition of the cell wall in contrast to the nakedness of animal cells, or the motility of cells in different organisms will have an effect on neoplastic progression.

As a basis for further evaluation of the problem let us first summarize the main ways of tumor spreading in the mammal.

VARIATIONS IN METASTATIC SPREADING IN THE MAMMALIAN BODY

1. Direct spreading without separation from the primary growth during progression of the process.
2. Metastasis
   (1) Spreading via tissue spaces
   (2) Hematogenous spreading via the channels of the circulatory system
   (3) Spreading via the lymphatic system, including the thoracic duct
   (4) Transcoelomic metastasis and by way of serous membranes
   (5) Spreading via implantation at epithelial surfaces
   (6) Metastasis from teratomas.

The following selected factors of the host are important for the spread of secondary neoplastic growth:
1. Tissue spectrum and phylogenetic age of tissues
2. Differences in the body fluids of animals and plants

3. Possibility of neoplastic spread in various eumetazoan groups
4. Possibility of spreading in acoelomates
5. Spreading in pseudocoelomates
6. Spreading in coelomates
7. Spreading in animals with no circulatory system
8. Spreading in animals with open circulatory system
9. Spreading in animals with mixed circulatory system
10. Spreading in animals with closed circulatory system
11. Immune system
12. Endocrine systems
13. Species–specific life span
14. Continued or catastrophic ontogenetic development
15. Chronobiologic factors (rhythms)
16. Genetic factors
17. Angiogenesis

The following selected factors of malignant cells are important for secondary growth:
1. Cell membrane or cell wall
2. Cell biochemistry
3. Mobility of cells
4. Cell consistency
5. Enzyme destruction of tissues
6. Detachment of neoplastic cells
7. Invasion of malignant cells

The following selected factors of both host and malignant cells are important in spreading:
1. Cell membrane
2. Tumor pressure

Abnormal growth processes have been observed in many species of animals and plants; most have been found in man. They may be diagnosed as curiosities if found unexpectedly in rarely observed species.

For an understanding of the genesis of these tumors and tumor-like structures the comparative pathologist needs to know about some aspects of comparative cytology and histology as well. An understanding of the composition of the different body plans of organisms is a precondition for a meaningful evaluation of growth processes which have produced tumors or tumor-like structures. In this chapter, selected examples of comparative oncology will be interpreted. Questions such as angiogenesis and others have been discussed in depth in other chapters.

H. E. Kaiser (ed.), Comparative aspects of tumor development.

Table 1. Distribution of tissues by number of phyla and species.

Type of Tissue	Number of Phyla	Approximate No. of Species
1. Simple squamous epithelium	10	1,200,000*
2. Stratified squamous epithelium	2	45,000
3. Simple cuboidal epithelium	20	1,200,000**
4. Simple columnar epithelium	26	1,203,000**
5. Pseudostratified columnar epithelium	2	45,250
6. Stratified cuboidal epithelium	1	45,000
7. Stratified columnar epithelium	1	45,000
8. Transitional epithelium	1	45,000
9. Sebaceous and sweat glands	1	5,000
10. Mammary glands	1	5,000
11. Salivary glands	10	1,154,000
12. Liver and hepatic portion of hepatopancreas	6	1,151,000
13. Exocrine portion of pancreas and pancreatic portion of hepatopancreas	3	1,145,000
14. Islets of Langerhans	1	less than 45,000
15. Pineal gland	1	less than 45,000
16. Pituitary gland	1	less than 45,000
17. Thyroid gland	1	less than 45,000
18. Parathyroid/ultimobranchial gland	1	less than 45,000
19. Adrenal cortex and medulla	1	less than 45,000
20. Testis	32	1,500,000
21. Ovary	32	1,500,000
22. Optic gland (cephalopoda)	1	600
23. Y-organs (crustacea)	1	20,000
24. Androgenic glands (crustacea)	1	20,000
25. Corpora allata (insecta)	1	1,000,000
26. Thoracic glands (insecta)	1	1,000,000
27. Ventral glands (insecta)	1	1,000,000
28. Desmal epithelium	19	1,167,000
29. Desmal epithelia/synovial origin	1	45,000
30. Mesenchyme	11	1,185,000
31. Spinocellular connective tissue	1	10,000
32. Reticular connective tissue	20?	1,200,000
33. Gelatinous connective tissue	1+	10,000+
34. Loose connective tissue	30	1,300,000
35. Fibrous connective tissue	5+	50,000+
36. Melanogenic system	30	1,300,000
37. Adipose tissue	20	1,200,000
38. Chordal tissue	4	50,000
39. Chondroid tissue	7+	100,000?
40. Cartilage	4+	1,100,000
41. Bone	1	45,000
42. Myoepithelial tissue	5	59,400
43. Smooth musculature	20	?
44. Helically striated musculature	7+	?
45. Transverse striated musculature	7	1,000,000–7,000,000
46. Cardiac musculature	2	50,000
47. Neurons of the central nervous system	4	1,154,000
48. Neurons of the peripheral nervous system	31	1,500,000?
49. Autonomous nervous system and chromaffin tissue	?	?
50. Meninges	?	?
51. Choroid tissue	?	?
52. Central glia	4	+800,000?
53. Peripheral glia	±25	+1,000,000?
54. Neurosecretory cells/tissue	31	1,500,000
55. Neurohemal structures of nemertinea	1	?
56. Cerebrovascular complex (annelida)	1	9,000
57. Neural perineum (mollusca)	1	100,000
58. Organ juxtacomissural (amphineura, polyplacophora)	1	?
59. Organesjuxtaganglionaires (proso- and opisthobranchia)	1	?
60. Dorsal bodies and comparative structures (pulmonata)	1	?
61. Neurohemal organs of arachnida	1	?
62. Sinus glands (crustacea)	1	20,000
63. Postcommissural organs (crustacea)	1	20,000

Table 1. *Continued*

Type of Tissue	Number of Phyla	Approximate No. of Species
64. Pericardial organs (crustacea)	1	20,000
65. Cerebral glands (chilopoda, diplopoda)	1	
66. Corpora cardiaca of insecta	1	1,000,000
67. Perisympathetic organs of insecta	1	(1,000,000)
68. Plectenchymata	2	20,000 ±
69. Pseudoparenchymata	?	
70. Phylloid, cauloid, or rhizoid true tissues	1	20,000 ±
71. True tissues of bryophyta	1	
72. Apical meristems	1	251,000 +
73. Lateral meristem	1	250,000 +
74. Meristemoids	1	250,000 +
75. Succeeding meristems	1	251,000 +
76. Phellogen	1	250,000 +
77. Phytoepidermis	1	251,000 +
78. Rhizodermis	1	251,000 +
79. Collenchyma	1	251,000 +
80. Sclerenchyma	1	250,000 +
81. Xylem	1	251,000 +
82. Phloem	1	251,000 +
83. Periderm	1	250,000 +
84. Secretory structures	1	250,000 +

After Kaiser, 1981. (p. 653)

SELECTED FACTORS OF THE HOST

1. The tissue spectrum (Table 1)

Phylogenetically, animal tissues are older than plant tissues. According to the fossil content of respective layers, true animal tissues were present in the Cambrian period as proven by the index fossils of trilobites which belong to the arthropods. True plant tissues did not appear before the Silurian/Devonian periods.

Not only does the phylogenetic age of tissues vary in organisms but the distribution in genera and species is also dissimilar. The mesenchymatic stem cell in flatworms is able to produce only more differentiated connective tissue cells, whereas the mesenchymatic stem cell in certain annelids is able to produce only more differentiated connective tissue cells, and, additionally, also cartilage. In the chordates chondroid tissue is a new potential addition. The mesenchymatic stem cell has its highest potential in vertebrates and especially in mammals, where it also produces bone. The distribution of some tissues can be explained by the phylogenetic age of the organisms concerned. The theoretical spectrum indicating which neoplasms can be expected to occur in a number of species varies drastically. The insects with the highest species number have striated musculature; thus, the theoretical tumor potential of rhabdomyosarcoma is very large because of the many species which have transverse striated musculature. Cartilage, in contrast, is distributed in more phyla but in a smaller species number, being present in molluscs, annelids, arthropods, and several phyla of chordates. The theoretical tumor spectrum of cartilage is more diffused in the phyla but more rare in the species number. Chordal tissue is restricted to the chordate phyla. As the phylogenetically youngest tissue, bone occurs only in oste-

ichthyes, amphibians, reptiles, mammals, and birds. To date neoplasms have not yet been found in all the taxonomic units where they may occur potentially. The value of the theoretical tumor spectrum lies in the fact that it tells us in which phyla and species a tumor may not occur, simply because neoplasms develop by differentiation from tissues only present in phyla and species.

2. Body fluids

In animals and man, body fluids are very important for the spreading of cancer. In plants, body fluids play no role whatsoever. Their movement can be compared to two parallel one-way streets, running in different directions. Plant body fluids (with a few exceptions, such as in the milk of the coconut), contain no floating cells. The circulatory systems in animals also show distinct variations, but basically, they can be compared to a circle. In animals and man, the body fluids contain floating cells among the metastatic tumor cells which are distributed like leukocytes (see Chapter 15/Vol IV).

3. Vessels

Where present, vessels in animals are always composed of living tissues which exhibit permeability for certain cells, like plasma cells. The vascular system of the plants is composed of xylem and phloem, both of which are divided into several types of cells, either alive or nonliving. The vessels of vascular plants differ from those of animals through the thickness of the cell walls, thus preventing penetration by other cells.

Table 2. Review of circulatory types in animals and plants.

	Animals
Type of circulation	*Selected animal phyla*
Missing circulatory system	Platyhelminthes, Acanthocephala, Tardigrada
Open circulatory system	Mollusca, Arthropoda, Echinodermata
Mixed circulatory system	Mollusca: Pulmonata, Cephalopoda
Closed circulatory system	Nemertinea, Annelida, Vertebrata

Plants	
The vascular system of plants is composed of two "one-way" systems	*Plant groups*
Xylem (water conduction)	vascular plants
Phloem (food conduction)	vascular plants

Source:

Esau, K. (2nd ed.). *Plant Anatomy*, New York–London–Sydney: Wiley & Sons, Inc., 1965.

Strasburger, E. (31st edition). *Lehrbuch der Botanik*, Jena: Gustav Fischer 1978.

4. The possibility of neoplastic spreading in acoelomates

It is not easy to distinguish between regenerative or possible neoplastic processes in these small animals. The organs of acoelomates are embedded in connective tissue and they have no space between body wall and internal organs. Neoplastic dissemination could take place only by a process as we know it of plasma cells in their body. Circulating neoplastic cells cannot occur. If present in these phyla, the simplest type of neoplastic distribution, tissue invasion, would be evident.

5. The pseudocoelom

In the animals of the pseudocoelomate phyla, a space exists between the body wall and the internal organs (Entoprocta, Acanthocephala, Rotifera, Gastrotricha, Kinorhyncha, Nematoda, Nematomorpha). In contrast to the coelomates, they do not have an epithelial layer covering the wall of the internal organs and the inside of the body wall. Neoplastic cells could be distributed, possibly by the pseudocoelomic fluids, in addition to movements between different cells of the body.

6. The coelom

The coelomic cavity, present in the majority of animals, develops as a space between the internal organs and the body wall of the organism; but the surfaces of the internal organs and the internal surface of the body wall are characterized by an epithelial lining. Tumors deriving from desmal epithelium are possible only in the coelomates; they include malignant mesothelioma, Kaposi's disease, hemangiothelioma (angiosarcoma), lymphangioendothelioma, and chemodectoma.

7. Eumetazoan animals without a circulatory system

Animals belonging in this group are either rather primitive or very small. Tumor distribution is only possible via tissue invasion.

8. Eumetazoan animals with an open circulatory system

These animals, as, for example, the arthropods, display a circulatory system which is, in general, composed of a vessel-like heart and sinuses. Their dorsal artery (heart) could exhibit diseases similar to the vessels in animals with a closed circulatory system. Otherwise, movement of floating cells occurs and a circulation of metastatic cells would be possible.

9. Eumetazoan animals with a mixed circulatory system

This type of circulatory system is present only in pulmonate and cephalopod molluscs and can be considered as an intermediate stage between the open and the closed circulatory systems in animals. It is composed of a general vessel (heart), sinuses, and additional vessels in other specific portions of the body. Metastasis via the circulatory sinuses and the vessels is possible.

10. Closed circulatory system in eumetazoan animals

Man is a representative of these species and metastasis, circulation of malignant cells, and detachment and attachment of malignant cells have been described in detail in other chapters.

11. The immune system

The phylogenetic development of the animals as indicated by current taxonomic classification shows a step-by-step development of the immunologic structures and functions. In low forms, immunologic compounds occur together with simple cells with phagocytic capability. Development leads to such complicated structures as the reticular endothelial system and the lymphatic system in vertebrates, especially mammals. Table 3 reviews the several taxonomic units.

12. The endocrine system

Endocrine structures occur in animals as well as in plants. In the latter, they are involved in such processes as bud development. In invertebrates, a wide variety of endocrine structures have been described together with their neurosecretory and hormonal actions. Best known are the corpora cardiaca, the corpora allata and the thoracic glands or their equivalents. The endocrine system of invertebrates and vertebrates is reviewed in Table 4.

Table 3. Immune systems in the various animal phyla.

Phylum	Immunologic characteristics
Coelenterata (Cnidaria)	primordial cell-mediated immunity
Ctenophora (Ctenaria)	antibiotic properties, cancer inhibiting factors
Platyhelminthes (flatworms)	transplantation immunity, resistance to x-rays
Nemertinea (ribbon worms)	nothing known
Gnathostomulida	nothing known
Entoprocta or Camptozoa	nothing known
Acanthocephala (thorny-headed worms)	scattered remarks in the literature
Rotifera (wheel animalcules)	response to dietary alpha-tocoprol
Gastrotricha	immunity reaction are unknown
Kinorhyncha (Echinodera)	no data reported
Nematoda (round worms)	immunity of nematodes against drugs and other effects*
Nematomorpha (horse-hair worms)	not investigated
Priapulida	not investigated
Mollusca	phagocytic cells, effects against ionizing radiation, thermal resistance, and immune response to chemicals**
Sipunculida	immune reactions and immunologic properties of coelomic fluid***
Echiurida	nothing known
Annelida (segmented worms)	rates of rejection, cell recognition, formation of antibodies, acclimatization to environmental changes****
Onychophora	immunity and placentation
Pentastomida (tongue worms)	nothing known
Tardigrada (water bears)	nothing known
Arthropoda	immune to chemicals, reaction to antigens, invertebrate agglutinins, immune receptors, humoral immunity, hemolymph coagulation, genetic aspects, immunologic comparison of hemocyanins, encapsulation of foreign material, application of immunofluorescence methods, serological responses against infections, etc.*****
Phoronida	unknown
Ectoprocta (moss animals)	unknown
Brachiopoda (lamp shells)	unknown
Echinodermata (echinoderms)	protective actions of embryos against chemical antagonists; response to ionizing radiation, to transplants; heterotransplantation of echinoderm organs; immunologic effects of lipids; pressure tolerance. Different types of hemocytes.
Chaetognatha (arrow worms)	unknown
Pogonophora (beard worms)	unknown
Hemichordata	unknown
Tunicata (sea squirts)	hemagglutinins, allogenic inhibition, immune response to vertebrate tissues******
Cephalochordata (lancelets)	unknown
Vertebrata	see chapter 2/V

Sources: Ref. 35: * p. 76; ** p. 94, *** p. 96, **** p. 107, ***** p. 148, ****** p. 168.

13. Species specific life span

The life span of animals and plants exhibits a very wide variation. Members of gymnosperm plants, such as *Pinus aristata*, have the longest life span, about 4,000 years. The continued growth and almost endless life span of mosses and similar lower plants cannot be considered because the earlier portion of the plant rotts away and is replaced by a new plant portion. The smallest life span is that of microorganisms such as bacteria. Table 5 reviews the life span of selected animals and plants of various taxonomic units.

14. The species specific size of animals and plants

The size of animals and plants shows two facts which are important for comparative oncology: on one side, small species exhibit a short life span and, parallel with it, a small size (rotifers and water bears); on the other side, phyla such as the nematodes or molluscs, with the same body plan, bring forth species of very small and very large size. In nematodes, a great number of species have a size of only millimeters, but the largest species reach a size of more than 8 m and a diameter of $2\frac{1}{2}$ cm, as in the female *Placentonema gigantissima*. Molluscs range in size from a few millimeters to several meters. In cephalopod molluscs, the pigmy squid, *Idiosepius*, is not longer than 15–20 mm whereas the giant squid, the cephalopod *Architheutis princeps*, has a body length of 6.6 m and, with arms of 18 m, is the largest mollusc and, indeed, the largest invertebrate.

15. Continued or catastrophic development

Animals develop either continuously, that is, the organs built in early life continue to exist, or catastrophically, in which case several organs or structures are discarded by histolysis and replaced by new structures deriving from cells with embryonal potential. Catastrophic development is best known from holometabolic insects.

16. Chronobiologic rhythms

The rhythms of the life functions of animals and plants are variable. Since man is a daylight creature, incorrect to compare the rhythms of man with the rhythms of such nocturnal animals as mouse or owl.

Table 4. Endocrine systems of vertebrates and invertebrates, including main functions.

Phylum	Endocrine structures	Main function
Cnidaria	nettle cells and neurosecretion	
Ctenophora		neurosecretion ?
Platyhelminthes	neurosecretory cells in brain, and near ovaries and testes	neurosecretion
Nemertinea	cerebral organ, neurohemal organ	neurosecretion
Gnathostomulida, Entoprocta, Acanthocephala, Rotifera, Gastrotricha, Kinorhyncha, Nematoda, Nematomorpha, Priapulida	neurosecretory cells	neurosecretion
Mollusca	neurosecretory cells, neurosecretory glands, neurohemal organs, neuroendocrine glands, independent endocrine glands, in particular: organes juxtacommissural in polyplacophora; organes juxtaganglionaires in prosobranchia and opisthobranchia; dorsal bodies in pulmonates. Neurosecretory cells occur in all ganglia of pelecypods Optic glands of cephalopods	control of genetic
Sipunculida	neurosecretory cells, neurohemal organs and neurosecretory glands	
Echiurida	neurosecretory cells, neurosecretion	
Annelida	neurosecretory cells, cerebrovascular complex, infracerebral glands	
Onychophora	neurosecretory cells (glands)	neurosecretion
Pentastomida	unknown	unknown
Tardigrada	unknown	neurosecretion may be assumed
Arthropoda	neurosecretory cells, neurosecretory glands, neurohemal organs, neuroendocrine glands, and independent endocrine glands, in particular: neurosecretory cells in CNS in merostomata; cerebral neurosecretory cells and neurohemal organs in arachnida; epithelial endocrine glands, the Y-organs, androgenic glands.	
	Neurohemal organs are: sinus glands, postcommissural organs and pericardial organs; X-organs in crustaceans. Protocerebral neurosecretory cells and the cerebral glands occur in myriapods. Neurosecretory cells in the brain; the corpora cardiaca; transformed ganglia; the corpora allata; the thoracic glands and/or ventral glands are known.	
Phoronida, Ectoprocta, Brachiopoda	Neurosecretory cells ?	Neurosecretion ?
Echinodermata	Neurosecretory cells	Neurosecretion
Chaetognatha	Neurosecretory cells, gonads ?	Neurosecretion
Pogonophora	Neurosecretory cells	Neurosecretion
Hemichordata	Neurosecretory cells and cells of gonads	
Tunicata	Neurosecretory cells and cells in gut and esophagus	Neurosecretion
Cephalochordata	Neurosecretory cells and cells of gonads	Neurosecretion

Table 4. Continued

Phylum	Endocrine structures	Main function
Vertebrata	Single endocrine cells are found in various organs of vertebrates. The islets of Langerhans appear phylogenetically first time in osteichthyes. Cyclostomes possess an adeno- and neurohypophysis, a thyroid gland and adrenocortical cells. From the pituitary only chondrichthyes show a pars ventralis. The ultimobranchial bodies are paired and associated with the thyroid gland in cartilaginous and bony fishes. Adrenal cortex and medulla are separated in cartilaginous fishes and intermingled in bony fishes.	The hormones of endocrine cells, tissues and organs of vertebrates attain the highest development of endocrine function, be compared with the action of hormones in highest invertebrates (special arthropods and molluscs – as in the case of ecdyson) and vascular plants. Separation into these three groups is justified as can be seen by their different hormone-producing structures. Single cells may be comparable whereas the end-organs of invertebrates form distant organ-complexes. Such vertebrate hormones as insulin, thyroxin, gonadotropin, adrenalin, progesterone, and testosterone are well known. Some interrelationships between the three groups are known, e.g. between vascular plants and invertebrates (ecdyson). In placental mammals, the placenta produces hormones also.
	The adenohypophysis of amphibians has three cell types and occurs in a pars intermedia and neurohypophysis. The thyroid plays an important role in frog metamorphosis. The parathyroid tissue changes seasonally. Adrenals are more or less definite organs.	
	The pituitary of reptiles lacks a pars tuberalis. The pars intermedia is very large, the thyroid gland is single and only two parathyroids occur in some lizards. The adrenals show great varieties in reptiles.	
	In birds, the pituitary lacks a pars intermedia but exhibits anterior and posterior lobe and pars tubularis. The thyroid gland consists of two unconnected oval organs. Parathyroids contain only chief cells. The ultimobranchial body is comparable to fishes, the adrenals' position similar to the mammal. The islets of Langerhans comprise three cell types. The pineal gland presents in young mammals perineal neuroglia and epithelioid cells; the amount of brain sand increases in older organisms. The hypophysis of mammals consists of adeno- and neurohypophysis. The pars intermedia may be absent and is small in certain aquatic mammals. The thyroid gland exhibits two lobes and an isthmus. Mainly four parathyroids are present. The paired adrenal glands are composed of cortex and medulla. In the ovary, endocrine cells occur, as in the testes.	

17. Genetic factors

Genetic factors play an important part in the development of different species and consequently, in oncology. Genetic tumors occur in both animals and plants, the best known being the genetic plant tumors originating from crossing of different subspecies of the tobacco plant *Nicotiana sp.* or the genetic tumors of the fish *Xiphophorus*. Chromosome abnormalities are known from many tumors (Chapter 15/vol. III).

18. Angiogenesis

Angiogenesis is a necessity for metastatic neoplastic growth. A neoplasm still *in situ* or having not yet penetrated the basement membrane, may push aside the surrounding cells through its malignantly transformed cells. An outgrowth of vessels (angiogenesis) from the host's circulatory system is needed to nourish a cancer *in situ* and to permit the cells of such a tumor to penetrate the vessels and to spread by way of hematologic distribution.

Selected elements of malignant cells important for secondary growth are discussed below:

1. Cell membrane or cell wall
The most important difference between animal and plant cells is that plants, in general, have non-protoplasmic cell walls while animals generally do not. A typical exception in vascular plants is the sexual cells. The nonprotoplasmic plant cell walls exhibit a relationship to the functional non-living plant cells, which may be found in the sclerenchyme, but also in vessels of vascular plants.

2. Cell biochemistry
The most important difference between animal and plant cells is the presence of cellulose in the cell wall of plants, the mantle of the urochordates being a rare exception in animals.

3. Mobility of cells
Plants exhibit movement quite different from what we consider movement in animals. Most easily comparable are the cell movements of cilia and flagella, whose structure is generally similar in plants and animals. Movement in plant cells, such as plasmatic streaming, and of cell organelles is, to some extent, comparable to movement in animals, but the free movement of whole plants, including that of plant organs, as found in tropisms and nastias, is incomparable to that of animals. Endogenous plant movements as produced by turgor, wetness and cohesion are controlled by totally different forces than in the movement of animals.

4. Cell consistency and nonliving cells

This phenomenon is present in animals such as rotifers and water bears, or in our own neurons. It is evident that tumor growth and activity cannot occur in animals which exhibit cell consistency or in nonliving plant tissues. Only the precursor stages of these cells in both animals and plants are able to induce neoplastic growth.

5. Enzyme destruction of tissues

Destruction of tissues by enzymes occurs in both, animals and plants, but the chemistries involved are different.

6. Detachment of neoplastic cells

This process does not occur in plant cells, but is very important for neoplastic (especially secondary) growth in animals.

7. Invasion by malignant cells

This occurs in both animals and plants. Selected factors which affect both host and malignant cells are:

1. *Cell membrane.* The nonprotoplasmatic cell membrane, lacking free movable cells in plants such as the free connective tissue cells in animals and the makeup of the vessel walls make metastasis in plants impossible. This phenomenon is the most important difference between malignant tumors in animals and plants.

2. *Tumor pressure.* This can be developed by two components: the tumor parenchyma and the growing of tumor stroma, which is stimulated by the cells of tumor parenchyma. In plants, tumor pressure may develop from the parenchyma alone. Angiogenesis in the plant neoplasms is impossible.

Justification for the designation "malignant" can be found in both, animal and plant neoplasms. Under these circumstances it is necessary to change the terminology relating to malignant characteristics, to mammalian tumors as the typical representative of animals. The important difference between malignant animal and plant neoplasms is the fact that neoplasms of vascular plants are unable to metastasize. This inability occurs due to the variation of normal animal and plant cells and the variation in the normal make-up of the systems of body fluids in animals and plants. These differences, explained earlier in the text, are not due to variations in the basic pathological process. Malignancy has to be determined by inferiority of the neoplastic cells when compared to the normal cells of which they derive, continued growth after cessation, increase of growth potential, transplantability, and spreading. Rarely does spontaneous regression occur. Metastasis is a characteristic type of spreading of malignant animal neoplasms, especially sophisticated in mammals at its highest level where the circulatory system, including the lymphatic system with its lymph nodes, is very highly developed. There are even human cancers that rarely metastasize or which we may think of as dormant neoplasms.

Similarities of malignant neoplastic growth in animals and plants

1. Similar causes of neoplastic initiation in animals and plants.

Causes	Animals	Plants
Chemical compounds	experimental tumors in mice	experimental swellings in Norway spruce
Physical agents	tumor initiation by x-rays	
Radioactive emissions	lesions in mice, survivors of Hiroshima	
Virus	Rous'sarcoma of chicken	wound tumor virus disease of clover
Genetic initiation	genetic diseases and familiar occurrence of neoplasms in man	genetic tumors in tobacco hybrids
Parasites	*Cysticercus* induced bladder cancer in man and rat	
Bacteria	tumors in fish	crown gall disease in vascular plants

2. Similar inferiority of neoplastic cells in animals and plants.
3. Value of topographic location: certain neoplasms in animals and plants exhibit a variation in aggressiveness at different locations whereas in other tumors such differences based on location are lacking.
4. Malignant transformation at the initial stage of malignancy.
5. Increase of growth potential of neoplastic cells.
6. Continued growth on cessation of stimulus.
7. Transplantability of malignant animal and plant neoplasms
8. Spreading of animal and plant neoplasms.
9. Regression in animal and plant neoplasms.

REFERENCES

1. Highham KC, Hill L: *The Comparative Endocrinology of the Invertebrates* (2nd edition). Baltimore: University Park Press, 1977
2. Kaiser HE: Studies on species-specific carcinogenesis in different phyla: studies regarding the reaction in coelenterates and echinoderms after implantation and feeding of polycyclic hydrocarbons. *Arch f Geschwulstforsch* Berlin, 1965
3. Kaiser HE: Pre-carcinogenesis and secondary facts of carcinogenesis in different species. *Amer Zoologist* Abstract #150, 5:2, 1965
4. Kaiser HE: The phylogenetic adaptation of aquatic mammals to their environment. *Amer Zoologist* Abstract #158, 5:2, 1965
5. Kaiser HE: Species bound evolutinary differences of comparative oncology and potential therapeutic application. *J Nat'l Med Association* 58(2):114, 1966
6. Kaiser HE: New perspectives on cancer with species specific reactivity. *J Nat'l Med Assn* 58:275, 1966
7. Kaiser HE, Bartone JC: A plea for the analysis of the formation of cancer and allied diseases into separable multiphase processes. *J Nat'l Med Assn* 58:5, 1966

8. Kaiser HE, Bartone JC: Suggestions and general principles of comparative oncology. *Fed Proc* 25:2, Part 1, 1966

9. Kaiser HE, Bartone JC: Different reactions of chemical and physical carcinogens in specific area of mouse skin. *ASB Bulletin* 13:2, 30, 1966

10. Kaiser HE, Bartone JC: Microscopic observations of the specific responses of invertebrates to chemical carcinogens. The Royal Microscopical Society, Royal Charter Centenary, 151, 1966

11. Kaiser HE, Theisz J, Bartone JC: Species specific differences of absorption as a variation of stage one (contact) of multiphase carcinogenesis. *Bull of the Virginia Acad of Sci* 1966

12. Kaiser HE: The importance of the distribution of chemical compounds in living organisms for comparative cancer studies. 152nd meeting *Amer Chem Soc* Abstract #205, 1966

13. Kaiser HE: Differences in absorption of 3.4 benzopyrene by various plant and animal species, *Amer Chem Soc* Abstract 215 154th meeting ACS, Chicago, 1967

14. Kaiser HE: Distribution of chemical compounds in living organisms from the comparative pathological viewpoint. Seventh Internat'l Congr. of Biochemistry, Tokyo. Abstract I-268, 1967

15. Kaiser HE: Cytogenetic behavior of 3.4 benzopyrene and 1.2 benzopyrene in several species in the initial stage of multiphase carcinogenesis. *Amer Zool* vol. 7, Abstract #340, 1966

16. Kaiser HE: Application of combined experimental methods in comparative oncology *Fed Proc* 27:2, Abstract #1831, 542, 1968

17. Kaiser HE: The body covering of animals and plants as a promising comparative goal for cytochemical studies in regard to neoplastic changes, occurring at short-term intervals. Summary report. Third Internat'l Congr. of Histochemistry and Cytochemistry, 122, 1968

18. Kaiser HE: Comparative studies of the cytology (cytochemistry and histochemistry) of developing cancer cells. Third Internat'l Congr. of Histochemistry and Cytochemistry, pp. 123/124. Summary report, 1968

19. Kaiser HE: Behavior of regeneration area cells in annelids and echinoderms under the influence of 1.2 and 3.4 benzopyrene. Annual AIBS meeting, Abstract #1029, 1968

20. Kaiser HE: The integuments of animals and plants as challenging model for comparative pathological research with species reference to problems of oncology. *SIP Newsletter*, I:6, Soc. for Invertebrate Pathology, 1969

21. Kaiser HE: The integuments of plants and animals as a general model for experimental pathology with special reference to histologic comparability. 53rd Annual Meeting of the Amer. Soc. for Exp. Path., *Fed Proc* 28:2, Abstract #2020, 1969

22. Kaiser HE: The advantages of pathological and oncological research with invertebrates II. Annual Meeting, Soc. of Invertebrate Pathology, *Newsletter* II:2, 27, 1969

23. Kaiser HE: The histologic comparability of plant and animal tissues from a functional point of view. Abstracts, XI. *Internat'l Botanical Congr* 105, 1969

24. Kaiser HE: Comparability of the effect of carcinogenic compounds upon widely separated species of both kingdoms. Abstract of papers. 162nd ACS Nat'l Meeting, Biol 130, 1971

25. Kaiser HE: Phylogenetic age and recent distribution of normal true animal and plant tissues – A comparative basic question of oncology. *Archivos mexicanos de Anatomia* Ano 13:39, 22, 1972

26. Kaiser HE: Histology of larval forms and histology of aging, with stressing electron microscopy – a comparison, *Anat Rec* 172:2, 339, 1972

27. Kaiser HE: Larval tissues as experimental model in comparative oncology. *Fed Proc* 31:2, Abstract #4060, 928, 1972

28. Kaiser HE, Nordmann M: The potential contribution of comparative pathology to laboratory medicine and clinical pathology. Seventh Internat'l Congr. of Clinical Pathology and Laboratory Medicine, Abstract of papers, 1972

29. Kaiser HE: The application of chemical carcinogens to plants. *Fed Proc* 33:3, 595, Abstract #2166, 1974

30. Kaiser HE: Reaction of plant tissues to mammalian carcinogens. XII. Internat'l Cancer Congress, Florence, 1974

31. Kaiser HE, Heatfield BN, Kahng MW: The value of comparative chronobiology in experimental pathology and toxicology. Chronobiologia, Suppl. 1, Abstracts. XII. Internat'l Conf., Internat'l Soc. for Chronobiology, Abstract #70, Il Ponte, Milano, 1975

32. Kaiser HE: A new approach to histology: a functional comparison of animal and plant tissues. *Anat Rec* 184:440, 1976

33. Kaiser HE: The relationship of limited and unlimited abnormal growth processes in animals and plants. *Fed Proc* 37:3, 1978

34. Kaiser HE: Review of species-specific metabolic pathways of carcinogenic polynuclear aromatic hydrocarbons in marine organisms. EPA Symposium; Carcinogenic polynuclear aromatic hydrocarbons in the marine environment, July 1982. Keynote address presented 1978

35. Kaiser HE: *Species-specific Potential of Invertebrates for Toxicological Research.* Baltimore: University Park Press, 1980

36. Kaiser HE: *Neoplasms – Comparative Pathology of Growth in Animals, Plants, and Man*, Baltimore: Williams & Wilkins, 1981, chapters 2–4, 6, and 13

37. Kaiser HE: Principles of comparative functional histology. Gegenbaurs morph. Jahrb., Leipzig 129:2, 137–180, 1983

38. Kaiser HE: Comparative pathologic aspects of neoplastic growth with special consideration of the lymphatic system. Keynote address at the Annual Meeting of the German Soc. of Lymphology, University of Goettingen, Sept. 18, 1981 (unpublished)

39. Kaiser HE: Functional Comparative Histology. 2. Communication Organismic Taxonomy (Plant and Animal Taxonomy). Gegenbaurs morph. Jahrb. Leipzig 131:5, 643, 1985

40. Siewing R: *Lehrbuch der vergleichenden Entwicklungsgeschichte der Tiere.* Hamburg and Berlin: Paul Parey, 1969

41. Willis RA: *The Spread of Tumours in the Human Body.* 3rd edition Butterworths, 1973

2

REVIEW OF SELECTED ASPECTS OF NEOPLASTIC PROGRESSION IN THE MAMMALIAN ORDERS

H.E. KAISER

Progression of neoplastic diseases seems to be highest developed and most diversified in mammals. This is due to the diverse body structure and the great variation in this class of vertebrates, in comparison for example to the other class of warm-blooded animals, the birds. In taxonomy, the mammals are considered to be the highest step in phylogenetic development. We know, however, from paleontology that the last group to appear on earth were the birds. They appeared in the Jurassic, whereas the mammals had already evolved in the Triassic. The body plan from small birds to large ones is very similar in structure and arrangement, whereas the body plan of mammals exhibits great diversification. Also the size of the different groups of birds varies much less than that of mammals. The same is the case with the life span. Variation among mammalian types becomes readily clear if one compares the four smallest mammals found in the insectivores and bats. The pigmy shrew, *Microsorux crawfordi* with a length of 51 to 61 mm and a weight of 2.1 to 6.3 gr, and the shrews *Suncus etruscus* and *Sorex minutus* of similar length and body weight are among the smallest; the bat *Craseonycteris thonglongyai* is also very small, with a length of 29 to 33 mm and a weight of about 2 grams. The largest terrestrial mammal is the African elephant, *Loxodonta africana* with a length of 600 to 750 cm and a weight of 2200 to 7500 kg. The tallest mammal is the giraffe, *Giraffa camelopardalis*, of which the record height is 5880 mm, the average weight 800 kg. The largest marine mammal is the blue whale, *Balaenoptera musculus*, the largest animal ever known to have existed, with a maximum length of 30 m and about 160 000 kg. From the above mentioned species it becomes clear that mammals are adapted to flying (order Chiroptera, bats), to aquatic environments (the orders Cetacea, whales; Sirenia, sea cows; Pinnipedia, walrusses, seals; Carnivora, river, giant, sea otters) as well as to terrestrial life, as is the case with the majority of orders.

Neoplasms may occur in all metazoans and vascular plants as well as in a few taxonomic splinter groups. The neoplasms of mammals, especially man, have to be considered the most complex appearance of neoplasms particularly if we think on the progression of neoplastic processes. Kaiser (1952) (5) stated that pathologic structures and function are preceded by the normal phylogenetic development of structures and functions. Diseases therefore can be considered as a secondary development in phylogeny. Beside the plant tissues there are a few other types of tissues not known in the mammal. These are listed in Table 1.

Table 2 lists some selected types of organs and functions varying from the adult mammal.

The majority of tissues listed in Table 1 such as the sinus glands in crustaceans or the corpora cardiaca in insects can be considered as a counterpart for such mammalian structures as the pituitary or the adrenals. Therefore, only the helically striated musculature is a structure with no comparative counterpart in the mammal because the plectenchymata in fungi can only be compared to all mammalian tissues and the same holds true for the phylloid, cauloid or rhizoid true tissues of lower plants, the true plant tissues of mosses or the true tissues of vascular plants.

In table 3 aspects of mammalian neoplastic progression are compared with other organismic groups.

A short review of neoplastic spreading in members of the mammalian orders gives the following picture:

In this review not all cases of malignant neoplastic growth have been listed but only those selected cases in which the neoplastic spreading has been properly documented.

SELECTED CASES OF NEOPLASTIC SPREADING IN MAMMALS

Order Monotremata. The order comprises three genera and three species. Cases indicating neoplastic progression such as metastases have not been observed in Monotremata.

Table 1. Tissues not present in mammals.

Tissue	Taxonomic group where present
helically striated musculature	Nematoda
neurohemal structures	Nemertinea
cerebrovascular complex	Annelida
neural perineum	Mollusca
organ juxtacomissural	Aiaphineura, polyplacophora
organes juxtaganglionaires	Proso- and opisthobranchia
dorsal bodies	Pulmonata
neurohemal organs	Arachnida
sinus glands	Crustacea
postcommissural organs	Crustacea
pericardial organs	Crustacea
cerebral glands	Chilopoda, Diplopoda
corpora cardiaca	Insecta
perisympathetic organs	Insecta
plectenchymata	Fungi
phylloid, cauloid or rhizoid true tissues	Plants
true plant tissues	Bryophyta (mosses)
true tissues	vascular plants

H. E. Kaiser (ed.), Comparative aspects of tumor development.
© 1989, Kluwer Academic Publishers, Dordrecht. ISBN-13:978-0-89838-994-4

Table 2. Types of organ variation of mammals as compared to those structures and functions not present in the mammal.

Organ system	Deviations from the mammalian type
Body coverings	No hairs or mammary glands in other groups than mammals
Structures of digestion	Missing in several phyla
Structures of gaseous exchange	Gills (e.g., in arthropods, molluscs and fishes), tracheids (in tracheates) and other special structures
Structures of excretion and waste	Different types of nephrons
Hormonal structures	Other organs, especially arthropods and molluscs as in table 1
Structures of sensitivity	e.g., facet eyes of insects, eyes of spiders
Structure of motion	Helically striated musculature and various endo- and exoskeletons
Systems of body fluids	Various types of circulation
Interstitial tissues	Other types of secreted structures of endo- and exoskeletons

Order Marsupialia. Marsupials are divided in 71 genera and 258 species; they are one of the orders exhibiting neoplasms quite frequently. Spreading of malignancy has been observed occasionally. One tasmanian devil (*Sarcophilus harrizi*) exhibited an adenocarcinoma of the perianal glands with metastasis in the liver, and another one had a metastasizing mammary carcinoma, with additional sebaceous gland adenoma and thyroid hyperplasia or adenoma (4). A Parama wallaby (*Macropus parma*), with a squamous cell carcinoma of the uterine cervix and vagina, exhibited metastasis to regional lymph nodes (4). Canfield found benign neoplasms composed of a mixture of cartilage and bone appearing in four koalas (*Phascolarctos cinereus*) (2).

Order Insectivora. There are 60 genera and 379 species. A bronchial adenoma in the lungs of an East African hedgehog (*Erinaceus albiventris*) infiltrated the surrounding tissues (4). A fibrosarcoma of the abdominal wall with lung and lymph node metastases was seen in a *Tenrec ecaudatus*.

Order Dermoptera. One genus and two species belong to this order. Spread of malignancies in dermoptera has not been observed but undoubtedly occur. The lack of knowledge is due to the rarity of these animals in captivity.

Order Chiroptera. The 175 genera of this order are divided into 942 species. Chiroptera contain the second largest number of species of all mammalian orders. Malignancies and their spreading only rarely have been observed.

Order Primates. This order, to which man belongs, comprises 56 genera divided into 203 species. In a report of 2,176 autopsies of nonhuman primates in a large colony 43 animals exhibited neoplastic growth and only 10 showed metastases. Metastases in nonhuman primates are not as rare as believed earlier. Skin: In a *Tupaia glis*, exposed to benzo(a)pyrene a subcutaneous sarcoma metastasizing to the lungs was seen. A tree shrew (*Tupia* sp.) exhibited a mammary ductile sclerosing adenocarcinoma, with nodules in both mammary glands (in tissues near the axilla and submandibular region), infiltrating adjacent tissues and metastasizing to lymph nodes and lung (4). A fibrosarcoma in a *Galagos* sp. metastasized to mesentery lymph nodes. A Diana guenon (*Cercopithecus d. diana*) suffered from a metastasizing biliary adenocarcinoma which penetrated the tissues of the liver. The location of the metastatic process was the lung (4). A hepatoma in a mangabey (*Cercocebus atys*) exhibited metastases to lung and omentum. Mesodermal sarcomas with liver metastases occurred in rhesus monkey treated with DMBA and ultraviolet light or DDB. Three basal cell carcinomas in rhesus monkeys were locally invasive but did not metastasize. The tumors showed the same behavior as the same tumor type in man. The same species

Table 3. Comparative aspects of mammalian neoplastic progression.

Spread in the mammal (man)	Possible in other phyla	Not possible in other phyla
Direct spread	Eumetazoans and vascular plants	
Local recurrence	in treated domestic, laboratory and zoo animals	not in untreated species
Metastasis via lymphatics	due to the distribution of lymph nodes, restricted in birds, reptiles and more restricted in amphibians and fishes	not in invertebrates
Spreading at thoracic duct	mammals only; but in comparative structures in other vertebrates	
Metastasis by blood stream	possible in animals with closed, mixed or open circulatory system	not in animals without circulatory system
Transcoelomic metastasis and secondary tumors of the serous membranes	can occur in coelomate phyla	not possible in acoelomates – restricted in pseudocoelomates
Metastasis by implantation of epithelial surfaces	possible in all eumatazoans	
Metastasis of teratomas	possible in all eumetazoans	
Metastasis from metastasis	possible in all eumetazoans	
Multiple primary neoplasms	possible in all eumetazoans and vascular plants	

also exhibited disseminated malignant lymphoma. *Macaca mulatta* showed in another study a disseminated endometriosis.

Organs of motion: A giant cell tumor of bone in the ulna of *Papio porcarius* resembled the giant cell tumor of bone in man and metastasized to the lungs, heart and muscle. Another baboon had an adenocarcinoma of undetermined origin with widespread metastases to the skeletal system. A fibrosarcoma of the forearm in a rhesus monkey metastasized to regional lymph nodes and a fibrosarcoma of the thigh in an animal, exposed to 320 rem irradiation 17 years before tumor development, metastasized to kidneys, diaphragm, liver and lungs.

Digestive tract. Four intestinal carcinomas in rhesus monkeys metastasized to regional lymph nodes and one to the liver, and another one to the lung. Liver and biliary tract: In the study by McClure (8) no primary neoplasms of the biliary system have been observed, a condition noteworthy due to the fact that primary neoplasms of the biliary tract and especially hepatic tract are very frequent and can be said to be characteristic of the ursidae, the bears. This frequent occurrence in the biliary tract of bears will be described below.

Respiratory system. Osteogenic sarcoma, fibrosarcoma of the thigh, intestinal carcinoma and malignant lymphoma of rhesus monkeys exhibited lung metastases. Salivary glands, pancreas and endocrine system: An undifferentiated carcinoma of the salivary glands in a baboon metastasized to regional lymph nodes. According to origin an unknown, perhaps adrenal cortical, carcinoma metastasized widely.

Genital organs and mammary glands. A 42-year-old male cebus monkey had an adenocarcinoma of the breast with metastases to intercostal muscles, lungs, lymph nodes and adrenal. Apes and monkeys are frequently used as zoo and circus animals that surely more cases of metastatic growth could be known if the animals would be permitted to live out their lives or if properly autopsies would be performed in all cases.

Order Edentata. Seventeen genera and 33 species belong to this order. Members of this order exhibit neoplastic growth but the spreading of malignancies was not observed. Since the armadillo is used widely in leprosy research more knowledge in this regard may accumulate.

Order Pholidota. The order contains one genus and seven species. Neoplastic spreading in members of this order has not been observed.

Order Lagomorpha. Eleven genera and 65 species belong to this order. Several cases of malignant neoplasms have been seen in wild species. The older world rabbit, *Oryctolagus cuniculus* has become a widely used domesticated and laboratory animal as well. There exists an extensive literature of neoplasms of this rabbit.

Order Rodentia. This largest order of mammals is composed of 380 genera and 1,687 species and has the largest number of species in the class of mammals. One prairie dog (*Ammos-*

permophilus sp.) had a squamous carcinoma of the mouth metastasizing to the kidney and another one had an adenocarcinoma of the stomach metastasizing to the liver (4). Spontaneous tumors in a number of those species are known, also with progressive spreading as in *Ondatra* sp. (osteosarcoma of tibia and fibula spreading to lung and kidney or primary osteosarcoma of rib and diaphragm spreading to lung, pericard, and myocard). In this huge order, only a few species have been investigated with regard to neoplastic malignancy, and fewer still with regard to malignant spreading. In contrast, four species of this order, namely the mouse, *Mus musculus*, the rat, *Rattus norwegicus*, the hamster, *Cricetus aureus*, and the guinea pig, *Cavia* sp. in this sequence used in laboratories have gained a tremendous importance for cancer research. The many inbred strains of the mouse and rat especially are the only species comparable to man himself regarding the development of neoplasms. Other species such as *Praomys natalensis*, the African soft-furred and the spiny mouse, and a few others are of lesser importance (see chapter 16 on species, racial and breed variations).

Order Cetacea. Thirty-nine genera and 79 species comprise this order. Of the five malignancies known in the cetaceans only Hodgkin's disease in the fin whale, *Balaenoptera physalus*, with a multicentric involvement of organs can be considered as a progressive stage of tumor development.

Order Carnivora. There are 92 genera and 238 species of carnivores. Single case reports have been collected in different types of wild carnivores of which some have indicated neoplastic progression as an adenocarcinoma of the thyroid gland of a red fox, *Vulpes vulpes*, metastasizing to the lungs. Also seen were a hypernephroma of the kidney with metastases in lung and thorax of a coyote, *Canis latrans*, a basal cell tumor of a wolf, *Canis lupus*, with metastasis to the lung, a secondary chondrosarcoma of the liver and an epithelioma of the neck with liver metastasis also in the wolf. A black backed jackal, *Canis mesomelas* suffered from metastasizing hemangiosarcoma and Indian golden jackals, *Canis aureus syriacus*, had an adenocarcinoma of sweat gland with metastasis in a 17-year-old individual with metastasis and an adenocarcinoma of the maxillary sinus with metastasis in another one (4). One maned wolf, *Crysocyon brachyurus*, indicated an osteofibrosarcoma with metastasis and another one, renal adenocarcinoma also with metastasis. An African hunting dog, *Lycaon pictus* exhibited a metastasizing hemangiosarcoma.

In *Felis concolor* an adenocarcinoma of the thyroid was metastatic to the lung and also an adenocarcinoma of the thyroid was metastatic to the lung in a lion, *Leo leo*.

Ursus thibetanus showed a malignant lymphoma in kidney, lymph node and small intestine. The family of ursidae is of particular interest to comparative oncology because the bears show a tendency to develop cancers of the biliary ducts and especially the extrahepatic one not found commonly in any other animal species. In different types of bears as in the Kodiak bear, *Ursus americanus middendorfi*, grizzly bear, *Ursus arctos* (*horribilis*), American black bear, *Ursus americanus*, Asian black bear, *Ursus thibetanus*, and sloth bear, *Ursus ursinus*, hepatomas and/or bile-duct cancers have been observed. A Montague island brown bear (*Ursus sheldoni*) was afflicted with a lymphosarcoma which showed also lesions besides the lymphopoietic system in liver and kidney (4). Extrahepatic bile-duct cancers are uncommon in man where they are found most often in males; they are also rare in the domestic and laboratory animals. Bile-duct cancer in *Helarctos malayanus*, the Malayan sun bear with metastases to diaphragm and uterus, adrenal glands, pancreas, portal and metastatic lymph nodes, and omentum was seen by Montali (10) in an approximately 28-year-old bear. Biliary cancers have been found in the grizzly bear, *Ursus horribilis*, sloth bear, *Melursus ursinus*, two other sun bears, *Helarctos malayanus* and five additional bears.

In *Mustela vison*, the American mink, a primary osteosarcoma of the rib metastasized to lung and liver. A lymphosarcoma with lymphocyte accumulations in most viscera occurred in the ferret (*Mustela* sp.) (4). A fisher, *Martes pennanti* exhibited an adenocarcinoma of the right parotid which metastasized to the right mandibular lymph node.

A widely spreading mammary carcinoma was seen in a binturong (*Arctictis binturong*) with metastasis to the ovary, vagina, kidney, spleen, lymph nodes, liver, and lung (4).

A cheetah (*Arcinonyx jubatus*) and an African lion (*Panthera leo*) had metastatic lymphosarcoma each. A metastatic lymphosarcoma in a Bengal tiger (*Panthera t. tigris*) and a metastatic squamous cell carcinoma were observed in a Canadian lynx (*Lynx canadensis*). A bobcat (*Felis rufus?*) showed a metastatic fibrosarcoma of the face (4).

In the order of carnivora also belong two species which have developed as the most beloved pets, dogs and cats. Of these animals many races have been bred which makes them even more valuable for comparative aspects among their different breeds and to other species (see chapter 16).

Order Pinnipedia. Eighteen genera and 34 species belong to this order. Neoplasms affecting the hematopoietic system are the most common malignancies. Seven lymphosarcomas exhibited in six pinniped species distribution in the viscera, including the spleen, liver, kidneys, heart, colon, etc. In *Zalophus californianus* a clear cell carcinoma of urogenital origin with metastases in kidneys, adrenals, lungs, lymph nodes, uterus, ovaries, and pancreas, and a squamous cell carcinoma metastasizing to lung, liver, pancreas, spleen, lymph nodes have been observed. Another California sea lion afflicted with malignant ocular melanoma which seems to have originated in the iris spread to surrounding soft tissues and the bony portion of the orbit and presented metastases in the brain.

Order Tubulidentata. Composed of one genus with one species. No reports about progressive development of malignant neoplasms are available.

Order Proboscidea. Two living genera and two species are known. No cases of progressive neoplasms with metastatic spreading are known in elephants. Benign and malignant tumors of course have been found.

Order Hyracoidea. This order comprises three genera and seven species. No metastatic or otherwise progressing cases in species of this order are known.

Order Sirenia. Two genera and four living species are

Also in sirenians progressing malignancies showing metastasis are not known.

Order Perissodactyla. Six genera and 17 species are known. The hoofed mammals, Odd-toed ungulates, comprise the equidae, the tapiridae and the rhinocerotidae, the horses, the tapirs, and the rhinos. Progressive stages of neoplastic diseases are not known from wild, including zoo animals. To this order also belong, included in the first family the domestic animals known as horse, donkey and mule. Especially the horse was developed in different races. Progressive cases of neoplastic growth are known from those domestic breeds. (See (11)).

Order Artiodactyla. This last order of mammals comprises 79 genera and 192 species. This order of hoofed mammals, even-toed ungulates, exhibits nine families of which the suidae (pigs), camelidae (llamas and camels), cervidae (deer) and bovidae (antilopes, cattle, goats and sheep) supplied important domestic species and additional species for hunting (deer). Many cases of disseminated neoplastic growth as well as metastasis have been observed in the domestic animals of this order. A few examples of neoplastic progression in wild species should be given. A disseminated lymphosarcoma was seen in Eld's deer (*Cervus eldi*). A pheochromocytoma in a *Cervus* sp. was metastasizing as well as an undifferentiated carcinoma in the giraffe, *Giraffa camelopardalis*. A squamous cell carcinoma involving portions of the oral mucosa and the maxillary sinus in a pronghorn (*Antilocapra americana*) metastasized to the adjacent lymphatics. (4). An Arabian oryx (*Oryx leucoryx*) exhibited a widely distributed lymphosarcoma (3). A uterine adenocarcinoma of an impala (*Aepyceros melampus*) originated perhaps in the vagina and metastasized to regional lymph nodes (4). A Creatan goat (wild goat), (*Capra aegagrus?*) presented with benign to malignant adenomas in the digestive tract which may have metastasized to the lung (4).

SUMMARY AND CONCLUSIONS

This review of selected cases of neoplastic progression in species of the mammalian orders is incomplete, but shall give a review of neoplastic spreading as it occurs in the mammalian orders. The material is based on zoo animals, which is a somewhat artificial selection, because zoo animals reach in general higher ages than wild counterparts. Housing and food cannot be considered as exactly natural, what holds especially true for the whole life style. For selected examples of free ranging mammals see chapter 26 by Williams & Thorne. There are whole mamalian orders of which we know nothing about neoplastic progression.

REFERENCES

1. Ashley DJB: *Evans' Histological Appearances of Tumours* (3rd edition) vols. 1 and 2, Edinburgh, London and New York: Churchill Livingstone, 1978
2. Canfield PJ, Perry R, Brown AS, McKenzie RA: Cranio-facial tumours of mixed cartilage and bone in koalas (Phascolarctos cinereus). Aust Vet J 64(1):20–2, 1987
3. Dellmann H-D Brown EM: *Textbook of Veterinary Histology*

(2nd edition) Lea & Febiger, Philadelphia, 1981

4. Griner LA: *Pathology of Zoo Animals.* San Diego: Zoological Society of San Diego, 1983

5. Kaiser, HE. Die Entwicklung der Osteomyelitis seit dem Perm. Monatshefte Veterinarmedizin, 7. Jg. (14):275–279, 1952.

6. Kaiser HE (ed.): *Neoplasms – Comparative Pathology of Growth in Animals, Plants, and Man,* chaps. 43 and 48, Baltimore, London: Williams & Wilkins, 1981

7. Klös H-G, Lang EM: *Handbook of Zoo Medicine,* translated by G. Speckmann. New York a.o.: Van Nostrand Reinhold Company, 1982

8. McClure HM: Tumors in nonhuman primates: Observations during a six-year period in the Yerkes Primate Center Colony. Am J Phys Anthrop 38:425–430, 1973

9. Montali RJ, Migaki G (eds.): *The Comparative Pathology of Zoo Animals* Washington, D.C.: Smithsonian Institution Press, 1980

10. Montali RJ, Hoopes PJ, Bush M: "Extrahepatic biliary carcinomas in asiatic bears", NCI, vol. 66, no. 3, pp. 603–608, 1981

11. Moulton JE (ed.): *Tumors in Domestic Animals.* Berkeley, Los Angeles, London: University of California Press, 1987

12. Nowak RM, Paradiso JL (eds.): *Walker's Mammals of the World* (4th edition). Baltimore and London: The Johns Hopkins University Press, 1983

13. Priester WA, McKay FW: *The Occurrence of Tumors in Domestic Animals.* NCI Monograph 54. NIH Publication no. 80-2046, U.S. Department of Health and Human Services, 1980

14. Reznik G, Stinson SF: *Nasal Tumors in Animals and Man.* Vols. 1 and 2. Boca Raton, FLA: CRC Press, Inc. 1983

15. Turusov VS (ed.): *Pathology of Tumours in Laboratory Animals.* Vol. 1, Pts. I and II: Tumours of the Rat, Vol. 2: Tumours of the Mouse Vol. 3: Tumours of the Hamster. Lyon: WHO (International Agency for Research on Cancer), 1973–1982

16. Willis RA: *The Spread of Tumours in the Human Body* (3rd edition). London: Butterworth, 1973

NEOPLASTIC PROGRESSION IN PLANTS

WILLIAM L. PENGELLY

1. INTRODUCTION

Neoplastic transformation to the fully virulent state is not accomplished in a single step, but occurs gradually and progressively during tumor development. This phenomenon is known as neoplastic progression and, in both plants and animals, is marked by increased anaplasia and growth rate. The basic problem for the oncologist is to find out how transformed cells of common origin can express different capacities for neoplastic growth.

Fundamental differences in development distinguish the course of neoplastic progression in plants from that in animals. Plant cells are limited by cell walls and fixed in position. There are no morphogenetic movements in plant development, and the migratory (invasive) cell is not part of the plant's developmental repertoire. Thus, secondary tumors are relatively rare in plants (29), and their occurrence may be attributed to the systemic spread of an oncogenic pathogen such as a virus (16) or bacterium (90), or to the transfer of oncogenic potential from cell to cell in the absence of the pathogen (56). Secondary tumors, therefore, result from separate inductive events and not from the spread of tumor cells with new and more virulent properties. For this reason, studies of tumor progression in plants have focused on the growth of primary tumors and cells derived from them.

A second characteristic of plants is their high capacity for regeneration, and the formation of organized structures such as roots or shoots is a common feature of plant tumor diseases. Since the differentiation of complex structures implies some degree of normal development, organogenic tumors are considered to be less advanced than tumors which grow in a chaotic and unorganized fashion. This may seem backwards at first because the absence of an organized vascular system should weaken the tumor and limit its growth. Nevertheless, the most rapidly growing tumors are generally unorganized, a fact that undoubtedly reflects the high degree of nutritional autonomy that plant cells can achieve. Rapidly growing, unorganized tumors are the most disruptive with respect to normal plant structure, and generally represent the greatest danger to survival.

The best-studied plant tumor diseases are the genetic tumors which arise spontaneously in certain interspecies hybrids (7, 79), the wound tumor disease caused by the phytoreoviruses (16), and the crown gall disease caused by a soil bacterium (26). In this review I will concentrate on the crown gall disease because its molecular biology is the best known, and because it was with this system that the definitive studies of tumor progression were performed.

2. THE CROWN GALL DISEASE

Smith and Townsend (80) were the first to identify the causal agent of a neoplastic disease when they discovered that crown-gall tumors were induced by the soil bacterium *Agrobacterium tumefaciens*. The true neoplastic nature of the disease was demonstrated by Armin Braun who isolated in culture tumor cells which retained their neoplastic properties in the absence of bacteria (30). This led Braun to conclude that a tumor-inducing principle must be transferred from the bacterium to the plant cell (28). It is now known that *A. tumefaciens* contains tumor-inducing (Ti) plasmids and that a segment of plasmid DNA (T-DNA) is transferred to the host and integrated into nuclear DNA (reviews: (9, 11, 45, 63)).

Genes of the T-DNA code for the formation of unusual amino acids called opines (e.g., octopine, nopaline, lysopine, etc.) which are not metabolized by the host, but which may serve as a sole carbon and nitrogen source for *A. tumefaciens* (reviews: (81, 82)). Several strains of *A. tumefaciens* have been identified which contain Ti plasmids that differ somewhat in DNA sequence and organization, and which may be categorized by the type of opine production encoded by the plasmid. However, within the T-DNA of all strains examined is a highly conserved sequence which is required for oncogenesis (38). Thus, the apparent strategy of the pathogen is to engineer plant cells for opine production, and to select for opine-producing cells by neoplastic transformation. This same strategy is used by *A. rhizogenes* which causes the hairy root disease. This bacterium contains root-inducing (Ri) plasmids which transfer T-DNA genes for oncogenesis and opine biosynthesis (see 96).

A characteristic feature of crown-gall cells is their autonomy for the growth hormones auxin and cytokinin (22). It has now been demonstrated that oncogenes in the highly conserved T-DNA sequence code for the biosynthesis of these hormones. One gene codes for an isopentenyl transferase which catalyzes the first step of cytokinin biosynthesis (1, 5, 34), and two others code for enzymes which produce the auxin indole-3-acetic acid (IAA). The product of one gene converts tryptophan to indoleacetamide (IAM) (85), and the product of the second gene converts IAM to IAA (76, 84). Other T-DNA genes in Ti and Ri plasmids are known to affect tumor growth and morphology (39, 41, 50, 96). The functions of these additional genes remain to be characterized.

The importance of the auxin and cytokinin genes in oncogenesis has been demonstrated by insertion and deletion mutagenesis. The mutation of both the cytokinin gene and

H. E. Kaiser (ed.), *Comparative aspects of tumor development.*
© 1989, Kluwer Academic Publishers, Dordrecht. ISBN-13:978-0-89838-994-4

one of the auxin genes leads to a loss of virulence (70), whereas a mutation in only one of the three oncogenes leads to an attenuated response characterized by a slow tumor rate and/or the formation of shoots (auxin gene mutants) or roots (cytokinin gene mutants) (39, 41, 64). It is well known that the formation of roots and shoots by normal cells in culture can be controlled by the relative amounts of auxin and cytokinin in the growth medium (78). Analysis of hormones in crown-gall tumors varying in morphology have shown auxin-cytokinin ratios predicted by hormone-feeding experiments (2, 3, 92). Thus, an important aspect of tumor transformation is the abnormal production of auxin and cytokinin directed by T-DNA genes, and the degree of virulence depends on the activities of at least three different oncogenes.

An additional consequence of auxin and cytokinin production by transformed cells arises from the fact that these low molecular weight substances can move in plant tissues by diffusion or via specific transport systems. Early studies on crown gall documented abnormal development which occurred at some distance from the tumor site and which could be attributed to the secretion of auxin by the tumor (53, 62). More recently, studies based on the clonal analysis of primary tumor tissues have revealed that less than half of the cells in the tumor are actually transformed by T-DNA (13, 93). It appears, therefore, that growth substances secreted by transformed cells can induce proliferation in surrounding tissues. Thus, tumor virulence depends upon the growth rate of the tumor cell as well as the extent to which the tumor cell can induce hyperplastic growth in healthy cells.

3. TUMOR PROGRESSION IN CROWN GALL

Riker (72) found that tomato plants inoculated with *A. tumefaciens* did not form tumors when grown at temperatures greater than 30°C, despite the fact that both the plant and bacteria grew well at this temperature. Using this principle of thermal inactivation, Braun (17, 18, 19) established that host cells were only susceptible to transformation between 1 and 5 days after wounding. He also found that tumor growth rate was affected by thermal inactivation during this period of inception. Plants provided only 36 hours of permissive temperature produced slow-growing tumors, whereas plants provided about 50 hours of permissive temperature produced tumors with a moderate growth rate. The growth rates of the tumors were stable, and isolated tissues maintained their slow, moderate, or rapid growth rates for many years in culture (23). Thus, crown-gall transformation is a progressive process requiring several days.

Braun (23) examined the physiological basis for tumor progression by studying the nutritional requirements of cultured tumor tissues. In addition to White's basic medium, non-transformed cells also required auxin, cytokinin, glutamine, asparagine, *myo*-inositol, and cytidylic and guanylic acids to proliferate at a rate comparable to that of fully virulent tumor cells. Slow-growing tumor tissues required all of these supplements except cytokinin to show rapid proliferation, whereas tumor tissues showing a moderate growth rate required only glutamine, *myo*-inositol and auxin

as supplements. These studies support the view that several biosynthetic systems are progressively activated in the host during tumor inception and are required for expression of the fully virulent phenotype. These findings take on renewed interest in view of our current knowledge of bacterial oncogenes, for they indicate that growth systems other than auxin and cytokinin biosynthesis are required for maximum virulence. They also show that two functions encoded by the T-DNA, i.e., auxin and cytokinin autonomy, appear at very different times in the inception period.

4. BACTERIAL FACTORS AND TUMOR PROGRESSION

The thermal sensitivity of crown gall transformation depends in part on the strain of *A. tumefaciens* (8, 35, 73), implying that bacterial factors play a role in tumor progression. The most probable thermal-sensitive processes are the transfer and expression of T-DNA genes.

4.1 Transfer of T-DNA

Temperatures greater than 30°C inhibit the conjugative transfer of Ti plasmids in *Agrobacterium* (83). Assuming that the mechanism for T-DNA transfer is similarly sensitive, one can describe a simple model for progression based on the initial number of transformed cells. The ultimate size of a crown-gall tumor is known to be proportional to the size of the initial wound site (29) and, presumably, to the number of cells transformed by bacteria. Therefore, when high temperatures are applied early in the inception phase, only a few cells are transformed and the resulting tumor is small.

This simple model would not appear to provide an adequate explanation of progression, however, since tumor tissues maintained their characteristic slow, moderate, or rapid growth rates for many years in culture (23). Therefore, progression cannot be explained solely by the number of initial transformation events, but must also involve properties of the transformed cells themselves. Thus, models for progression based on T-DNA transfer would have to include some change in the transformation event. This may be viewed in terms of gene dosage, where the number of T-DNA copies transferred determines the degree of virulence, or may involve the transfer of a truncated sequence in which some oncogenic functions are missing.

Hybridization studies have shown that the number of T-DNA copies may vary in tumor cells (9), but there does not appear to be a correlation between copy number and virulence. Tumors may form with as little as one T-DNA copy per cell (36, 46, 51, 60, 86), suggesting that gene dosage does not account for tumor progression. However, it is not known whether some plant species require multiple T-DNA copies to show a virulent response. Unfortunately, there is a paucity of molecular studies with *Vinca rosea* (also *Catharantus roseus*) which was used by Braun in his detailed analysis of tumor progression.

Since mutations in the T-DNA can attenuate the tumor response, the transfer of truncated T-DNA fragments provides a possible explanation for tumor progression. According to this hypothesis, the interruption of T-DNA transfer at different times results in the transmission of T-DNA fragments of varying size. The major difficulty with this proposal is the fact that progression occurs over a period of 3 to 4 days, and it is difficult to imagine how part of the T-DNA can be transferred after 1 day while other portions are not transferred for several more days. This problem is underscored by the fact that auxin and cytokinin genes are closely linked in the T-DNA (63), whereas auxin and cytokinin autonomy appear at very different times during the inception phase (23). Nevertheless, with current molecular methods it would be possible to directly test whether or not thermal inactivation and subsequent tumor attenuation are associated with a change in the T-DNA sequence in the tumor cell.

4.2 Expression of T-DNA genes

Regulation of oncogene expression provides an attractive hypothesis for tumor progression since it is possible to visualize, in principle, how variable gene expression could account for gradual changes in tumor virulence. A discussion of T-DNA gene expression is included in this section because the topic concerns the fate of bacterial oncogenes. It should be remembered, however, that the bacterial contribution to tumor formation is fixed in the T-DNA sequence, and that expression of these genes in the nucleus of the plant cell must also be considered part of the host contribution to tumor virulence (see Section 5).

Considerable evidence is accumulating showing that variable expression of T-DNA genes does occur in the tumor cell. In a clonal analysis of tobacco crown-gall tumors, Van Slogteren et al. (93) obtained cell lines which varied in hormone autonomy and production of the opine, octopine. Hormone autotrophic clones were obtained, some of which showed octopine synthase activity (Ocs$^+$) and some of which did not (Ocs$^-$). Northern blot analysis of these cell lines showed the presence of the expected T-DNA hormone transcripts, but only the Ocs$^+$ lines showed substantial amounts of the octopine synthase transcript. The absence of the Ocs transcript was not due to the absence of the Ocs T-DNA sequences and, moreover, an Ocs$^+$ subclone was obtained from the Ocs$^-$ clone. These results show that expression of T-DNA genes can vary in a reversible fashion in the tumor cell. More importantly, they show that T-DNA genes can be regulated independently.

The selective expression of T-DNA oncogenes has also been demonstrated in tobacco tumor tissues. By cloning unorganized tumor tissues transformed by the virulent B6 strain of *A. tumefaciens*, Amasino et al. (4) obtained cell lines which retained the unorganized phenotype, but which also produced sectors capable of forming shoots. Although Southern blot analysis of DNA from the two sectors showed a similar T-DNA sequence, Northern blot analysis of RNA revealed strikingly different patterns of transcription. The unorganized tissues produced transcripts for most of the T-DNA genes including the two auxin genes, but produced no detectable RNA homologous to the cytokinin gene. On the other hand, only transcripts for the cytokinin gene were detected in the shoot-forming sector.

The expression of T-DNA genes has been associated with DNA methylation. Southern blot experiments using isoschizomer endonucleases have shown reduced T-DNA methylation to be related to increased transcriptional activity, and complementary experiments have further shown that transcriptional activity can be increased with 5-azacytidine treatment (4, 43).

The important question that arises is whether oncogene expression accounts for the progressive activation of growth during tumor inception. Evidence to support this view was obtained by Toothman (88) who showed that the accumulation of octopine in primary tumors was progressive and increased well after the appearance of tumorous growth, suggesting that oncogenes were activated in advance of opine synthesis. However, these studies are difficult to interpret since primary tumors include both transformed and non-transformed cells, and changes in opine synthesis may reflect in part changes in the distribution of normal and tumor cells. While it is becoming clear that recovery from the tumor state is associated with the loss or reduced expression of T-DNA genes, it is not known whether full expression of these genes is sufficient to induce a fully virulent response.

5. HOST FACTORS AND TUMOR PROGRESSION

Studies of the nutritional requirements of cultured tumor tissues reflecting different stages of tumor inception indicate that several biosynthetic systems must be activated for rapid tumor growth (23). There is increasing evidence that the state of the host cell plays an important role in the tumor response (review: 11). One of the most important requirements for tumor formation is wounding of the host.

5.1 The wound response

Early experiments showed that exposure of plant cells to virulent bacteria resulted in tumor formation only when such treatment was accompanied by wounding (66, 69, 71). The importance of wound-induced changes in susceptibility, known as conditioning of the host, was shown by Braun (20). By applying bacteria at some time after wounding, he found that the minimum exposure time required for tumor formation could be shortened. Thus, conditioning involved changes in the host independent from the action of the pathogen.

One possible explanation for conditioning is the exposure of cell surface binding sites, which are known to be important in transformation (52), or the appearance of other changes in the host necessary for T-DNA transfer. On the other hand, the time course of wound-induced susceptibility to crown-gall transformation follows very closely the sequence of events associated with wound healing (29). Biochemical studies of the wound response have revealed the progressive activation and transient activity of several biosynthetic systems (review: 49). Perhaps the most important effect of the wound response with respect to progression is the dedifferentiation and subsequent proliferation of cells surrounding the wound site. Thus, tumor progression may reflect the progressive activation of host growth systems associated with wound healing (25). This hypothesis implies that oncogenes do not encode sufficient information to induce the fully virulent tumor state, but are sufficient to prevent the return to normalcy once rapid growth is initiated. This view is attractive since one can, in principle, explain tumorous growth with a minimum amount of transferred DNA.

Wounding is also associated with the formation of Kostoff genetic tumors (7) and with the wound tumor disease caused by the phytoreoviruses (16). More recently, wounding has been found to be important for tumor formation in chickens infected with Rous sarcoma virus (40). Thus, wound-induced activation of growth may account for progression in a wide variety of neoplastic diseases and may help to explain the general role of irritation in the promotion of tumor growth.

5.2 Tumor suppression

Braun (24) was the first to demonstrate the reversible suppression of neoplastic growth. By serially grafting teratomatous shoots of single cell origin onto healthy hosts, Braun obtained shoots that were phenotypically normal. The process was fully reversible, and tissues would revert to the tumorous state in culture (31, 91), showing that the capacity for neoplastic growth was not lost. Clonal analysis of suppressed shoots indicates that most, if not all, of the cells may be potentially tumorous (14, 98). The phenomenon of tumor suppression shows that transformed cells can regain control of growth and undergo normal development.

One would like to know whether suppression is caused by altered expression of T-DNA genes (see Section 4.2 above) or by a change in host response. Suppressed shoots produce opines (97) and typically cannot be rooted, suggesting that at least the cytokinin gene is expressed. Other T-DNA functions may be involved, however, and further studies on the activities of T-DNA genes in suppressed plants are warranted. Nevertheless, it is clear that the tumor response depends on the state of the host cell. Since tumor suppression and progression represent reverse processes, the mechanisms which underlie these phenomena may be similar. (For a more detailed discussion of tumor suppression in plants, see (89), and Chapter 8, volume IV in this series by Meins).

5.3 Host range and host response

The host range of crown gall is very wide with at least 643 species belonging to 331 genera being susceptible to transformation (37). Most of the host plants are dicotyledonous, although many gymnosperms are also susceptible. On the other hand, very few monocotyledonous plants respond to infection by *A. tumefaciens*. Some support has been obtained for the hypothesis that host range is limited by T-DNA transfer. Evidence showing the lack of bacterial binding sites in the cell walls of monocotyledonous plants has provided a reasonable explanation for the resistance of these plants to crown-gall infection (52).

However, a more complex situation was indicated by the discovery that some bacteria show a limited host range. For example, a strain of *A. tumefaciens* was isolated which would only form tumors on grapevine (65), whereas another strain isolated from grapevine would form tumors on other test species, but not on *Kalanchoë*, which served as a suitable host for several other strains (47). More recently, cells at inoculation sites of monocotyledonous plants have been found to produce opines even though no tumors formed (48), indicating that T-DNA was transferred; and opine-producing tumor cells of asparagus have been obtained by infecting cultured stem segments (44). These studies suggest that host range is determined by the host response to transformation and not necessarily by the ability to transfer T-DNA.

The transfer of Ti plasmids to different chromosomal backgrounds showed that the host range of *A. tumefaciens* is directed by the plasmid (54, 87). Further analysis of the limited host range plasmid pTiAg63 showed that functions determining host range lie in the T-DNA region (32, 33). The limited host range of pTiAg63 was found to result in part from an altered cytokinin gene, and a broader host range could be restored to pTiAg63 by insertion of the cytokinin gene from the wide host range plasmid pTiA6. The role of other host factors was also indicated by the fact that pTiAg63 derivatives would induce tumors on some inbred lines of sunflower but not others (33).

Variation in the host response to crown-gall transformation may occur between species and in different tissues of the same plant (review: 11). For example, Braun (21) showed that strain T37 could induce either unorganized or shoot-forming tumors (teratomas) on tobacco plants depending on the site of inoculation. Ooms et al. (64) found that plasmids carrying mutant auxin genes induced small tumors on *Kalanchoë* stems, but were avirulent on leaves. Strong, indirect evidence suggests that tumor formation in response to plasmids with mutant oncogenes depends on the auxin content of the plant (27) or on the position of the inoculation site relative to the direction of auxin transport (6, 74). However, not all species show an attenuated response or position effects with mutant strains. In a limited survey of the genus *Nicotiana*, Binns (11) showed that several species gave a fully virulent response to Ti plasmids with mutations in either an auxin or cytokinin gene, whereas other species showed an attenuated response to these mutant plasmids. Studies of this type show that the physiological state of the host is an important determinant of virulence. Variation in the hormone requirements of the host cell appears to play an important role in determining both host range and host response.

5.4 Hormone autonomy

Cultured plant cells may spontaneously lose their requirement for growth hormones and thereafter proliferate indefinitely on hormone-free growth medium. This stable and heritable change in hormone requirement is known as habituation, and in some cases habituated tissues may form tumors when transplanted to a healthy host (review: 57). Thus, normal plant cells may show the potential for neoplastic growth without transformation by a pathogen, and the expression of this potential may be an important factor determining the host response to crown-gall transformation.

The hormone requirement of cultured cells can be estimated by comparing their growth rate on basal medium with that on medium supplemented with growth hormones.

Since plant tissues show a biphasic dose-response to auxins and cytokinins, the ratio of growth obtained with (+H) and without (−H) hormone supplements provides a measure of hormone autonomy (12). Hence, tissues which grow well without added hormone but show inhibited growth with hormone supplements are considered to be highly habituated (−H/+H > 1), whereas hormone-dependent cells only grow well when hormone is provided (−H/+H ≃ 0). Clonal analysis of tobacco tissues habituated for cytokinin revealed that cells may vary markedly in degree of autonomy (12). The response of cell lines to exogenous cytokinin ranged from large growth promotion to severe growth inhibition. One cell line which showed a low degree of autonomy (−H/+H = 0.19) was followed for many months in culture (58). The analysis of habituation over this period revealed a gradual increase in cytokinin autonomy (−H/+H increasing to 1.5). Thus, habituation involves the type of graded changes in growth autonomy which could account for tumor progression (58).

The competence of tobacco cells for cytokinin habituation is tissue specific (59). Cells isolated from leaves or stem pith normally require cytokinin for growth in culture, whereas primary explants of stem cortex are invariably habituated. The interaction of habituation with T-DNA determinants of hormone autonomy was studied by Binns (10). He was able to regenerate plants from cells transformed by a mutant derivative of pTiT37 which contained an insertion in the cytokinin gene, but an intact auxin locus. Primary leaf explants from these regenerated plants were found to be autotrophic for auxin but cytokinin-requiring, whereas primary cortical explants showed the reverse phenotype, being autotrophic for cytokinin and auxin-requiring. The phenotype of the leaf tissues was stable in culture, but cortex tissues became fully autotrophic for both auxin and cytokinin after an initial passage on growth medium containing auxin. These results demonstrate two important points: first, the expression of T-DNA-directed growth autonomy (in this case auxin autonomy) can differ with cell type; and second, the tissue-specific expression of habituation (in this case cytokinin autonomy) can substitute for missing oncogenes and contribute to the autonomous state of the transformed cell.

The simplest explanation for habituation is the activation of host pathways for hormone biosynthesis. Measurements of auxin and cytokinin content by several workers support the view that habituated tissues indeed produce the hormone for which they are habituated (see 57). However, recent analysis of a cloned cytokinin-habituated cell line failed to detect any cytokinins (42). Thus, either the production of unusual cytokinins accounts for habituation in some cases, or habituation can occur without hormone production.

Recent results obtained in our laboratory provide further evidence that hormone autonomy may be separated from hormone production (68). In studies using cells transformed by wild type or mutant strains of *A. tumefaciens*, we found that a high degree of auxin autonomy can occur without T-DNA-directed auxin biosynthesis. Normally tobacco cells transformed by the virulent A6 strain show rapid and unorganized growth *in situ* and in culture, whereas tumors induced by the mutant A66 strain produce numerous shoots (13). The genetic basis for the A66 mutation is the inactivation of gene 2 of the auxin locus by a 2.7 Kb insertion element (13, 55, 77, 94). As expected, tobacco tumors induced by auxin mutants show high cytokinin and relatively low auxin levels (2), conditions which promote the regeneration of shoots (78). However, when Janaki Vijayaraghavan grew an A66-transformed tobacco cell line for long periods in total darkness, she found that the tissue lost its capacity to form shoots. When returned to the light, the tissue continued to grow rapidly on hormone-free medium and

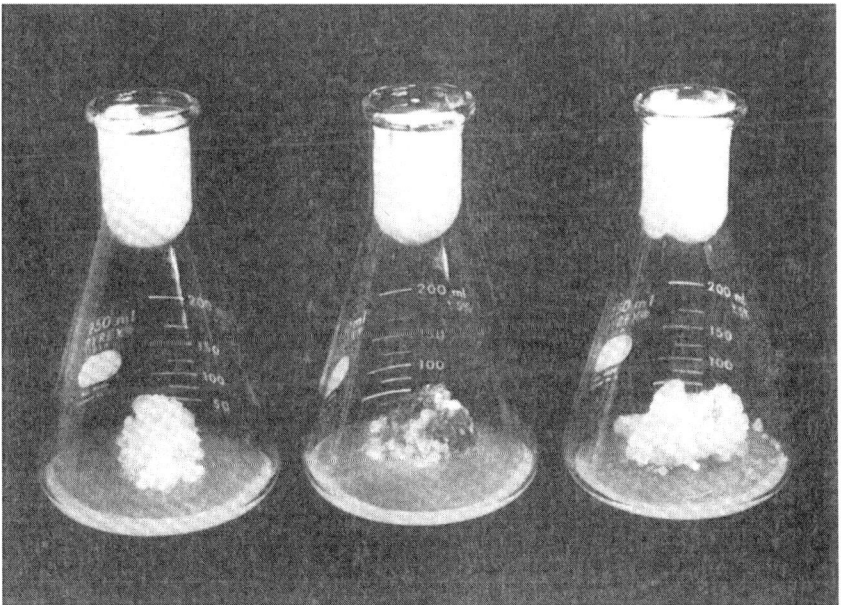

Figure 1. Crown-gall tissues of tobacco cultured on hormone-free growth medium. Right: Cloned cell line TA6-5 transformed by the wild-type A6 strain of *A. tumefaciens*. Center: Cloned cell line TA66C3-78 transformed by the auxin mutant A66 strain. Left: Line TA66-D1 derived from TA66C3-78 after dark treatment. TA6-5 and TA66C3-78 were isolated by A.N. Binns (13).

showed an unorganized phenotype which was indistinguishable from a cell line transformed by the wild-type A6 strain (Fig. 1). The unorganized phenotype was stable, and this tissue has been maintained for over a year in continuous light without reverting to the shooty phenotype.

Since the unorganized phenotype indicates a high auxin content (3, 4), we examined the auxin requirement of the dark-treated tissue. Growth of this tissue line (TA66-D1) was inhibited by treatment with the synthetic auxin, α-naphthaleneacetic acid (NAA) (Fig. 2). The high sensitivity of TA66-D1 to auxin treatment was similar to the A6-transformed cell line (TA6-5), whereas the shooty cell line (TA66C3-78) showed a low degree of sensitivity, and growth was usually promoted slightly at moderately high auxin doses. Therefore, the change in phenotype from shooty to unorganized growth was accompanied by an increase in auxin sensitivity.

We wanted then to find out whether increased auxin sensitivity in TA66-D1 resulted from changes in the T-DNA, i.e., reversion of the A66 mutation, or from changes in the host. Using Southern blot analysis, Daniela Sciaky of the Brookhaven National Laboratory showed that all three cell lines contained about one T-DNA copy per genome and, more importantly, that T-DNA of line TA66-D1 still contained the insertion sequence in gene 2 (68). This showed that the auxin system encoded in the T-DNA was still mutated, and suggested that host systems for auxin biosynthesis were activated instead. To our surprise, however, we

found that IAA levels in TA66-D1 were low (10^{-9} to 10^{-8} mol/kg fresh wt) and comparable to the IAA content of the shooty line TA66C3-78, whereas IAA levels in the wild-type tumor line TA6-5 were considerably higher (10^{-6} mol/ kg fresh wt). It appears, therefore, that a change in auxin sensitivity occurred without a corresponding change in auxin production.

Although IAA is the major auxin in higher plants, there are other naturally occurring auxins such as phenylacetic acid, indolepropionic acid and indolebutyric acid (75) which would not have been detected with our specific immunoassay for IAA (67). We tested for the production of other auxins indirectly by studying ethylene biosynthesis. It is well known that auxins of different types increase ethylene production by stimulating the biosynthesis of the ethylene precursor 1-aminocyclopropane-1-carboxylic acid (ACC) (review: 99). We have also shown that cells transformed by the wild-type A6 strain contain much higher levels of ACC than cells transformed by the mutant A66 strain, and that tumor tissues generally show increased ACC levels when fed auxin (61). However, our analysis of ACC correlated well with our IAA measurements and failed to detect other sources of auxin activity. The level of ACC in both TA66C3-78 and TA66-D1 was low (10^{-6} mol/kg fresh wt) compared to TA6-5 (10^{-4} mol/kg fresh wt). Thus, neoplastic progression occurred *in vitro* without the contribution of a hormone believed to be essential for virulent tumor growth. Either some change in hormone reception or transduction made the cells more sensitive to auxin, or the cells no longer required auxin stimulation for rapid and unorganized growth. Although a role for other T-DNA genes in this process cannot be excluded at the present time, these results strongly suggest that a change in the hormone requirement of the host cell was responsible for the switch in phenotype.

6. CONCLUSIONS

Tumor transformation in crown gall is a progressive process occurring over a period of several days. Transformation is caused by the transfer of bacterial oncogenes, some of which code for the production of naturally occurring plant growth hormones. The crown-gall problem is therefore analogous to tumor transformation in animals by retroviruses which contain oncogenes homologous to normal genes in the host (reviews: 15, 95). The important question is how oncogenes of pathogen or host origin convert the normal cell to the tumor cell. Progress on this problem will undoubtedly come from further identification of oncogene functions. However, in cases where the functions of retroviral oncogenes are known, it is still not clear how tumor transformation occurs. Nor is it known how auxin and cytokinin induce cell proliferation in plants. Studies on tumor progression in crown gall implicate host factors as important determinants of oncogene virulence. In some cases the activation of host pathways for hormone biosynthesis may be involved, but it is becoming increasingly clear that other factors associated with hormone requirement are also important. Those host systems which contribute to crown-gall transformation appear to be activated by wounding, and wound-induced growth may play an important role in neoplastic diseases generally (25). Future studies on the interaction of on-

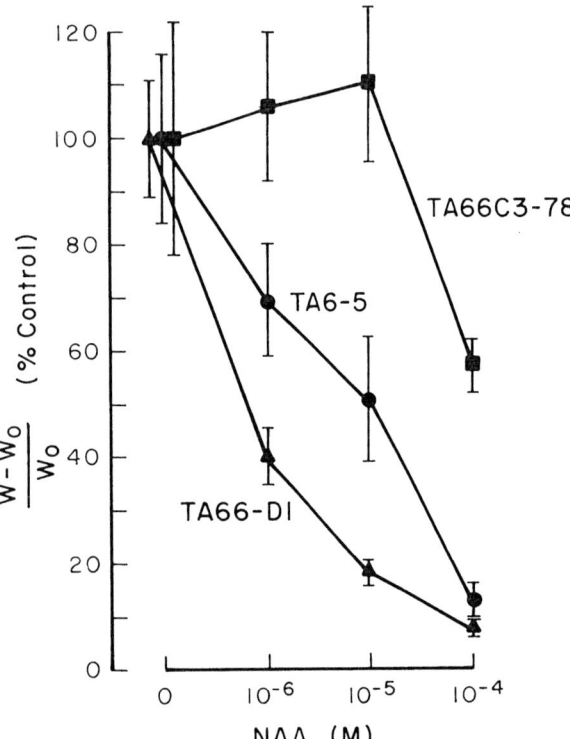

Figure 2. The effect of the auxin α-naphthaleneacetic acid (NAA) on the growth of crown-gall tumor tissues after 2 weeks in culture. Growth was calculated as $(W - W_0)/W_0$, where W and W_0 are the final and initial fresh weights of the explant. Bars indicate standard error for 5 replicates.

cogenes with host systems should contribute greatly to our understanding of tumor progression and to our general knowledge of growth and development.

7. ACKNOWLEDGEMENTS

The author would like to thank several colleagues who provided unpublished results and manuscripts in press. Support for work in the author's laboratory by the National Science Foundation (DMB-8417087) is gratefully acknowledged.

REFERENCES

1. Akiyoshi DE, Klee H, Amasino RM, Nester EW, Gordon MP: T-DNA of *Agrobacterium tumefaciens* encodes an enzyme of cytokinin biosynthesis. *Proc Natl Acad Sci USA* 81:5994–5998, 1984
2. Akiyoshi DF, Morris RO, Hinz R, Mischke BS, Kosuge T, Garfinkel DJ, Nester EW: Cytokinin/auxin balance in crown gall tumors is regulated by specific loci in the T-DNA. *Proc Natl Acad Sci USA* 80:407–411, 1983
3. Amasino RM, Miller CO: Hormonal control of tobacco crown gall tumor morphology. *Plant Physiol* 69:389–392, 1982
4. Amasino RM, Powell ALT, Gordon MP: Changes in T-DNA methylation and expression are associated with phenotypic variation and plant regeneration in a crown gall tumor line. *Mol Gen Genet* 197:437–446, 1984
5. Barry GF, Rogers SG, Fraley RT, Brand L: Identification of a cloned cytokinin biosynthetic gene. *Proc Natl Acad Sci USA* 81:4776–4780 1984
6. Barton KA, Binns AN, Matzke AJM, Chilton M-D: Regeneration of intact tobacco plants containing full length copies of genetically engineered T-DNA, and transmission of T-DNA to R1 progeny. *Cell* 32:1033–1043, 1983
7. Bayer MH: Genetic tumors: Physiological aspects of tumor formation in interspecies hybrids. In: Molecular Biology of Plant Tumors. Kahl G, Schell JS, eds. Academic Press, New York, pp. 33–67, 1982
8. Beiderbeck R: Überwindung der thermosensitiven Phase der Crown-Gall-Induktion durch eine Wirt-Bakterien-Kombination. *Z Pflanzenkr Pflanzenschutz* 90:173–177, 1983
9. Bevan MW, Chilton M-D: T-DNA of the *Agrobacterium* Ti and Ri plasmids. *Annu Rev Genet* 16:357–384, 1982
10. Binns AN: Host and T-DNA determinants of cytokinin autonomy in tobacco cells transformed by *Agrobacterium tumefaciens*. *Planta* 158:272–279, 1983
11. Binns AN: The biology and molecular biology of plant cells infected by *Agrobacterium tumefaciens*. In: Oxford Surveys of Plant and Molecular and Cell Biology. Miflin BJ, ed. Clarendon, Oxford, pp. 133–160, 1984
12. Binns AN, Meins F Jr: Habituation of tobacco pith cells for factors promoting cell division is heritable and potentially reversible. *Proc Natl Acad Sci USA* 70:2660–2662, 1973
13. Binns AN, Sciaky D, Wood HN: Variation in hormone autonomy and regenerative potential of cells transformed by strain A66 of *Agrobacterium tumefaciens*. *Cell* 31:605–612, 1982
14. Binns AN, Wood HN, Braun AC: Suppression of the tumorous state in crown gall teratomas of tobacco: a clonal analysis. *Differentiation* 19:97–102, 1981
15. Bishop JM: Cellular oncogenes and retroviruses. *Annu Rev Biochem* 52:301–354, 1983
16. Black LM: Wound tumor disease. In: Molecular Biology of Plant Tumors. Kahl G, Schell JS, eds. Academic Press, New York, pp. 69–105, 1982
17. Braun AC: Studies on tumor inception in the crown-gall disease. *Am J Bot* 30:674–677, 1943
18. Braun AC: Thermal studies on the factors responsible for tumor initiation in crown gall. *Am J Bot* 34:234–240, 1947
19. Braun AC: Cellular autonomy in crown gall. *Phytopathology* 41:963–966, 1951
20. Braun AC: Conditioning of the host cell as a factor in the transformation process in crown gall. *Growth* 16:65–74, 1952
21. Braun AC: Bacterial and host factors concerned in determining tumor morphology in crown gall. *Bot Gaz* 114:363–371, 1953
22. Braun AC: The activation of two growth-substance systems accompanying the conversion of normal to tumor cells in crown gall. *Cancer Res* 16:53–56, 1956
23. Braun AC: A physiological basis for autonomous growth of the crown-gall tumor cell. *Proc Natl Acad Sci USA* 44:344–349, 1958
24. Braun AC: A demonstration of the recovery of the crown-gall tumor cell with the use of complex tumors of single-cell origin. *Proc Natl Acad Sci USA* 45:932–938, 1959
25. Braun AC: The Cancer Problem. A Critical Analysis and Modern Synthesis. Columbia University Press, New York, 1969
26. Braun AC: Plant tumors. *Biochim Biophys Acta* 516:167–191, 1978
27. Braun AC, Laskaris T: Tumor formation by attenuated crown-gall bacteria in the presence of growth promoting substances. *Proc Natl Acad Sci USA* 28:468–477, 1942
28. Braun AC, Mandle RJ: Studies on the inactivation of the tumor inducing principle in crown gall. *Growth* 12:255–269, 1948
29. Braun AC, Stonier T: Morphology and physiology of plant tumors. *Protoplasmatologia* 10(5a):1–93, 1958
30. Braun AC, White PR: Bacteriological sterility of tissues derived from secondary crown-gall tumors. *Phytopathology* 33:85–100, 1943
31. Braun AC, Wood HN: Suppression of the neoplastic state with the acquisition of specialized functions in cells, tissues, and organs of crown gall teratomas of tobacco. *Proc Natl Acad Sci USA* 73:496–500, 1976
32. Buchholz WG, Thomashow MF: Comparison of T-DNA oncogene complements of *Agrobacterium tumefaciens* tumor-inducing plasmids with limited and wide host ranges. *J Bacteriol* 160:319–326, 1984a
33. Buchholz WG, Thomashow MF: Host range encoded by the *Agrobacterium tumefaciens* tumor-inducing plasmid pTiAg63 can be expanded by modification of its T-DNA oncogene complement. *J Bacteriol* 160:327–332, 1984b
34. Buchmann I, Marner F-J, Schröder G, Waffenschmidt S, Schröder J: Tumor genes in plants: T-DNA encoded cytokinin biosynthesis. *EMBO J* 4:853–860, 1985
35. Charest PJ, Dion P: The influence of temperature on tumorigenesis induced by various strains of *Agrobacterium tumefaciens*. *Can J Bot* 63:1160–1167, 1985
36. De Beuckeleer M, Lemmers M, De Vos G, Willmitzer L, Van Montagu M, Schell J: Further insight on the transferred-DNA of octopine crown gall. *Mol Gen Genet* 183:283–288, 1981
37. De Cleene, M, De Ley J: The host range of crown gall. *Bot Rev* 42:389–466, 1976
38. Depicker A, Van Montagu M, Schell J: Homologous DNA sequences in different Ti plasmids are essential for oncogenicity. *Nature* 275:150–152, 1978
39. Depicker A, Van Montagu M, Schell J: Plant cell transformation by *Agrobacterium* plasmids. In: Genetic Engineering in Plants: An Agricultural Perspective. Kosuge T, Meredith CP, Hollaender A, eds. Plenum, New York, pp. 143–176, 1983
40. Dolberg DS, Hollingsworth R, Hertle M, Bissell MJ: Wounding and its role in RSV-mediated tumor formation. *Science* 230:676–678, 1985

41. Garfinkel DJ, Simpson RB, Ream LW, White FF, Gordon MP, Nester EW: Genetic analysis of crown gall: Fine structure map of the T-DNA by site-directed mutagenesis. *Cell* 27:143–153, 1981

42. Hansen CE, Meins F Jr, Milani A: Clonal and physiological variation in the cytokinin content of tobacco-cell lines differing in cytokinin requirement and capacity for neoplastic growth. *Differentiation* 29:1–6, 1985

43. Hepburn AG, Clarke LE, Pearson L, White J: The role of cytosine methylation in the control of nopaline synthase gene expression in a plant tumor. *J Mol Appl Genet* 2:315–329, 1983

44. Hernalsteens J-P, Thia-Toong L, Schell J, Van Montagu M: An *Agrobacterium*-transformed cell culture from the monocot *Asparagus officinalis. EMBO J* 3:3039–3041, 1984

45. Holsters M, Hernalsteens JP, Van Montagu M, Schell J: Ti plasmids of *Agrobacterium tumefaciens*: The nature of the TIP. In: Molecular Biology of Plant Tumors. Kahl G, Schell JS, eds. Academic Press, New York, pp. 269–298, 1982

46. Holsters M, Villarroel R, Van Montagu M, Schell J: The use of selectable markers for the isolation of plant-DNA/T-DNA junction fragments in a cosmid vector. *Mol Gen Genet* 185:283–289, 1982

47. Hooykaas PJJ, Schilperoort RA, Rorsch A: *Agrobacterium* tumor inducing plasmids; potential vectors for the genetic engineering of plants. *Genet Eng* 1:151–179, 1979

48. Hooykaas-Van Slogteren GMS, Hooykaas PJJ, Schilperoort RA: Expression of Ti plasmid genes in monocotyledonous plants infected with *Agrobacterium tumefaciens. Nature* 311:763–764, 1984

49. Kahl G: Molecular biology of wound healing: The conditioning phenomenon. In: Molecular Biology of Plant Tumors. Kahl G, Schell JS, eds. Academic Press, New York, pp. 211–267, 1982

50. Leemans J, Deblaere R, Willmitzer L, De Greve H, Hernalsteens JP, Van Montagu M, Schell J: Genetic identification of functions of TL-DNA transcripts in octopine crown galls. *EMBO J* 1:147–152, 1982

51. Lemmers M, De Beuckeleer M, Holsters M, Zambryski P, De picker A, Hernalsteens JP, Van Montagu M, Schell J: Internal organization, boundaries and integration of Ti-plasmid DNA in nopaline crown gall tumours. *J Mol Biol* 144:353–376, 1980

52. Lippincott JA, Lippincott BB: Cell walls of crown-gall tumors and embryonic plant tissues lack *Agrobacterium* adherence sites. *Science* 199:1075–1078, 1978

53. Locke SB, Riker AJ, Duggar BM: Growth substance and the development of crown gall. *J Agric Res* 57:21–59, 1938

54. Loper JE, Kado CI: Host range conferred by the virulence specifying plasmid of *Agrobacterium tumefaciens. J Bacteriol* 139:591–596, 1979

55. Machida Y, Sakurai M, Kiyokawa S, Ubasawa A, Suzuki Y, Ikeda J: Nucleotide sequence of the insertion sequence found in the T-DNA region of mutant Ti plasmid pTiA66 and distribution of its homologues in octopine Ti plasmid. *Proc Natl Acad Sci USA* 81:7495–7499, 1984

56. Meins F Jr: Evidence for the presence of a readily transmissible oncogenic principle in crown gall teratoma cells of tobacco. *Differentiation* 1:21–25, 1973

57. Meins F, Jr: Habituation of cultured plant cells. In: Molecular Biology of Plant Tumors. Kahl G, Schell JS, eds. Academic Press, New York, pp. 3–31, 1982

58. Meins F, Jr, Binns AN: Epigenetic variation of cultured somatic cells: Evidence for gradual changes in the requirement for factors promoting cell division. *Proc Natl Acad Sci USA* 74:2928–2932, 1977

59. Meins F Jr, Lutz J: Tissue-specific variation in the cytokinin habituation of cultured tobacco cells. *Differentiation* 15:1–6, 1979

60. Merlo DJ, Nutter RC, Montoya AL, Garfinkel DJ, Drummond MH, Chilton M-D, Gordon MP, Nester EW: The boundaries and copy numbers of Ti plasmid T-DNA vary in crown gall tumors. *Mol Gen Genet* 177:637–643, 1980

61. Miller AR, Pengelly WL: Ethylene production by shoot-forming and unorganized crown-gall tumor tissues of *Nicotiana* and *Lycopersicon* cultured *in vitro. Planta* 161:418–424, 1984

62. Nemec B: Bakterielle Wuchsstoffe. *Ber Deut Botan Ges* 48:72–74, 1930

63. Nester EW, Gordon MP, Amasino RM, Yanofsky MF: Crown gall: A molecular and physiological analysis. *Annu Rev Plant Physiol* 35:387–413, 1984

64. Ooms G, Hooykaas PJJ, Moolenaar G, Schilperoort RA: Crown-gall plant tumors of abnormal morphology, induced by *Agrobacterium tumefaciens* carrying mutated octopine Ti plasmids; analysis of T-DNA functions. *Gene* 14:33–50, 1981

65. Panagopoulos CG, Psallidas P: Characteristics of Greek isolates of *Agrobacterium tumefaciens* (Smith & Townsend) conn *J Appl Bacteriol* 36:233–240, 1973

66. Patty FA: Some experiments with crown gall bacteria. *Phytopathology* 20:856, 1930

67. Pengelly WL, Meins F Jr: A specific radioimmunoassay for nanogram quantities of the auxin, indole-3-acetic acid. *Planta* 136:173–180, 1977

68. Pengelly WL, Vijayaraghavan SJ, Sciaky D: Neoplastic progression in crown gall in tobacco without elevated auxin levels. *Planta* 169:454–461, 1986

69. Rack K: Untersuchungen über die Bedeutung der Verwundung und über die Rolle von Wuchsstoffen beim bakteriellen Pflanzenkrebs. *Phytopathol Z* 21:1–44, 1953

70. Ream LW, Gordon MP, Nester EW: Multiple mutations in the T region of the *Agrobacterium tumefaciens* tumor-inducing plasmid. *Proc Natl Acad Sci USA* 80:1660–1664, 1983

71. Riker AJ: Some relations of the crown gall organism to its host tissue. *J Agric Res* 25:119–132, 1923

72. Riker AJ: Studies on the influence of some environmental factors on the development of crown gall. *J Agric Res* 32:83–96, 1926

73. Rogler CE: Strain-dependent temperature-sensitive phase of crown gall tumorigenesis. *Plant Physiol* 68:5–10, 1981

74. Ryder MH, Tate ME, Kerr A: Virulence properties of strains of *Agrobacterium* on the apical and basal surfaces of carrot root discs. *Plant Physiol* 77:215–221, 1985

75. Schneider EA, Kazakoff CW, Wightman F: Gas chromatography-mass spectrometry evidence for several endogenous auxins in pea seedling organs. *Planta* 165:232–241, 1985

76. Schröder G, Waffenschmidt S, Weiler EW, Schröder J: The T-region of Ti plasmids codes for an enzyme synthesizing indole-3-acetic acid. *Eur J Biochem* 138:387–391, 1984

77. Sciaky D, Thomashow MF: The sequence of the tms transcript 2 locus of the *A. tumefaciens* plasmid pTiA6 and characterization of the mutation in pTiA66 that is responsible for auxin attenuation. *Nucl Acids Res* 12:1447–1461, 1984

78. Skoog F, Miller CO: Chemical regulation of growth and organ formation in plant tissues cultured *in vitro. Symp Soc Exp Biol* 11:118–131, 1957

79. Smith HH: Plant genetic tumors. *Prog Exp Tumor Res* 15:138–159, 1972

80. Smith EF, Townsend CO: A plant tumor of bacterial origin. *Science* 25:671–673, 1907

81. Tempé J, Goldmann A: Occurrence and biosynthesis of opines. In: Molecular Biology of Plant Tumors. Kahl G, Schell JS, eds. Academic Press, New York, pp. 427–449, 1982

82. Tempé J, Petit A: Opine utilization by *Agrobacterium*. In: Molecular Biology of Plant Tumors. Kahl G, Schell JS, eds. Academic Press, New York, pp. 451–459, 1982

83. Tempé J, Petit A, Holsters M, Van Montagu M, Schell J: Thermosensitive step associated with transfer of the Ti plasmid during conjugation: Possible relation to transformation in crown-gall. *Proc Natl Acad Sci USA* 74:2848–2849, 1977

84. Thomashow LS, Reeves S, Thomashow MF: Crown-gall on-

cogenesis: evidence that a T-DNA gene from the *Agrobacterium* Ti plasmid pTiA6 encodes an enzyme that catalyzes synthesis of indoleacetic acid. *Proc Natl Acad Sci USA* 81:5071–5075, 1984

85. Thomashow MF, Hughly S, Buchholz WG, Thomashow LS: Molecular basis for the auxin-independent phenotype of crown-gall tumor tissues. *Science* 231:616–618, 1986

86. Thomashow MF, Nutter R, Postle K, Chilton M-D, Blattner FR, Powell A, Gordon MP, Nester EW: Recombination between higher plant DNA and the Ti plasmid of *Agrobacterium tumefaciens*. *Proc Natl Acad Sci USA* 77:6448–6452 1980

87. Thomashow MF, Panagopoulos CG, Gordon MP, Nester EW: Host range of *Agrobacterium tumefaciens* is determined by the Ti plasmid. *Nature* 283:794–796, 1980

88. Toothman P: Octopine accumulation early in crown gall development is progressive. *Plant Physiol* 69:214–219, 1982

89. Turgeon R: Suppression of, and recovery from, the neoplastic state. *Int Rev Cytol Suppl* 13:59–81, 1981

90. Turgeon R: Teratomas and secondary tumors. In: Molecular Biology of Plant Tumors. Kahl G, Schell JS, eds. Academic Press, New York, pp. 391–414, 1982

91. Turgeon R, Wood HN, Braun AC: Studies on the recovery of crown gall tumor cells. *Proc Natl Acad Sci USA* 73:3562–3564, 1976

92. Van Onckelen H, Rudelsheim P, Hermans R, Horemans S, Messens E, Hernalsteens J-P, Van Montagu M, De Greef J: Kinetics of endogenous cytokinin, IAA, and ABA levels in relation to the growth and morphology of tobacco crown gall tissue. *Plant Cell Physiol* 25:1017–1025, 1984

93. Van Slogteren GMS, Hoge JHC, Hooykaas PJJ, Schilperoort RA: Clonal analysis of heterogenous crown gall tumor tissues induced by wild-type and shooter mutant strains of *Agrobacterium tumefaciens*-expression of T-DNA genes. *Plant Mol Biol* 2:321–333, 1983

94. Waldron C, Hepburn AG: Extra DNA in the region of crown gall Ti plasmid pTiA66. *Plasmid* 10:199–203, 1983

95. Weinberg RA: The action of oncogenes in the cytoplasm and nucleus. *Science* 230:770–776, 1985

96. White FF, Taylor BH, Huffman GA, Gordon MP, Nester EW: Molecular and genetic analysis of the transferred DNA regions of the root-inducing plasmid of *Agrobacterium rhizogenes*. *J. Bacteriol* 164:33–44, 1985

97. Wood HN, Binns AN, Braun AC: Differential expression of oncogenicity and nopaline synthesis in intact leaves derived from crown gall teratomas of tobacco. *Differentiation* 11:175–180, 1978

98. Wullems GJ, Molendijk L, Ooms G, Schilperoort RA: Retention of tumor markers in F1 progeny plants from *in vitro* induced octopine and nopaline tumor tissues. *Cell* 24:719–727, 1981

99. Yang SF, Hoffman NE: Ethylene biosynthesis and its regulation in higher plants. *Annu Rev Plant Physiol* 35:155–189, 1984

4

SELECTED ASPECTS OF NEOPLASTIC PROGRESSION IN MOLLUSKS

C. AUSTIN FARLEY

INTRODUCTION

An extensive literature on molluscan neoplasia has developed since the late 1960's. A few have emphasized naturally occurring, presumably malignant epizootic disease (1, 2, 4, 6, 8–12, 14, 17, 18, 20, 21). Most lesions were characterized as sarcomas with many showing leukemic features. These epizootics exclusively affected marine bivalve mollusks. These observations do not necessarily imply that estuarine bivalve mollusks are the only group where neoplasms exist but probably reflect the intensive efforts in molluscan pathology spent studying severe oyster mortalities which affected Atlantic coast oysters since the late 1960's (13). A correlation was found by Mix (21) between neoplasm prevalence and polynuclear aromatic hydrocarbons in mussels in Yaquina Bay, Oregon, but only Khudolei and Sirenko (19) have presented experimental evidence of inducibility by carcinogenic compounds.

This discussion is restricted to those episodes of epizootic neoplasia with which I am most familiar particularly as they relate to progression of the disease. Relatively high prevalences of neoplasms were discovered in populations of oysters (*Ostrea lurida*) and blue mussels (*Mytilus edulis*) in Yaquina Bay, Oregon in 1969 (12, 20, 21) and in British Columbia (9). Since in most species and in most locations neoplastic disease is reportable only in cases per thousand (1/5000 in Chesapeake Bay oysters (10), any prevalence measured in whole percentage numbers is considered to be an epizootic level of involvement. A second epizootic site was discovered in Chesapeake Bay and involved duck clams (*Macoma balthica*) (6). The third and most extensive epizootic was found in soft-shell clams (*Mya arenaria*) which included two distinct types of neoplasms (24) that were found in numerous sites throughout New England in the 1970's (4). More recently the disease has apparently spread into Chesapeake Bay populations (16).

These epizootics have a number of features in common which should be considered in assessing disease progression in this group. Prevalences vary from 10% to 90% in a few sites. Lesions are most commonly found from October through April. Neoplasms appear to progress to more advanced lesions through the winter months and disappear in the spring presumably because of mortality. The cytology of neoplastic cells is characterized by anaplasia, hyperchromatic enlarged nuclei which are often lobed and contain large sometimes multiple nucleoli. A decreased nuclear cytoplasmic ratio is evident and cells in all of the above lesions are probably polyploid. Mitotic rates are variable but mitotic

figures are always present at some stage of the disease. Neoplastic cells always invade hemolymph spaces where proliferation results in sinuses that become densely packed with these cells. This feature is true regardless of whether or not cell origin is hematopoietic or epithelial. The duck clam lesion appeared histologically to be a leukemia but was found to be a gill carcinoma by electron microscopy (15).

Until recently studies on progression of these diseases were limited to histologic evaluation of static material after the animal had been sacrificed (6, 11, 20). Interpretations were based on apparent changes seen by sequential sampling of populations. Using this method, apparent early lesions (Plate 1c) consist of rare isolated neoplastic cells inhabiting blood and connective tissue spaces such as the typhlosole region (Plate 1a) of the intestine or blood sinuses in the gill or plycate organ. Intermediate lesions (Plate 1e) show focal collections of neoplastic cells in the same sites mentioned above. Advanced lesions (Plate 1g, i) consist of densely packed collections of neoplastic cells throughout the connective tissue and blood spaces of the animal. Cooper (7) was the first to develop and evaluate an *in vivo* bleeding technique for diagnosing and staging molluscan neoplasms. Permanent preparations were made using Wright's stain and staging was done by live cell haemocytometer counts.

PROGRESSION OF DISEASE IN SOFT-CLAM SARCOMA

Recent studies on the new occurrence of epizootic sarcoma in Chesapeake Bay soft-shell clams (16) has led to the initiation of new approaches in methods of studying this disease in field and laboratory experiments. (Earlier studies of this disease in New England clam populations suggested a relationship with oil pollution or other contaminants (5, 18, 23, 24) but Brown (3) demonstrated transmissibility *via* a waterborne agent and experimental studies by Oprandy (22) suggested that the agent was filterable. Reinisch (23) recently implied that prevalence was enhanced by PCB's and other contaminants in New Bedford Harbor, Massachusetts. Evidence for a relationship between this disease in soft-shell clams and pollution is tenuous at best based on the sum of knowledge from past and present studies.

Long term periodic surveys of soft-shell clams in Chesapeake Bay which began in 1969 demonstrated that populations were sarcoma-free until 1979. Only rare cases were found until late 1983 when prevalences above 40% were detected. The new epizootic was closely monitored by

24

H. E. Kaiser (ed.), Comparative aspects of tumor development.
© 1989, Kluwer Academic Publishers, Dordrecht. ISBN-13:978-0-89838-994-4

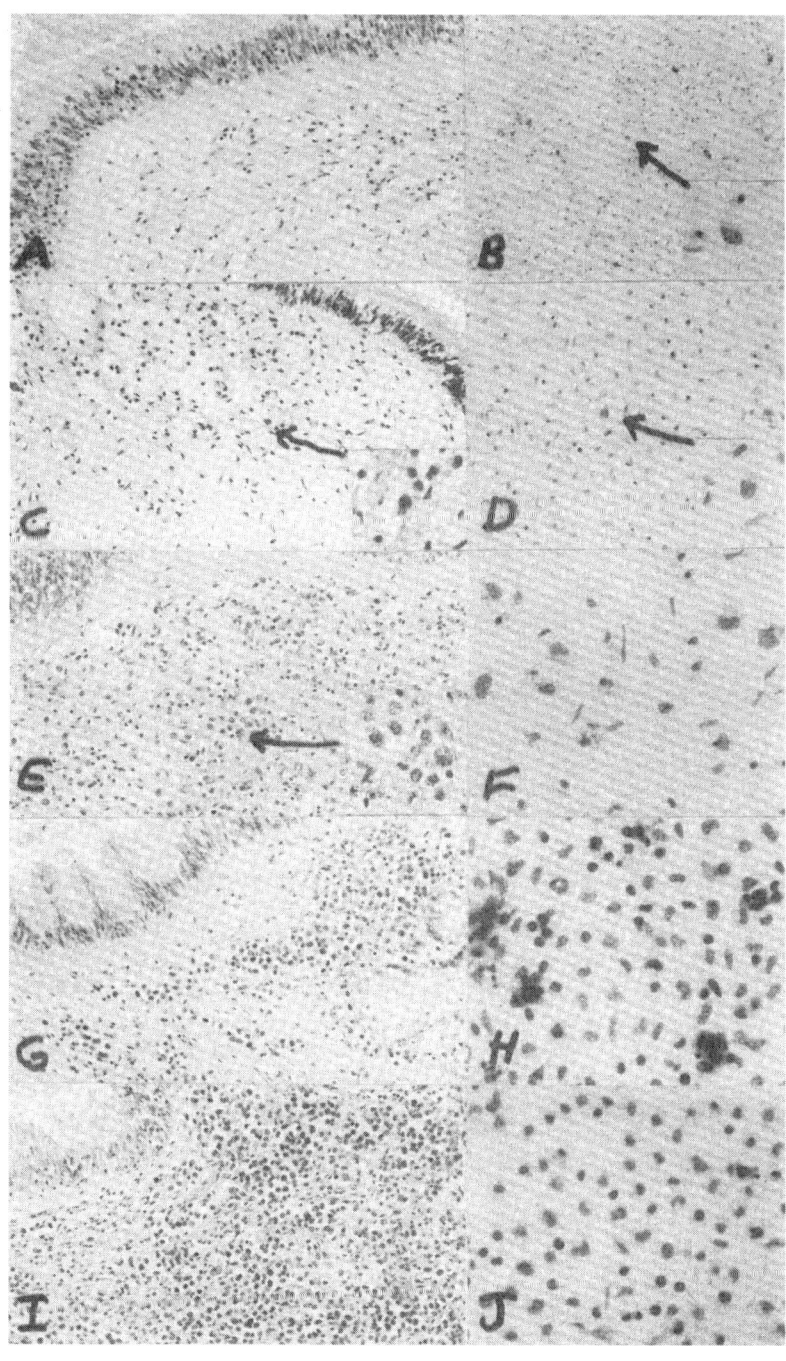

Plate 1. Comparison of histologic and histocytologic preparations. All histologic sections are through the typhlosole region. Photomicrographs of sections are at 200 ×, inserts showing sarcoma cells are 1000 ×. Staining of all material is by the Feulgen-picromethyl-blue method (10). A. Clam TIM-840615-30 typhlosole is normal. Sarcoma cells were rare elsewhere. B. Histocytologic preparation shows stage 1 involvement with one cell present in 100 × field. C. Clam POM-840705-26 has a very early neoplasm. One sarcoma cell is visible in the typhlosole region. The hemolymph preparation (D) is a stage 2 lesion. One cell is visible in a 200 × field of view. E. Clam TIM-850615-26 has an intermediate neoplastic lesion. Nests of sarcoma cells can be seen in the typhlosole region. F. Shows the stage 3 hemolymph preparation with a number of neoplastic cells evident in the 400 × field. G. TIM-840619-21 is an early advanced case. Neoplastic cells are abundant in the typhylosole. H. The hemolymph preparation is a stage 4 lesion clumps are still present (400 ×). I. TIM-840615-66 is a terminal advanced neoplasm. Necrosis is evident and neoplastic cells are very abundant throughout the tissues. J. Shows the hemolymph preparation from this animal. Normal hemocytes are rare and pyknosis is evident in many nuclei (400 ×).

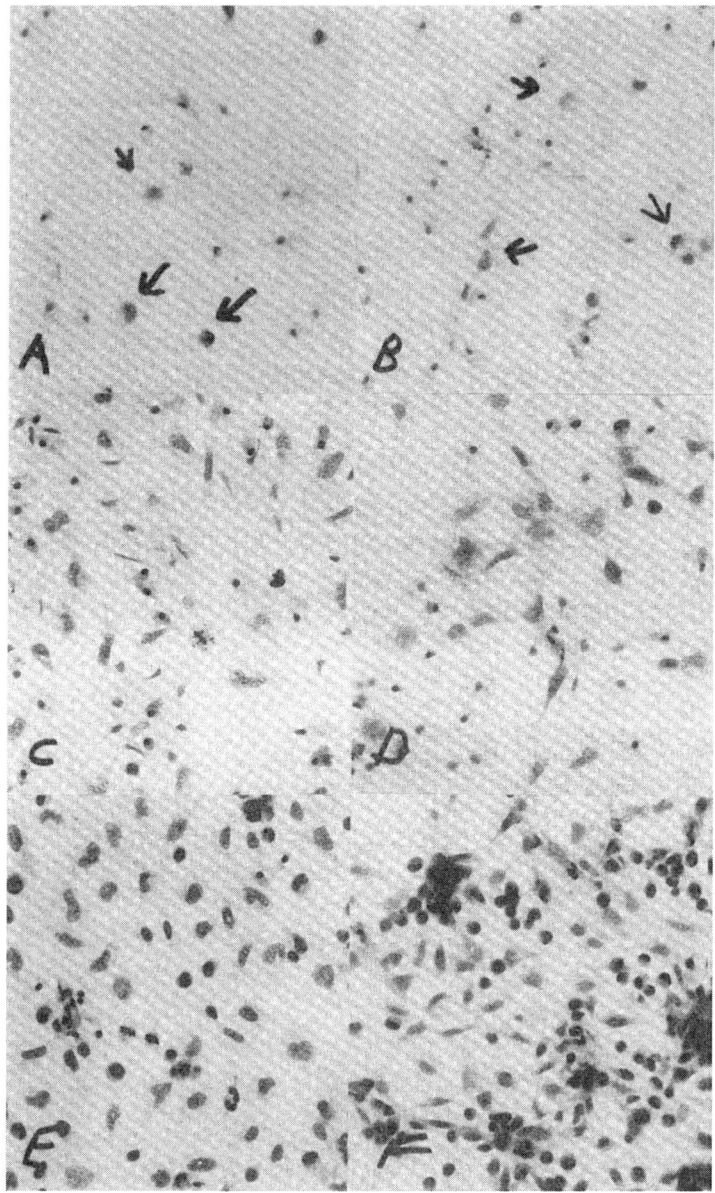

Plate 2. Clinical progression of sarcoma in clam OXC-2 (see Table 1) over time. Stain is by the Feulgen-picromethyl blue method. Magnification is 400 ×. A. Histocytologic preparation made December 13, 1983. Diagnosed stage 3. B. Histocytologic preparation made December 19, 1983 (stage 3). C. Histocytologic preparation made January 3, 1984 (late stage 3). D. Histocytologic preparation made January 19, 1984 (late stage 3). E. Histocytologic preparation made January 30, 1984 (early stage 4). F. Histocytologic preparation made February 2, 1984 (late stage 4). (Mitotic figures are evident in (C) and (E).)

periodic sampling of key sites for more than a year (16). Following the lead of Cooper (7) an *in vivo* bleeding method called "histocytology" was developed using living animals, thus permitting repeated diagnosis in individual specimens. The permanent stained monolayer preparations were found to be more accurate than histology for early stages of the disease. Using this method the disease could be followed clinically in individual animals. This approach produced a means of categorizing stages of the disease by cell ratios (Table 1) (Plate 1b, d, f, h, j) and following its progression clinically (Table 1, Plate 2) (16).

LABORATORY STUDIES

Demonstration of clinical progression and malignancy

Thirty clams were diagnosed by histocytology for sarcomas (Table 1). The disease stage was assessed by determining the sarcoma cell/blood cell ratio. Repeated periodic diagnosis of all individuals over a 6 month period demonstrated that the disease progressed from early to advanced stages and resulted in a fatal outcome within 5 months of all of the sarcomatous animals. Although mortality was high in non-affected

Table 1. Sarcoma progression in individual, laboratory-held soft clams: Dec 1983–June 1984. Whole numbers = percent ratios of neoplastic cells to hemocytes and numbers in parentheses = stages of disease. Stages: Early – (1) = 0.01–0.09% and (2) = 0.1–0.9%; Intermediate – (3) = 1–49%; Advanced – (4) = 50–89% and (5) = 90–100%. (Diagnosed from Feulgen-stained cytologic preparations.) (Farley, 1986).

Date	Specimen Data							Sample Data			Neoplastic clams: % Advanced Cases (N = 10)	% Cumulative Mortality (N = 10)	Normal clams: % Cumulative Mortality (N = 20)
	OXC 1	OXC 2	OXC 4	OXC 8	OXC 10	OXC 11	OXC 13	OXC 1	OXC 18	EBC 6			
6 Dec 83	70(4)	0.5(2)	0.01(1)	(0)	0.02(1)	12(3)	0.5 (2)	0.1(2)	(0)	–	14	0	0
12 Dec 83	76(4)	6 (3)	–	0.03(1)	–	10(3)	0.96(2)	–	–	5(3)	11	0	0
19 Dec 83	Died	11 (3)	29 (3)	0.9 (2)	0.1 (2)	Died	1 (3)	0.8(2)	(0)	62(4)	14	20	5
3 Jan 84		33 (3)	16 (3)	2 (3)	8 (3)		33 (3)	0.9(2)	(0)	50(4)	14	20	15
16 Jan 84		40 (3)	50 (4)	8 (3)	8 (3)		25 (3)	0.1(2)	0.1(2)	67(4)	25	20	15
30 Jan 84		80 (4)	50 (4)	10 (3)	2 (3)		17 (3)	0.8(2)	0.1(2)	57(4)	38	20	20
22 Feb 84		90 (5)	80 (4)	53 (4)	2 (3)		70 (4)	5 (3)	0.1(2)	95(5)	63	20	25
3 Apr 84		95 (5)	90 (5)	85 (4)	40 (3)		92 (5)	8 (3)	10 (3)	95(5)	63	20	25
13 Apr 84		Died	98 (5)	99 (5)	Died		98 (5)	12 (3)	62 (4)	99(5)	83	40	40
May 84			Died	–			Died	–	Died	Died	–	70	50
Jun 84				Died				Died			–	100	55

Table 2. Epizootiology of sarcomas in lab held populations June–Aug 1985.

Pop. Data	Date	Stage 0	Stage 1	Stage 2	Stage 3	Stage 4	Stage 5	Prevalence	Mortality
Swan Point	27 Jun 85	N = 25	5	5	4	0	0		collection date
Juveniles	% in Pop.		13%	13%	10%	0	0	36%	
35–50 mm	% Sarcoma		36%	36%	29%	0	0		
N = 39									
	16 Aug 85	N = 12	6	2	8	8	1		5%
	% in Pop.		16%	5%	22%	22%	3%	68%	
	% Sarcoma		24%	8%	32%	32%	4%		
	27 Aug 85								3%
									8% (cum.)
Replicate 1									
Swan Point	13 Aug 85	N = 19	7	1	5	17	6		collection date
Juveniles	% in Pop.		13%	2%	9%	30%	11%	65%	
35–50 mm	% Sarcoma		20%	3%	14%	46%	17%		
N = 55	27 Aug 85								33%
Replicate 2	16 Aug 85	N = 11	3	3	3	11	6		collection date
Juveniles	% in Pop.		8%	8%	8%	30%	16%	70%	
35–50 mm	% Sarcoma		12%	12%	12%	42%	23%		
N = 37	27 Aug 85								37%

X^2 Evaluation of mortality-sarcoma stage relationships in August collections from Swan Point

# Live Clams	N = 38	10	13	15	13	1	146	
# Dead Clams	10	2	2	8	21	13	Observed (O)	
% Mortality	21%	17%	13%	36%	62%	92%		
Expected Mortality	18	5	6	9	13	5	Expected (E)	
	−8	−3	−4	−1	8	8	Difference = (O–E)	
	3.56	1.8	2.67	0.111	4.92	12.8		

$$X^2 = \frac{(O-E)^2}{E}$$

Sum of X^2 = 25.86 with 5° of Freedom P = 0.001
0 – Stage 3 comprised 22% of the mortality (N = 93)
Stages 4 and 5 comprised 71% of the mortality (N = 48).

animals, a 55% survival was noted in this group. Ten clams were positive and 20 were negative throughout the study.

A second laboratory observational experiment was performed to determine if a relationship existed between mortality and sarcoma stages. A sample of Swan Point juvenile clams was collected in June 1985 (Table 2). A prevalence of 36% was noted and sarcoma stages were early to intermediate. When these individuals were examined 1 month later the prevalence had increased to 68% and sarcomas were found in all stages of development (these animals were held in a charcoal filtered recirculated seawater aquarium at 14°C). Additional replicate samples were collected fresh from Swan Point on August 13, 1985. Prevalences were 65% and 70% respectively but advanced stages predominated in both replicates (ambient Bay water temperatures from June through August ranged between 22 and 27°C.)

All three groups were closely monitored for mortality until the end of August and each individual was recorded by date along with its disease stage at last diagnosis. The experiment showed the close similarity between field and laboratory data and demonstrated a clear progressive relationship between advanced disease stages and mortality. Animals in stages 4 and 5 were three times as likely to die as stage 0, 1, 2 or 3 animals. The Chi square evaluation (Table 2) and regression analysis (Plate 3) demonstrated a 99.9% proba-

bility that these differences were real. This experiment clearly demonstrated that stages as described (16) are valid as indicators of a clinically progressive malignant disease in soft-shelled clams.

Demonstration of transplantability

A sample of clams obtained from a commercial source was diagnosed by histocytology for sarcomas. An initial prevalence of 23% was noted and neoplastic clams were removed from the population. Forty clams were held for a period of 3 months in aquaria with recirculated seawater. All remained negative for sarcomas through 3 monthly diagnostic examinations. Temperature was maintained at between 11° and 14°. All clams were diagnosed monthly for sarcomas. Stage 4 and 5 donor clams were selected from several samples and neoplastic cells were harvested and cell density determined. Recipient clams were injected via the musculature of the siphon by the following protocol: Clams (KNC 3, 5, 8, 11, and 13) were injected with 245,000 cells each from stage 5 donor OXC-2; clams (KNC 17, 21, 26, 30, and 43) were injected with 300,000 cells each from stage 5 donor EBC-6; clams (KNC 53, 55, 57, 59, and 61) were injected with 250,000 cells each from stage 5 donor KNC-36;

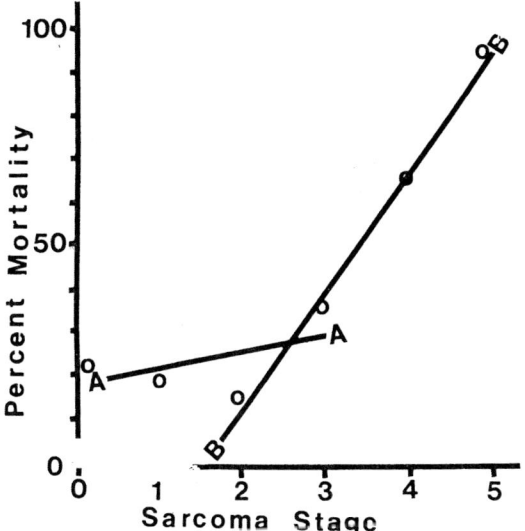

Plate 3. Linear regression of sarcoma stages and percent mortality

Sarcoma stage (X)	Frequency (F)	Percent mortality (Y)
0	48	21%
1	12	17%
2	15	13%
3	23	36%
4	34	62%
5	14	92%

A-A = regression of stages 0, 1, 2, and 3 and mortality (N = 98). The slope suggests that there is no relationship. B-B = regression of stages 2, 3, 4, and 5 and mortality (N = 83). The correlation coefficient is 0.9997 and the R test indicates that the regression is significant at the 99.99% level.

and clams (KNC 63, 66, 68, 70, and 73) were injected with 250,000 cells each from stage 4 donor OXC-4 on April 1, 1984.

Results of this experiment appear in Table 3. On May 17 (47 days post-injection) 75% of the injected animals were diagnosed positive. Three were stage 4, 11 were stage 3, and 1 was stage 2. By May 17, 90% were positive; 4 were stage 4, 8 were stage 3, 2 were stage 2 and 4 were stage 1. Prevalence reached 90% in injected clams by June 21 (82 days post-injection), 2 were dead, 6 were stage 4, 5 were stage 3, 3 were stage 2, and 2 were stage 1. At the termination of the experiment on July 9, 95% of the injected clams had sarcomas with 2 dead, 2 stage 5, 8 stage 4, 3 stage 3, 2 stage 2, and 1 stage 1 sarcomas diagnosed. Only a few possible early cases were seen in the control group. These could be explained as early spontaneous cases. The appearance of stage 3, 4 and 5 cases in injected clams clearly demonstrates massive increases in numbers of neoplastic cells. The results of this experiment strongly suggest that the sarcomas were transferred by transplantation of cells rather than by virus transmission because of the shortness of the incubation period, the high prevalence attained in this short period of time, and their first appearance as relatively advanced lesions (14/20 were stage 3 or higher in 1½ months). In other transmission experiments Brown (3) first observed sarcomas 4 months post-injection (4/12 positive) and Oprandy (22) found sarcomas after 2 months in the highest titer group (6/36 positive). (My transplantation experiment also provided another example of clinical disease progression as determined by advancing stages over time in individual animals). The fact that 4 different donors were used with no apparent differences would indicate that infectious agents were in a very high titer or that the transplantability features of this system were consistent in regard to neoplastic cell

Table 3. Transplantation experiment – soft-shell clam sarcoma.

Injected clams Specimen Code	February 2	22	April 3	May 17	May 23	June 21	July 9	Control clams Specimen Code	February 2	22	May 17	July 13
KNC 3	−	−	−	+3	+3	+3	+4	KNC 4	−	−	−	−
5	−	−	−	+4	+4	+4	+5	6	−	−	−	−
8	−	−	−	−	−	−	−	10	−	−	−	−
11	−	−	−	+4	+4	(DIED)		12	−	−	+	−
13	−	−	−	+3	+3	+3	+4	14	−	−	−	−
17	−	−	−	+3	+3	+4	+4	18	−	−	−	−
21	−	−	−	+3	+3	+4	+5	20	−	−	−	−
26	−	−	−	+3	+4	+4	+4	22	−	−	−	−
30	−	−	−	+3	+3	+?	+4	27	−	−	−	−
43	−	−	−	+4	+4	+4	+3	45	−	−	−	−
53	−	−	−	+3	+3	+3	+5	51	−	−	−	−
55	−	−	−	+3	+2	+1	+4	54	−	−	−	−
57	−	−	−	+3	+2	(DIED)		56	−	−	−	−
59	−	−	−	−	+	+2	+1	58	−	−	−	−
61	−	−	−	+2	+1	+2	+2	60	−	−	−	+
63	−	−	−	−	+1	+2	+3	62	−	−	−	−
66	−	−	−	−	+1	+1	+2	65	−	−	−	+
68	−	−	−	+3	+3	+3	+4	67	−	−	−	+1
70	−	−	−	−	+1	+3	+3	69	−	−	−	−
73	−	−	−	+3	+3	+4	+4	71	−	−	−	−

Clams (*Mya arenaria*) were injected *via* siphon muscle with 245,000 to 300,000 sarcoma cells on April 3, 1984. Four donors were used in four sets of 5 clams each. Donors were – OXC-2, EBC-6, KNC-36, and OXC-4. Initial prevalence in the KNC sample was 23%. (Positive animals were eliminated from the experiment prior to injection of experimental animals.)

Table 4. Epizootiology of soft clam sarcoma in Chesapeake Bay sites.

Date	Live Clams	Empty Intact Shells	Dead Clams	Swan Point – Chesapeake Bay								
				Obs. Mort	Corr. Mort	Cum. Mort	% Stg 1, 2	% Stg 3	% Stg 4, 5	% Prev	Samp. Time	Den. sq/yd
23 Oct 84	52	0	0	0	0	0	3/60	5/60	7/60	25%	11 min	0.35
4 Jan 85	60	0	6	9%	9%	9%	7/65	4/55	26/65	59%	16 min	0.31
30 Mar 85	99	1	0	1%	1%	10%	11/57	3/57	22/57	58%	31 min	0.32
23 Apr 85	73	24	3	27%	24%	34%	–	–	4/25	–	28 min	0.20
8 May 85	83	15	2	17%	13%	47%	0	0	10/52	20%	27 min	0.30
22 May 85	76	15	9	24%	13%	60%	0	3/67	10/67	19%	25 min	0.22
6 Jun 85	52	46	2	48%	19%	79%	2/51	4/51	16/51	44%	22 min	0.17
25 Jun 85	63	35	2	37%	8%	87%	5/60	7/60	7/60	32%	27 min	0.18
13 Aug 85	44	10	1	20%	3%	90%	11/43	16/43	9/43	91%		
16 Sep 85	97	2	1	3%	3%	90%	8/30	4/30	6/30	47%		

viability and host compatibility. It would appear that at least under the conditions of this experiment immunologic factors were not evident. If this is indeed transplantation, it is the first real proof that true neoplasia exists in mollusks.

FIELD STUDIES

Samples and population data were collected periodically in cooperative studies with the Maryland Department of Natural Resources from October 1984 to October 1985. Table 4 presents these data. Swan Point is a site in the northeast part of Chesapeake Bay which was a productive commercial clamming site prior to the sarcoma epizootic. Clams were collected using a Hanks hydraulic conveyer belt dredge. (Mortality was estimated by counting live clams, dead clams, and boxes (empty shells with both valves intact) and determining the ratio of live versus dead – % observed mortality = dead clams + boxes/live clams × 100; corrected mortality = % observed mortality × estimated % of population surviving × 0.01; cumulative mortality = sum of corrected mortality). In the year under study clams at this site experienced very high mortality which correlated with initial high prevalence of sarcoma and subsequent decreases concomitant with mortality. Also evident was the increasing catch effort based on time and decreasing density of clams (Table 4). Advanced stages were most prevalent just prior to major mortality periods. The field data correlate well with laboratory data and confirm the malignant nature of this disease. The high prevalences and widespread occurrence in Chesapeake Bay clam populations indicate the potential for severe impact on the population and ultimately the production of marketable clams. This trend is already apparent. Swan Point is no longer commercially clammed. The production of clams for the state of Maryland declined in half from 1983 to 1985 and price per bushel doubled during this time.

SUMMARY

Presumed malignant neoplasms were discovered in mollusks in the late 1960's. Epizootics were identified in mussels, oysters, and several species of clams from sites on both coasts of the United States but early histologic studies of static collections from the field left large gaps in our knowledge regarding etiology, clinical progression, malignancy, and heritable changes in neoplastic cells. Recent studies have helped to answer some of these questions and provided documentation for clinical progression of the disease and malignancy in soft-shelled clams by developing a means of staging the disease cytologically in living animals. Experimental *in vivo* studies in individual animals have shown that stages as defined demonstrate that sarcomas in clams progress over time clinically and result in death of the animal. Other studies have shown that this diagnostic method can be related to the accepted method of diagnosis (histology) but is actually more sensitive for early stages. Coordinated studies between laboratory-held animals and field-collected animals exhibit similar results regarding progression and mortality. Finally, experimental studies have demonstrated tentatively that these lesions are transplantable.

REFERENCES

1. Alderman DJ, Van Banning P, Perez-Colomer A: Two European oyster (*Ostrea edulis*) mortalities associated with an abnormal haemocytic condition. *Aquaculture* 10:335–340, 1977
2. Barry MM, Yevich PP: The ecological, chemical and histological evaluation of an oil spill site: Part III. Histopathological studies. *Mar Pollut Bull* 6:171–173, 1975
3. Brown RS: The value of the multidisciplinary approach to research on marine pollution effects as evidenced in a three-year study to determine the etiology and pathogenesis of neoplasia in the soft-shell clam, *Mya arenaria*. *Rapp P-v Reun Cons Int Explor Mer* 179:125–128, 1980
4. Brown RS, Wolke RE, Saila SB, Brown CW: Prevalence of neoplasia in 10 New England populations of the soft-shell clam (*Mya arenaria*). *Ann N Y Acad Sci* 298:522–534, 1977
5. Brown RS, Wolke RE, Brown CW, Saila SB: Hydrocarbon pollution and the prevalence of neoplasia in New England soft-shell clams (*Mya arenaria*). In *Animals as Monitors of Environmental Pollutants*. pp. 41–51. National Academy of Sciences, Washington, D.C, 1979
6. Christensen DJ, Farley CA, Kern FG: Epizootic neoplasms in the clam *Macoma balthica* (L.) from Chesapeake Bay. *J Natl Cancer Inst* 52:1739–1749, 1974
7. Cooper KR, Brown RS, Chang PW: Accuracy of blood cytological screening techniques for the diagnosis of a possible hematopoietic neoplasm in the bivalve mollusc, *Mya arenaria*. *J Invertebr Pathol* 39:281–289, 1982a
8. Cooper KR, Brown RS, Chang PW: The course and mortality

of a hematopoietic neoplasm in the soft-shell clam, *Mya arenaria. J Invertebr Pathol* 39:149–157, 1982b

9. Cosson-Mannevy MA, Wong CS, Cretney WJ: Putative neoplastic disorders in mussels (*Mytilus edulis*) from southern Vancouver Island waters, British Columbia. *J Invertebr Pathol* 44:151–160, 1984

10. Farley CA: Probable neoplastic disease of the hematopoietic system in oysters, *Crassostrea virginica* and *Crassostrea gigas. Natl Cancer Inst Monogr* 31:541–555, 1969a

11. Farley CA: Sarcomatoid proliferative disease in a wild population of edible mussels (*Mytilus edulis*). *J Natl Cancer Inst* 4:509–516, 1969b

12. Farley CA: Proliferative diseases of hemocytes, endothelial cells and connective tissue cells in mollusks. *Bibl Haematol* 36:610–617, 1970

13. Farley CA: Epizootic and enzootic aspects of *Minchinia nelsoni* (Haplosporida) in the American oyster *Crassostrea virginica J Protozool* 15:585–599, 1975

14. Farley CA: Proliferative disorders in bivalve mollusks. *Mar Fish Rev* 38:30–33, 1976a

15. Farley CA: Ultrastructural observations on epizootic neoplasia and lytic virus infection in bivalve mollusks. *Prog Exp Tumor Res* 20:283–294, 1976b

16. Farley CA, Otto SV, Reinisch CL: New occurrence of epizootic sarcoma in Chesapeake Bay soft shell clams (*Mya arenaria*). *Fish Bull* 84:851–857, 1986

17. Green M, Alderman DJ: Neoplasia in *Mytilus edulis L.* from United Kingdom waters. *Aquaculture* 30:1–10, 1983

18. Harshbarger JC, Otto SV, Chang SC: Proliferative disorders in *Crassostrea virginica* and *Mya arenaria* from Chesapeake Bay and intranuclear virus-like inclusions in *Mya arenaria* with germanomas from a Maine oil spill site. *Haliotis* 8:243–248, 1977

19. Khudolei VV, Sirenko OA: Tumor development in the bivalve mollusk *Unio pictorum* induced by n-nitroso compounds. *Bull Exp Biol Med* 83:684–686, 1977

20. Mix MC: Haemic neoplasms of bay mussels, *Mytilus edulis L* from Oregon: occurrence, prevalence, seasonality and histopathological progression. *J Fish Dis* 6:239–248, 1983

21. Mix MC, Schaffer RL, Hemingway SJ: Polynuclear aromatic hydrocarbons in bay mussels (*Mytilus edulis*) in Oregon. In *Phyletic Approaches to Cancer*, (Dawe CJ, Harshbarger JC, Kondo S, Sugimura T, Takayama S, eds.), pp. 167–177. Japan Scientific Societies Press, Tokyo, 1981

22. Oprandy JJ, Chang PW, Pronovost AD, Cooper KR, Brown RS, Yates VY: Isolation of a viral agent causing hematopoietic neoplasia in the soft-shell clam, *Mya arenaria. J Invertebr Pathol* 38:45–51, 1981

23. Reinisch CL, Charles AM, Stone AM: Epizootic neoplasia in soft shell clams collected from New Bedford Harbor. *Haz Waste* 1:73–81, 1984

24. Yevich PP, Barszcz CA: Neoplasia in soft-shell clams (*Mya arenaria*) collected from oil-impacted sites. *Ann NY Acad Sci* 298:409–426, 1977

LEUCOSES IN INVERTEBRATES

H.E. KAISER

Leukemias and lymphomas are a distinct group of neoplasms in man and other mammals, they are the predominant type of neoplasms in birds and deriving from reticular connective tissues including free connective tissue cells. In the adult mammal one of the important producers of the responsible cells is the bone marrow, in birds, the bursa of Fabricius, and in fishes the posterior kidney. In embryonal life extramedullary (liver, kidney, spleen . . .) hematopoiesis occurs. The variation of the production of hematogenic tissues in vertebrates, as shown above, already is impressive. In invertebrates different hematopoietic organ systems occur and also various types of hematogenic/lymphocytic cells. To evaluate the few leucoses of invertebrates properly it is advisable to review briefly the hematogenic organs and the hematopoietic cells in invertebrates in the following table 1. Leucoses comparable to those in mammals can only occur in a type of animal with a circulatory system as briefly summarized in the table.

The table has shown what a tremendous arsenal to study spontaneous and experimental hematogenous invertebrate neoplasms as up-to-date unused. In the following hematogenic neoplasms described to date the two major invertebrate phyla of mollusca and arthropoda shall be discussed. Besides the chordate phyla, hemichordata, urochordata, cephalochordata, and vertebrata hemic neoplasms are only known from the two largest invertebrate phyla, the mollusca and arthropoda. The knowledge of these tumors is collected in less than 200 scientific papers and approximately 70 species of invertebrates have been considered.

Mollusca, class pelecypoda. Bivalve molluscs exhibit chemical and viral routes in the development of hemic neoplasms. Interaction of both routes may exist. These neoplasms have been found in oysters, clams and mussels derived from five continents.

Bivalve molluscs

Mytilus edulis. This animal is able to concentrate polynuclear hydrocarbons up to 1.32 ng/g in its tissues and also to metabolize these carcinogens. Such carcinogens have been found in the tissues of this species, together with hemic neoplasms.

Unio pictorum. After exposure to nitrosodimethylamine and nitrosodiethylamine. This species developed neoplasms, characterized by hyaline hematocytes.

Crassostrea virginica. Inbreeding led to 8% of hemic neoplasms in this species in contrast to 0.07% in wild oysters.

Mya arenaria. Hemic neoplasms of this species seem to be viral induced.

Insect arthropods:

Drosophila melanogaster. Neoplasms in this animal are genetic because they result from the mutation of a single gene on the first or second chromosome. These mutations result in the production of neoplastic plasmatocytes. In the mutation of the first chromosome the production of plasmacytes is uncontrolled and during the third larval instar the hematopoietic organs release highly differentiated plasmacytes into the hemolymph. The cells continue to divide and produce 10 to 15 times the amount of cells than normal. These lysosome rich cells are immunologic active and highly destructive to host tissues.

The cells resulting from the mutations of the second and third chromosomes are characterized by poor differentiation not as much by poor regulation. Hematopoietic organs disintegrate into widely distributed blood cell centers which produce enormous numbers of immature plasmacytes (Harshbarger, 1982). These plasmacytes are in situ destructive but do not destroy other host tissues. The nuclei of all these mutant cells contain virus-like particles.

Ecdyonorus lateralis
Rhithrogena semicolorata
Symbiocladius rhithrogenae
Mayfly naiads of the first two species are ectoparasitized by the third species, a chironomid wasp. The wasp is an exclusive hemophage feeding on host blood cells.

To understand the complex relationship of these diseases which run under different names, such as leukemia, lymphomas or leukoses (see Table 3) in an organismic frame it is valuable to discuss the terms used in the invertebrate papers as related to medicine and to try to establish a classification of the whole group of diseases dealing with neoplastic development of leukocytes and related cells of body fluid (Table 4).

Comparative definition of neoplasms developing from or related to the hematopoietic system
At the present scientific situation a cellular comparison is the only possible method. Phagocytic or leukocytic cells in dif-

H. E. Kaiser (ed.), Comparative aspects of tumor development.

Table 1. Review of circulatory systems, hematogenic organs, cells in body fluids and species with hemic neoplasms

Phylum	Type of Circulatory system	Hematogenic organ	Cells in body fluids	Species with hemic neoplasms	References
4. Nemertinea	closed		Nucleated cells		
13. Priapulida	open		Round cells		
14. Mollusca	open (mixed (Pulmonata, Cephalopoda	Pericard? Branchial gland? (*Octopus* sp.)	Blood cells vary in the species. Amebocytes, pore cells in freshwater snails	*Mytilus edulis, Unio pictorum, Crassostrea virginica, Mya arenaria*, a.o.	
15. Sipunculida	open	Coelom?	Body fluid: red corpuscles, hyaline amebocytes, granulocytes, floating urns and multinucleated cells.		
16. Echiurida	closed		Circulatory system: phagocytic amebocytes Coelomic cavity: erythrocytes and leukocytes		
17. Annelida	closed		Earthworm coelomocytes with 5 subtypes: basophils, acidophils, neutrophils, granulocytes, and chloragogen cells.		34, 316
18. Onychophora	open		free amebocytes		
19. Pentastomida	open?		One type of blood cell		
21. Arthropoda Merostomata (*Limulus* sp. Arachnida:	open		One type of blood cell		
Aranea	Circular musculature of heart	Various blood cells			
Scorpiones	"Lymphatic organs"	Various blood cells			
Crustacea (*Callinectes sapidus*)			Hyaline cells, intermediate cells, granulocytes		
Insecta			Hemocytes with functional or developmental stages: Prohemocytes, blasmocytes, granular cells, spherule cells, cystocytes, oenocytoids, thrombocytoid cells (easy fragmentation as in mammalian platelets). Larvae exhibit special conditions	*Drosophila melanogaster* *Ecdyonurus lateralis, Rhithrogena semicolorata*	
22. Phoronida			nucleated blood cells		
23. Ectoprocta	only coelom		ameboid cells		
24. Brachiopoda	open		no blood cells, but sometimes coelomocytes		
25. Echinodermata	three open systems		various amebocytes		
26. Chaetognatha	open		not well known		
27. Pogonophora	closed				
28. Hemichordata	open		floating cells		
29. Tunicata	open		several types of blood cells		
30. Cephalochordata	closed				

Table 2. Brief review of the immunologic aspects of metazoan invertebrates*.

Phylum	Immunologic aspects		Characterization of immunologic system	Remarks
	+	−		
Placozoa		−		
Mesozoa		−		
Porifera	+		Cells of different species do not mix.	
Coelenterata	+		quasi-immuno-recognition or primordial cell-mediated immunity	Lack of lymphoid cells
Ctenophora	+		Antibiotic properties of *Beroe cucumis*, cancer inhibiting factors	
Platyhelminthes	+		Antigens, transplantation immunity, resistance to x-rays and vertebrate species	
Nemertinea		−		
Acanthocephala	?			
Rotifera	?			
Gastrotricha		−		
Kinorhyncha		−		
Nematoda	+		Antigens	
Nematomorpha		−		
Priapulida		−		
Mollusca	+		Diversified immunologic responses, phagocytic cells are known since 1914	
Sipunculida			Immune reactions in *Dendrostomum zostericolom*, immunologic properties of coelomic fluid	
Annelida	−	+	Antibodies	
Onychophora	+			
Pentastomida		−		
Tardigrada		−		
Arthropoda	+		Antibodies, immunology to chemicals, agglutinins, humoral immunity, encapsulation of foreign particles, phagocytosis as cellular immune response, serological responses, cell-mediated immunity in parasitic infections.	
Phoronida		−		
Ectoprocta		−		
Brachiopoda		−		
Echinodermata	+		Protective action of embryos, responses to transplants, immunologic effects of lipids	
Chaetognatha		−		
Pogonophora		−		
Hemichordata		−		
Tunicata	+		Hemagglutinins, allogeneic inhibition, immune response to vertebrate tissue, colony specificity, graft-versus-host relationship	
Cephalochordata		−		

* Invertebrates produce no immunoglobulin antibodies as vertebrates do.
+ Definite data are available
− The situation is unknown
? Positive and negative results in members of this phylum have been obtained
Reference: H.E. Kaiser: Species-specific Potential of Invertebrates for Toxicological Research. Baltimore, University Park Press, 224 pp, 1981.

ferent phyla may vary from one phylum to the other, and it is therefore useful to add the name of the phylum when describing such abnormalities or neoplasms. The circulatory systems and "leukemic" cells of the various animal phyla are diversified (Table 1). We find open, mixed and closed systems of body fluid. Echinoderms, for example, have three systems of body fluids. The immunologic system of the different phyla exhibit a similar diversity at a different level of development. The best known classification of neoplasms and related diseases deriving from the reticular connective tissue, leukemias and lymphomas alike, exists from man. A comparative classification of leukemias and lymphomas, perhaps under the umbrella term of leukosis, in man, other

vertebrates and invertebrates alike, can only be based on the comparison of parent cells of the lesions. The significance of follicular structure as employed in the NCIS classification of non-Hodgkin's lymphomas cannot be employed because the specific data are lacking in invertebrates where various terms such as leukosis, leukemia, lymphoma, hematogenous neoplasms, hemic neoplasms, hyaline hemocyte neoplasms, neoplastic plasmatocytes and undifferentiated mesenchymal cells have been employed but a proper classification is still lacking.

At the present time I suggest a taxonomy for these pathologic lesions based on the character of the parent cells from which the neoplastic cells derive and additional mentioning

Table 3. Terms used in publications about organismic (mainly invertebrates) leukemias, lymphomas, and leukoses*.

Terms found in literature on invertebrates	Meaning in Medical Use
Mesenchyme	Primordial embryonic tissue giving rise to mesodermal tissues during ontogency
Leukemia	Progressive proliferation of abnormal leukocytes – specific lesion named after dominant cell type and speed of progression to fatal end: acute and chronic
Leukosarcoma	Variant of malignant lymphoma in which immature cells of the lymphocytic series occur in large numbers in the circulating blood beside the additionally present lymphosarcoma involving the lymph nodes and other tissues and organs
Leukosis	Abnormal proliferation of one or more leukopoietic tissues. Avian leukosis (leukemia of fowls): subtypes: lymphoid, erythroid, myeloid 1. – caused by closely related viruses – transmissible.
Hemic (hematic) neoplasms	Neoplasms related to or involved with blood (unusual term in medicine)
Hematogenous neoplasms	Neoplasms derived from, produced from or transported by the blood.
Plasmacyte	Plasma cell
Plasmatocyte	Combining cell denoting plasma
Lymphoma	Malignant neoplasm of lymph and reticulo-endothelial tissues presenting as circumscribed solid tumors, composed of primitive appearing cells resembling lymphocytes, plasma cells or histiocytes. L. appear with high frequency in normal sites of lymphoreticular cells and lymph nodes or spleen. Especially lymphocytes lymphomas may invade the blood stream and manifest as leukemias. Classification according to cell types.
Lymphosarcoma	A diffuse lymphocytic sarcoma.

*Illustrated Stedman's Medical Dictionary – 24th Edition – Williams and Wilkins – Baltimore, Maryland – 1982.

Table 4. Leukoses in Invertebrates*.

1. Leukoses in mollusca/bivalvia	*Mytilus edulis* chemically induced *Unio pictorium* chemically induced *Crassostrea virginica* chemically induced *Mya arenaria* virus (nucleosis)
2. Leukoses in arthropods/insects	*Drosophila melanogaster* plasmacytes**; genetic virus *Ecdyonurus lateralis* blood cells (leukoses is mixture of lymphomatype at beginning, leading to fatal type of leukemia; parasitized by *Symbiocladius rhithrogenae* *Rhithrogena semicolorata* blood cells (leukoses is mixture of lymphomatyupe at beginning, leading to fatal type of leukemia; parasitized by *Symbiocladius rhithrogenae*

*Invertebrates have cells comparable to lymphatic cells in vertebrates but no homologous organs, such as thymus, spleen or bone marrow. Lymph glands in insects (2) can be considered analogous to lymph nodes in mammals but are in no way homologous. It is therefore more cautious to place the lesions of invertebrates somewhat separated and can call them leukose, to underline the variation to vertebrate lesions. Certain abnormalities in arthropods resemble lymphosarcomas in vertebrates but the comparison remains unsecured.
**The highly enlarged mutant lymph glands, in contrast to normal conditions release constantly new blood cells into the hemolymph causing increased cell counts. The cell involved in the pathologic process is known as plasmacyte and these mutant cells have lost their capacity to recognize self from non-self. The encapsule and melanize larval tissues, invade the imaginal discs, the muscles and the fat body. The mutant pathologic plasmacytes exhibit all major characteristics of malignant neoplastic cells (2).

of the phylum or phylum and class concerned under the main heading of organismic leukosis to be divided into mammalian vertebrate leukemias and lymphomas, non-mammalian vertebrate leukemias, lymphomas and leukosis, and invertebrate leukosis.

The best knowledge on this disease group exists in the diseases of man followed by certain laboratory and domestic animals. For man I follow the classification of the World Health Organisation (WHO) concerning leukemias and the Hodgkin's lymphomas. Regarding the non-Hodgkin's lymphomas it is best to accept the NCI classification of 1982 and Jaffe and Green (4). In human subject the normal immunologic activities are of high importance to the progression of the diseases. The invertebrates, nearly uninvestigated in regard to leukoses and related diseases have to be considered a tremendous, until now unused, potential. They may be used especially as model organisms for specific questions. Of course, these invertebrate leukoses are not directly related to vertebrate leukemias and lymphomas but they are part of the phylogeny of these neoplastic processes.

REFERENCES

1. Cohen WD: (ed.) *Blood Cells of Marine Invertebrates: Experimental Systems in Cell Biology and Comparative Physiology*, MBL Lectures in Biology, Vol. 6, New York: A. R. Liss, Inc, 1985
2. Gateff E: Malignant blood cell neoplasms of genetic origin in *Drosophila melanogaster. J Cell Biol* 70(2/Part 2):6a, 1976
3. Harshbarger JC: Epizootiology of leukemia and lymphoma in poikilotherms. *Advances in Comparative Leukemia Research* 39, 1982
4. Jaffe ES, Green I: Neoplasms of the immune system. In: *Mechanisms of Tumor Immunity*, edited by Green I, Cohen S, McCluskey RT, New York: John Wiley & Sons, Inc, 1977
5. Kaiser HE: *Species-specific Potential of Invertebrates for Toxicological Research*. Baltimore: University Park Press, 1980
6. Kaiser HE: Distribution of true (real) tissues in organisms: A preliminary condition of neoplastic growth. In: *Neoplasms – Comparative Pathology of Growth in Animals, Plants, and Man*, edited by Kaiser HE, Baltimore: Williams & Wilkins, pp. 43–88, 1981
7. Kaiser HE: The species-specific spectrum of neoplasms. In: *Neoplasms – Comparative Pathology of Growth in Animals, Plants, and Man*, edited by Kaiser HE Baltimore: Williams & Wilkins, pp. 649–721, 1981
8. Kaiser HE: Animal neoplasms – A systematic review. In: *Neoplasms – Comparative Pathology of Growth in Animals, Plants, and Man*, edited by Kaiser HE, Baltimore: Williams & Wilkins, pp. 747–812, 1981
9. Mathe G, Rappaport GH, in collaboration with O'Conor GT, Torloni H: Histological and cytological typing of neoplastic diseases of hematopoietic and lymphoid tissues. WHO Internat'l Histological Classification of Tumours No. 14, Geneva, 1976
10. National Cancer Institute Sponsored study of Classification of Non-Hodgkin's Lymphomas. Cancer, vol. 49: 2110–2135, 1982

6

METASTASIS OF INVERTEBRATE NEOPLASMS

KEITH R. COOPER

INTRODUCTION

The ability to demonstrate metastasis in an invertebrate is a difficult problem for several reasons: (1) many invertebrates have no circulatory system (2) the majority of invertebrates that do have a circulatory system is based on an open system with large blood sinuses (3) many invertebrates have non discrete organ systems (4) relatively few neoplasms have been reported in invertebrates and (5) the majority of neoplasms that have been described are anaplastic in appearance. Metastases are the occurrence of tumor implants arising independently from the primary tumor or a secondary metastasis. In invertebrates that do not have a circulatory system the ability of neoplastic cells to migrate to secondary sites is restricted. The majority of neoplasms that have been described in invertebrates (see Chap. 8, Vol. V) are anaplastic in appearance and are believed to arise from hematopoietic tissues. Because of the open sinusoidal blood systems it is difficult if not impossible to distinguish areas where the neoplastic cells perculate through the tissues and metastasize. Because of the above reasons it may be incorrect or at least difficult to use the term metastasis for invertebrate neoplastic progression. It should also be pointed out that the proposed examples described below may not be metastasis in the mammalian sense, but are believed to be the closest examples to mammalian metastasis within invertebrate species.

METASTASIS IN INVERTEBRATES

Wolf (11, 12) described a papillary epithelioma from the Sydney Rock oyster, *Crassostrea commercialis* from Australia. Based on the descriptions and histological findings in these animals the neoplasm would be considered malignant by most pathologists. Sparks (10) suggested that the occurrence of two discrete neoplastic growths in one of the oysters could be interpreted as an example of metastasis. An alternative hypothesis could be the occurrence of two independent neoplasms.

Christensen, Farley and Kern (1) described a gill carcinoma in *Macoma balthica* from the Chesapeake Bay. The neoplastic cells arose from cells within the gill and spread throughout the animals by the open circulatory system. The anaplastic cells did lodge in sinusoids in other tissues resulting ultimately in the death of the animal.

Yevich and Barscz (13) described a gonadal neoplasm in the soft shell clam, *Mya arenaria* in which they reported metastasis in 40% (73/182) of the animals. The gonadal follicles of the clam were the primary site of the neoplasm and the cells which metastasized were believed to have arisen from the follicle. Once the cells were no longer maintained in the gonadal follicle they were distributed throughout the animal by the open circulatory system. The sites of metastasis were those areas where the cells were trapped in the sinuses and began to divide rapidly. In many instances these cells displaced the normal organ systems and resulted in the death of the animal.

Although some researchers have reported metastasis in animals with a hematopoietic type neoplasm, this cannot be accepted due to the nature of the animals' circulatory system. Because of the open circulatory system and hematopoietic nature of the neoplasm there would be no way to distinguish the primary neoplasm from the metastatic sites. (Distribution of *Monuli linfermines*).

CONCLUSIONS

As stated in Chapter 84/107 there are very few invertebrate neoplasms that have been reported and even fewer that have been adequately studied. It is generally accepted that to prove metastasis also in an invertebrate the primary neoplasm must be separated from the sites of metastasis. Based on this criteria there would appear to be only three examples that meet these requirements.

REFERENCES

1. Christensen DJ, Farley CA, Kern FG: Epizootic neoplasms in the clam, *Macoma balthica* (L) from the Chesapeake Bay. *J Nat Cancer Inst* 52:1739, 1974
2. Farley CA: "Neoplasms in estuarine mollusks and approaches to ascertain causes". *Annals of the New York Academy of Sciences* 298:225, 1978
3. Kaiser HE: *Species Specific Potential of Invertebrates for Toxicological Research*. Baltimore: University Park Press, 1980
4. Kaiser HE: "Species-specific Spectrum of Neoplasms" in: *Neoplasms-Comparative Pathology of Growth in Animals, Plants, and Man* edited by Kaiser HE, Chap. 43, pp. 649–724. Baltimore: Williams & Wilkins, 1981
5. Krieg K: "Experimentelle Kanzerogenese bei Mollusken; 2. Transplantationsversuche mit einem bei der La-Plata-Apfelschnecke *Ampullarius austris* d'Orbigny (gastropods, prosobranchia) chemisch induzierten Adenopapillom." *Arch Geschwulstforsch* 33:18–30, 1969
6. Krieg K: "Experimental carcinogenesis in molluscs; 3. Further

H. E. Kaiser (ed.), Comparative aspects of tumor development.
© 1989, Kluwer Academic Publishers, Dordrecht. ISBN-13:978-0-89838-994-4

studies on tumor formation in the La-Plata apple snail *Ampullarius australis* d'Orbigny (gastropods, prosobranchia) with special attention to methylcholanthrene." *Arch Geschwulstforsch* 33:255–267, 1969

7. Krieg K: "Experimental carcinogenesis in mollusca and comparative studies of cancerogenesis in land snails and water snails." *Arch Geschwulstforsch* 35:109, 1970

8. Krieg K: *Invertebraten in der Geschwulstforschung* Beitr. Krebsforsch. Steinkopff, Dresden. Includes a shorter English version of text, 1973

9. Pflugfelder O: "Geschwulstbildung bei Wirbellosen und niederen Wirbeltieren." *Strahlentherapie* 93:181–195, 1954

10. Sparks AK: *Invertebrate pathology, Non-Communicable Diseases.* Academic Press, New York, 1972

11. Wolf PH: "Neoplastic growth in two Sydney rock oysters, *Crassostrea virginica. Nat'l Cancer Inst Monogr* 31:563–573, 1969

12. Wolf PH: "Unusually large tumor in a Sydney rock oyster." *J Nat'l Cancer Inst* 46:1079–1084, 1971

13. Yevich PP, Barsczc DA: Gonadal and hematopoietic neoplasms in *Mya arenaria. Marine Fish Rev* 38:42–43, 1976

SELECTED ASPECTS OF NEOPLASTIC GROWTH IN ARTHROPODS

H.E. KAISER

1. INTRODUCTION

Crustaceans, insects, cephalopod molluscs, and vertebrates are the four highest developed animal groups. These four groups of animals exhibit endocrine glands and hormonal control of life function. Concerning the insects which comprise approximately 1 million known species which are described and 5 to 7 million species which are assumed to be alive in *Blatta, Blattella* and *Periplaneta* the capability of learning and recollection are proven (A. Kaestner, Lehrb. d. Spe. Zoologie (1973) vol. I, pt. 3, Insecta B p. 365). Circadian rhythms of activity (depending on light and temperature) are known from *Blattella orientalis, Blatta germanica, Periplaneta americana* and *Leucophaea* sp.

Vertebrates and vascular plants are organisms where neoplasms have been found most frequently but they have also been found in molluscs and arthropods because these animals too display highly developed organs and tissues. Insects outnumber totally all other animal classes together by species number. They are the most successful animal class. Their investigated tumors comprise only a very small number of pathologic structures, nearly nothing if compared with the number of species. But they offer the scientist dealing with them a tremendous reservoir of unknown data. They have advantages for experiments such as small size, reasonable costs for purchase and maintenance, high reproduction power. Also in regard to ethical aspects to save our usual laboratory animals of the class of mammals, they may be preferred for several types of experiments. These experiments could also illuminate questions of agricultural and forest protection.

2. BASIC ASPECTS

1. Types of arthropod development - catastrophic development and neoplasms.

An opportunity for cancer research in arthropods, and as yet less exploited, is the investigation of developmental aspects of insects; and the opportunities lying therein. In regard to oncogenes, response to radiation and chemical carcinogens in insects can be compared to vertebrates. Insects show comparable tissues such as cross-striated musculature, etc. The endocrine system differs but is in principle comparable.

The ontogeny of insects reaches from comparable direct development as it occurs in the apterygota or ametabola with direct development to this one of pterygota with gradual or abrupt (catastrophic) development. The insects therefore offer the unique opportunity to study tissues, even organs, under this gradual variation as, for example, gill epithelia and species direct development, hemimetabolic development and under conditions of holometabolic development including histolysis of certain tissues. The implications of these processes for an understanding of neoplastic regression are described in chapter 9/Volume V.

Comparable larval development occurs also in crustaceans in form of the cypris with histolysis.

2. Oncogenes in insects

The formation of oncogenes during neoplastic development has also been observed in insects.

Transcription of the *Drosophila melanogaster* homologs of the *abl* and *src* cellular oncogenes termed D*ash* and D*src*, respectively, was investigated by Levy (30). On one hand D*ash* and D*src* share sequence homology, on the other they have distinct pattern of transcription during development. The relative amount of each of the three D*src* transcripts changes during the different stages of tumor development. The Dash transcript, 6.2 kilobases long, is found in maternal RNA stored in unfertilized eggs and in embryos up to 4 h after egg laying. D*src* transcripts are 3.2, 4.8, and 5.2 kilobases long.

Rous sarcoma virus (RSV) is an acutely oncogenic avian retrovirus which induces sarcomas in animals and transforms fibroblasts in cell culture. Genetic analysis indicated that the viral *src* gene (*v-src*) mediates neoplastic transformation. The viral *src* gene is derived from a cellular gene (*c-src*) which also encodes a 60,000 MW phosphoprotein (pp60c-*src*) with tyrosine-specific protein kinase activity. Both birds and mammals are known to possess *c-src*. Shilo and Weinberg (44) have reported that the genome of the

Table 1. Ontogenetic aspects of the main insect group.

Class: Insecta, hexapoda
    Subclass: Apterygota (Ametabola) – direct development
    Subclass: Pterygota, Metabola with gradual or abrupt (catastrophic) metamorphosis
        Paleoptera
        Neoptera
            Paurometabola
            Paraneoptera
            Holometabola, endopterygota, with abrupt or catastrophic development with larvae, pupa and adult (imago) (660 100 species)

H. E. Kaiser (ed.), Comparative aspects of tumor development.

fruit fly, *Drosophila melanogaster*, contains nucleotide sequences that are homologous to *v-src*. Simon and co-workers (45) report here the molecular cloning and chromosomal mapping of three loci from the *Drosophila* genome that contain such sequences. It should be possible to identify the precise locus that encodes a *src*-specific protein kinase in *Drosophila*, and to explore the role of *c-src* in the growth and development of *D. melanogaster*.

Drosophila melanogaster genomic sequences that hybridize with *v-myc* have been reported by Shilo and Weinberg. Madhaven (31) and coworkers have detected *Drosophila* RNA sequences that also hybridize with *v-myc*. It seems unlikely that the mRNA sequences or the genomic sequences that have been isolated by hybridization with *v-myc* represent homologs of the vertebrate *myc* gene Polyadenylic acid-containing transcripts of 2.7, 2.2, and 1.7 kilobases (kb) in embryos, pupas, adults, and Kc cells and an additional 1.4-kb transcript in adults were complementary to the *Drosophila* genomic clones and to *v-myc*. These results suggest that the transcripts in early embryos are of maternal origin.

Drosophila melanogaster DNA clones are homologous to vertebrate oncogene: evidence for a common ancestor to the *src* and *abl* cellular genes (20) cloned *Drosophila* sequences, D*ash* and D*src*, were previously isolated by hybridization to the viral oncogenes *v-abl* and *v-src*. Hoffmann et al. (21) report that the *Drosophila* DNA sequences are more than 50% homologous to 700 base pairs of the vertebrate oncogenes that are essential for kinase activity of the *v-abl* and the *v-src* gene products. Comparison of the *Drosophila* and vertebrate sequences identifies amino acids that may be essential for the distinct functions of the *c-src* and the *c-abl* gene products and places the gene duplication event that has generated the two genes prior to the chordate-arthropod divergence.

Three *Drosophila* genes homologous to the Ha-*ras* probe were isolated and mapped to positions 85D, 64B, and 62B on chromosome 3. Two of these genes (termed D*ras* 1 and D*ras* 2) were sequenced. Alignment of the amino acid sequence of D*ras* 1 with the vertebrate Ha-*ras* protein shows that at the amino terminus and central portion (residues 1-121 and 137-164) the two proteins are remarkably similar, and have an overall homology of 75%. The D*ras* 2 gene lacks significant homology to the vertebrate counterpart at the extreme amino terminus and is homologous only between positions 28-120 and 139-161 (overall homology of 50%). At the carboxy terminus, the major region of variability among the vertebrate *ras* proteins, the two *Drosophila* sequences also display considerable variability (39).

Moser et al. (38) cloned a *Drosophila melanogaster ras* gene (Dm*ras*64B) on the basis of its homology to the *ras* oncogene from Harvey murine sarcoma virus. This gene mapped at chromosomal position 64B on the left arm of the third chromosome. Sequencing of Dm*ras*64B revealed extensive amino acid homology with the proteins encoded by the human and *Saccharomyces cerevisiae ras* genes. Dm*ras*64B encodes three different RNAs (1.6, 2.1, and 2.6 kb long) that are constantly expresed throughout the development of the fly.

The proto-oncogene *c-myb* was isolated from *Drosophila melanogaster* by Katzen et al. (25). The gene may encode a protein with a molecular weight of at least 55,000 that shares a domain with *c-myb* (chicken) in which 91 of 125 (or 73%) of the amino acids are identical in the *Drosophila* and chicken genes. These findings represent the first rigorous identification of a *Drosophila* proto-oncogene that can encode what may be a nuclear protein, and they set the stage for a genetic analysis of how *c-myb* serves the normal organism.

3. Cell transformation in arthropods is similar as in mammals.

4. Tissue culture in insects in relation to neoplastic growth provides similar opportunities as in mammals.

TN-368 lepidopteran insect cells display a multiphasic survival response in both air and nitrogen. In each case the survival curve is characterized by an initial small-shouldered component having a steep slope, a plateau or broad-shouldered region near the 0.1 survival level, and finally a shallow slope component. In addition, the survival of cells which had previously been irradiated with a dose well into the logarithmic region of the more resistant shallow slope portion of the curve retained a multiphasic response (27a).

3. COMPARATIVE ASPECTS OF NEOPLASTIC PROGRESSION BETWEEN ARTHROPODS AND VERTEBRATES

3.1. Theoretically impossible neoplastic types in insects/mammals

a. According to tissue types of primary tumors
The appearance of the primary tumor is always dependent upon the parent tissue from which it is derived. In this regard differences are present if insects and mammals are compared.

Table 2. Comparison of the spectrum of tissues in insects and mammals.

Insects: Lacking tissues	Mammals: Lacking tissues
Stratified squamous epithelium	Corpora allata
Pseudostratified columnar epithelium	Thoracic glands
Stratified cuboidal epithelium	Ventral glands
Stratified columnar epithelium	Corpora cardiaca
Transitional epithelium	Perisympathetic organs of insecta
Sebaceous and sweat glands	
Mammary glands	
Islets of Langerhans	
Pineal gland	
Pituitary gland	
Thyroid gland	
Parathyroid gland	
Chordal tissue	
Chondroid tissue	
Cartilage	
Bone	
Myoepithelial tissue	
Smooth musculature	
Helically striated musculature	
Cardiac musculature	

Table 3. Theoretical differences between arthropods and mammalian vertebrates.

Phylum	Class	Development	Circulation	Lymphatic system	Direct spread	Hematogenous metastasis	Lymphatic metastasis	Coelomic spreading	Metastasis of teratomas	Unusual metastasis	Metastasis from metastasis
Arthropoda	Chelicerata		open	−	+	+	−	+	+	+	+
	Arachnida		open	−	+	+	−	+	+	+	+
	Crustacea		open	−	+	+	−	+	+	+	+
	Myriapoda		open	−	+	+	−	+	+	+	+
	Insecta		open	−	+	+	−	+	+	+	+
	Entotropha										
	Ectotropha										
	Pterygota										
	Holometabola										
Vertebrata	Mammalia		closed	+	+	+	+	+	+	+	+

In insects functional differences occur in the comparative tissues insofar as the testis and ovary have no endocrine function as in the mammal. Variations also exist between mammals and crustaceans or arachnids but will not be elaborated upon here (see Kaiser, (23), Table 43.1.). The comparisons in the above table indicate clearly the supreme multiplicity of tissues in the mammals mentioned in earlier chapters. Tissue distribution and topographic distribution (especially of secondary neoplasms) varies as well between other animal groups. However, a detailed description of these would be beyond the scope of this chapter.

b. Variations according to the type of secondary distributions

Table 3 indicates that lymphatic metastasis is not probable in arthropods and that hematogenic differences will prevent a direct comparison between neoplastic distribution of a closed circulatory system in mammals and an open one in arthropods. Another difference is presented by various types of development and the occurrence of larvae with normal tissue autolysis in the majority of arthropods, the holometabolic insects. In aquatic larvae with gills or tracheid gills "blood" hemoglobin to be replaced by tracheids acting without body fluid is exhibited in the imago. Even more important are the different types of development as in chelicerata and other major groups of the arthropods, where a continued development or a catastrophic one in a large number of variations may occur. Crustacea show life cycles with many larvae as well as direct development of abbreviated type. Similar conditions occur in insects where we must only think on hemimetabolic or holometabolic development. From these growth conditions the comparative oncologists may learn about basic growth processes on a normal background to understand abnormal growth processes in the progression or regression of neoplasms.

3.2. Other comparative aspects

a. Variation among circulatory systems

Insects have an open type circulatory system while mammals have a closed type with a remnant of the open system in the form of the sinuses in the spleen. Both animal classes exhibit several types of cells in their body fluid which are comparable but not equal. In mammals, the leukocytes or white blood cells, the erythrocytes in man without a nucleus and the thrombocytes (which may represent this discarded nucleus) are relatively well known by biologists. In insects

hemocytes are found in which case six developmental or functional stages may be distinguished: prohemocytes, blastocytes, granular cells, spherule cells, cystocytes, and oenocytoids. In both classes, phagocytic activity can be seen in movable cells. The most important difference between the system of body fluids in both classes is that insects have no lymphatic system, therefore no lymph vessels and especially no lymph nodes. This variation between both classes has a very wide ranging effect on the comparability of neoplastic distribution in mammals and insects. Most mammalian solid cancers disseminate predominantly via the lymphatic system in which case the lymph nodes play a highly important, not yet fully understood role. Table 4 reviews briefly neoplastic distribution and regression in insects and mammals.

b. Preneoplastic changes are comparable

Preneoplastic changes are comparable between arthropods and vertebrates in the development of neoplasms and related diseases.

Table 4. Neoplastic secondary distribution and regression in insects and mammals.

Insecta Neoplastic distribution and regression	Mammals Neoplastic distribution and regression
Direct spread	Direct spread
Hematogenous spread*	Hematogenous spread*
−	Lymphatic spread
−	Spreading through cancerous thoracic duct
Spreading on coelom**	Spreading on coelom**
Metastasis of teratomas	Metastasis of teratomas
Unusual metastasis***	Unusual metastasis***
Metastasis from metastasis****	Metastasis from metastasis****
Neoplastic regression based on normal ontogenetic histolysis	Neoplastic regression is a phenomenon of pathologic recovery

*Due to the open and closed circulatory systems in both classes variations in the distribution of neoplastic cells must be assumed.
**Spreading on coelomic surfaces may be more prominent in mammals than in insects because the coelom in insects is restricted.
***Unusual metastasis in the mammal is described in chapter 7/Vol. VII. whereas in the insects no specifics are known regarding metastasis in this class.
****The value of metastasis from metastasis in the mammal seems to have been underestimated (chapter 15/Vol. 1) and in the insects the question was nevery properly addressed.

Table 5. Virus-induced hematopoietic neoplasm in *Tipula paludosa*

Stage	Characteristics
1 Proliferation stage	The number of hemocytes increases nearly 100 times
2 Hypertrophy stage	The hemocytes double in size, primarily by enlargement of the nucleus
3 Virogenic stage	Formation of nuclear vacuole, followed by virogenic stroma and finally the development of polyhedra. (The virogenic stage is composed of three substages)

The inducing virus is a DNA nuclear polyhedrosis virus.

c. Stagewise progression in both insects and mammals

Progression may vary between remodeling in the holometabolic insects ontogeny when compared to the non-holometabolic Ectotropha (Paleoptera, Neoptera, Paurometabola and Paraneoptera) in which some may have less pronounced developmental stages because of catastrophic development during the processes of histolysis while undergoing ontogenetic development. During the histolytic process of tissue discarding, neoplasms of these tissues will also be discarded if no dissemination has occurred before. These developmental differences between insects and mammals may be reflected, at least in some differences of neoplastic progression.

The nymphs of the mayflies of *Rhithrogena semicolorata* and *Heptagenia lateralis* when parasitized by larvae of the chironomid wasp *Symbiocladius rhitrog* showed two stages; an inflammatory process and then neoplastic development. These two stages can be divided into substages and examples of stagewise neoplastic development in other arthropods could be added (16). A tumor-like hemocytic proliferation in the European cranefly, *Tipula paludosa*, is characterized by the three distinct stages shown in Table 5.

d. Loss of nourishment

The growth of neoplasms depends in insects as well as in mammals on the presence of necessary nourishment. Nothing is known of a possible or comparative angiogenesis during the development of insect neoplasms. In the mayflies parasitized by the chironomid wasp during the developmental stage, two large masses of tumor tissues astride the dorsal vessel appeared. Then centers of the tumors became degenerated and the cells vacuolated. The peripheral cells remained mitotically activated, invading muscular and adipose tissues during tissue advancement. In the final instar, the tumor cells became leukemic, spreading through the hemocoel, and causing death.

4. CANCER CAUSING AGENTS IN ARTHROPODS

With the exception of bacterial initiation as neoplasm causing agents known to arise in plants, the usual causes of neoplasms also occur in insects and other arthropods.

4.1. Chemical carcinogens

The exposure of arthropods to the chemical carcinogens of mammals does not necessarily lead to neoplastic growth.

Sometimes the shorter life span of insects is thought to be the cause, but the same magnitude of difference exists between the longevity of mammalian species (Blue whale and mouse) to the life span between mouse and insect. Clarification of this question may be derived from the comparative use of mammalian and insect tissue culture. But growth abnormalities can be induced as shown in Table 5. The chemical compounds were polycyclic hydrocarbons, nitrosamines and aflatoxins from the fungus *Aspergillus flavus*. The statement of J. Harshbarger (16) is still valid: "Chemicals carcinogenic for mammals are generally mutagenic for *Drosophila melanogaster* and are generally toxic for insect tissues". Neoplasms have not been produced in insects, but under some experimental conditions excessive mitotic activity for regenerative cells has been reported.

4.2. Radiation

The information on the effect of radiation on arthropod tissues is scarce. Direct damage of the cells by interaction with the molecules or damage of molecules by the ionization of the cytoplasmic sap are the two modes of radiation damage. It is assumed that the latter is more pronounced. In the nucleus both ways of damage occur either as chromosomal aberration with chromosome damage and unnatural repair, e.g. unnatural ways of rejoining of chromosomal fragments or by point mutations in which case nucleids of the DNA strand are added, deleted, transposed or replaced. The most important damage of the cytoplasm are the changes of the enzyme activity. As in invertebrates rapidly growing cells such as embryonic cells and others are more sensitive to radiation than mature cells which show a much slower pace of growing. Especially sensitive to radiation are also the dividing cells. Insect embryos exhibit a resistance to radiation of approximately 100 R which is raised to several 100 000 R for imagines. This has to do that, with exception of germinal tissues, adult insects exhibit nondividing fully differentiated cells. These conditions are most pronounced in those insect species where the imagines live only hours are unable to drink or feed and undergo only sexual activity. A few studies exist in which abdominal cells of certain insects treated were examined by light and electron microscopy as of gnotobiotic diapausing *Melanoplus differentialis* embryos by Talmisian (1971) (cited after (16)). The embryos showed in a 56 day period: (a) an increase in oxygen uptake and cytochrome exidase; (b) a negative growth to about 50% of normal size; (c) a gradual loss of recognizable features; and, (d) a continual increase in the ratio of abnormal to normal cells. Irradiated insects in preimaginal insects do not properly develop but linger instead for longer periods of time or until death, in which case no imagines are developed. Radiation seems to have an influence on insect immunity and it may lower the resistance to infectious agents. New studies are necessary to understand better the complicated immunologic and other functions in the body of insects and other arthropods before we learn more about the neoplastic potential of this largest phylum of animals. M. Berrios and coworkers (2) identified in *Drosophila* with virtual identical mobility on sodium dodecyl sulfate-polyacrylamide gels as the major photolabeled species in fractions from the nuclear envelope obtained from chickens, opossums, rats, and guinea pigs. The following table 6 summarizes some recent

Table 6. Effects of mammalian chemical carcinogens in arthropods

Procambarus clarkii	N-nitrosodimethylamine	Degeneration of antennal gland Hyperplasia of tubular cells in hepatopancreas	Harshbarger, J.C.; G.E. Cantwell; M.F. Stanton (1971)
Artemia salina nauplii	Aromatic hydrocarbons		Morgan & Warshawsky, 1977 (3558)
Tetraclita squamosa rubescens, Mitella polymerus	Polycyclic hydrocarbons	Without effect	Shimkin, Koe, Zechmeister, 1951 (4653)
Drosophila cl tu	C.I. Direct Blue tetrasodium salt	50% tumors, 65.2% in 5th generation contr.	Baroche, C., 1968 (342)
Drosophila cl tu	Aminopterin	100% tumors in larvae; no descendants	Baroche, C., 1968 (342)
Drosophila cl tu	Aminopterin	87.7% tumors, 48.6% in contr., no descendants	Baroche, C., 1968 (342)
Drosophila cl tu	Aminopterin	72.5% tumors, no descendants	Baroche, C., 1968 (342)
Drosophila cl tu	N,N-Dinitrosopentamethyl-enetetramine	1 hepatic tumor, 1 pit tumor	Boyland et al., 1968 (342)
Drosophila cl tu (first generation)	Thalidomide	14% tumors, 49.5% in contr	Baroche, C., 1968 (342)
Drosophila cl tu (second generation)	Thalidomide	67.9% tumors, 63.5% in contr.	Baroche, C., 1968 (342)
Drosophila cl tu (third generation)	Thalidomide	80.4% tumors, 64.2% in contr.	Baroche, C., 1968 (342)
Drosophila cl tu (fourth generation)	Thalidomide	84.2% tumors, 60.9% in contr.	Baroche, C., 1968 (342)
Drosophila cl tu (fifth generation)	Thalidomide	85.9% tumors, 55.5% in contr.	Baroche, C., 1968 (342)
Drosophila cl tu (12th generation)	Thalidomide	79.5% tumors, 53.2% in contr.	Baroche, C., 1968 (342)
Drosophila antibes VIII 55 strain	Thalidomide	No tumors	Baroche, C., 1968 (342)
Drosophila mutant cardinal strain	Thalidomide	No tumors	Baroche, C., 1968 (342)
Drosophila mutant strain	Thalidomide	Tumors appear but no quantitative results available due to contamination of culture	Baroche, C., 1968 (342)
Drosophila melanogaster	Aflatoxin B 1, rubratoxin B, patulin, diacetoxyscirpinol		Reiss, 1975 (4205)
Drosophila melanogaster	Aflatoxin B 1		
Drosophila melanogaster	N-nitroso compounds	Somatic mutagenesis	Shabad et al., 1976 (4616)
Blattella germanica (larvae)	Azo dyes	Without effect	Noland & Baumann, 1949 (3733)
Periplaneta americana	Aflatoxin B		Llewellyn et al., 1976 (3155)
Periplaneta americana	Apholate	Tumorlike growth	Saxena & Aditya, 1976 (4496)
Periplaneta americana	Farnesylmethyl-ether	Large genital tumors	O'Farrell & Stock, 1964 (3769)
Periplaneta americana	Methylcholanthrene	Aggregation of hemocytes	Schlumberger, 1952 (4546)
Periplaneta americana	Methylcholanthrene, 2-fluorenamine, N, N-dimethyl-p-azoanilin benzo(a)pyrene	Unspecific changes	Sutherland, 1969 (4921)
Cockroaches	20-Methylcholanthrene crystals	No tumors	Schlumberger, 1952 (4546)
Musca domestica (larvae)	9,10-dimethyl-1,2-dibenzan-thracene, 1,2,5,6-dibenzan-thracene benzo(a)pyrene	Same changes resembled *Drosophila* tumors	Cantwell et al., 1966 (810) Shortino et al., 1963 (4667)

after (22)

Table 7. Radiation and arthropods.

Phylum	Class	Species	Influence of Radiation	Effect	Reference
Arthropoda	Insects	–	Photoperiodic influence	Hormonal regulation	(42)
Arthropoda	Merostomata	*Limulus* sp.	P-like peptide	Photosensitivity in circadian rhythms	(33)
		Limulus sp.	substance P	Light-responsive	(32)
		Limulus sp.	Light induced decrease in potassium current	Light-responsiveness	(24)
		Limulus sp.	Control mechanisms	Burst of shedding of light sensitive membranes (rhabdoms) in lateral Eye	(7)
		Limulus sp.	Receptor potential evoked by light (comparable to conditions with cat motoneuron)	Light adaptation	(48)
	Arachnida	*Rhipicephalus sanguinis, R.* and *R. guilhoni* ticks	Light	Behavioral response	(14)
	Crustacea		Laser irradiation of ova	Effect on larval morphology and fertilization	(3)
		Daphnia magna	Lighting regime simulation of sunset and sunrise	Increasing phototactic response rates	(13)
		–	Illumination of retinal field of eyestalk	Identification of intercellular response of neurosecretory cells identified by lucifer yellow injection	(12)
Arthropoda	Insecta	–	Effects of microwave irradiation on cuticle, fat body, muscles, reproductive organs and eggs	Values compare well to similar effects in mammals	(40)
		Leptinotarsa decemlineata (Say) (Colorado potato beetle) (O.:Coleoptera)	Photoperiod and starvation	Light influence controlled through juvenile hormone of corpus allatum	(26)
		Apis mellifera (O.:Hymeoptera)	Light induction	Changes in extracellular volumes of retina	(41)
		Galleria mellonella (O.:Lepidoptera)	Photo and UV-enhanced reactivation	Repair of nuclear polyhedrosis-virus by insect cells	(50)
		Drosophila melanogaster, embryos (O.:Diptera)	Ultraviolet irradiation (300 nm) of egg surface	Arrest of intravitelline mitosis	(47)
Drosophila melanogaster	Gamma-ray-radiation	Mutation in male germ cells c 3 g strain	(36)		
		Drosophila melanogaster	light	Isoelectric point (pI) changes in three classes of retina-specific polypeptides (80, 49 and 39 kilodaltons)	(34)
		Drosophila melanogaster	Treatment of long-wave length UV light	Contact of the eggs 4–5 hrs after the contact with cis-dehydromatricaria ester showed highest enhancement of the chemical toxicity	Lagam. ;094
		Culiseta incidens	Constant light	Differential effects of constant light	(9)
Arthropoda	Insecta	*Acricotopus lucidus*	Millimeter wave radiation	Effect on puffing of giant chromosomes	(27)
		Smittia sp.	Ultraviolet light	Inhibition of pole cell formation (UV peak at 260 nm)	(4)
		Musca domestica wild type	Illumination of flye photoreceptors	Induced endocytosis of dye lucifer yellow, without loss of viability	(49)
		Aedes caspius Pallas	Photoperiod	Diapause induction	(1)
		Flies and mosquitoes	Light traps	Attraction of flies and mosquitoes	(51)

results of studies dealing with the influence of radiation on arthropod tissues.

4.3. Virus

The virus-induced (DNA nuclear polyhedrosis virus) proliferation of hemocytes in the European cranefly *Tipula paludosa* has been mentioned above.

A close relationship exists between long terminal repeats of avian leukosis-sarcoma virus and copia-like genetic elements of *Drosophila* sp. The avian leukosis sarcoma virus is believed to have been derived from infection of a progenitor *Drosophila* with a retrovirus (29). Also Shiba (43) reported retrovirus-like particles containing RNA homologous to the transparable element copia in *Drosophila melanogaster*. Genetic effects of injection of Rous sarcoma virus DNA into polar plasma of early *Drosophila melanogaster* embryos

Table 8. Abnormal growth in arthropods.

PHYLUM: ARTHROPODA
Class: Merostomata

Limulus polyphemus L.	Ectodermal lesion with articular enlargement	Hanstrom, 1926 (199); Krieg, 1973 (comments) (308)
	Class: Arachnida	
Phalangium opilio	Expansive growing neoplasms	Kolosvary, 1934 (299)
Mitella polymerus		Shimkin, Koe, Zechmeister, 1951 (505)
Tetraclita squamosa rubescens		Shimkin, Koe, Zechmeister, 1951 (505)
Lernaenicus radiatus	Parasitic fungi	Meyers, 1975 (209)
Crab? (Brachiura)+	Cellular growth	Fischer, 1928 (146); Krieg, 1973 (308)
Gigantocypris mueller	Physical injury(?)	Kornicker, 1975 (209)
Homarus vulgaris	Parasitic fungi	Alderman, 1977 (212)
Homarus sp.	Stomach neoplasm	McIntosh, 1884, 1885 (361)
Penaeus azetecus	Hamartomas	Overstreet and van Devender, 1977 (212)
	Epidermal hyperplasia	Lightner, 1977 (212)
	Class: Insecta Lesions of larvae	
Pygaera curtula	Neoplasms of trachea, rectum, hypoganglion, musculature, testis and coelomic fluid	White, 1921 (626)
Drosophila sp.	Malignant neuroblastoma. Semi-malignant and malignant imaginal disk neoplasms	Gateff, 1978 (155) Gateff, 1978 (155)
	Malignant neoplasms of larval hematopoietic system	Gateff, 1978 (155)
	Embryonal neoplasms	Gateff, 1978 (155)*
Gilpinia hercyniae	Proliferation of midintestinal epithelium	Bird, 1949 (36)
Gryllotalpa sp.	Cell proliferation in area of corpus	Palm, 1948 (415); Scharrer and Lochhead, 1950 (486) (comments)
	Lesions of imagines Order: Orthoptera	
Blattella germanica	Intestinal neoplasms	Schreiner and Johannson, 1966 (494)
Leucophaea maderae	Intestinal neoplasms (Cells with enlarged nuclei and abnormal mitoses (exp.))	Scharrer, 1953 (485) Matz, 1961 (343)
Locusta migratoria	Intestinal neoplasms	Matz, 1961 (343); Harshbarger and Taylor, 1968 (213) review
Orygia pseudotsugata	Developmental anomaly	Mattignoni and Iwai, 1977 (212) (AR)
Periplaneta americana	Tumorlike growth	Llewellyn et al., 1976 (324)
	Large genital tumors	O'Farell and Stock, 1964 (407)
	Aggregation of hemocytes	Schlumberger, 1952 (489)
	Unspecific changes	Sutherland, 1969 (561, 562, 563)
	Proliferation	Baerwald and Boush, 1969 (15)
	Order: Hymenoptera	
Apis mellifera	Connective tissue growth near second thoracic ganglion	Federlay, 1935, 1936 (137, 138)?
	Growth of vacuolized giant cells	Orösi-Pal, 1937 (411)
Bombus terrestris	Adenoma-like growth of pharyngeal glands with hypersection and regressive changes	Palm, 1949 (416)
	Order: Coleoptera	
Phydecta variabilis	Abnormal growth of pro-thorax	Kirby and Spencer, 1826 (292) Balazuc, 1948 (17)
Other species of coleoptera	Development abnormalities	Kraatz, 1881 (301); Pantel, 1898 (417); Balazuc, 1948 (17); Krieg, 1973 (308) (review)
	Order: Diptera	
Musca domestica	Melanotic tumors with sclerotizations	Bodnaryk, 1968 (38) (exp.)
Drosophila sp.	Benign neoplasms in the sclerotizations	Gateff, 1978 (155)*

*See also Chapter 30 by Burdette in Kaiser 1981.

Table 9. Selected spontaneous growth abnormalities, including neoplasms in insects.

Species	Growth Abnormality
Rhitrogena semicolorata	Hematopoietic neoplasms
Heptagenia lateralis	Hematopoietic neoplasms
Tipula paludosa	Hematopoietic neoplasm
Drosophila melanogaster	Imaginal disc neoplasms
Drosophila melanogaster	Hereditary melanotic tumors
Drosophila melanogaster	Tumorous head
Drosophila melanogaster	Ovarian tumors
Drosophila melanogaster	Invasive neuroblastoma

similar: as when foreign DNAs were introduced into a mouse germ line, mutations were induced (11). Mutations induced by DNA of oncogenic viruses seem to be of the insertion type. Gazarian (10) induced mutations, generally unstable with the injection of RNA-containing Rous sarcoma virus plasmid pBR322 inserted by kDNA R8V (pPrC11) and Sa7 adenovirus DNA into the polar region of *Drosophila melanogaster*. In certain populations of flies, RSV provirus was found incorporated into cellular DNA, and in one mutant family of *Drosophila melanogaster*, the disintegrated form of plasmid DNA was identified (46). Some evidence of mechanical transmission of reticoloendothelioseis virus by mosquitoes (*Culex annulirostris*) was described by Motha in 1984. The role of the insect *Stomoxys calcitrans*, *Haematobia irritans*, *Chrysops* sp. and *Tabanus atratus* in the transmission of bovine leukosis virus were studied. Infection depends much on the feeding behavior of these insects. Infection occurred after bites of *Chrysops* and *Tabanus*; *Haematobia irritans* acted negative. *Stomoxys* did not infect when interrupted during feeding (6). Mellor and coworkers 1984 recorded the first isolation in the Sudan from arboviruses from *Culicoibes* sp., with identification of a BTV serotype and the presence of a member of the EHD (genus arbovirus, family reoviridae) serogroup.

4.4. Trauma

Traumatic lesions of abnormal growth can be produced in such insects as *Leucophaea maderae* or *Periplaneta americana* by nerve severance, or by sealing the anus with methyl-2-cyanocrylate (35). In the latter case, tumor-like lesions develop after normal feeding of 2 weeks. It is known from dogs that fractures of bone are often followed by neoplastic development.

4.5. Brief review of arthropod neoplasms

(See table 8.)

5. SUMMARY AND CONCLUSION

Neoplasms have been observed in the three most important animal phyla, of arthropoda, mollusca and vertebrata. Comparative aspects of these three phyla, morphologic, physiologic, genetic, pathologic embryologic and many still unknown characteristics of the huge phylum of arthropoda with approximately 1 000 000 described species explain two things: (1) how little we know about abnormal growth in this huge phylum and (2) what a vast number of species awaits scientific exploitation in regard to abnormal growth in general and neoplasms in particular.

REFERENCES

1. Abdel-Rahman AM, Adham FK: The effect of photoperiod on diapause induction in *Aedes caspius* Pallas (Diptera: Culicidae) *J Egypt Soc Parasitol* 13(2):343, 1983
2. Berrios M, Blobel G, Fisher PA: Characterization of an ATPase/dATPase activity associated with the *Drosophila* nuclear matrix-pore complex-lamina fraction. Identification of the putative enzyme polypeptide by direct ultraviolet photoaffinity labeling. *J Biol Chem* 258(7):4548, 1983
3. Brand GW, Troup GJ, Rumble S, Ninio F: Laser irradiation of crustacean ova: effects on larval morphology and fertilization. *Australas Phys Eng Sci Med* 6(1):38, 1983
4. Brown PM, Kalthoff K: Inhibition by ultraviolet light of pole cell formation in *Smittia* sp (Chironomidae, Diptera) action spectrum and photoreversibility. *Dev Biol* 97(1):113, 1983
5. Burdette WJ: Aberrant tissue in *Drosophila*, pp. 461–465, In: Neoplasms – Comparative Pathology of Growth in Animals, Plants, and Man edited by Kaiser HE, Baltimore: Williams & Wilkins, 1981
6. Buxton BA, Hinkle NC, Schultz RD: Role of insects in the transmission of bovine leukosis virus: potential for transmission by stable flies, horn flies, and tabanids. *Am J Vet Res* 46(1):123, 1985
7. Chamberlain SC, Barlow RB Jr: Transient membrane shedding in *Limulus* photoreceptors: control mechanisms under natural lighting. *J Neurosci* 4(11):2792, 1984
8. Chinn K, Lisman J: Calcium mediates the light-induced decrease in maintained K = current in *Limulus* ventral photoreceptors. *J Gen Physiol* 84(3):447, 1984
9. Clopton JR: Mosquito circadian flight rhythms: differential effects of constant light. *Am J Physiol* 247(6 Pt 2):R960, 1984
10. Gazarian KG, Nabirochkin SD, Shakhbazian AK, Shibanova EN, Tikhoneko TI: Induction of unstable mutations in *Drosophila melanogaster* by the microinjection of oncogenic viruses and their DNA into early embryos. *Genetika (Moskva)* 20(8):1237, 1984
11. Gazaryan KG, Nabirochkin SD, Tatosyan AG, Shakhbazyan AK, Shibanova EN: Genetic effects of injection of Rous sarcoma virus DNA into polar plasm of early *Drosophila melanogaster* embryos. *Nature* 311(5984):392, 1984
12. Glantz RM, Kirk MD, Ar'echiga H: Light input to crustacean neurosecretory cells. *Brain Res* 265(2):307, 1983
13. Grover PB Jr, Miller RJ: Effects of crepuscular photoenvironment on light-induced behavior of *Daphnia*. *Physiol Behav* 33(5):729, 1984
14. Hafez M, Bishara SI: Behavioural responses of *Rhipicephalus sanguineus*, *R. turanicus* and *R. guilhoni* ticks to relative humidity, light and host odour. *J Egypt Soc Parasitol* 14(2):623, 1984
15. Harshbarger JC, Cantwell GE, Stanton MF: Effects of N-nitrosodimethylamine on the crayfish, *Procambarus clarkii*. Proc. of the Fourth Internat'l Colloquium on Insect Pathology with the Soc. for Invertebrate Pathology, pp. 425, 1971
16. Harshbarger JC: Radiation, Neoplasms, Carcinogenic Chemicals, and Insects. In: Insect Diseases, Cantwell GE, (ed.). vol. 2, iii+. New York: Marcel Dekker, 1974
17. Harshbarger JC: Role of the Registry of Tumors in Lower Animals in the Study of Environmental Carcinogenesis in Aquatic Animals. Annal of the N.Y. Acad. of Sciences, vol. 298, pp. 280–89, 1977
18. Harshbarger JC: Neoplasms in Zoo Poikilotherms Emphasizing Cases in the Registry of Tumors in Lower Animals. Symp.

of the Nat'l Zoological Park: *The Comparative Pathology of Zoo Animals.* Montali RJ, Migaki G, (eds.), pp. 585–591. Smithsonian Institution Press, Washington, D.C, 1980

19. Harshbarger JC: Epizootiology of Leukemia and Lymphoma in Poikilotherms. Advances in Comparative Leukemia Research. Yohn DS, Blakeslee JR, Amsterdam: Elsevier North-Holland, Inc, 1982

20. Hoffman-Falk H, Einat P, Shilo BZ, Hoffmann FM: *Drosophila melanogaster* DNA clones homologous to vertebrate oncogenes: evidence for a common ancestor to the src and abl cellular genes. *Cell* 32(2):589, 1983

21. Hoffmann FM, Fresco LD, Hoffman-Falk H, Shilo BZ: Nucleotide sequences of the *Drosophila* src and abl homologs: conservation and variability in the src family oncogenes. *Cell* 35(2 Pt 1):393, 1983

22. Kaiser HE: *Species-Specific Potential of Invertebrates for Toxicological Research.* Baltimore: University Park Press, 1980

23. Kaiser HE: Animal Neoplasms – A Systematic Review. In: *Neoplasms – Comparative Pathology of Growth in Animals, Plants, and Man.* Kaiser HE, (ed.). Baltimore: Williams & Wilkins, 1981

24. Kagan I, Kolyvas CP, Lam J: The ovicidal activity of cis-dehydromatricaria ester: time-dependence of its enhancement by UV light. *Experientia* 15:40(12):1396, 1984

25. Katzen AL, Kornberg TB, Bishop JM: Isolation of the Proto-oncogene c-myb from *D. melanogaster.* *Cell* 41(2):449, 1985

26. Khan MA, Koopmanschap AB, de Kort CA: The relative importance of nervous and humoral pathways for control of corpus allatum activity in the adult Colorado potato beetle, *Leptinotarsa decemlineata* (Say). *Gen Comp Endocrinol* 52(2):214, 1983

27. Koschnitzke C, Kremer F, Santo L, Quick P, Poglitsch A: A non-thermal effect of millimeter wave radiation on the puffing of giant chromosomes. *Z Naturforsch(C)* 38(9–10):883, 1983

27a. Koval TM: Multiphasic survival response of a radioresistant lepidopteran insect cell line. *Radiat Res* 98(3):642, 1984.

28. Krause J, Kohler W: Dispersal behavior of photonegative selection lines of *Drosophila melanogaster.* *Behav Genet* 14(3):269, 1984

29. Kugimiya W, Ikenaga H, Saigo K: Close relationship between the long terminal repeats of avian leukosis-sarcoma virus and copia-like movable genetic elements of *Drosophila.* *Proc Natl Acad Sci USA* 80(11):3193, 1983

30. Levy Z, Leibovitz N, Segev O, Shilo BZ: Expression of the src and abl cellular oncogenes during development of *Drosophila melanogaster* *Mol Cell Biol* 4(5):982, 1984

31. Madhavan K, Bilodeau-Wentworth D, Wadsworth SC: Family of developmentally regulated, maternally expressed *Drosophila* RNA species detected by a v-*myc* probe. *Mol Cell Biol* 5(1):7, 1985

32. Mancillas JR, Selverston AI: Neuropeptide modulation of photosensitivity. II. Physiological and anatomical effects of substance P on the lateral eye of Limulus. *J Neurosci* 4(3):847, 1984

33. Mancillas JR, Brown MR: Neuropeptide modulation of photosensitivity of a substance P-like peptide in the lateral eye of *Limulus.* *J Neurosci* 4(3):832, 1984

34. Matsumoto H, Pak WL: Light-induced phosphorylation of retina-specific polypeptides of *Drosophila* in vivo. *Science* 223(4632):184, 1984

35. Mellor PS, Osborne R, Jennings DM: Isolation of blue-tongue and related viruses from *Culicoides* spp. in the Sudan. *J Hyg* (*Lond*) 93(3):621, 1984

36. Miyamot T: Gamma-ray-induced mutations in male germ cells of a recombination-defective strain (c3G) of *Drosophila melanogaster.* *Mutat Res* 120(1):27, 1983

37. Motha MX, Egerton JR, Sweeney AW: Some evidence of mechanical transmission of reticuloendotheliosis virus by mosquitoes. *Avian Dis* 28(4):858, 1984

38. Mozer B, Marlor, Parkhurst S, Corces V: Characterization and developmental expression of a *Drosophila* ras oncogene. *Mol Cell Biol* 5(4):885, 1985

39. Neuman-Silberberg FS, Schejter E, Hoffman FM, Shilo BZ: The *Drosophila* ras oncogenes: structure and nucleotide sequence. *Cell* 37(3):1027, 1984

40. Ondr'a'cek J, Brunnhofer V: Dielectric properties of insect tissues. *Gen Physiol Biophys* 3(3):251, 1984

41. Orkand RK, Dietsel I, Coles JA: Light-induced changes in extracellular volume in the retina of the drone, *Apis mellifera.* *Neurosci Lett* 45(3):273, 1984

42. Photoperiodic regulation of insect and molluscan hormones. *Ciba Found Symp* 104:1, 1984

43. Shiba T, Saigo K: Retrovirus-like particles containing RNA homologous to the transposable element copia in *Drosophila melanogaster.* *Nature* 302(5904):119, 1983

44. Shilo, B–Z, Weinberg, RA: DNA sequences homologous to vertebrate oncogenes are conserved in *Drosophila melanogaster.* Proc Nat Acad Sci 78: 6789, 1981.

45. Simon MA, Kornberg TB, Bishop JM: Three loc related to the src oncogene and tyrosine-specific protein kinases activity in *Drosophila.* *Nature* 302(5911):837, 1983

46. Tatosyan AG, Nabirochkin SD, Shakhbazyan AK, Gazaryan KG, Kisseljov FL: Detection of virus-specific sequences in *Drosophila melanogaster* mutants induced by injection of RSV DNA into early embryos. *Nature* 311(5984):394, 1984

47. Togashi S, Okada M: Arrest of intravitelline mitoses in *Drosophila* embryos by u.v. irradiation of the egg surface. *J Embryo Exp Morphol* 80:43, 1984

48. Wang LT, Wasserman GS: Direct intracellular measurement of non-linear postreceptor transfer functions in dark and light adaptation in *Limulus.* *Brain Res* 328(1):41, 1985

49. Wilcox M, Franceschini N: Illumination induces dye incorporation in photoreceptor cells. *Science* 225 (4664):851, 1984

50. Witt DJ: Photoreactivation and ultraviolet-enhanced reactivation of ultraviolet-irradiated nuclear polyhedrosis virus by insect cells. *Arch Virol* 79(1–2):95, 1984

51. Yang JQ: Comparison of six insect light-traps with various spectral colors in attracting mosquitoes and flies. *Chung Hua Yu Fang I Hsueh Tsa Chih* 18(1):15, 1984

8

METASTASES IN FISH

S.V. MACHOTKA, B.B. McCAIN and M. MYERS

Nearly all comparable tumors of mammals and fish have been found in both classes of vertebrates. Differences exist mainly due to variations of body structures, most notably those regarding the respiratory organs in mammals and fishes (lungs in mammals, gills or "lungs" in fishes). Another variation is the appearance of the osteoid substance of Kölliker besides bones in teleosts, though not in mammals. Hairs and mammary glands are characteristic of mammals, but not of fish, many of whom have scales and swim bladders not occurring in mammals. This list could be extended (13).

Some tumors develop in fish, but not in mammals. Similarly, mammals may develop tumors which cannot occur in fish. The following exceptions should be noted: the skin of mammals lacks guanophores, cells which contain guanine.

Guanine

Guanophores are present in some cold blooded vertebrates, especially fishes, thus giving the animals a metallic luster. Neoplasms of these cells are known as guanophoromas. Fish lack sebacious and sweat glands, mammary glands and salivary glands and therefore do not have neoplams of these tissues. The presence of chondroid tissue in osteichthyes is questionable. Certain fish, such as the carangidae, exhibit the "Osteoid substance of Kölliker" (15). The cartilaginous chondrichthyes lack bone, as do the lampreys and hagfishes. Fish also lack myoepithelial tissue.

In contrast to primary tumors, secondary tumors are very rare in fishes. In explaining the rarity of secondary tumors, we must first consider the different avenues of tumor spreading, in which the body fluid system plays the most important role in tumor distribution in the mammal. Of less importance are such types of spreading as via the coelomic covers, from teratomas, metastatic implantation of epithelial surfaces, and by a few rare special types of metastatic spreading. The spread by the circulatory system, the basis for spread via the body fluids, shows interesting differences. These differences point to the special role of the lymph nodes, especially regarding so-called solid tumors, on one hand, and the "lymphatic cells" in lymphomas and leukemias on the other. Table 1 compares the circulatory systems of fishes and mammals.

In the mammal, the lymph, before returning to the blood (via the veins), passes through one or more lymphnodes, which filter the lymph. We know from mammalian metastasis via the body fluids that metastatic cells must overcome many hostile influences when entering the vessels, when traveling in the body fluids (as killer cells do), and when re-entering the new tissue where they settle as metastasis. It appears plausible that the metastatic cells, unfiltered by lymphnodes, may be destroyed in another phase of their travel. This fact may suggest one reason why neoplasm metastases in fishes are so rare. The question remains, how-

Table 1. Comparison of the circulatory systems in fish and mammals.

A. THE CIRCULATORY SYSTEM IN FISHES

1. The circulatory system in cyclostomata (hagfishes, lampreys)

Heart	Blood vessels	Lymphatic system
Heart composed of ventricle and atrium	Arteries with intima, media adventitia. Veins simple. Way of blood in fish from heart to respiratory organs and from there to body and heart. Blood cells: granulocytes, agranulocytes, erythrocytes. Distinction between erythrocytes and leukocytes well established.	No distinct system of lymphatic channels — lymphocytes

48

H. E. Kaiser (ed.), Comparative aspects of tumor development.
© 1989, Kluwer Academic Publishers, Dordrecht. ISBN-13:978-0-89838-994-4

Table 1. Contd.

A. THE CIRCULATORY SYSTEM IN FISHES

2. The circulatory system in chondrichthyes (cartilaginous fish)

Heart	*Blood vessels*	*Lymphatic system*
Heart (sinus venosus, atrium, ventricle and conus arteriosus)	Blood flows through arteries (muscular and elastic walls) — in shark no pulse — gills, arteries, capillaries, veins, heart. Blood cells: erythrocytes and several types of leukocytes (large and small lymphocytes, neutrophilic granulocytes, eosinophilic granulocytes, hemocytoblasts, thrombocytes, and certain immediate stages. Basophilic granulocytes are lacking.	Lymphatic system poorly developed — no lymph nodes. Interstitial fluid is collected. Spleen, Organ of Leydig.

3. The circulatory system in osteichthyes (bony fish)

Heart	*Blood vessels*	*Lymphatic system*
Heart (sinus venosus, atrium, ventricle)	Arteries exhibit poor development of smooth muscle. Blood cells: erythrocytes and leukocytes are known. Of the latter especially eosinophils and neutrophils are characterized by remarkable species specificity.	Many teleosts have a well-developed lymphatic system with vessels beneath the skin and within viscera and glands. Lymph hearts and considerable amounts of lymphocytic tissue occur in certain species. Lymph nodules in the spleen but no lymph node hematopoiesis occurs in connective tissue, kidneys, and subcapsular areas of liver and spleen.

B. THE CIRCULATORY SYSTEM IN MAMMALS

1. The circulatory system in mammals

Heart	*Blood vessels*	*Lymphatic system*
Heart: 2 atria, 2 ventricles. Endocardium, myocardium, pericardium. Heart skeleton — node of Aschoff-Tawara, Sinus node of Keith-Flack	Arteries: Intima, media, adventitia. Veins: as arteries but not as pronounced. Capillaries. Blood Cells: Erythrocytes, leukocytes (with subtypes)	The lymphatic system, most pronounced in all animals is a oneway system, starting with lymph capillaries, found in nearly all tissues and characterized in certain regions by dilated walls. Most of the lymph returning to the circulatory system via lymph vessels passes through one or more of the abundant lymph nodes exhibiting age changes. Other lymphatic organs are: the tonsils, thymus, spleen, and diffuse lymphatic tissue as in the intestine. Bone marrow is the major area of hematopoiesis.

(adapted after 1 (W. Andrew and CP Hickman))

Table 2. A review of neoplasm metastasis in fish

Species	Primary Tumor	Metastasis	Reference
Sea lamprey (*Petromyzon marinus*)	Melanoma, skin, subcutis	Gill, kidney	(8)
Rainbow trout (*Salmo gairdneri*)	Liver, hepatocellular carcinoma	Kidney	(3)
Crucian carp (*Crassius crassius*)	Kidney, nephroblastoma	Pancreas	(10)
Northern spiky dogfish (*Squalous blainvilli*)	Mesentery, probable neurilemmoma	Liver	(9)
Croaker (*Nibea mitsukurrii*)	Skin/subcutis, malignant melanoma	Spleen	(11)
Coalfish (*Teragra chalcogramma*)	Rectal gland, adenocarcinoma	Stomach, small intestine, liver, spleen, urinary bladder, swim bladder	(28)
Goldfish (*Carassius auratus*)	Pancreas, adenocarcinoma	Mesentery	(21)
Goldfish (*Carassius auratus*)	Ovary, carcinoma	Cerebrum	(5)
Northern pike (*Esox*)	Lymphosarcoma	Numerous other organs: kidney, liver, spleen	(20)
Rainbow trout (*Salmo gairdneri*)	Hepatoma liver	Gills, esophagus, stomach, pancreas, intercaecal fascia, hematopoietic kidney, excretory kidney and ovary	(2)

ever, why other types of tumor spread, such as direct spreading, spreading on coelomic surfaces, spreading on surface epithelia, metastasis of teratomas and unusual metastasis, are also so rare. Perhaps heterogeneity and specialization of metastatic cells, which remain in animals running at a very low survival rate, may not be so highly developed in fish. It should be considered that other vertebrate classes, such as birds, show a lesser development of the metastatic process than mammals, perhaps at least partially due to the fact that birds have fewer epithelial neoplasms (an exception are ovarial tumors) than mesenchymal ones, such as leukemias and lymphomas, e.g. Marek's disease, etc. However, other causes of rare incidence of secondary tumors in fish to be considered are that we are generally left to examine feral animals that become weak and are easily trapped or die before a metastasis can occur, so this occurrence of low incidence of metastasis may partially be low due to sampling error, not inability to produce and grow metastasis by fish, amphibians, reptiles or birds. Selected examples of neoplasms in fish that have metastasized are presented in Table 2.

A model for the similarities of neoplastic spreading of neoplasms in organs present in mammals and fish is exemplified by the spreading of malignant liver neoplasms of selected marine fish.

Metastatic Hepatic Neoplasms in Teleost Species

Metastatic hepatic tumors in teleost species have been reported in hatchery-reared rainbow trout (*Salmo gairdneri*) exposed to aflatoxins (2, 6, 12, 24, 31, 32) and dimethylnitrosamine (4), in feral Atlantic tomcod (*Microgadus tomcod*) from the Hudson River estuary (26) and feral English sole

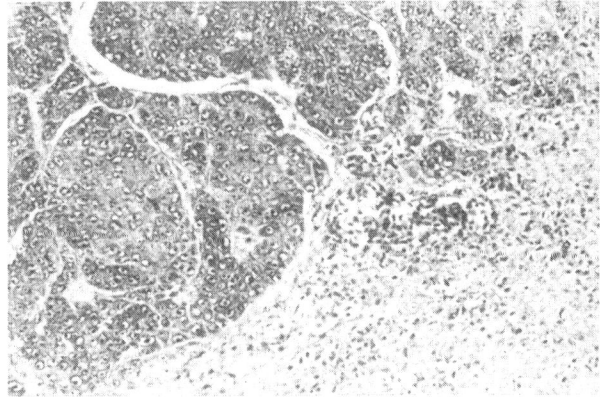

Figure 1. Metastases of hepatocellular carcinoma in feral Atlantic tomcod to the spleen. (H & E) × 272 (reduced).

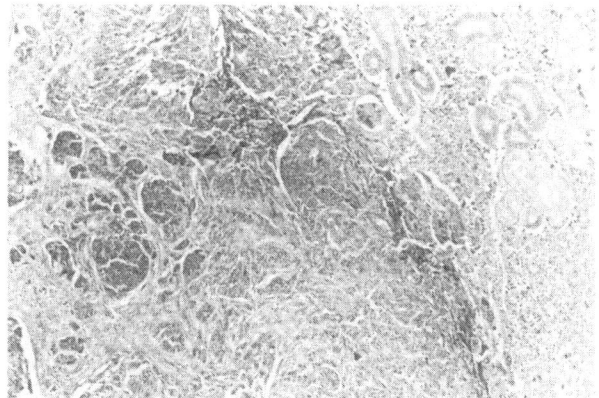

Figure 2. Metastases in the kidney from hepatocellular carcinoma of feral Atlantic tomcod. (H & E) × 136 (reduced).

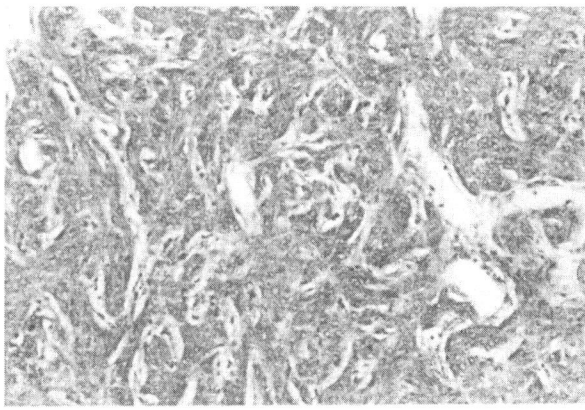

Figure 5. Higher magnification of primary cholangiocellular carcinoma of English sole. (H & E) × 270 (reduced).

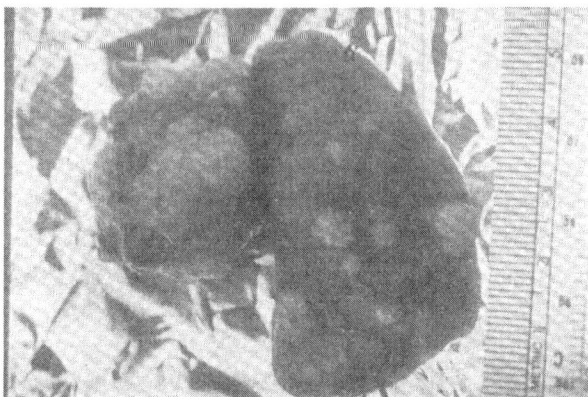

Figure 3. Cholangiocellular carcinoma in English sole; macroscopic picture.

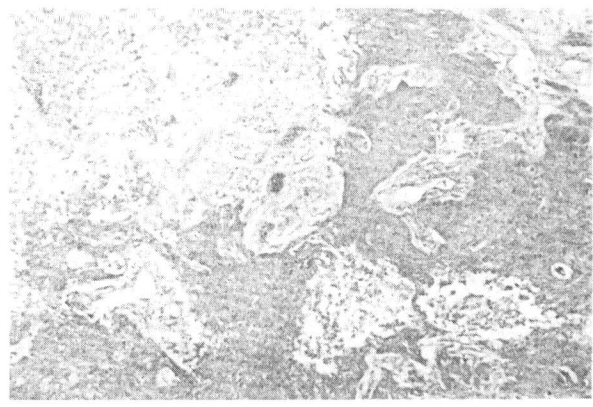

Figure 6. Ischemic and hemorrhagic necroses in primary cholangiocellular carcinoma of English sole. (H & E) × 135 (reduced).

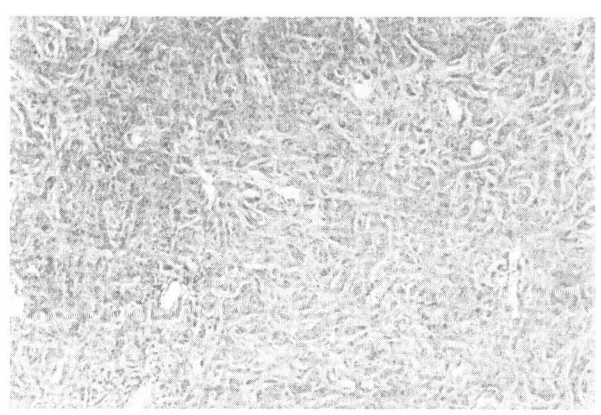

Figure 4. Lower magnification of primary cholangiocellular carcinoma of English sole. (H & E) × 135 (reduced).

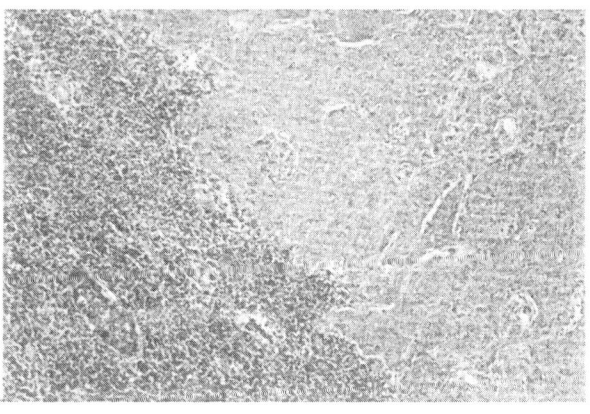

Figure 7. Metastasis of cholangiocellular carcinoma in spleen of English sole. (H & E) × 135 (reduced).

from the Duwamish Waterway in Puget Sound, WA (19).

The metastatic lesions in rainbow trout are derived strictly from primary hepatocellular carcinomas in adult, hatchery-reared fish. Although affected individuals are usually 3–6 years of age (12), tumor emboli and vascular invasion are detectable in fish 12–18 months in age, and trout as young as 18–20 months have been shown to contain extrahepatic metastases of hepatocellular carcinoma (4, 32). The frequency of metastasis in this species is generally low, but in older animals (4 yrs.), up to 30% of tumor-bearing trout

Figure 8. Metastasis of cholangiocellular carcinoma in spleen of English sole. (H & E) × 135 (reduced).

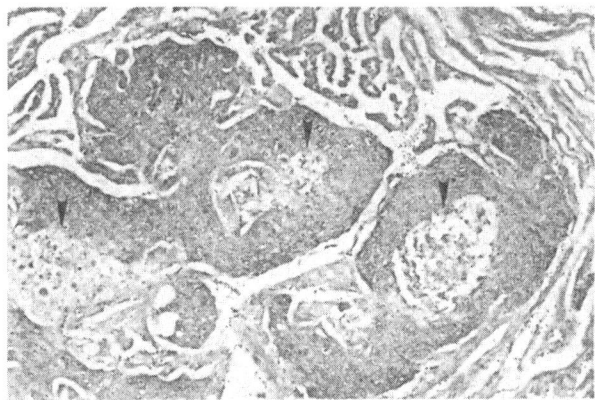

Figure 10. Lower magnification of metastasis of cholangiocellular carcinoma in ventricular myocardium of English sole. (H & E) × 270 (× 189 reduced).

have been shown to have metastatic hepatocellular carcinoma (2). The most common organs for metastatic dissemination are the spleen (infrequent site of metastasis in mammals), kidney and gills (2, 6, 12, 24, 31, 32), with metastatic foci of this tumor type also reported in the heart (6), stomach (2, 6, 24), pyloric caecae (2, 4, 6, 24), esophagus (2), pancreas (2, 4), intestine (4) and ovary (2, 4). Spread to the gill, heart, kidney and spleen appears to occur primarily through the hematogenous route, while metastasis to the pyloric caecae, stomach, intestine, pancreas and ovary are the result of direct intraabdominal extension of the tumor, followed by invasion of serosal surfaces (4, 24).

Metastatic hepatocellular carcinomas in feral Atlantic tomcod from the Hudson River estuary in New York have also been demonstrated (C.E. Smith, pers. comm.). The prevalences of hepatocellular carcinoma in this species have been determined primarily by gross findings with supportive histopathologic diagnoses, therefore, complete necropsies have not been performed on all tumor-bearing specimens. However, of the approximately 20 tumor-bearing tomcods which have been necropsied fully and subjected to histopathologic examination, two specimens exhibited metastases in the spleen (Figure 1) and kidney (Figure 2). These fish were adults two years of age.

Microscopically, these metastases were composed of irregular trabeculae of anaplastic, pleomorphic hepatocytes, within a prominent fibrous stroma. It is a very unique condition that biliary proliferation was also present within the metastases. This may imply that the biliary epithelium also was malignant. Substantial proportions of the spleen and kidney were replaced by the invasive metastases from the primary hepatocellular carcinoma, and a rapid growth rate was suggested by numerous zones of ischemic and hemorrhagic necrosis within the metastases.

The single case of a metastatic hepatic tumor detected in English sole (19) from Puget Sound was in an eight-year-old female from the Duwamish Waterway (Figure 3). The anterior portion of the liver consisted primarily of a firm, white mass of tissue which was multinodular and contained cystic, hemorrhagic zones. The total diameter of the area affected by these nodules was approximately 40 mm. The posterior region of the liver also contained multiple, white, firm nodules ranging from 1–7 mm in diameter. Within the spleen was a firm white nodule approximately 10 mm in diameter, with several smaller nodules 1–3 mm in diameter within the splenic parenchyma. Visible within the trunk kidney was a large (7 mm) white, firm spherical nodule in the anterior portion of this organ.

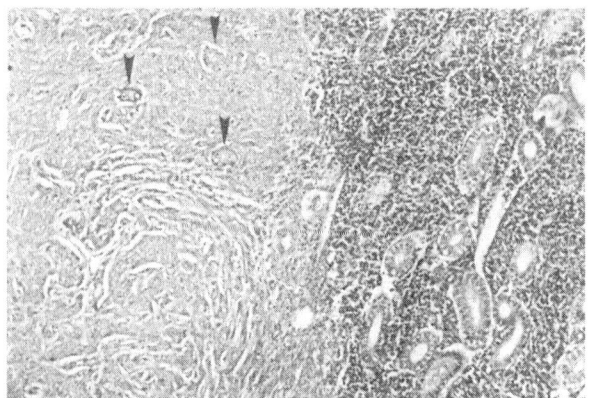

Figure 9. Metastasis of cholangiocellular carcinoma in kidney of English sole. (H & E) × 135 (reduced).

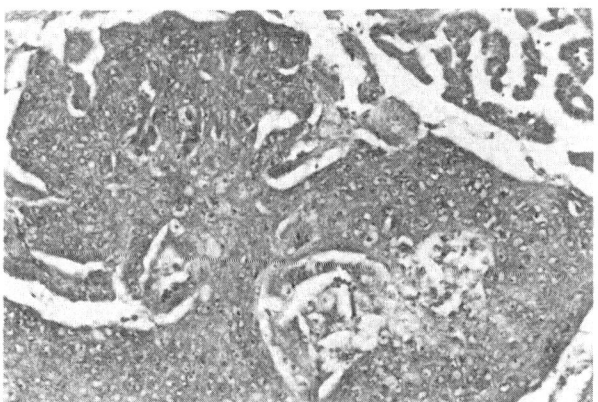

Figure 11. Higher magnification of cholangiocellular carcinoma in ventricular myocardium of English sole. (H & E) × 540 (× 370 reduced).

Microscopically, the primary hepatic tumors were characterized by a disorganized proliferation of cholangiolar epithelium, occasionally assuming a faintly detectable tubular pattern (Figures 4 and 5). The borders of the nodules were irregular, with fungiform, finger-like extensions invading the surrounding hepatic parenchyma. The stroma was composed of fibroblasts and collagen (a typical desmoplasia of biliary carcinoma). The cell of origin in this neoplasm was biliary epithelium based on the following features: the small, ovoid nuclei lacking a prominent nucleolus; the eosinophilic cytoplasm, and the occasional presence of ductal structures. The primary neoplasm had almost entirely replaced the anterior region of the liver, and had outgrown the available blood supply, resulting in massive areas of ischemic and hemorrhagic necrosis (Figure 6). Diagnostic features of this neoplasm were consistent with a cholangiocellular carcinoma. Other hepatic lesions detected in the liver were liver cell adenoma, hepatocellular carcinoma, eosinophilic and clear cell foci of cellular alteration (putative preneoplastic lesions), hepatocellular coagulation necrosis and hepatocellular regenerative islands. The most significant findings, however, were metastases from the primary cholangiocellular carcinoma to the spleen (Figures 7 and 8), kidney (Figure 9) and ventricular myocardium (Figures 10 and 11). In all affected organs the metastatic neoplasms were actively invading and replacing the adjacent tissue elements. The organs which the primary neoplasm had seeded to, especially the heart, suggested a purely hematogenous route of dissemination.

Summary and Conclusion

The spreading of neoplastic growth of fish was discussed, using selected examples, showing that:
1. Fish and mammals exhibit many similar tissues, though others are lacking in one or the other group, limiting a particular tumor appearance.
2. The anatomy of both groups provides differences in the systems of body fluids which may influence tumor spreading and early death due to primary disease.
3. Spreading of selected neoplasms (e.g. hepatic) into certain organs of fish and mammals seems to be similar.
4. Future investigations will surely reveal more details and similarities of neoplastic spreading in the phylum of vertebrates as compared to the phyla of invertebrates.

Acknowledgements

The furnishing of the histologic slides and figures by Dr. C.E. Smith is highly appreciated.

References

1. Andrew W, Hickman CP: Vertebrate Histology. St. Louis, MO.: C.V. Mosby, 1972
2. Ashley LM, Halver JE: Multiple metastases of rainbow trout hepatoma. *Trems Am Fish Soc* 92:365, 1963
3. Ashley LM: Histopathology of rainbow trout aflatoxicosis. *Res Rep U.S. Fish Wildl Serv* 70:103, 1965
4. Ashley LM, Halver JE: Dimethylnitrosamine-induced hepatic cell carcinoma in rainbow trout. *J Nat'l Cancer Inst* 41:531, 1968
5. Ceretto F: Carcinoma di tipo psammornatoso in *Carassius auratus*. Riv. ital. Piscis. Ittiopat. (A.) 3:37, (transl. – Carcinoma of the psammomatype in the goldfish.) 1968
6. Cudkowicz G, Scolari C: Un tumore primitive epatico a diffusione epizootica nella trota iridea di allevamento (*Salmo irideu*). Tumori 41:524, 1955
7. Haddow A, Blake I: Neoplasms in fish: A report of six cases with a summary of the literature. *J Path & Bact* 36:41, 1933
8. Harshbarger JC: Activities Report, Registry of Tumors in Lower Animals, 1965–1973. Washington, DC: Smithsonian Institution, 1974
9. Harshbarger JC (1975). Activity Report, Registry of Tumors in Lower Animals. Suppl. Washington, DC: Smithsonian Institution, 1975
10. Harshbarger JC: Activity Report, Registry of Tumors in Lower Animals, 1975. Supplement. Washington, DC: Smithsonian Institution, 1976
11. Harshbarger JC (1978). Activity Report, Registry of Tumors in Lower Animals, 1977. Suppl. Washington, DC: Smithsonian Institution, 1978
12. Hendricks JD, Meyers TR, Shelton DW: Histological progression of hepatic neoplasia in rainbow trout (*Salmo gairdneri*). *Nat'l Cancer Inst Monogr* 655:321, 1984
13. Kaiser HE: Distribution of True (Real) Tissues in Organisms: A Preliminary Condition of Neoplastic Growth. In: *Neoplasms – Comparative Pathology of Growth in Animals, Plants, and Man*. 43, Baltimore: Williams & Wilkins, 1981
13a. Kaiser HE: Species specific spectrum of neoplasms. In: *Neoplasms – Comparative Pathology of Growth in Animals, Plants, and Man*. 649. Baltimore: Williams & Wilkins, 1981
14. Kaiser HE: Animal neoplasms – a systematic review. In: *Neoplasms – Comparative Pathology of Growth in Animals, Plants, and Man*. Baltimore: Williams & Wilkins, 1981
15. Kolliker A: Ueber verschiedene Typen in der mikroskopischen Struktur des Skelettes von Knochenfischen. *Verhdl. Wuerzburger phys.-med. Ges.* 9, 1859
16. Lucke B: Am. J. Cancer 20:352, 1934
17. Lucke B: Am. J. Cancer 34:15, 1938
18. Machotka SV: Progression of leucoses and lymphomas in reptiles and fish. In: Lymphocytic neoplasms in reptiles and fish. In *Cancer Growth and Progression*, HE Kaiser (ed), this volume, 1988
19. McCain BB, Myers MS, Varansi U et al: Pathology of two species of flatfish from urban estuaries in Puget Sound. EPA Interagency Energy/Environment, Research and Development Program Report (EPA 600/7-81-001), pp. 1–100, 1982
20. Mulcahy MF: Lymphosarcoma in the pike, *Esox lucius* L. (Pisces; Esocidae) in Ireland, Proc. R Ir Acad (B) 63:103, 1963
21. Otte E: Eine boesartige Neubildung in der Bauchhoehle eines Goldfisches (*Carassius auratus* L.). Wien tieraerztl. Mschr 51:485, (transl. A malignant formation in the abdomen of a goldfish), 1964
22. Pick L: Deutsche med. Wschr. 31:1817, 1905
23. Plehn M: Travaux de la deuzième conference internat. p. l'étude du cancer, Paris; F. Alcan, 1911, p. 221
24. Scarpelli DG, Greider MH, Frajola WJ: Observations on hepatic cell hyperplasia, adenoma and hepatoma of rainbow trout (*Salmo gairdneri*). Cancer Research 23:848, 1963
25. Schwab M, Anders A: Carcinogenesis in *Xiphophorus* and the role of the genotype in tumor susceptibility. In: *Neoplasms – Comparative Pathology of Growth in Animals, Plants, and Man*. Baltimore: Williams & Wilkins, edited by HE Kaiser, pp 451, 1981
26. Smith CE, Peck TH, Klauda RJ, McLaren JB: Hepatomas in Atlantic tomcod *Microgadus tomcod* (Walbaum) collected in the Hudson river estuary in New York. J Fish Dis 2:313, 1979
27. Stegeman JJ: In vitro metabolism of polynuclear aromatic

hydrocarbons in deep-sea fishes. In: *Neoplasms – Comparative Pathology of Growth in animals, Plants, and Man,* edited by HE Kaiser, Baltimore: Williams & Wilkins, pp. 361, 1981

28. Takahashi K: Studie ueber die Fischgeschwuelste. Ztschr. f. Krebsforsch. 29:1–73, 1929

29. Thomas L: Les tumeurs des poissons (Étude anatomogie et pathogenique). (transl.: Tumors of fish (an anatomical and pathological study). Bull. Assoc. franc. p. l'étude du cancer 20:703, 1931

30. Wood EM, Larson CP: Hepatic carcinoma in rainbow trout. *Arch Path* 71:471, 1961

31. Yasutake WT, Rucker RR: Nutritionally induced hepatogenesis of rainbow trout. *US Fish Wildlife Serv Res Rep* 70:39, 1967

9

METASTASES IN AMPHIBIANS

MIRIAM R. ANVER

Metastatic tumors, in general, are uncommon in amphibians. With the exception of the Lucké renal adenocarcinoma, a herpes-virus-associated spontaneous neoplasm of *Rana pipiens* (the leopard frog), the majority of spontaneous metastasizing tumors involve single animals (case reports). There are, however, several experimental systems which allow study of metastatic epithelial and hematopoietic neoplasms. These systems will be discussed in more detail in this chapter.

Table 1 is a summary of metastatic tumors reported in anurans (frogs, toads) and urodeles (salamanders, newts, axolotls). Wherever possible, references are secondary source citations, which include comprehensive reviews of amphibian neoplasms of Balls and Clothier (1), Harshbarger (3) and Marcus (10).

"Lymphosarcomas" of *Xenopus laevius* and *Cynops pyrroghaster* are not listed in Table 1 because the preponderance of scientific evidence at this time indicates that the lesions represent a granulomatous inflammatory response to mycobacteria (13).

Lucké renal adenocarcinoma

Metastatic growth of the Lucké tumor in leopard frogs is influenced by the nutritional status of the frog (occurring at an accelerated rate in well-fed frogs), and by tumor size, with large tumors more likely to metastasize (14). Ambient environmental temperature of the frogs also plays a critical role, with a high proportion (77%) of tumor-bearing frogs having metastatic Lucké tumor foci when held at 28°C versus 6% or less when held at cool (18°C or below) temperatures (15).

The mechanisms of temperature-dependent metastatic capability of the Lucké tumor are being studied *in vitro* with tumor cell explants and *in vivo* by injecting disaggregated tumor cells into the dorsal lymph sac of outbred frogs immunosuppressed with Cyclosporin-A. Issues addressed are temperature-related changes in blood viscosity and their role in reducing metastases at restrictive temperatures, stimulation of tumor cell collagenase synthesis at permissive temperatures, and disappearance of organized cytoplasmic microtubular complex in tumor cells at restrictive temperatures (7°C) (15).

Adenocarcinoma in Xenopus borealis

An experimental system somewhat analogous to the Lucké tumor has been developed in *Xenopus borealis* (11). In this system, an euploid, epithelioid cell line derived from a *Xenopus borealis* tadpole was transformed to a hypotetraploid cell line following incubation in N-methyl-N'-nitro-N-nitrosoguanidine (NMNG). Transformed cells were inoculated into the dorsal lymph sac of partially histocompatible *Xenopus borealis* adults housed at 22°C. Primary tumors developed in the dorsal lymph sac; these had the appearance of adenocarcinoma, with anaplastic epithelial cells arranged in sheets, tubules or acini. Histologic evidence of metastasis was found in 63% of the animals (Table 1).

Skin carcinomas in Triturus cristatus

A third experimental system has been studied in the newt, *Triturus cristatus* (17). If this amphibian is housed in the laboratory at 22–25°C and not allowed to hibernate, a collagenolytic system is activated in the dermis. Spontaneous or wound-induced epithelial tumors (derived from stratified squamous epithelium or dermal glands) then display marked metastatic activity. This is in contrast to other reported cutaneous tumors in urodeles (with the exception of melanomas) and anurans, where invasion of deeper tissues may be present but metastasis rarely occurs (2, 4, 6, 7, 16).

Lymphosarcoma in axolotls

This is the sole reproducible hematopoietic neoplasm in amphibians. The neoplasm originally arose in a skin graft in an *Ambystoma mexicanum* and was perpetuated by transplantation in the histocompatible C^{wis} strain or in other strains thymectomized within 65 days of spawning. Following transplantation to susceptible animals, tumor cells proliferated rapidly at the graft site, metastasized to the liver and spleen, and were present in peripheral blood (leukemic phase) in the terminal stage of the cancer. If the experimental skin graft was removed prior to invasion and metastasis of tumor cells, the host would reject a subsequent graft and disseminated lymphosarcoma would not occur.

H. E. Kaiser (ed.), Comparative aspects of tumor development.

Table 1. Metastatic tumors in amphibians

Species	Tumor type	Primary site	Metastatic site(s)	Comments	Reference
Anurans					
Rana pipiens	Adenocarcinoma	Kidney	Liver, lungs, coelom, ovaries, pancreas, urinary bladder retrocoelomic tissues, other sites	Induced by herpesvirus	(14)
				Viral particles in metastatic tumors	(9)
	Carcinoma	Not specified	Fat body, lung		(1)
	Liposarcoma	Not specified	Spleen, urinary bladder, body wall		(1)
	Lymphosarcoma		Widely disseminated in visceral organs		(1)
Rana catesbiana	Adenocarcinoma	Kidney	Metastases following tumor cell transplant	Enhanced by cortisone treatment	(1)
Xenopus borealis	Cholangiocarcinoma	Liver	Kidney	Induced by 400 ppm N-nitro-dimethylamine in aquarium water	(8)
Xenopus borealis	Adenocarcinoma	Transformed tadpole cell line	Liver, kidney, lung, spleen	Cell line transformed by N-methyl-N'-nitro N-nitrosoguanidine	(11)
Xenopus laevius	Anaplastic carcinoma	Intestine	Stomach, pancreas, kidney, urinary bladder		(1)
Ceratophrys ornata	Fibrosarcoma	Leg	Liver		(1)
Dendrobates pumillo	Erythrophoroma	Not specified	Viscera, skin		(1)
Urodeles					
Ambystoma mexicanum	Lymphosarcoma	Skin	Liver, spleen, peripheral blood	Transplanted by skin graft into histocompatible C^{wis} strains or strains thymecto-mized within 65 days of spawning	(5)
Ambystoma tigrinum	Carcinoma	Pancreas	Coelom		(5)
	Malignant melanoma	Skin	Viscera	Neotenic sala-manders in sewage lagoon	(12)
Necturus maculosus	Undifferentiated neoplasm	Kidney		"Probably metastatic"	(3)
Triturus cristatus	Squamous cell carcinoma, mucous gland carcinoma	Skin	Liver, lung, kidney, other viscera	Associated with decreased dermal collagen content and increased collagenolytic activity	(17)

References

1. Balls M, Clothier RH: Spontaneous tumors in amphibia. A review. *Oncology* 29:501–519, 1974
2. Delanney L, Chang SC, Harshbarger J, Dawe C: Mast cell tumors in the caudate amphibian, *Ambystoma mexicanum. Adv Comp Leuk Res Proc Int Symp 9th, 1979* 221–222, 1980
3. Harshbarger JC: Activities Report. Registry of Tumors in Lower Animals. Smithsonian Institution, Washington, DC (supplements issued annually), 1965–1981
4. Harshbarger JC: Epizootiology of leukemia and lymphomas in poikilotherms. *Adv Comp Leuk Res, Proc Int symp, 11th, 1981* 39–46, 1982

5. Harshbarger JC, Dawe CJ: Hematopoietic neoplasms in invertebrate and poikilothermic vertebrate animals. In: *Unifying Concepts of Leukemia,* Bibl, haemat. No. 39. RM Dutcher and L Chieco-Bianchi, eds., pp. 2–25. Karger, Basel, 1973
6. Harshbarger JC, Roe FL, Cullen LJ: Histopathology of skin, connective tissue, pigment cell and liver neoplasms in neotenic *Ambystoma tigrinum* from a sewage lagoon. *Second International Colloquium on Pathology of Reptiles and Amphibians,* Sept. 16–19, 1984. Proceedings *in press,* University of Angers Press
7. Khudoley VV, Mizgireuv IV: On spontaneous skin tumors in amphibia. *Neoplasm* 27:289–293, 1980
8. Khudoley VV, Picard JJ: Liver and kidney tumors induced by

N-nitrosodimethylamine in *Xenopus borealis* (Parker). *Br. J. Cancer* 25:679–683, 1980

9. McKinnell RG, Cunningham WP: Herpesviruses in metastatic Lucké renal adenocarcinoma. *Differentiation* 22:41–46, 1982
10. Marcus LC: *Veterinary Biology and Medicine of Captive Amphibians and Reptiles*. pp. 198–210. Lea & Febiger, Philadelphia, Pennsylvania, 1981
11. Picard JJ, Afifi A, Pays A: An oncogenic cell line inducing transplantable metastasizing adenocarcinoma in *Xenopus borealis*. *Carcinogenesis* 4:739–743, 1983
12. Rose FL, Harshbarger JC: Neoplastic and possibly related skin lesions in neotenic tiger salamanders from a sewage lagoon. *Science* 196:315–317, 1977
13. Squire RA, Goodman DG, Valerio MG, Frederickson TN, Strandberg JD, Levitt MH, Lingeman CH, Harshbarger JC, Dawe CJ: Tumors. In: *Pathology of Laboratory Animals*. K. Benirschke, FM Garner and TC Jones, eds. Vol. 2, Chapter 12, pp. 1255–1257. Springer-Verlag, Berlin and New York, 1978
14. Stewart HL, Snell KC, Dunham LJ, Schlyen SM: *Transplantable and Transmissible Tumors of Animals*. pp. 208–217. Armed Forces Inst. Pathol., Washington, DC, 1959
15. Tarin D, McKinnell, RG, Nace GW: Artificially induced metastasis by cells from spontaneous Lucké renal adenocarcinoma. *Invasion Metastasis* 4:198–208, 1984
16. Van der Steen ABM, Cohen BJ, Ringler DH, Abrams GD, Richards CM: Cutaneous neoplasms in the leopard frog (*Rana pipiens*). *Lab. Anim. Sci.* 22:216–222, 1972
17. Wirl G: Collagenolytic activity and carcinogenesis in the skin of the newt *Triturus cristatus*. Arch. Geschwulstforsch. 40:111–115, 1972

10

SELECTED ASPECTS OF NEOPLASTIC PROGRESSION IN REPTILES

S.V. MACHOTKA and E.R. JACOBSON

Reptiles first appear in the Mississipian (upper Paleozoic) during the history of the earth. They are the ancestral stock of mammals and birds. The mammals appeared before the birds in the Triassic (Mesozoic) and the birds followed as the last group of vertebrates in the Jurassic (Mesozoic). Reptiles are therefore phylogenetically an important group in regard to the last diversification of the vertebrates. Neoplasms of mesozoic reptiles were described by R.L. Moodie (30).

Comparative pathology is the basis for new progress in the study of diseases of various species with different taxonomic position and the comparison of the different classes of vertebrates may shed new light on the tissue and organ susceptibility to primary or metastatic growth. Cell types from nearly every determined system in reptiles, amphibians and fish are capable of neoplastic transformation (16). Without mentioning certain papillomas in turtles and lizards (21) Jacobson counts 195 reports of neoplasms in reptiles, 28 in Chelonia (11 malignant), four in Crocodilia (1 malignant), 30 in Sauria (12 malignant) and 97 in Serpentes (68 malignant). There is no report in Rhynchocephalia (*Sephenodon punctatus*). In turtles, 17 species were involved, 3 in crocodilians, 23 in lizards, and 45 in snakes.

A look at the circulatory system in regard to neoplastic spreading is in order because the circulatory system is so important for tumor spreading (38). The separation of oxygenated and unoxygenated blood has almost been achieved in reptiles due to the anatomy of the heart exhibiting incomplete separation of the single ventricle by a septum and a division of the conus (if present) to its base to the wall of the ventricle. Separation of oxygenated and unoxygenated blood has nearly been achieved in the reptile (1). Actually, crocodilians have a true fourth-chambered heart, with moving via a foramen in the aorta. *Karge arterues* exhibit little collagenous tissue, cutaneous veins are lacking. Lymphatic vessels are well developed with thoracic ducts present and terminating into the innominate veins in the neck region. Posterior lymph hearts may be present and pump lymph into the iliacs. The spleen resembles that of mammals and birds. Lymph sinuses are scarce. It is assumed that lymph nodes first appear phylogenetically in the mesentery of crocodiles (1); but there is also much debate whether true lymph nodes are present in reptiles. The main lymphatic vessel forms a sheet around the dorsal aorta in some snakes (5).

Tumor spreading may be direct, in which case the secondary tumors invade for example a vein and continues to growth therein. The secondary tumor remains connected with the primary tumor. In distant tumor spreading known as metastasis, there is lymphohematogenous spreading, seeding on the coelomic surfaces and spreading by implantation on epithelial surfaces. R. Willis, (38), considered metastasis from teratomas as a separate type of spreading. Direct spread as of a liver cell carcinoma in the lizard *Eumeces fasciatus* and metastatic spreading of various neoplastic types in turtles, crocodiles and lizards have been observed (21). Spreading on coelomic surfaces, on epithelial surfaces, and metastasis from teratomas can be assumed to occur also; nevertheless they have not been reported. The collection of the Zoological Society of San Diego studied by Effron and Benirschke (8) revealed neoplasia of 2.19 percent of 1,233 necropsies of reptiles. Lymphosarcomas occurred with high frequency in reptiles and birds. It is noteworthy that no neoplasia were detected among 198 amphibian necropsies. Ermoschenkov and Khudoley (11) reported two tumors in 34 reptiles found among 50 neoplasms of 716 animals which had died and autopsied between 1930 and 1974 in the Leningrad Zoo.

Viruses have been found associated with neoplastic growth processes in reptiles (21). Recent findings concerning the distribution of nucleotide sequences related to cDNAsarc in viral genomes as well as cell nucleic acids are summarized by Stehelin and Roussel (35) who postulated that all upper vertebrates contain in their DNA nucleotides sequences related to cDNAsarc. The values of annealing observed, if standardized to 100% for chicken DNA, decrease to 73% for primitive birds, 38% for mammals and reptiles, 26% for fishes. The tumorigenicity of Rous sarcoma virus (RSV) was studied in 22 reptile species representing 10 families of the orders Chelonia and Squamata by Tubcheninova et al. (36). RSV did not induce tumors in 13 inoculated species. In nine species, RSV induced polymorphous sarcomas with spindle-shaped (fibroblast-like), round, and polynuclear cells. Chromosome analysis indicated that the tumors originated in the reptile cells. Tumors were induced in adult reptiles with a patent period of only 1–3 mo by inoculation with a 30% cell-free homogenate of Schmidt-Ruppin strain RSV ($4 \times 10^{**}7$ sarcomagenic doses per snake; $10^{**}6$–$10^{**}7$ sarcomagenic doses per lizard). The case of tumor induction suggests that reptiles are more susceptible to this strain of RSV than mice, rats, guinea pigs, rabbits, and monkeys. The tumors of two snakes were tumorigenic in chickens. Since RSV is oncogenic for a wide range of birds and mammals as well as reptiles and since these three classes belong to the tetrapods the pathogenicity of RSV for these animals appears to be predetermined by evolution.

H. E. Kaiser (ed.), Comparative aspects of tumor development.

An adenovirus-like cytopathic agent, designated frog adenovirus 1 (FAV-1) was recovered by Clark, H.F. et al. (6) from turtle (TH-1) cell cultures inoculated with cells of a granuloma-bearing kidney of a leopard frog, *Rana pipiens*. Virus replication, as indicated by cytopathic effect (including intranuclear inclusions) was limited to TH-1 cells. A variety of other cell types from amphibians, reptiles, fish, and mammals were refractory to infection. FAV-1 appears to be an 'orphan' virus, and the first described adenovirus from apoikilothermic vertebrate. It has a host range in cell culture, antigenic composition, and temperature requirement for replication that are unique among members of the adenovirus group.

Herpes-viruses are the only DNA viruses associated with lymphoid tumors, namely animal lymphosarcomas in molluscs, fish, reptiles and mammals (13).

Corticotropin-releasing factor (CRF)-containing cells have been shown to be present in the pancreas of representative species of fishes, amphibians, reptiles, birds, and mammals including man. Light and electron microscopic

Table 1. Neoplasm metastasis in reptiles.

Reptilian order	Family	Species	Primary neoplasm	Metastasis with location	Author	Year
A. Chelonia (turtles)	Pelomedusidae	*Pelusius subniger*	Carcinoma of stomach	Metastases to kidney	Cowan	1968
	Testudinidae	*Geomyda trijuga*	Carcinoma of thyroid	Metastases to mediastinum	Cowan	1968
		Emys orbicularis	Oral squamous cell carcinoma	Metastasis to liver	Billups, Harshbarger	1976
		Terrapene carolina	Adenocarcinoma of kidney	Metastases to liver	Ippen	1972
B. Crocodilia (crocodiles)	Crocodylidae	*Crocodylus porosus*	Round cell sarcoma of liver	Metastases to cerebellum and heart	Scott, Beattie	1927
C. Squamata: Sauria (lizards)	Agamidae	*Hydrosaurus amboinensis*	Malignant lymphoma (kidneys?)	Metastases all vital organs	Zwart, Harshbarger	1972
	Lacertidae	*Lacerta sicula zetti*	Malignant lymphoma, neck	Metastases to all major organs	Lawson	1962
		Lacerta sicula	Mesenchymal, sarcoma (fibrosarcoma), forleg	Metastases to mediastinum, mesentery, aorta, stomach and lungs	Elkan, Cooper Harshbarger	1976 1975
	Scincidae	*Eumeces fasciatus*	Liver cell carcinoma	Direct spread into body cavity	Ippen	1972
	Varanidae	*Varanus komodoensis*	Carcinoma of colon	Metastatic adenocarcinoma in spleen[1]	Harshbarger	1976
		Varanus exanthematicus	Leiomyosarcoma (intestine)	Metastasis to liver[1]	Harshbarger	in preparation
D. Squamata: Sepentes (snakes)	Boidae	*Eunectes murinus*	Lymphosarcoma	Diffuse metastasizing lung, liver, kidneys	Frank, Schepky	1969
		Python sebae	Ovarian adenocarcinoma		Bland-Sutton	1885
		Python molurus	Oral carcinoma	Metastases to liver	Wilhelm, Emswiller	1977
		Python molurus	Mucinous adenocarcinoma of the liver	liver, intestine, kidney	Billup, Harshbarger (AFIP)[2]	1976
		Constrictor constrictor	Adenocarcinoma, mesentery	Cervical	Elkan, Cooper	1976
	Colobridae	*Pituophis melanoleucus*	Malignant melanoma, skin of tail	Metastases to liver	Ball	1946
		Pituophis melanoleucus	Sarcoma, (leiomyosarcoma?) abdominal	Liver, pancreas, celiac area	Cown	1968
		Matrix stolata	Hemangioendothelioma (hepatic or splenic origin)	Pulmonary, cardiac and renal metastases	Ippen	1972
		Lampropeltis getulus getulus	Lymphosarcoma	Metastasis in all major organs	Jacobson et al.	1981
		Elaphe obsoleta rossalleni	Melanoma	Local spread and metastasis via blood stream into most organ systems	Elkan	1974
		Elaphe guttata guttata	Fibrosarcoma of skin	Metastatic to liver	Harshbarger	in preparation
		Heterodon platyrhinos	Lymphosarcoma	Metastasizing to lung, kidney	Cowan	1968
	Elapidae	*Naja melanoleuca*	Carcinoma of Poison gland	Metastases to cervical region	Hill	1952
		Naja naja	Lymphosarcoma	Metastatic to heart and liver	Cowan	1968
		Naja naja	Rectal leiomyosarcoma	Metastasis to liver	Harshbarger	1974
		Naja nigricollis	Osteochondrosarcoma	Metastatic to kidney and spleen		in preparation[1]
	Viperidae	*Bitis arietans*	Adenocarcinoma	Metastasizing	AFIP[2]	
		Bitis arietans	Granulosa cell tumor	Renal metastasis	Onderka, Zwart	1978
		Bitis nasicornis	Lymphosarcoma	Metastasizing to liver, kidneys, adrenal glands, spleen, gut wall	Cowan	1968

[1] See text figures.
[2] Armed Forces Institute of Pathology, Registry of Veterinary Pathology, Washington, D.C.

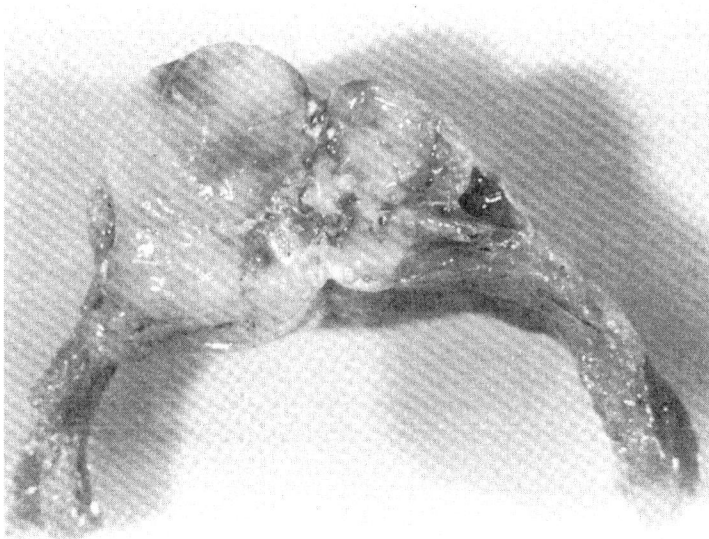

Figure 1

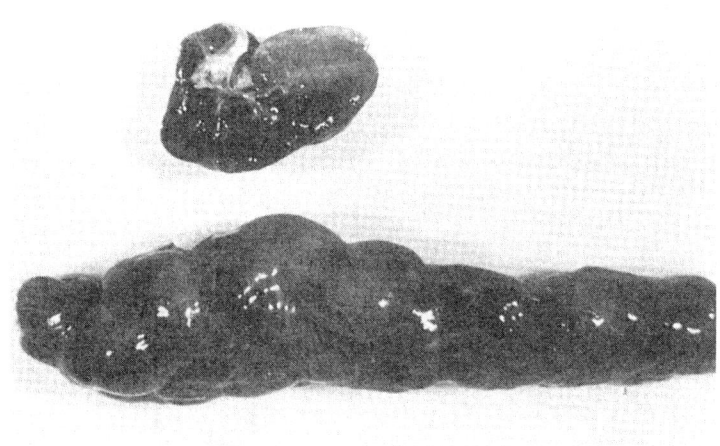

Figure 2

Figure 1. Osteochondrosarcoma in the spinal column of a spitting cobra, *Naja nigricollis* (RTLA 2474).

Figure 2. Kidney and spleen with metastatic osteochondrosarcoma (RTLA 2474)

Figure 3. Spleen from Komodo dragon, *Varanus komodoensis* with metastatic mucinous adenocarcinoma primary in the colon. H&E X293 (RTLA 1166).

Figure 4. Osteochondrosarcoma in the spinal column of a spitting cobra, *Naja nigricollis*. H&E X29 (RTLA 2474).

Figure 5. Higher magnification of vascular embolus of specimen above. H&E X80 (RTLA 2474)

Figure 6. Kidney with metastatic osteochondrosarcoma in interstitium (note glomeruli and tubules). H&E X47 (RTLA 2474)

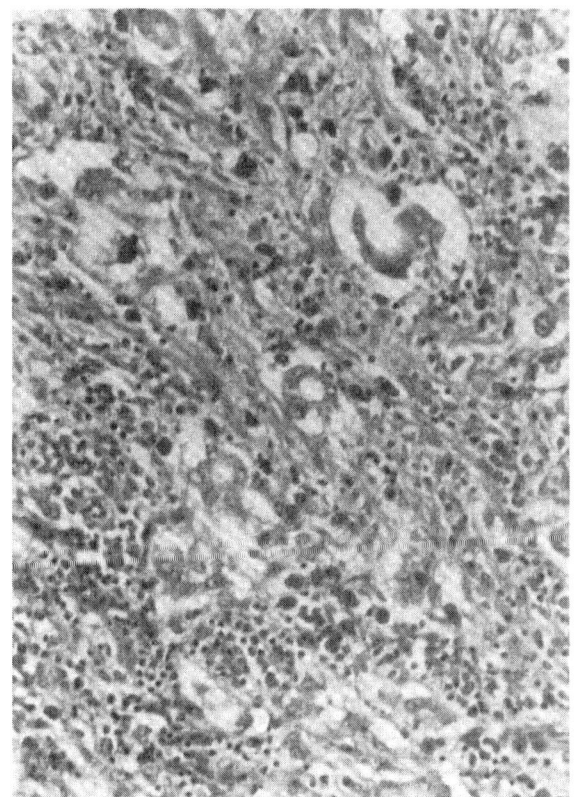

Figure 3

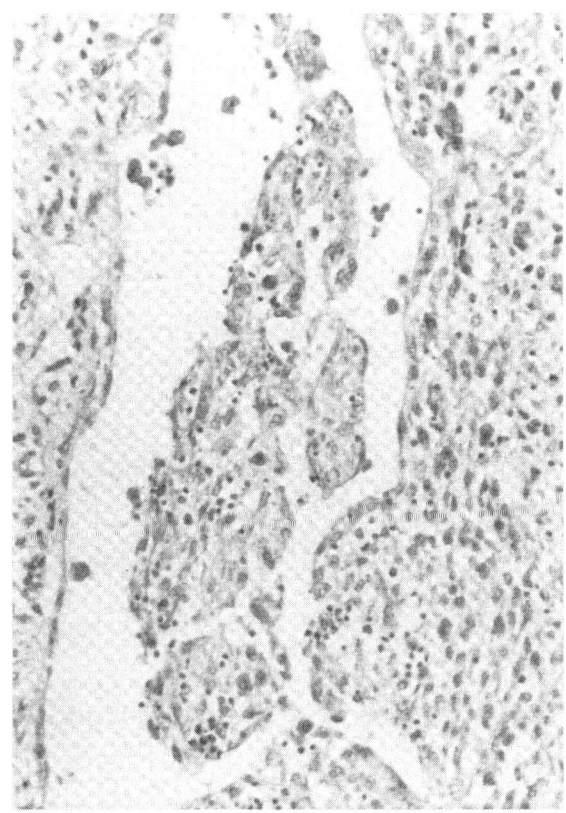

Figure 5

Figure 4

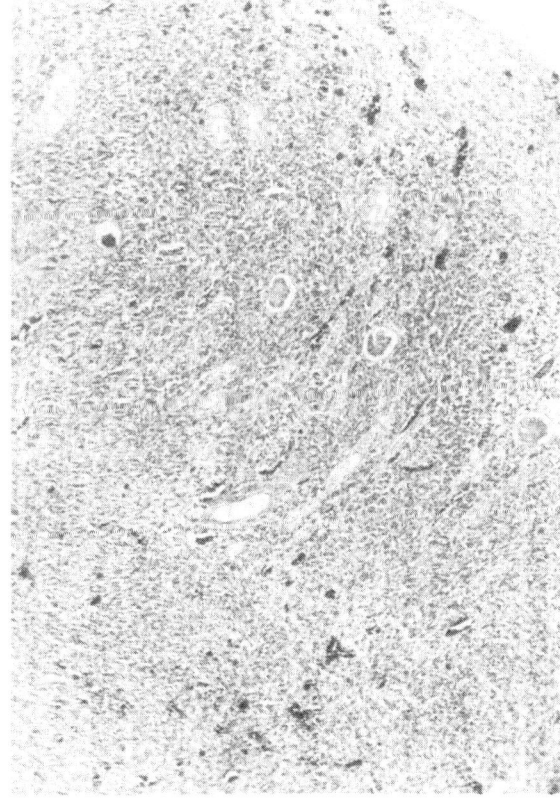

Figure 6

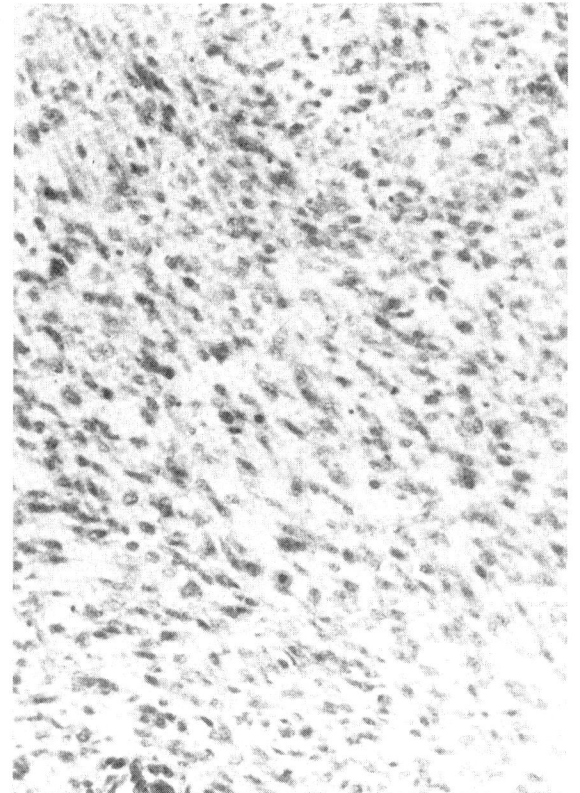

Figure 7

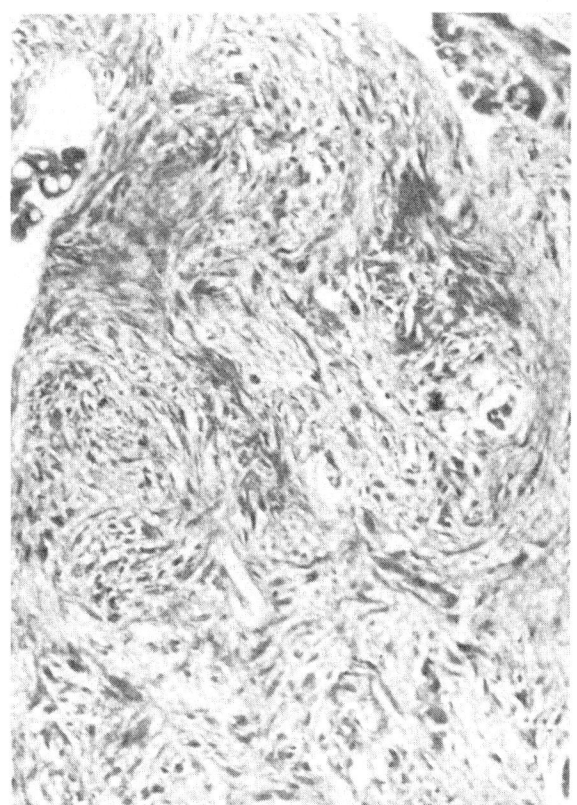

Figure 9

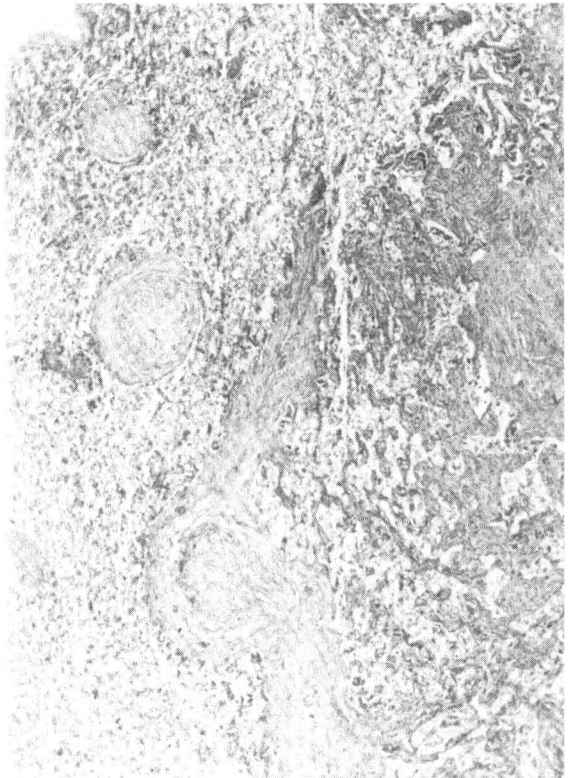

Figure 8

Figure 7. High magnification of Figure 3 demonstrating spindling and streaming of tumor cells. H&E X293 (RTLA 2474)

Figure 8. Liver containing intravascular nodules and intrasinusoidal cords/sheets of metastatic leiomyosarcoma primary in the intestine from a Savannah monitor, Varanus exanthematicus. H&E X47 (RTLA 2518).

Figure 9. High magnification of specimen above. H&E X293 (RTLA 2518).

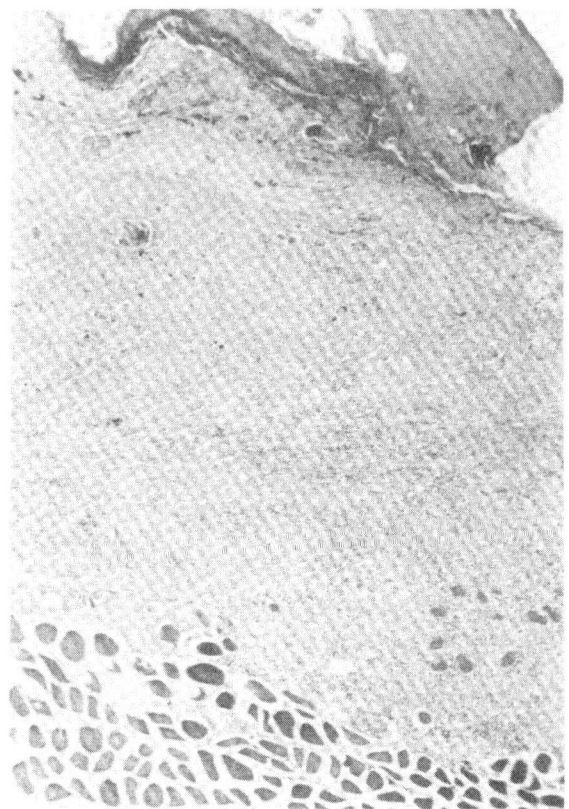

Figure 10

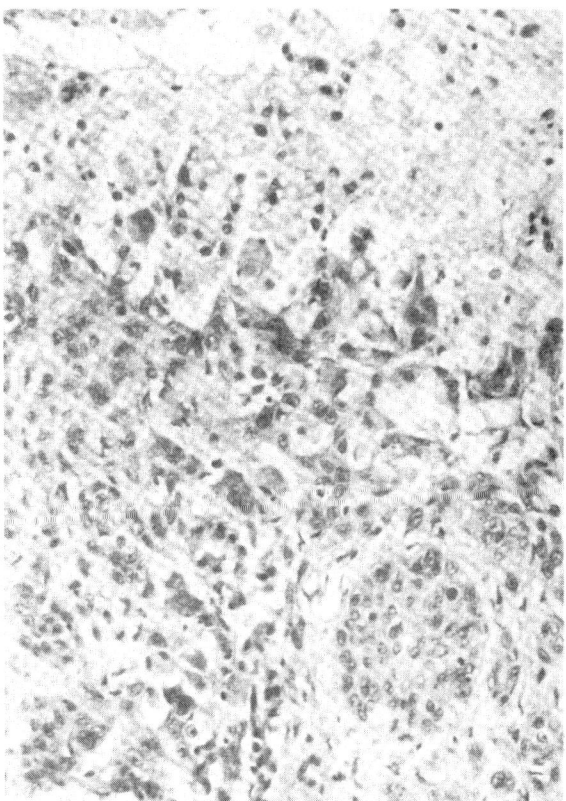

Figure 12

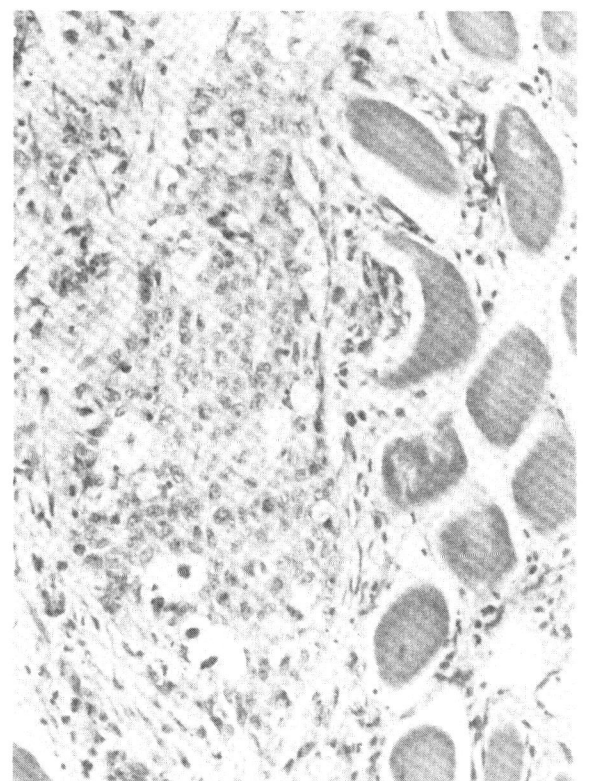

Figure 11

Figure 10. Skin from leopard geko, *Eublepharis maculatus*, with squamous cell carcinoma producing necrosis and ulceration of epidermis and extension of neoplasm through dermis with incorporation of subcutaneous muscle fibers. H&E X47 (RTLA 2774).

Figure 11. High magnification of specimen above, showing cluster of neoplastic epithelial cells, some with ballooning degeneration. H&E X293 (RTLA 2774).

Figure 12. Liver-degenerate hepatocytes (left 1/3rd of photo), vascular embolus (right corner) and sinusoidal infiltration of metastatic squamous cell carcinoma. H&E X293 (RTLA 2774).

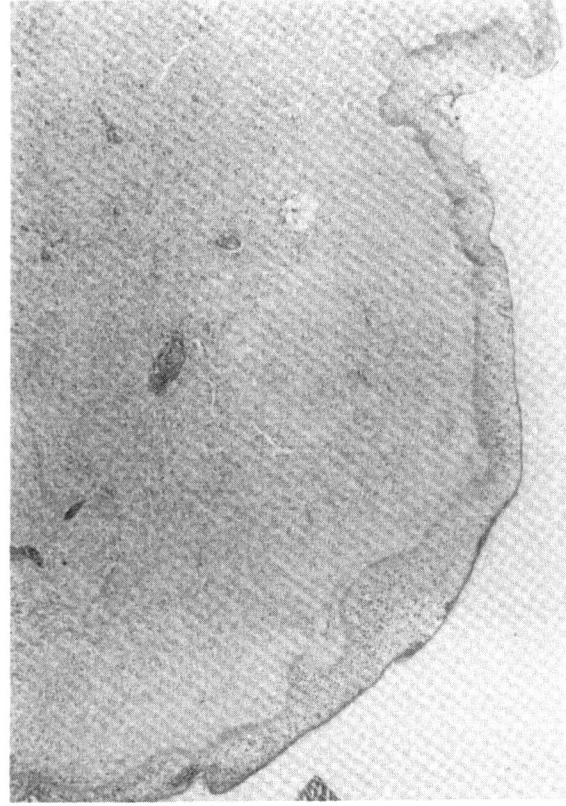

Figure 13

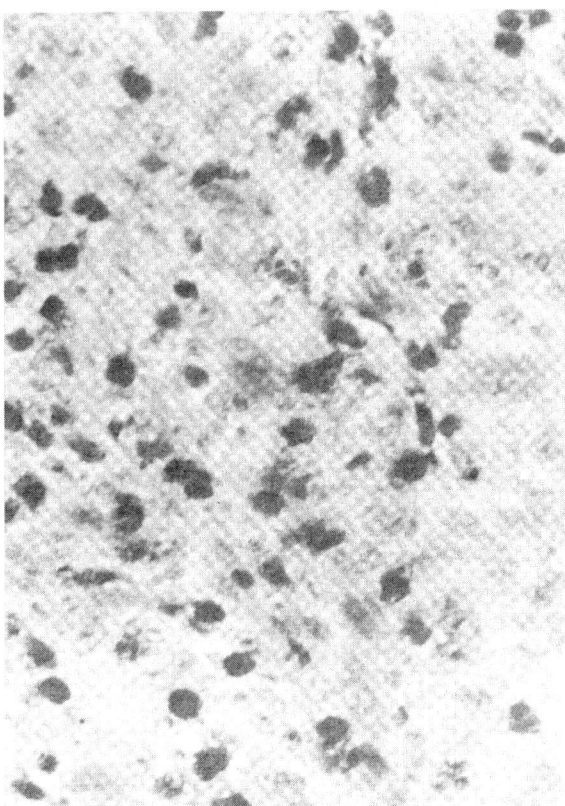

Figure 15

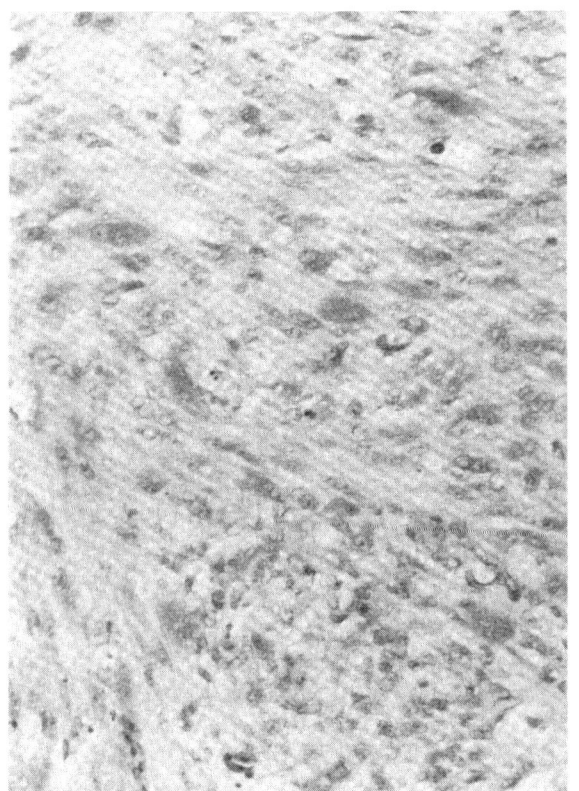

Figure 14

Figure 13. Skin from corn snake, *Elaphe guttata guttata*, containing a fibrosarcoma. Mass abuts basement membrane of epidermis but does not penetrate it. H&E X29 (RTLA 2808-1).

Figure 14. High magnification of specimen above, demonstrating packets/bundles and cords of plump, oval-to-spindle shaped nuclei. H&E X293 (RTLA 2808).

Figure 15. Higher magnification of same specimen, demonstrating numerous eosinophils within neoplasm (eosinophils are commonly numerous in reptilian skin but their presence in mammals is thought to be a significant host response to neoplasia). H&E X469 (RTLA 2808).

Figure 16. Liver with metastatic fibrosarcoma. H&E X47 (RTLA 2808).

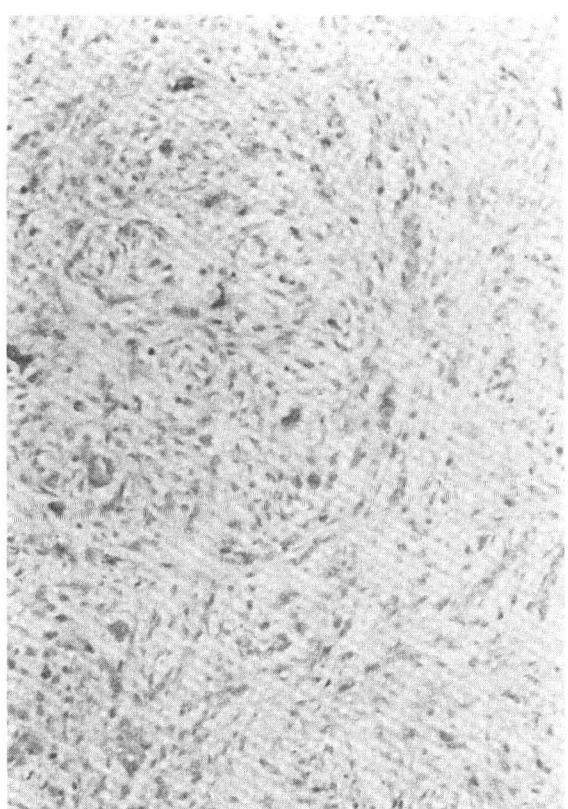

Figure 17. Higher magnification of 4 showing swirling pattern and a few trapped hepatocytes/bile duct epithelium. H&E X117 (RTLA 2808).

observations indicate that the CRF-containing cells in the endocrine pancreas are similar to glucagon (A) cells both in their morphology and distribution. Observations indicate that they are widely distributed in peripheral tissues and may represent a new tumor marker (32). Tumor markers seem to be present in reptiles as in other classes of vertebrates.

Etiology and epidemiology of cancer in mammals (primates, rodents and lagomorphs), birds, and reptiles were discussed by Kollias (27). Diagnosis and treatment of non-domestic animals will allow a more regional approach in cancer therapy in zoological medicine. The viral aspects of etiology may be important in progression/metastasis of neoplasia in reptiles.

Attempted therapy of neoplastic diseases in reptiles has included such methods as surgery and chemotherapy. The techniques of verterinary cryotherapy, for example, and its use in dogs, cats, horses, cattle, and reptiles were reviewed by Podkonjak (33).

The secondary neoplasms of reptiles found today are summarized in Table 1 followed by photographs of selected tumors demonstrating their macroscopic and/or microscopic appearance.*

---

*Histologic sections of the photographed neoplasms are on file at the Registry of Tumors in Lower Animals (RTLA), Smithsonian Institution, Washington, D.C. and were made available by the registries Director, John C. Harshbarger, Ph.D.

References

1. Andrew W, Hickman CP: *Histology of the Vertebrates.* St. Louis, C.V. Mosby, 1974
2. Ball HA: Melanosarcoma and rhabdomyoma in two pine snakes (*Pituophis melanoleucus*). *Cancer Res* 6:134, 1946
3. Billups LH, Harshbarger J: Reptiles. In: *Handbook of Laboratory Animal Science.* E.C. Melby and N.H. Altman (eds.), CRC Press, Cleveland, 1976
4. Bland-Sutton J: Tumors in animals *J Anat Physiol* 19:415, 1885
5. Borghese E: Ricerche sul' apparecchio linfatico dei Rettili. II. I vasi linfatici paravertebrali degli Ofidi. Arch. Ital. Anat. Embriol. 43/2:139, 1940
6. Clark HF, et al: An adenovirus, FAV-1, isolated from the kidney of a frog (*Rana pipiens*). *Virology* 51(2):392, 1973
7. Cowan DF: Diseases of captive reptiles. *J Amer Vet Med Ass*, 153:848, 1968
8. Effron M, Griner L, Benirschke K: Nature and rate of neoplasia found in captive wild mammals, birds, and reptiles at necropsy. *JNCI*, 59(1):185, 1977
9. Elkan E: Malignant melanoma in a snake. *J Comp Pathol*, 84:51, 1974
10. Elkan E, Cooper J: Tumors and pseudotumors in some reptiles. *J Comp Pathol*, 86:337, 1976
11. Ermoschenkov VS, Khudoley VV: Tumors registered in animals of the Leningrad zoo. *Vopr Onkol*, 22(5):78, 1976
12. Frank W, Schepky A: Metastasierendes Lymphosarkom bei einer Riesenschlange, *Eunectes murinus* (Linnaeus, 1758). *Pathol Vet*, 6:437, 1969

13. Hardy WD: Epidemiology of primary neoplasms of lymphoid tissues in animals. *Compr Immunol*, vol. 4, 1978

14. Harshbarger JC: *Activities Report Registry of Tumors in Lower Animals*, 1965–1973. Smithsonian Inst., Washington, D.C., 1974

15. Harshbarger JC: *Activities Report Registry of Tumors in Lower Animals*, 1975 Supplement. Smithsonian Inst., Washington, D.C., 1976

16. Harshbarger JC: Role of the registry of tumors in lower animals in the study of environmental carcinogenesis in aquatic animals. *Ann NY Acad Sci*, 298:280, 1977

17. Harshbarger JC: *Activities Report, Registry of Tumors in Lower Animals, 1982–1986*. Supplement. Smithsonian Inst., Washington, D.C., (in preparation)

18. Hill WCO: *Report of the Society's Prosector for the Year 1951*. Proc. Zool. Soc. London, 122:515, 1952

19. Ippen R: Ein Beitrag zu den Spontantumoren bei Reptilien. XIV. Internationales Symposium über die Erkrankungen der Zootiere. *Akademie der Wissenschaften der DDR*, Berlin, 1972

20. Jacobson ER, Seely J, Novilla MN: Lymphosarcoma associated with virus-like intranuclear inclusions in a California king snake (Colubridae: *Lampropeltis*). *J. Nat. Cancer Inst.*, 65:577, 1980

21. Jacobson ER: Virus associated neoplasms of reptiles. In: *Phyletic Approaches to Cancer*, C.J. Dawe et al. (eds.), Japan Sci. Soc. Press, Tokyo, 1981

22. Jacobson ER, Calderwood MB, French TW, Iverson W, Page D, Raphael B: Lymphosarcoma in an eastern king snake and a rhinoceros viper. *J. Amer. Vet. Med. Association*, 179(11): 1231, 1981

23. Jacobson ER: Neoplastic diseases. In: *Diseases of Reptilia*. J.E. Cooper and O.F. Jackson (eds.) New York: Academic Press, 1982

24. Kaiser HE: Distribution of true (real) tissues in organisms: A preliminary condition of neoplastic growth. In: H.E. Kaiser (ed.) *Neoplasms — Comparative Pathology of Growth in Animals, Plants, and Man*. Baltimore: Williams & Wilkins, pp. 43, 1981

25. Kaiser HE: The species-specific spectrum of neoplasms. In: H.E. Kaiser (ed.) *Neoplasms — Comparative Pathology of Growth in Animals, Plants and Man*. Baltimore: Williams & Wilkins, pp. 649, 1981

26. Kaiser HE: Animal neoplasms — A systematic review. In: H.E. Kaiser (ed.), *Neoplasms — Comparative Pathology of Growth in Animals, Plants, and man*. Baltimore: Williams & Wilkins, pp. 747, 1981

27. Kollias GV: Tumors in zoo animals and wildlife. In: *Veterinary Cancer Medicine*. G.H. Theilen, B.R. Madewell (eds.). Philadelphia: Lea & Febiger, 1979

28. Lawson R: A malignant neoplasm with metastases in the lizard, *Lacerta sicula cetti* Cara. *British J. Herpetol.*, 3: 22, 1962

29. Machotka SV: Neoplasia in reptiles. In: *Diseases of Amphibians and Reptiles*. Hoff, Jacobson and Frye (eds.). New York: Plenum Publishers, 1984

30. Moodie RL: *Paleopathology, An Introduction to the Study of Ancient Disease*. Urbana, Ill.: University of Illinois Press, 1923

31. Onderka DK, Zwart P: Granulosa cell tumor in a gartr snake (*Thamnophis sirtalis*) J. Wildlife Dis., 14: 218, 1978

32. Petrusz P, et al: Corticotropin-releasing factor (CRF)-like immunoreactivity in the gastro-entero-pancreatic endocrine system. *Peptides* (Fayetteville), 5 Suppl. 1: 71, 1984

33. Podkonjak KR: Veterinary cryotherapy-2. A. comprehensive look at uses, principles, and successes. *VM Sac*, 77(2): 183, 1982

34. Scott HH, Beattie J: Neoplasm in a porose crocodile. *J. Pathol. Bacteriol.*, 30: 61, 1927

35. Stehelin D, Roussel M: Studies on the origin and evolution of the transforming gene of avian sarcoma viruses. Fourth meeting of the European Association for Cancer Research, at Université de Lyon, Sept. 13–15, 1977

36. Tubcheninova LP, et al.: Body temperature and tumor virus infection. I. Tumorigenicity of Rous sarcoma virus for reptiles. *Neoplasms*, 24(1): 3, 1977

37. Wilhelm RS, Emswiler B: Intraoral carcinoma in a Burmese python. *Vet. Med. Small Animal Clin.*, 72: 272, 1977

38. Willis R: The spread of tumours in the human body. (edition 3). London: Butterworths, 1973

39. Zwart P, Harshbarger JC: Hematopoietic neoplasms in lizards: Report of a typical case in *Hydrosaurus amboiensis* and of a probable case inf *Varanus* salvator. *Int. J. Cancer*, 9: 538, 1972

11

LYMPHOCYTIC NEOPLASMS IN REPTILES AND FISH

S. V. MACHOTKA

INTRODUCTION

More than one and three quarter centuries, ago, in 1802, The Medical Committee of the Society for Investigating the Nature and Cure of Cancer was established in Edinburgh. This committee drew up thirteen queries, the tenth of which asked "Are brute creatures subject to any disease resembling cancer in the human body?" When considering fish, that question has long ago been answered affirmatively, (11, 94, 108). The continued search for similarities between various neoplasms in animals and man has gone on with the hope that such efforts will enable researchers to better understand the phenomenon we call cancer and subsequently lead to effective treatment and possibly prevention. Germane to this concept is the visualization of the phylogenetic tree which demonstrates the key positions fish and reptiles play as ancestral stock in the evolution of the mammalia, (Figure 1, (58)).

As recently as 1969, only three cases of lymphocytic neoplasms had been reported in reptiles (14, 33, 75). And though more information has been collected in neoplasms of blood cell origin in fish than any other single class of cold-blooded vertebrate, as of 1969 only seventeen reports were in the literature (16, 78, 106, 107). In the succeeding fifteen years various reviews or tabulations of neoplasms in reptiles and fish have been published (61, 80–83, 128). One paper has dealth strictly with hematopoietic neoplasms (52). With cold-blooded vertebrates there are large gaps in our knowledge about how their neoplasms conform to what is known about neoplasms in mammals. In many, if not most, cases we were not fully aware of their morphologic course, relation to host-regulating mechanisms and transplantability or transmissability. To help alleviate some of these deficiencies, a workshop on comparative pathology of hematopoietic and lymphoreticular neoplasms was conducted in May of 1971 at the National Cancer Institute, Bethesda, Maryland. Study sets representing leukemias and lymphomas in animals and man were discussed and are available on a loan basis from the Registry of Experimental Cancers of the National Cancer Institute by contacting Margaret Deringer. The relevant cases in this study set are listed in Table 1. Many additional cases are available for review at the Registry of Tumors in Lower Animals (RTLA), Smithsonian Institution, Washington, D.C. which is directed by John Harshbarger.

In 1969 John W. Berg wrote in the preface to the NCI Monograph 32, Comparative Morphology of Hematopoietic Neoplasms ". . .different backgrounds have engendered. . . quite different vocabularies. Different, incompatible – even conflicting – terminologies have concealed both analogies and provocative species differences," (6). J.W. Berg summarizes my interest in presenting the lymphocytic neoplasms in reptiles and fish in a comparative manner; to point out similarities and dissimilarities when known. These neoplasms are discussed from a comparative standpoint regarding anatomy and hematopoiesis, classification, etiology, diagnosis, and therapy. In addition, a section reviewing selected cases from the literature and submissions to the RTLA is presented. The preceding information is then discussed and summarized with some suggestions for further investigation.

Comparative aspects

Anatomy and hematopoiesis

We know that the blood forming organs and tissues in reptiles and fish are not morphologically or functionally directly comparable to those in mammals (Table 2, modified from (70)). Lymph nodes as defined in the mammalian body are sparsely represented in reptiles. The pharyngeal tonsils, thymus and the spleen are organs of this nature (5). The thymus in lizards and snakes is represented by paired glands which are situated in the neck, one pair on each side which are placed one behind the other (1). Bone marrow and lymph nodes are absent entirely in most fish and do not play a major role in lymphocytopoiesis in reptiles. Unlike reptiles or mammals, the mesonephros or head kidney is a major site of lymphocytopoiesis in fish. As an aside, in some ganoid fish (e.g. sturgeon, long nose gar, bowfin) the connective tissue of the meninges, particularly that of the choroid plexus of the fourth ventricle, corresponds to mammalian bone marrow, which here in the ganoids makes its first appearance in the vertebrata (105). Though lymphocytes are seen in reptiles and fish, their relative numbers in the white blood count vary (13, 23, 35), and there is a variation in the occurrence of other hemic and reticular cells (Table 3, modified from (52)). Additional information on the normal anatomy, histology, and hematology of reptiles and fish is available (1–5, 39, 54, 70).

Classification of lymphocytic neoplasms

There is some difficulty in presenting the material since much controversy regarding the selection of a scheme for the classification of hematopoietic neoplasms in man exists. "But try anyway; no man knows what is possible" as

H. E. Kaiser (ed.), Comparative aspects of tumor development.

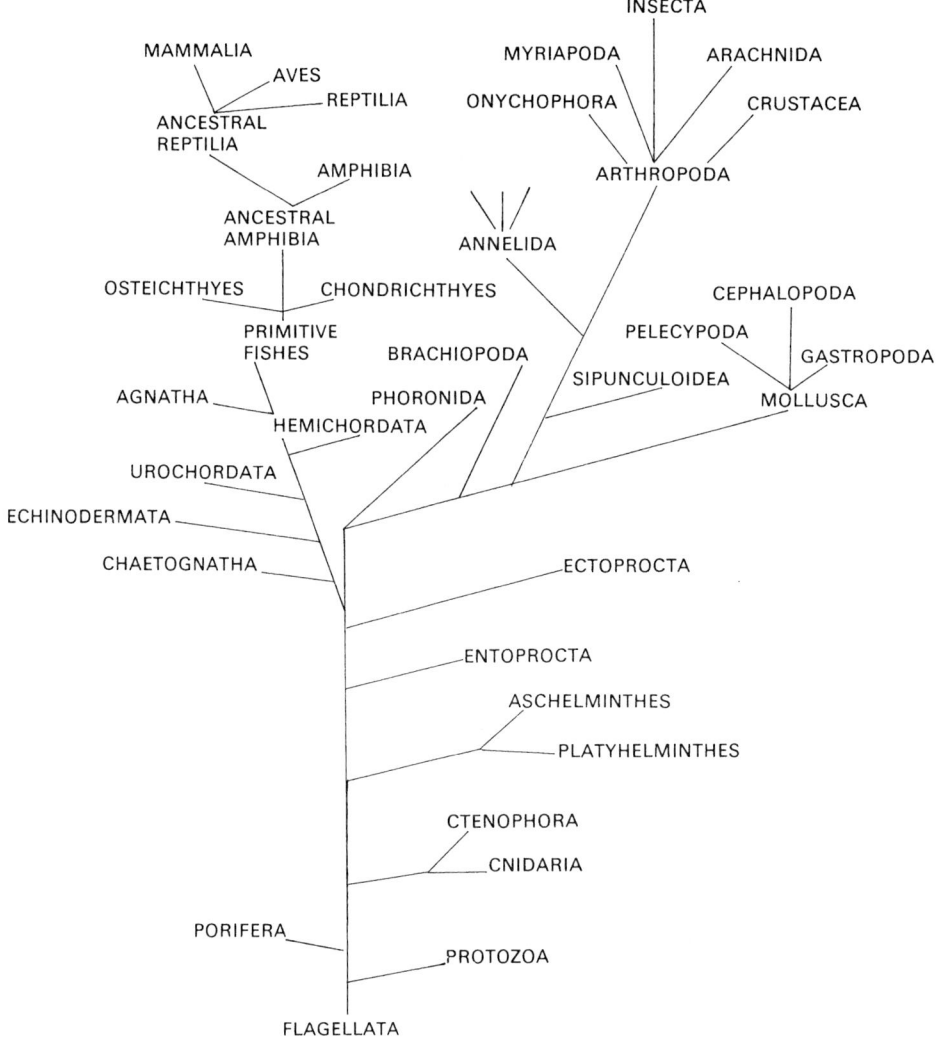

Figure 1. Phylogenetic tree of the animal kingdom. (Modified from (58)).

Table 1. Pertinent case material in comparative pathology of hematopoietic and reticular neoplasms study set available at the Registry of Experimental Cancers, National Cancer Institute, Bethesda, MD. (Modified from (52)).

Host Animals	Disease	Contributor
Northern pike, *Esox lucius*	malignant lymphoma, hemocytoblastic type	MF Mulcahy, Univ College, Cork, Ireland
Muskellunge, *Esox masquinongy*	malignant lymphoma, lymphoblastic type	R Sonstegard, Univ of Guelph, Ontario, Canada
Brook trout, *Salvelinus fontinalis*	malignant lymphoma, with leukemia	RL Herman, Owens-Illinois, Inc, Castalia, OH
Cutthroat trout, *Salmo clarki*	malignant lymphoma, with leukemia	CE Smith, Fish Cultural Day Center, US Dept of the Interior, Bozeman, MT
Timber rattlesnake, *Crotalus horridus horridus*	lymphoid leukemia	LA Griner, Zoological Garden, San Diego, CA

Table 2. Sites of blood-cell formation in a reptile, various fish and man. (Modified from (70)).

	Erythrocyte	Granulocyte	Lymphocyte	Thrombocyte
Reptilia				
lizard	spleen bone marrow	bone marrow intestine	spleen thymus intestine bone marrow liver	spleen bone marrow
Agnatha				
hagfish	spleen (gut) circulation	spleen	spleen thymus ±	spleen circulation
lamprey	spleen (spiral valve of intestine) circulation	spleen intestine	spleen thymus	spleen circulation
Chondrichthyes				
shark	spleen mesonephros	intestine ± gonads	spleen mesonephros intestine thymus	spleen mesonephros circulation
Osteichthyes				
bowfin	spleen circulation meningeal myeloid tissue	intestine ± mesonephros meningeal myeloid tissue	spleen mesonephros intestine thymus meningeal myeloid tissue	spleen circulation
trout	spleen mesonephros liver	mesonephros intestine	spleen mesonephros intestine thymus	spleen mesonephros circulation
Mammals				
man	bone marrow	bone marrow	spleen bone marrow thymus lymph nodes intestine	bone marrow (megakaryocytes and platelets)

Michael Faraday advised (15). Traditionally, neoplasia has been classified by its cell of origin, morphology, pattern of distribution and behavior so that the non-Hodgkin lymphomas were for example considered nodular (follicular) and diffuse lymphomas/lymphosarcomas of various cell types, malignant lymphoma-unclassified, and composite lymphomas, or the less common Burkitt's lymphoma, immunoblastic sarcoma, or mycosis fungoides-Sezary syndrome (97, 98). More recent approaches utilize the cytochemical, immunocytochemical, and electron microscopic characteristics of B and T lymphocytes, and the monocytic/histiocytic series in conjunction with more traditional criteria (76, 79). Baseline data concerning the normal blood profile, the nature of cells regarding immunological characteristics, cytochemical characteristics, etc. are still incomplete or lacking entirely though some studies have been

Table 3. Presence (+) or absence (−) of varieties of hemic and reticular cells in reptiles, fish and mammals. (Modified from (52)).

	Reptilia	Agnatha	Chondrichthyes	Osteichthyes	Mammalia
Erythrocytes	+	+	+	+	+
Hemoblasts	+	+	+	+	−
Lymphocytes	+	+	+	+	+
Plasma cells	+	+	+	+	+
Monocytes	+	+	+	+	+
Spindle cells	−	+	−	−	−
Thrombocytes	+	+	+	+	+
Megakaryocytes	−	+	−	−	+
Eosinophiles	+	+	+	+	+
Neutrophiles/Heterophiles	+	+	+	+	+
Basophiles	+	+	+	+	+

reported (13, 18, 28, 73). As of 1978 there had been very little evidence allowing conclusions as to the existence of functional populations analogous to B and T lymphocytes in reptiles and fish, though humoral and cell mediated immunity are well developed at this level of phylogeny (28).

Katharine C. Snell has stated that it sometimes seems difficult for us ". . .to agree upon a diagnosis for hematopoietic neoplasms because of our lack of agreement on the definition of such terms as "leukemia", "lymphocytic neoplasms", "malignant tumor of the lymphoreticular system", or "malignant lymphoma" (112). In this chapter I have chosen to present the neoplasms in reptiles and fish based purely on morphology and distribution since so little work has been done in fish and even less in reptilian immunology and immunocytochemistry of lymphocytes. Lymphocytic neoplasms that have no malignant white cells in the blood can be diagnosed as lymphosarcomas and those that have malignant white cells in the blood can be diagnosed as lymphocytic, lymphoblastic, or stem cell leukemias. Future reports of lymphocytic neoplasms in reptiles and fish, one would anticipate, will contain thorough descriptions with more sophisticated attempts to further identify the cell type involved.

Etiology

In considering the etiology of cancer, genetic factors, radiation, chemicals, and oncogenic viruses come to mind. However, the environment and geographic location of the victim also have a role. For example, the high incidence of stomach cancer in Japan versus that seen in the United States (55). More germane, perhaps, is the occurrence of Burkitt's lymphoma in Africa (10). A possible correllary is the large number of northern pike (*Esox lucius*) from Ireland, Scandinavia, Canada, and the northern United States (85) and muskellunge (*Esox masquinongy*) from the ponds and lakes of the United States and Canada (102, 106, 115) with lymphosarcomas.

Genetic factors of lymphocytic neoplasia in man have been established. Many distinctive nonrandom chromosomal abnormalities (mostly translocations) have been identified with a high frequency in several B cell lymphomas other than Burkitt's tumor (136). In most of these chromosome 14 is involved. Additionally, basal cell nevus and xeroderma pigmentosum of man are known to have a genetic basis (55). In poikilothermic vertebrates, there is a primary genetic influence on the development of melanomas in fish *Xiphophorus* sp. (113). It may be that the previously mentioned lymphosarcoma in Esocid fish have some genetic basis (82). Dunbar implied that there may be a genetic predisposition of brook trout (*Salvelinus fontinalis*) to lymphosarcoma and that it was transmitted to splake (hybrids of brook and lake trout) in which he reported lymphosarcomas (19).

Survivors of acute radiation syndrome have a high risk of developing leukemia. The induction of leukemia in experimental animals and man by exposure to external ionizing radiation is well documented (123). Radiation exposure of reptiles and fish with production of lymphosarcomas of leukemias have not been reported.

"Of the causes of cancer in man, chemicals are the most important. Reasonable estimates are that more than 5% of human cancer is due to viruses, and less than 5% to radia-

tion. Some 90% of cancer in man is therefore due to chemicals" (8). Though these statements are a bit simplistic, it is probably true that chemicals comprise the bulk of carcinogens. Although chemicals are suspected as etiologic agents in chronic granulocytic leukemia, clear-cut associations have been difficult to make. Benzene, chloramphenical, and phenylbutazone have been associated with acute myelogenous leukemia (74). Acute lymphocytic leukemia has not been associated with specific chemical insults. Some patients given maintenance doses over long periods of time of immunosuppressive drugs have developed tumors, usually leukemias or sarcomas but rarely solid cancers (95).

Viruses have been implicated in the etiology of neoplasia in man. There is an association of the Epstein–Barr Virus (EBV), a herpes virus, with two cancers in man, Burkitt's lymphoma, and nasopharyngeal carcinoma (29). The evidence that Burkitt's lymphoma may be caused by EBV is particularly strong (30). A neoplasm of the lymphoreticular system, Hodgkin's disease, has often been suspected to have a viral etiology. Some forms of herpes virus have been implicated in its causation (118). In animals several oncogenic RNA viruses are known to induce leukemias or sarcomas, such as avian leukemia virus, murine and feline leukemia viruses (MuLV, FeLV), Murine mammary tumor virus, the Rous sarcoma virus and the murine and feline sarcoma viruses. In 1908, Ellerman and Bang provided the first demonstration of viral induced leukemia in chickens with cell-free filtrates (27). Proof of the viral causation of leukemias in other animals eluded investigators until it was demonstrated by Gross in 1951 that murine leukemia could be transmitted with cell-free filtrates (40). Feline leukemia viruses have been isolated (65, 72, 101), and leukemia has been transmitted in newborn puppies with cellular material (84). The aforementioned viruses not only produce tumors in their natural hosts but also in a wide range of other vertebrates as is the case with Rous sarcoma virus which when injected into various reptiles, including turtles, lizards, and snakes, produces sarcomas (119, 122, 124). Viruses have been shown to be associated with the pathogenesis of various neoplasms in reptiles (60). Though leukemias and lymphosarcomas in reptiles and fish have not been shown to be virally induced, lymphosarcoma associated with virus-like intranuclear inclusions has been reported in a California king snake (*Lampropeltis getulus californiae*) (63). Additionally, it is suspected that the lymphosarcomas of Esocid fish are of viral etiology (89). Thus far, however, attempts to identify and isolate an infectious agent have been unsuccessful.

Diagnosis

Difficulties arise in the attempt to diagnose reptile and fish lymphocytic neoplasia that do not trouble the medical pathologist. Specimens are not so readily available or submitted in a well-preserved state. Feral poikilotherms that become diseased are soon eliminated from the population by natural forces and not available for examination. Neoplasia is generally considered to be a condition of adult or aged populations and many fish species, being world-wide food sources, are harvested before attaining sufficient age to develop neoplasia, thereby reducing what may be a higher incidence of neoplasia. Reptile specimens are usually obtained from zoos and private collections. These offer excellent opportunities for more advanced study and should be thoroughly investigated. Since the clinical presentation of lymphocytic neoplasms often does not suggest neoplasia to the veterinary clinician, complete hematology and clinical chemistries are frequently not obtained. Obtaining a bone marrow biopsy from fish is not possible as they lack bone marrow and is made difficult in snakes and other reptiles by the generally small amount available for sampling. Consequently, the diagnosis of neoplasia is often left solely to the pathologist at necropsy and following microscopic evaluation of the tissues. Complicating the diagnostic process is the fact that lymphocytes and histiocytes are the predominate cell types involved in inflammatory process of reptiles and fish which can resemble the appearance of lymphomas (26). A proliferative disease of the hemic cells in the turbot (*Scopthalmus maximus*) closely resembles malignant lymphoma but seems to be a reaction to intracellular parasitism by a protozoan (31). Blood profiles fluctuate with age, seasons, nutritional state, and salinity in the case of marine species. For example, the range of leukocytes in the carp (*Cyprinus carpio*) has been reported as being 32,000 to 146,000 per cubic mm (7). Coupled with these variations is the fact that immature or primitive blood cells are commonly found in circulating blood of fish and reptiles (3, 35, 39). The lymphocyte count in reptilian species is highly variable with counts of 15 to 89 per cent of the total white blood cells being recorded (35). Within many species, the lymphocyte count is markedly elevated during moulting (23). Differences in terminology of fish blood cells as in the classification of lymphocytic neoplasms is also complicated by the differences between species. Various texts and papers are available for additional information (64, 125–127). The phylogeny of blood cells has been interpreted by Catton (13) and an excellent overall text of comparative hematology has been prepared by Andrew (3).

Therapy
The discussion of therapy is necessarily limited since the literature is virtually devoid of attempts to treat lymphocytic neoplasms in reptiles and fish. Unless a therapeutic approach is undertaken for purely scientific purposes or it can be shown to have some economic benefit, it will be financially prohibitive. From a practical point of view it should be pointed out that there are no vessels readily available for IV treatment of reptiles and fish, and the erratic uptake of medicaments from the gastrointestinal tract makes oral treatment impractical. The fact that fish are aquatic further complicates therapeutic approaches. Little information is available for calculating the appropriate dosage of drugs for reptiles or fish. Using body weight or body surface area are both unsatisfactory primarily because these animals are poikilotherms and their metabolic rate fluctuates with changes in the environmental temperature. Consequently, few attempts at therapy are undertaken. Recently, however, a report mentions the treatment of a rhinoceros viper (*Bitis nasicornis*) with a lymphosarcoma utilizing the chemotherapeutic agent cystosine arabinoside (62). The snake was given a dose of 30 mg/kg body weight, divided into two doses administered subcutaneously, with a plan of once weekly treatment (53). Due to the severe renal tubular necrosis resulting from prior gentamicin administration, the margin of safety was reduced and the snake died within 24 hours of the first treatment. One other report discusses the unsuccessful treatment of a Indian python (*Python molurus*) with an intraoral lymphosarcoma using cobalt (103). Some reference has already been made to the similarities of lymphosarcoma in pike, which appear to regress spontaneously (116), muskellunge, and Burkitt's lymphoma in African children. The experience with chemotherapy applied to Burkitt's tumor, which responds spectacularly (9, 135), might be utilized in studies of Esox lymphosarcoma. In another paper, Rasquin and Hafter in 1951 reported on the response of lymphosarcomas in Mexican characins to mammalian ACTH (99).

Case reviews

Comprehensive reviews of tumors in reptiles and fish have been written (61, 78, 80–83). In most published reports, the classification of lymphocytic neoplasms has been based almost entirely on the histomorphology of the cell types involved and rarely have electron microscopy, cytochemistry, immunocytochemistry, or even peripheral blood smears been utilized in the diagnostic process. This section details selected published reports of lymphocytic neoplasms in reptiles and fish. Also presented are tables listing reports in the literature and cases on file at the Registry of Tumors in Lower Animals (RTLA).

Reptiles
Lymphocytic neoplasms of reptiles that have been reported in the literature and/or submitted to the RTLA are presented in Tables 4 and 5 respectively.

In 1977, Effron et al provided an interesting account of the nature and rate of neoplasia found at necropsy in captive reptiles held at the San Diego Zoo (24). The incidence of neoplasia was 27 of 1233 reptiles necropsied, or 2.19%. Of the 28 neoplasms (one snake had two tumors), 7 (25%) were lymphosarcomas, six occurring in snakes and one in a lizard.

Lymphoblastic lymphosarcoma has been described in a 320 g male Greek land tortoise or Herman's tortoise (*Testudo hermanii*) (59). The privately owned tortoise was dead when submitted. Following removal of the bottom shell, numerous amyloid, gray-white tumor nodules could be visualized. The liver was permeated with nodules up to the size of a pea. Similar processes appeared in the heart muscle, kidney, spleen, pancreas, and intestinal serosa. Cross sections of the shell also contained sharply delineated gray-white foci. In the lung there was a "walnut-sized" focus with the same dense consistency. Histologically, the liver contained localized accumulations primarily of large lymphoid cells with practically no cytoplasm and containing vesicular nuclei poor in chromatin. Small lymphoid and reticular cells were also present, but to a lesser extent. There was a distinct transition from the tumorous tissue to the little remaining liver tissue which showed fatty degeneration with large drops of fat. The tumorous tissue was penetrated by many capillaries which sometimes were lined by swollen endothelial cell nuclei. Neoplastic cells were particularly evident under the spleen capsule. Nearly identical accumulations of lymphoblasts also occurred in the lung, bone marrow, heart musculature, pancreas, and serous membranes of the body cavity. There was a distinct perivascular arrange-

Table 4. Lymphocytic neoplasms in reptiles published in the literature.

Taxonomic Classification/ Common name	Diagnosis	Reference
Chelonia (turtles) *Testudo hermanii* (Hermann's tortoise)	lymphoma, lymphoblastic	(59)
Crocodilia (crocodiles) *Crocodylus porosus* (saltwater crocodile)	round cell sarcoma (lymphosarcoma)	(107, 109)
Squamata:Saurina (lizards) *Hydrosaurus amboinensis* (water lizard)	malignant lymphoma, lymphoblastic	(137)
Uromastex acanthinurus (spring-tailed agamid)	lymphosarcoma	(24)
Lacerta sicula (Ruin lizard)	malignant lymphoma	(75)
Varanus salvator (Malayan water monitor)	lymphosarcoma	(137)
Squamata:Serpentes (snakes) *Constrictor constrictor* (*Boa constrictor*)	lymphatic leukemia	(36)
Eunectes murinus (anaconda)	lymphosarcoma	(33)
Python molurus (Indian python)	lymphoid leukosis	(32)
Heterodon platyrhinos (hognose snake)	lymphosarcoma	(14)
Lampropeltis getulus californiae (California king snake)	lymphosarcoma	(63)
Lampropeltis g. getulus (Eastern king snake)	lymphosarcoma	(62)
Naja naja (Egyptian cobra)	lymphosarcoma	(14)
Naja nigricollis (spitting cobra)	lymphosarcoma	(24)
Acanthophis antarcticus (death adder)	lymphosarcoma, leukemic	(24)
Bitis arientans (African puff adder)	lymphosarcoma, leukemic	(24)
Bitis nasicornis (rhinoceros viper)	lymphosarcoma	(14, 24, 62)
	lymphosarcoma, leukemic	(24)
Crotalus horridus horridus (timber rattlesnake)	lymphosarcoma, leukemic	(38)
	lymphoid leukemia	(24)

ment of the tumor tissue in the bone marrow. A round cell sarcoma was thoroughly described in a young saltwater crocodile (*Crocodylus porosus*) which was unable to rise and tended to fall on its right side (109). Upon necropsy, a tumor slightly larger than a cherry stone was observed on the ventral surface of the cerebellum. The mass consisted of small round cells and a few large, multinucleated cells. The right auricle of the heart was filled with cells that resembled those of the cerebellar mass and invaded the right ventricle and interventricular septum. Periportal clusters of these cells were also found in the liver. Though the author believed this to be a round cell sarcoma of hepatic origin, other authors, after examining photomicrographs, felt that the cells were of hemic origin, resembling those of a lymphosarcoma (107). In 1962, Lawson reported on an adult male Ruin lizard (*Lacerta sicula*) in which he diagnosed malignant lymphoma (75). The lizard, received from Holland, was kept in an indoor terrarium with other lacertids in California where it ate well and appeared to be thriving. After approximately one month a slight bulging on the right lateral aspect of the neck was noted. In the next three weeks this bulge increased in size and a second bulge began forming on the tail, which extended for about 10 mm along its length. About one week later the animal died. During the entire time of its captivity

Table 5. Lymphocytic neoplasms in reptiles on file at the Registry of Tumors in Lower Animals (RTLA), Smithsonian Institution, Washington, D.C. (42, 44, 45, 46, 49, 50).

Taxonomic Classification/Common name	Diagnosis	RTLA No/Contributor
Chelonia (turtles)		
Testudo hermanii (Herman's tortoise)	lymphoma, lymphoblastic	717, Ippen
Squamata:Sauria (lizards)		
Hydrosaurus amboinensis (water lizard)	malignant lymphoma, lymphoblastic	291, Zwart
Germosaurus sp. (plated lizard)	lymphoma, poorly-differentiated	2316, Heldstab
Iguana iguana (common iguana)	lymphoma, lymphocytic	1385, Frye
Varanus bengalensis (Bengal monitor)	lymphoblastic leukemia	1499, Shively
Varanus salvator (Malayan monitor)	lymphosarcoma	461, Zwart
	lymphoma, lymphocytic or plasmacytic	719, Ippen
Varanus exanthematicus albigularis (white-throated monitor)	lymphoma, lymphocytic, well-differentiated	2426, Zwart
Squamata:Serpentes (snakes)		
Python molurus (Indian python)	malignant lymphoma	1600, Robinson
Python reticulatus (reticulated python)	malignant lymphoma	1960, Heldstab
Lampropeltis getulus californiae (California king snake)	lymphosarcoma	1770, Jacobson
Lampropelis getulus getulus (eastern king snake)	malignant lymphoma	2240, Jacobson
Bitis nasicornis (rhinoceros viper)	lymphosarcoma	379, Griner
Crotalus horridus horridus (timber rattlesnake)	lymphoblastic,	378, Griner

the lizard was normally active and no abnormalities in behavior were noted except that it had not been seen to eat on the last four days preceding death. At necropsy the neck mass, which extended from 1 mm behind the external auditory opening almost to the shoulder, measured 10 × 9 × 4 mm. It was creamy white and moderately soft, with loose adherence to overlying skin and underlying tissues without encapsulation. Microscopic examination of sections from this mass revealed a mainly lymphoid cell composition. Peripheral to the mass, lymphoid cells had infiltrated between individual muscle bundles. The tail musculature was replaced by tumor cells, adjacent vessels were plugged with these cells, and muscles from many other parts of the body had been invaded as had the kidneys, spleen, and liver. The specific cell morphology was not described except to identify the tumor cells as lymphoid. Based on the difficulty of classifying the various malignant lymphomas, the author chose to use the inclusive term malignant lymphoma.

A diffuse lymphoblastic malignant lymphoma occurred in a female East Indian water lizard (*Hydrosaurus amboinensis*) from the Amsterdam Zoo (137). This animal was cachectic upon presentation and had become lethargic several weeks prior to its death. At necropsy, marked hepatosplenomegaly was found and the caudal two-thirds of the kidneys were swollen and pale. Approximately two-thirds of the liver volume consisted of interconnected masses of lymphoblasts which replaced much of the liver parenchyma and occupied the sinusoids. Cells comprising the masses and infiltrates were uniform in size and staining characteristics, had little cytoplasm, and were identifiable as poorly differentiated lymphocytes. Mitoses were fairly common. Necrosis was most conspicuous in the spleen and liver. Subendothelial collections of lymphoblasts were present and lymphoblastic cells had infiltrated muscle bundles of the myocardium at multiple foci. A subepicardial plaque of lymphoid cells was found at the heart base. In the spleen, proliferation of lymphoblasts completely obscured the normal architecture. Intracapsular infiltrations and extracapsular extension were also found. Lymphomatous accumulations were present throughout the kidneys, particularly in the caudal portions.

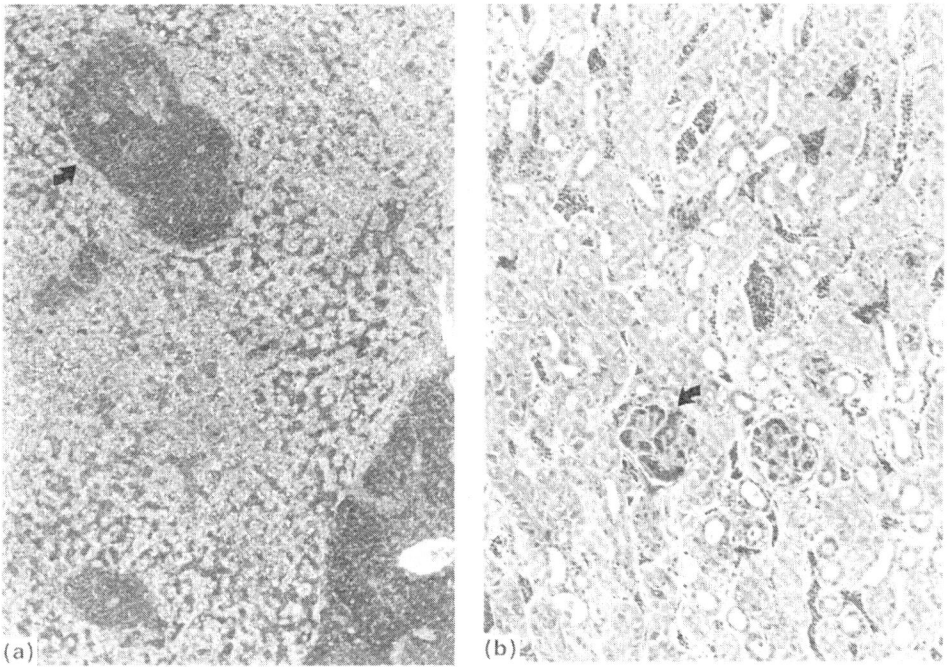

Figure 2. Lymphocytic lymphoma in a white-throated monitor (*Varanus exanthematicus albigularis*) (RTLA-2426, Zwart).
A. Liver containing periportal nodular accumulations (arrow), and sinusoids packed with neoplastic lymphocytes. H&E × 47.
B. Kidney with interstitial, intravascular, and intraglomerular (arrow) foci of neoplastic lymphocytes. H&E × 117.

Tubules were destroyed and glomeruli contained hyalin thickening of their basement membranes. The lungs generally contained diffuse infiltrations of the lymphoblasts with some focal accumulations. The histopathological features closely resemble those described for lymphoid neoplasms in mammals (20, 131), birds (71), and fish (16). The same report contains descriptions of a probable lymphosarcoma in a male Malayan monitor lizard (*Varanus salvator*). This animal died several months after being placed in the zoological collection even though it was in a good state of nutrition and no signs of illness were recognized prior to death. Dissection revealed a marked hepatosplenomegaly with the liver and spleen containing numerous circumscribed foci. The mucosa of the large intestine contained multiple deep ulcerations and necrotic pin-head sized foci were present in the myocardium. Densely cellular infiltrations of small, round, somewhat pleomorphic cells with scanty cytoplasm, whose cellular morphology ranged from lymphoid to plasmacytoid were present in the liver, spleen, kidneys, heart, testes, and other organs. Only a few mitoses were recognizable, possibly due to postmortem change. Regions of solid tumor tissue occupied about half of the liver and were concentrated around the portal triads. Veins, arteries, and bile ducts were enveloped by lymphoreticular tissue with infiltrations within vascular walls and lining the lumina. In the kidneys, lymphoid elements were predominantly located in the hilus, along peripheries of renal lobules, and around interlobular arteries. From solid foci of lymphoid cells came interstitial infiltrates. Some of the better preserved foci of lymphocytic cells infiltrated between fibers of heart muscle and were scattered throughout the lungs. In the testes, lymphoid cells had infiltrated the capsule and around arterioles. Lymphoid

aggregates also occurred in subcapsular areas of the adrenal glands, parafollicular foci of the thyroids, lamina propria of the gastric mucosa, and subepithelial zone of the urinary bladder. Though this animal also had concomitant bacterial infection and gastric parasites, the distribution of lesions and the morphology of the cellular constituents supported the diagnosis of malignant lymphoma. Lymphosarcoma in a spring-tailed agamid (*Uromastix acanthurinus*) has also been reported (24). The microscopic appearance of a diffuse lymphocytic lymphoma in a white-throated monitor (Varanus exanthematicus albigularis) obtained from the RTLA files is presented in Figure 2.

As noted previously, Effron et al also reported the occurrence of lymphosarcoma in six snakes: a female spitting cobra (*Naja nigricolis*); a male death adder (*Acanthopis antarcticus*); a female African puff adder (*Bitis arientans*); two female rhinoceros vipers (*B. nasicornis*); and a female timber rattlesnake (*Crotalus horridus horridus*) (24). Histopathology of the lymphosarcoma in the timber rattlesnake was depicted in photomicrographs. Each of the reptilian lymphosarcomas consisted predominantly of large, round mononuclear cells with prominent nucleoli and moderate to large amounts of cytoplasm. These cells were similar to the immature lymphoid or histiocytic cell type in mammalian lymphomas but the authors considered it inappropriate to assign such a term to the cells of these neoplasms because of their limited knowledge of reptilian cytology. The disease typically involved the lungs, liver, spleen, pancreas, gastrointestinal tract, and kidneys and in some instances, the heart, skeletal muscle, or skin. Four of the lymphosarcomas in snakes were accompanied by a leukemic blood picture.

Electron microscopy of snake lymphosarcoma cells did not verify the presence of virus particles.

The first description of lymphosarcoma in a snake was provided by Frank and Schepky in 1969 (33). The anaconda (*Eunectes murinus*) was 2.2 metres long and weighed 3.425 kg. The liver was considered to be the primary site of the tumor with secondary deposits occurring in the thyroid, spleen, pancreas, and kidneys. The lymphoblast was the predominant cell type. In the preceding year Cowan listed, without further description, lymphosarcoma in three snakes: an Egyptian cobra (*Naja naja*) involving the heart and liver; a hognose snake (*Heterodon platyrhinos*) affecting the liver, lungs, and kidneys; a river jack or rhinoceros viper (*B. nasicornis*) infiltrating the liver, kidneys, adrenal glands, spleen, and gut wall (14).

An Indian python (*P. molurus*), having a length of 2.98 metres and a weight of 16.33 kg and had been at the Sydney Zoo for approximately three and one-half years, died from complications of lymphoid leukosis (32). At necropsy a flat, pink, fleshy lesion of irregular shape, about 10 mm in diameter and 2 mm thick, was seen adjacent to the larynx in the pharyngeal cavity. Four similar, but smaller lesions were present in the mucosa of the esophagus, and two in the mucosa of the trachea. There was a diffuse, pale enlargement around the heart base. Within this enlargement was a 10 mm pinkish nodule. The right and left auricles also had nodular lesions approximately 5 mm in diameter. The liver was diffusely enlarged and its edges were thickened. A blood smear prepared from heart blood obtained several hours after death and stained with Leishman's stain, contained approximately 50% lymphocytic type cells, many of which were lymphoblasts. Infiltrations of uniformly shaped lymphoblasts with vesiculated nuclei containing nucleoli and a few mitotic figures were seen microscopically in the myocardium, primarily in periportal areas of the liver, throughout the spleen, perivascular areas of the lung, subcapsular and interstitial areas of the kidneys, trachea, esophagus, and stomach. Well vascularized lymphocytic nodular foci were present in the renal pelvis. The presentation of the disease in the python is similar pathologically to lymphoid leucosis of poultry and of the common domesticated animals, except for the greater vascularity of the nodules in the python.

Frye and Carney described acute lymphatic leukemia in an immature male South American boa constrictor (*Constrictor constrictor*) which was diagnosed upon examination of blood films prepared from cardiac blood and stained with Jenner–Giemsa stain (36). Necropsy revealed no gross abnormalities other than an absence of body fat deposits. The blood film contained large numbers of lymphocytes often demonstrating evidence of mitotic activity. Most lymphocytes were relatively rounded though some were somewhat elliptical. Many of the large prolymphocytes were characterized by irregularly shaped nuclei with prominent nucleoli, and scanty cytoplasm which was markedly blue-gray. The immature lymphocytes had a tendency to adhere to each other in "rafts". The kidneys, liver, lung, and bone marrow were considered normal microscopically. Lymphoid follicles with germinal centers were not found in the spleen (germinal centers in snake spleen are usually not well defined). Lymphoid elements in the spleen ranged from well-differentiated and mature lymphocytes to primitive reticulum cells. Lymphosarcoma has been described in a Cali-

fornia king snake (*Lampropeltis getulus californiae*) in 1980 (63), and in an adult male Eastern king snake (*Lampropeltis getulus getulus*) and in an adult make Rhinoceros viper (*B. nasicornis*) in 1981 (62). Major organs of the California king snake were infiltrated with lymphoblastic cells often containing Cowdry Type A intranuclear inclusions. Electron microscopy demonstrated intracytoplasmic virus-like particles in the neoplastic cells. The Eastern king snake was admitted due to a bloody discharge from the glottis that was noticed one week prior to presentation. The snake had bright skin and good muscle tone though the mucous membranes of the oral cavity appeared paler than normal and blood was seen in the trachea. Numerous lymphocytic cells and ciliated epithelial cells were observed in Wright–Giemsa stained smears of lung washings. Touch preparations of a biopsy stained with Wright–Giemsa stain from a liver nodule visualized radiographically contained a mixture of cells, most of which were immature lymphoid cells. These cells were generally large and somewhat variable in size with a moderate amount of basophilic, occasionally vacuolated cytoplasm. There was moderate chromatin clumping of the variably sized, round-to-oval nuclei which were occasionally indented. Nucleoli were not prominent and there were a few mitotic figures. The diagnosis rendered was prolymphocytic lymphosarcoma. Necropsy revealed the presence of numerous firm nodules throughout the lung, liver, kidneys, and gastrointestinal tract. Tumor cells in these lesions and in the lung septa had large round-to-oval, vesicular nuclei with marginated chromatin, infrequent mitotic figures, and moderate amounts of slightly granular, pale eosinophilic cytoplasm with indistinct borders resembling immature lymphocytes. These cells were arranged in sheets on a delicate reticular stroma with central necrosis of larger nodules. Though the Rhinoceros viper was originally presented with a history of mucous discharge from the nares which was determined to be secondary to verminous pneumonia, it subsequently developed a firm subcutaneous madd on its right side some distance anterior to the cloacal opening. Impression smears from this lesion were prepared and contained predominantly lymphoid cells with marked anisocytosis and nuclear pleomorphism. The nuclei were finely stippled with chromatin and contained frequent mitotic figures with occasional apparent multinucleation. Wright–Giemsa stained blood films contained occasional abnormal appearing lymphocytes. The cytologic diagnosis was prolymphocytic lymphosarcoma. Chemotherapy consisting of 30 mg of cytosine arabinoside/kg of body weight was divided into two doses to be administered once weekly via subcutaneous route. The margin of safety was reduced due to severe renal tubular necrosis resulting from prior administration of gentamicin and the snake died within 24 hours of the first treatment. At necropsy, a 9 × 6 × 4 cm cream-colored, firm mass located in the caudal coelomic cavity was seen to be attached by a pedicle to the subcutaneous tumor. The coelomic mass was composed of varied sized round cells with pleomorphic, large, round, cleaved or convoluted nuclei. The chromatin was coarsely clumped, nucleoli were occasionally prominent, mitotic figures were numerous, and many cells appeared multinucleated. The cytoplasm was pale-eosinophilic and cytoplasmic borders were distinct. The cells were often arranged in widely separated sheets on scanty stroma. Plaque-

Table 6. Lymphocytic neoplasms in fish published in the literature.

Taxonomic Classification/Common name	Diagnosis	Reference
Anguilliformes		
Conger conger (Conger eel)	lymphosarcoma	(130)
Clupeiformes		
Clupea harengus harengus (herring)	lymphosarcoma	(67, 68)
Salmoniformes		
Oncorhynchus gorbuschka (humpback salmon)	lymphosarcoma	(121)
Oncorhynchus keta (chum salmon)	lymphosarcoma	(57)
Salmo salar (Atlantic salmon)	lymphosarcoma	(41)
Salmo clarki (cutthroat trout)	lymphosarcoma	(110)
Salvelinus fontinalis (brook trout)	lymphosarcoma	(19)
Salvelinus namaycush (lake trout)	lymphosarcoma	(25)
S. fontinalis × *S. namaycush* (hybrid splake)	lymphosarcoma	(19)
Pleocoglossus altivelis	lymphosarcoma	(56)
Esox lucius (northern pike)	lymphosarcoma	(41, 85, 90, 93, 94)
Esox masquinongy (muskellunge)	lymphosarcoma	(102 cited in 106; 114, 115)
Cypriniformes		
Astyanax mexicanus (Mexican characin)	lymphosarcoma	(34, 93, 100)
A. mexicanus × *Anopthichthys jordani* (hybrid)	lymphosarcoma	(99)
Carassius auratus (goldfish)	lymphosarcoma	(96)
Rasbora lateristriata (yellow rasbora)	lymphosarcoma	(111)
Characiformes		
Pristellia riddlei (X-ray fish)	lymphosarcoma	(129)
Gadiformes		
Gadus morhua (cod)	lymphosarcoma	(134)
Pleuronectiformes		
Platichthus flesus (plaice)	lymphosarcoma	(66)
Psetta maeotica (flounder)	lymphosarcoma	(108)
Scophthalmus (Rhombus) *maximus* (turbot)	lymphosarcoma	(69)

like arrangement of similar cells were present in the heart, spleen, and portions of the pulmonary interstitium. The cells resembled immature lymphocytes. Electron microscopy confirmed that the nuclei were pleomorphic and often convoluted but true multinucleated cells or viral particles were not demonstrated.

Fish
Lymphocytic neoplasms of fish that have been reported in the literature and/or submitted to the RTLA are presented in Tables 6 and 7 respectively. Unlike reptiles, more information on neoplasia of blood cell origin has been collected from cases in fish than for any other class of poikilotherm. Most hematopoietic neoplasms in fish have been classified as lymphoma/lymphosarcoma regardless of degree and pattern of dissemination or evidence of leukemia. With the exception of the Northern pike (*Esox lucius*) and the muskellunge (*E. masquinongy*) in which the lymphomatous lesions are most prominent in the subcutaneous tissues or oral mucosa, lymphosarcoma in most species of fish are

Table 7. Lymphocytic neoplasms in fish on file at the Registry of Tumors in Lower Animals (RLTA), Smithsonian Institution, Washington, DC. (42, 43, 46, 47, 48, 49, 50, 51).

Taxonomic Classification/ Common name	Diagnosis	RTLA No/Contributor
Salmoniformes		
Oncorhynchus kitsutch (coho salmon)	lymphosarcoma	203, Boyce
Oncorhynchus tschawytscha (chinook salmon)	lymphoma	773, Bell; 1039, Hoskins
Salmo clarki (cutthroat trout)	leukemia	267, Smith
Salmo gairdneri (rainbow trout)	lymphosarcoma	901, Smith
	malignant lymphoma	1043, Hine; 1814, 2251, Smith
	lymphoma	630, 2129, Smith
Salvelinus fontinalis (brook trout)	lymphosarcoma	216, Dunbar
	lymphoma	2823, Morrison
Salvelinus namaycush (lake trout)	malignant lymphoma, lymphocytic	1046, Hnath
Esox lucius (northern pike)	lymphosarcoma	112, Mulcahy 127, Nigrelli
	lymphoma	1031–1035, Ljungberg 2276, Bogovski 2772, Stillman
Cypriniformes		
Abramis brama (common bream)	lymphosarcoma	1154, Boyce
Rutilus rutilus (roach)	malignant lymphoma	1878, Bucke
Siluriformes		
Ictalurus punctatus (channel catfish)	lymphoma, lymphocytic	2836, McCoy
Pimelodus clarias (barge pintado)	malignant lymphoma	2424, Urdaneta Ch
Antheriformes		
Cynolebias nigripinnis (blackfin pearl fish)	malignant lymphoma	1646, Blasiola
Oryzias latipes (medaka)	lymphoma	1850, Hitachi
	malignant lymphoma	2555, Wester
Perciformes		
Aequidens maronii (keyhole cichlid)	malignant lymphoma	511, Wolke
Micropterus salmonides (largemouth bass)	malignant lymphoma	2620, Blasiola
Pleuronectiformes		
Scophthalmus (Rhombus) *maximus* (turbot)	malignant lymphoma	842, Nightingale

thought to arise in the kidney or thymus. Lymphocytic neoplasms have not been reported in Chondrichthyes (cartilaginous fish). However, a reticulum cell sarcoma was reported in a sandbar shark (*Carcharhinus plumseus*) (17). This case and others have been well reviewed by Schlumberger (106), Schlumberger and Lucké (107), Dawe (16), and Wellings (128). Mawdesley-Thomas listed the taxonomic distribution of neoplasms, including lymphosarcomas, which had been reported in the literature up to that time (83). Review of these papers or a description of the lesions was not provided.

Lymphosarcoma appears to be a characteristic neoplasm among northern pike (*E. lucius*) (85, 90, 91, 93) and muskellunge (*E. masquinongy*) (102 cited in 106; 115, 116).

Although numerous reports have been published on lymphosarcomas in fish, comments here will be primarily restricted to those reported in the order Salmoniformes, specifically northern pike, muskellunge, salmon (*Salmo* sp.), and trout (*Salvelinus* sp.). Twelve pike housed in the New York Aquarium died during the summers of 1940 and 1941 from complications of lymphosarcoma (93). It was thought that the neoplasm originated in the posterior kidney with subsequent extension to the liver, spleen, and retroperitoneal tissues. The proliferating cells in the kidney were mainly of the large lymphoblast type supported by irregular strands of fibrous stroma and delicate reticulum. There was an occasional uninucleate or binucleate "giant" cell with hyperchromatic nuclei. Numerous mitotic figures were found throughout the masses. The lymphoid cells from the outer edge of the kidneys formed a nodular pattern as seen in follicular lymphoma. The outstanding feature in the spleen was the extensive development of "pulp cords". Nigrelli felt that metastasis to the liver probably took place through the portal system.

Lymphosarcomas reported by others in pike (41, 85, 90, 94) and in muskellunge (102 cited in 106; 114, 115) arise in the oral cavity or subcutaneous tissues with extension or metastasis to the trunk musculature, kidneys, spleen, and eventually liver with an accompanying leukemia. Some affected fish, less than 1%, do survive. The disease is contagious to muskellunge living in the same water with fish bearing the growth (115), and the tumor can be transplanted according to initial studies by Ritchie (102 cited in 106), there is epizootiological evidence of a viral etiology in these fish (117) and successful cell-free transmission of the disease in pike has been reported (89). The neoplastic cells in the pike were described by Mulcahy as having large, basophilic, round or oval nuclei (85). A few cells had more densely staining nuclei and slightly more cytoplasm. Usually there were many mitoses. Specimens from these fish were more thoroughly described by Dawe (16) and subsequently by Mulcahy in collaboration with Winqvist and Dawe (92). The neoplastic cells were uniform, highly undifferentiated and atypical in form. They often aligned themselves in contact with reticulin fibers of capillary walls. The nuclei were round or slightly indented with finely dispersed chromatin and a single, fairly large nucleolus. There was a juxtanuclear region which contained a Golgi complex and centrioles with a weakly positive periodic acid-Schiff reaction and strongly positive acid phospatase reaction. The cytoplasm, frequently containing a few fat droplets, was moderately abundant and smoothly basophilic and pyroninophilic. Mitochondria were numerous as were free ribosomes which were partly in polyribosomal aggregates. The endoplasmic reticulum was not as highly developed as it is in typical plasma cells, but some configurations were suggestive of protein secretory activity. The authors concluded that these cells are best classified as atypical hemocytoblasts (stem cells) or immunoblasts. Mulcahy has since reported on blood values in healthy adult pike (86) and blood changes associated with lymphosarcoma in pike (88). She found that changes in the blood of lymphoma-bearing pike were not associated primarily with white cells until late in the course of the disease. The red:white cell ratio was reduced, reflecting a drop in red cell count rather than a rise in the number of white cells. Consequently, the hematocrits and hemoglobin concentra-

tions were lowered. In fixed smears, many circulating red cells were considered immature because of their round shape and staining properties. There were also increased numbers of "ghost" cells. The serum total proteins were markedly decreased in pike with lymphomas though stress aggravated by leakage from tumors and perhaps by a disturbance of kidney function was probably the cause since there was a loss in the lower molecular weight protein, albumin.

Sonstegard has provided a detailed gross and histopathologic description of lymphosarcoma in muskellunge from the Kawartha Lake region of Ontario, Canada with comparisons to the disease in northern pike (115). The external lesions were found on the flank, fins, jaw, and head in descending order of occurrence. This is in some contrast to those reported in pike from Ireland by Mulcahy which occur on the jaws, head, gills, and flank in descending order of occurrence (85). Nigrelli found no external lesions in pike from the New York Aquarium (93). The tumor has an unicentric, subcutaneous origin producing a localized, nodular lesion. It metastasizes from the subcutis via intracellular spaces to involve the trunk musculature. Late in the disease, hematopoietic tissues of the spleen and kidneys become infiltrated simultaneously with leukosarcoma. The liver is also commonly involved but only after the kidney and spleen are infiltrated. The neoplastic cells resemble lymphocytes but are 1.5 to 2 times larger than the diameter of normal fish lymphocytes with the nuclei occupying most of the cell volume. The nucleus is typically round-to-oval with a distinct nuclear membrane. Some of the cells contain "bean shaped" or "horseshoe" appearing nuclei. A few mitotic figures and multinucleated cells are also observed. The moderately dense chromatin appeared to form a network of thick cords and was often clumped next to the nuclear membrane, not evenly dispersed throughout the nucleus. Hematoxylin and eosin, periodic acid-Schiff, Giemsa, or Wright stained preparations did not reveal the presence of nucleoli in the neoplastic cells. The thin, structureless rim of cytoplasm was primarily eosinophilic in H&E preparations, strongly basophilic with Giemsa stain, and was PAS negative. Giemsa stained smears of peripheral blood revealed large numbers of cells that resembled lymphoblasts. The "starry sky" effect, characteristic of various lymphoreticular neoplasms in man and domestic animals, was not found in muskellunge though Mulcahy did occasionally see this in the thymus of pike with lymphosarcoma (87). One of the interesting features of the neoplasm is its ability to infiltrate tissue spaces and cause atrophy without stimulating a fibroblastic or inflammatory response except in lesions which were in the process of healing. Despite this, the flank tumors frequently remain localized even though they have grown to enormous size. Scarpelli has mentioned the similarity of these neoplasms in pike and muskellunge to some examples in warm-blooded animals which are used as experimental models by oncologists (104). Those listed included the Murphy-Sturm, A-40, TT-8, and TT-10 lymphosarcomas, and the lymphocytic lymphoma No. 2.

Ljungberg has described skin sarcomas in about 10% of pike from brackish waters of certain areas in the Baltic (77). The results of electron microscopic evaluation of these sarcomas have in turn been reported (133). These authors felt that the skin sarcoma was probably not the same tumor

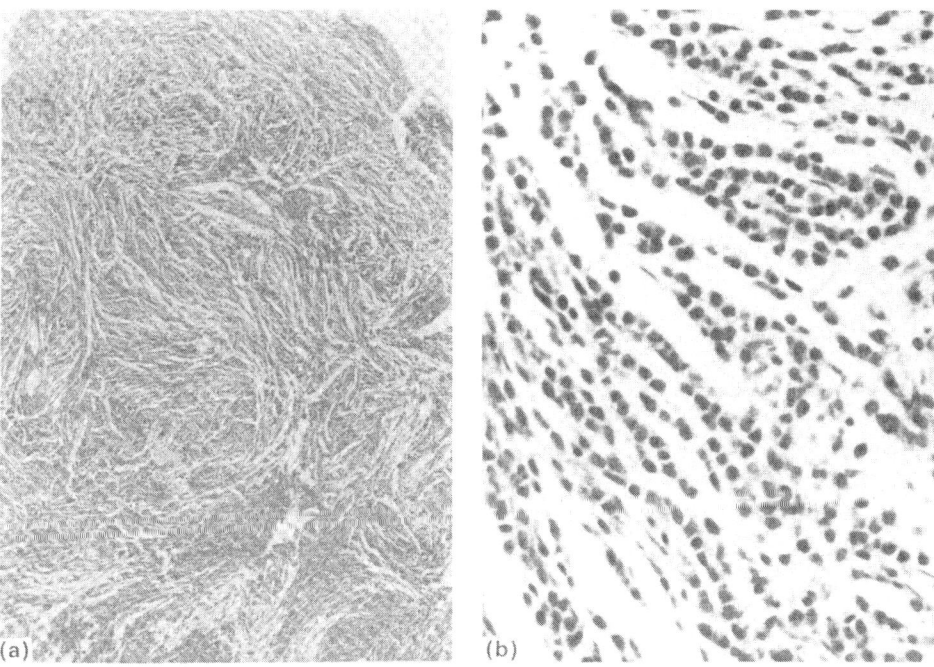

Figure 3. Malignant lymphoma in a black fin pearlfish (*Cynolebias nigripinnis*) (RTLA-1646, Blasiola).
A. Portion of large growth involving the left pectoral fin demonstrating the linear and swirling arrangement of the neoplastic cells. H&E × 47.
B. Higher magnification of the mass shows the linear arrangement of the small lymphoid cells on a delicate reticular stroma. H&E × 469.

as that described by Mulcahy since the skin sarcomas were restricted to the skin and underlying musculature. They commented, however, that from a morphological point of view, the tumors showed great similarities. In both cases the tumor is composed of round, poorly differentiated cells, though the skin sarcoma cells, in contrast, contained numerous lipid droplets. Also, a few virus-like particles of C-type were seen in the cytoplasm of the tumor cells from two cases. The relationship of these virus-like particles to the skin sarcoma is not established since epidermal proliferations containing numerous such particles occur in the same pike population (132).

The Salmonidae (salmon and trout) are another family in the order Salmoniformes from which lymphosarcomas have frequently been reported. Haddow and Blake, in 1933, reported a case of lymphosarcoma in a five year old, female Atlantic salmon (*Salmo salar*) (41). The entire kidney was involved and enlarged to such an extent that the hemal arch was occluded. The mesonephros, or head kidney, was thought to be the site of tumor origin. The precise tumor cell type cannot be determined as sufficient descriptive information was not provided. In 1969 Wellings (128) listed the report of Ehlinger in which several lake trout (*Salvelinus namaycush*) with lymphosarcoma involving the kidney were described (25). Lymphosarcoma of possible thymic origin in Salmonid fish has been reported by Dunbar (19). These cases include three yearling brook trout (*S. fontinalis*) and two splake (hybrids of brook trout crossed with lake trout). In the brook trout the neoplastic cells were characterized as large, round, uniform lymphoblasts with marginated or sometimes condensed chromatin. Nuclear membranes were

distinct and mitotic figures were numerous. The masses of cells filled much of the gill cavity, blood spaces, and invaded adjacent musculature, kidneys, and liver. The tumors in the splake consisted of small nodules generally lying under the operculum, suggesting a thymic origin. The tumor cells in the nodules were similar to those described in the brook trout except that they were slightly smaller. The appearance of this tumor in splake was thought to be due to transmission of a suspected genetic trait from the brook trout parent. The kidney or spleen was considered the origin of a neoplasm suggestive of lymphosarcoma in a 2-year-old cutthroat trout (*Salmo clarki*) reported by Smith in 1971 (110). The kidney tubules were replaced by "blastoid" cells that were large, round, and containing somewhat vesicular nuclei with some margination of chromatin. The spleen and liver were invaded by similar cells which were also present in the lumina of arteries and veins, thereby suggesting a leukemic progression. Malignant lymphoma involving the left pectoral fin of a black fin pearlfish (*Cynolebias nigripinnis*) obtained from the RTLA files is presented in Figure 3. The small lymphoid cells were arranged in a delicate swirling pattern (Figure 3A) on a delicate reticular stroma (Figure 3B). A diffuse lymphocytic lymphoma in a roach (*Rutilus rutilus*) obtained from the RTLA files is depicted in Figure 4. The malignant lymphocytes diffusely infiltrated the liver and kidneys which developed numerous small foci of necrosis (Figure 4A and B). The neoplastic lymphocytes generally contained small, round, uniform nuclei and a paucity of pale, eosinophilic cytoplasm (Figure 4C).

Lymphosarcomas have also been reported in various other Orders of fish including Anguilliformes, Clupeiformes,

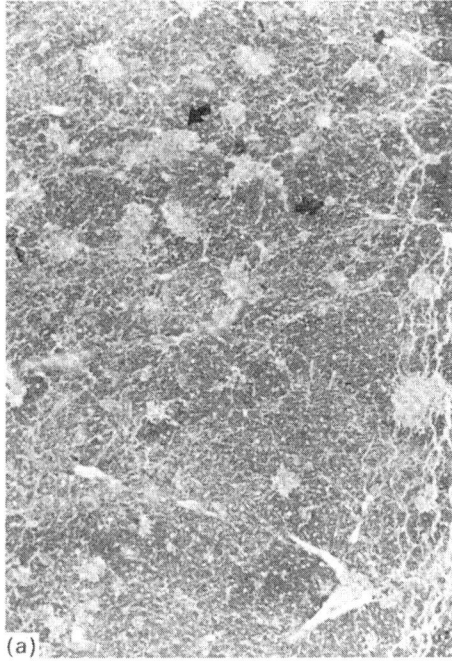

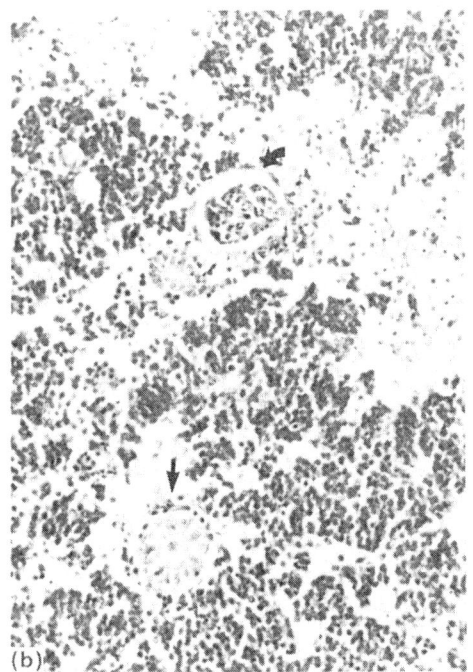

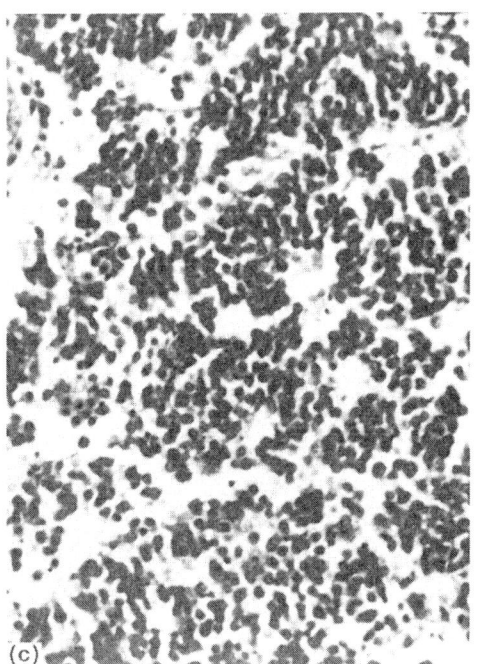

Figure 4. Malignant lymphoma in a roach (*Rutilus rutilus*) (RTLA-1878, Bucke).
A. The liver was diffusely infiltrated so that only an occasional bile duct, often surrounded by a zone of necrosis, is recognizable (arrow). H&E × 29.
B. The kidney was also diffusely infiltrated by small lymphocytes with foci of necrosis, leaving only a few glomeruli (curved arrow) and tubules (straight arrow). H&E × 293.
C. Higher magnification of malignant lymphocytes in the kidneys demonstrates the generally small, round, uniform nuclei and scanty cytoplasm. H&E × 469.

Characiformes, Gadiformes, and Pleuronectiformes (Table 6) with additional cases from the Orders Antheriformes, Siluriformes, and Perciformes submitted to the RTLA (Table 7).

Discussion and summary

The previous section on case reviews demonstrates that there are at least superficial similarities between reptilian and fish lymphocytic neoplasia and that described in mammals. However, insufficient effort has been put forth to identify more substantial similarities. Hematopoiesis in reptiles and fish has been studied in some detail, but to compare normal and neoplastic hemic cells to those in mammals, attempts to further characterize these cells must be made. Correlation of these neoplasms also depends on the acceptance of some classification scheme and determining if it can be applied to poikilotherms.

Identification and isolation of viruses associated with pike and muskellunge lymphosarcoma and transmission of the disease with cell-free filtrates have met with varied success (89, 117). Whether these tumors regress because of temperature mediated phenomenon linked to the inhibition of viral expression due to a temperature-sensitive reverse transcriptase is still to be determined and offers a significant area for further study. Production of sarcomas in various reptiles by the Schmidt–Ruppin strain of Rous sarcoma virus suggests that reptiles offer potential for experimental studies of virally induced hematopoietic neoplasms. The report of lymphosarcoma in a California king snake which contained intranuclear inclusions and virus-like particles in the neoplastic cells (63) lends additional support to the likelihood of a viral etiology in poikilotherms.

In their discussion of the lymphoid system, immunity, and malignancy, Good and Finstad relate thymic involution to cancer and suggest that a programmed involution of the thymus and thymus-dependent lymphoid system, probably under endocrine control, could be postulated (37). In rats and mice inoculated with murine leukemia viruses, cortical atrophy of the thymus often occurs prior to the appearance of lymphoid neoplasms (21, 22, 120). In the pike, thymic involution is associated with, and probably precedes, the development of lymphosarcomas (87). The thymus was thought to be the primary site of origin of lymphosarcomas described in Mexican characins (34, 93, 99, 100). Nigrelli mentioned that lymphoid hyperplasia of the thymus, which may progress to lymphosarcoma, occurs in those characins kept in the dark whereas Rasquin and Rosenbloom noted that marked involution of the thymus occurs when characins are kept in the dark. Rasquin and Hafter also reported on the effects of mammalian ACTH on lymphosarcomas in these fish. Friedman did attempt tissue culture studies on two lymphosarcomas of Astyanx but continuous cell lines were not established. The characins then seem to offer a good model to study the relationships hematopoiesis, immunology, and the development of lymphosarcomas.

Complete preparation of case material would add much to our current knowledge of reptilian and fish lymphocytic neoplasia. Clinical studies including evaluation of blood films, bone marrow and solid tumor biopsies, cytochemistry, immunocytochemistry, viral isolation, cell-free filtrate transmission, and therapy attempts are to be encouraged. If the animal should succumb to the neoplasm, a thorough necropsy procedure and complete microscopic evaluation along with electron microscopy and special stains are recommended to more completely characterize the cell type involved and enable further comparisons to mammalian lymphosarcomas.

Finally, familiarization with the literature, and review of case material available at the Registry of Experimental Cancers of the National Cancer Institute, Bethesda, Maryland and the Registry of Tumors in Lower Animals, Smithsonian Institution, Washington, D.C. would be of obvious use to investigators who wish to initiate studies.

REFERENCES

1. Adams WE: The cervical region of the Lacertilia, a critical review of certain aspects of its anatomy, *J of Anat* 74:57, 1939
2. Anderson BG, Mitchum DL: *Atlas of Trout Histology*, Bull No. 13, Cheyenne, Wyoming Game and Fish Department. 1974
3. Andrew W: Comparative Hematology, New York, Grune and Stratton. 1965
4. Ashley LM: Comparative fish histology In *The Pathology of Fishes*. WE Ribelin and G Migaki (eds), Madison, Univ of Wisconsin Press, pp. 3–30, 1975
5. Bellairs A d'A: *Reptiles*, London, Hutchison. 1957
6. Berg JW: Preface In *Comparative Morphology of Hematopoietic Neoplasms*, Nat Cancer Inst Monogr 32. 1969
7. Bond CE: Circulation, respiration, and the gas bladder In *Biology of Fishes, Sec 3*, Philadelphia, Saunders College Publishing, pp. 347–374. 1979
8. Boyland E: The correlation of experimental carcinogenesis and cancer in man In *Prog Exp Tumor Res*, vol II, Basel/N.Y., Karger, pp. 222–234. 1969
9. Burkitt D: Long-term remissions following one- and two-dose chemotherapy for African lymphoma, *Cancer* 20:756, 1967
10. Burkitt D: The African lymphoma – epidemiological and therapeutic aspects. In *Proceedings of the International Conference of Leukemia-Lymphoma*, C Zarafonetis (ed), Philadelphia, Lea and Febiger, pp. 194–206. 1968
11. Cameron AT, Vincent S: Notes on an enlarged thyroid occurring in an elasmobranch (*Squalus suckleyi*), *J Med Res* 27:251, 1915
12. Catton WT: Blood cell formation in certain teleost fishes. *Blood, J Hematol* 6:39, 1951
13. Conroy DA: Studies on the haematology of the Atlantic salmon (Salmo salar L.) In Diseases of Fish, LE Mawdesley-Thomas (ed) Symposia of the Zoological Society of London, No. 30, London, Academic Press, pp. 101–127. 1972
14. Cowan DF: Diseases of captive reptiles. *J Amer Vet Med Ass*, 153:848, 1968
15. Dawe CJ: Phylogeny and oncogeny In *Neoplasms and Related Disorders of Invertebrates and Lower Vertebrate Animals*, Nat Cancer Inst Monogr, 31:1, 1969a
16. Dawe CJ: Neoplasms of blood cell origin in poikilothermic animals – a review In *Comparative Morphology of Hematopoietic Neoplasms*, Nat Cancer Inst Monogr, 32:1, 1969b
17. Dawe CJ, Berard C: Workshop on comparative pathology of hematopoietic and lymphoreticular neoplasms, *J Nat Cancer Inst* 47:1365, 1971
18. Dorson M: Some characteristics of antibodies in the primary immune response of rainbow trout *Salmo gairdneri*. In *Diseases of Fish*, LE Mawdesley-Thomas (ed), Symposia of the Zoological Society of London, No. 30, London, Academic Press, pp. 129–140. 1972
19. Dunbar CE: Lymphosarcoma of possible thymic origin in salmonid fishes In *Neoplasms and Related Disorders of Invertebrates and Lower Vertebrate Animals*, Nat Cancer Inst Monogr, 31:167, 1969
20. Dunn TB: Natural and pathologic anatomy of the reticular tissue in laboratory mice, with a classification and discussion of neoplasms, *J Nat Cancer Inst* 14:1281, 1954
21. Dunn TB, Moloney JB: Pathogenesis of virus induced leukemia in rats In *The Morphological Precursors of Cancer*, Proc Int Conf Univ Perugia, pp. 259–268. 1961
22. Dunn TB, Moloney JB, Green AW, Arnold B: Pathogenesis of a virus-induced leukemia in mice, *J Nat Cancer Inst* 26:189, 1961
23. Duguy R: Number of blood cells and their variation In *Biology of the Reptilia, vol 3(C) Morphology*, New York, Academic Press, pp. 93–109. 1970
24. Effron H, Griner L, Benirschke K: Nature and rate of neoplasia in captive wild mammals, birds, and reptiles at necropsy, *J Nat Cancer Inst* 59:185, 1977
25. Ehlinger NF: Kidney disease in lake trout complicated by lymphosarcoma, *Prog Fish Cult* 25:3, 1963
26. Elkan E, Cooper J: Tumors and pseudotumors in some reptiles, *J Comp Pathol* 84:51, 1976
27. Ellerman E, Bang O: Experimentelle Leukemia bei Hühnern *Zentralbl Bakteriol* 46:595, 1908
28. Ellis AE: The immunology of teleosts In *Fish Pathology*, RJ Roberts (ed), London, Cassell Ltd, pp. 92–104, 1978
29. Epstein MA: Epstein–Barr Virus – discovery, properties and relationship to nasopharyngeal carcinoma. In *Nasopharyngeal Carcinoma: Aetiology and Control*, G DeThe, Y Ito, W Davis (eds), Lyon, IARC, p. 333–345. 1978
30. Epstein MA, Achong BG: (eds), In *The Epstein–Barr Virus*, Berlin, Springer, p. 321. 1976
31. Ferguson HW, Roberts RJ: Myeloid leucosis associated with sporozoan infection in cultured turbot (*Scophthalmus maximus L.*), *J Comp Pathol* 85:317, 1975
32. Finnie HEP: Lymphoid leukemia in an Indian python (*Python molurus*), *J Pathol* 107:1295, 1972
33. Frank W, Schepky A: Metastasierendes Lymphosarkom bei einer Riesenchlange, *Eunectes murinus (Linnaeus, 1758)*, *Pathol Vet* 6:437, 1969

34. Friedman LR: A study of normal and malignant thymus tissue of the teleost *Astyanax mexicanus* in tissue culture, *Bull Amer Mus Nat Hist* 124:69, 1962

35. Frye FL: Hematology of captive reptiles In *Zoo and Wild Animal Medicine*, ME Fowler (ed), Philadelphia, WB Saunders Co, pp. 146–150. 1978

36. Frye FL, Carney J: Acute lymphatic leukemia in a boa constrictor. *Vet Med Small Anim Clin* 68:653, 1973

37. Good RA, Finstad J: Essential relationship between the lymphatic system, immunity and malignancy In *Neoplasms and Related Disorders of Invertebrates and Lower Vertebrate Animals*, Nat Cancer Inst Monogr, 31:41, 1969

38. Griner LA: Hematopoietic neoplasia in animals of the San Diego Zoological Gardens, Int Symp Erkrankungen Zootiere, Berlin, Akademie der Wissenschaften der DDR. 1975

39. Grizzle JM, Rogers WA: Anatomy and Histology of the Channel Catfish, Auburn, Auburn Printing, Inc. 1976

40. Gross L: Pathogenic properties and "vertical" transmission of the mouse leukemia agent, *Proc Soc Expl Biol Med* 78:342, 1951

41. Haddow A, Blake I: Neoplasms in fish: A report of six cases with a summary of the literature. *J Path Bact* 36:41, 1933

42. Harshbarger JC: *Activities Report, Registry of Tumors in Lower Animals, 1965–1973*, Washington, DC, Smithsonian Inst. 1974

43. Harshbarger JC: *Activities Report, Registry of Tumors in Lower Animals, 1974 Supplement*, Washington, DC, Smithsonian Inst. 1975

44. Harshbarger JC: *Activities Report, Registry of Tumors in Lower Animals, 1975 Supplement*, Washington, DC, Smithsonian Inst. 1976

45. Harshbarger JC: *Activities Report, Registry of Tumors in Lower Animals, 1976 Supplement*, Washington, DC, Smithsonian Inst. 1977

46. Harshbarger JC: *Activities Report, Registry of Tumors in Lower Animals, 1977 Supplement*, Washington, DC, Smithsonian Inst. 1978

47. Harshbarger JC: *Activities Report, Registry of Tumors in Lower Animals, 1978 Supplement*, Washington, DC, Smithsonian Inst. 1979

48. Harshbarger JC: *Activities Report, Registry of Tumors in Lower Animals, 1979 Supplement*, Washington, DC, Smithsonian Inst. 1980

49. Harshbarger JC: *Activities Report, Registry of Tumors in Lower Animals, 1980 Supplement*, Washington, DC, Smithsonian Inst. 1981

50. Harshbarger JC: *Activities Report, Registry of Tumors in Lower Animals, 1981 Supplement*, Washington, DC, Smithsonian Inst. 1982

51. Harshbarger JC: *Activities Report, Registry of Tumors in Lower Animals, 1982–1983 Supplement*, Washington, DC, Smithsonian Inst. 1984

52. Harshbarger JC, Dawe C: Hematopoietic neoplasms in invertebrate and poikilothermic animals In *Unifying Concepts of Leukemia*, Bibl Haemat, No. 39, RM Dutcher and L Chieco-Bianchi (eds), Basel, Karger, pp. 1–25. 1973

53. Hess PW: Principles of cancer therapy, *Vet Clin North Amer* 7:21, 1977

54. Hickman LP, Andrew W: *Histology of the Vertebrate: A Comparative Text*, St Louis, CF Mosby Co. 1974

55. Hill HZ, Lin H: Carcinogenesis and tumor growth In *Clinical Pathology*, J Horton and GJ Hill (eds), Philadelphia, WB Saunders Co, pp. 1–33. 1977

56. Honma Y: Studies on the endocrine glands of the salmonoid fish, the ayu, *Plecoglossus altivelis* Temminck et Schlegal. VI. Effect of artificially controlled light on the endocrines of the pond-cultured fish, *Bull Jap Soc Scient Fish* 32:32, 1966

57. Honma Y, Hirosaki Y: Histopathology on the tumors and endocrine glands of the immature chum salmon, *Oncorhyn-chus keta*, reared in the Enoshima aquarium, *Jap J Ichthyol* 14:74, 1966

58. Hyman LH: The Invertebrates: Protozoa through Ctenophora, New York, McGraw Hill Book Co. 1940

59. Ippen R: Ein Beitrag zu den Spontantumoren bei Reptilien, 14th Int Symp Erkrankungen Zootiere, Berlin, Akademie der Wissenschaften der DDR. 1972

60. Jacobson ER: Virus associated neoplasms of reptiles In *Phyletic Approaches to Cancer*, CJ Dawe et al (eds), Tokyo, Japan Sci Soc Press, pp. 53–58. 1981

61. Jacobson ER: Neoplastic diseases In *Diseases of the Reptilia* CF Jackson, JC Cooper (eds), London, Academic Press, pp. 429–468. 1982

62. Jacobson E, Calderwood MB, French TW, Iverson W, Page D, Raphael B: Lymphosarcoma in an eastern king snake and a rhinoceros viper, *J Amer Vet Med Ass* 179:1231, 1981

63. Jacobson ER, Seely JC, Novilla MN: Lymphosarcoma associated with virus-like intranuclear inclusions in a California king snake (Colubridae: *Lampropeltis*), *J Nat Cancer Inst* 65:577, 1980

64. Jakowska S: Morphologie et nomenclature des cellules du sang des Teleosteens, *Rev Hematol* 11:519, 1956

65. Jarrett WFH, Martin WB, Crighton GW, Dalton RG, Stewart MM: Transmission experiments with leukemia (lymphosarcoma), *Nature* 202:566, 1964

66. Johnstone J: Internal parasites and diseased conditions of fishes, *Proc Trans Lpool Biol Soc* 26:103, 1912

67. Johnstone J: Diseased conditions in fishes. *Proc Trans Lpool Biol Soc* 38:183, 1924

68. Johnstone J: Malignant and other tumours in marine fishes, *Proc Trans Lpool Biol Soc* 40:75, 1926

69. Johnstone J: Diseased conditions in fishes, *Proc Trans Lpool Biol Soc* 41:162, 1927

70. Jordan HE: Comparative hematology In *Downey Handbook of Hematology*, vol 2, New York, Hoeber. 1938

71. Jungherr EL, Hughes WF: The avian leukosis complex In *Diseases of Poultry*, 5th ed, HE Biester, LH Schwarte (eds), Ames, Iowa State Univ Press, pp. 512–567. 1965

72. Kawakami TC, Theilen GH, Dungworth DL, Munn RJ, Beall SG: "C"-type viral particles in plasma of cats with feline leukemia, *Science* 158:1049, 1967

73. Klontz GW: Haematological techniques and the immune response in rainbow trout In *Diseases of Fish*, LE Mawdesley-Thomas (ed), Symposia of the Zoological Society of London, No. 30, London, Academic Press, pp. 89–99. 1972

74. Laskin S, Goldstein BD: (eds), *J Toxicol Environ Health*, Suppl. 2, Benzene Toxicity: A Critical Evaluation. 1977

75. Lawson R: A malignant neoplasm with metastases in the lizard, *Lacerta sicula cetti Cara.*, *Br J Herpet* 3:22, 1962

76. Lennert K, Mohri N, Stein H et al: The histopathology of malignant lymphoma, *Br J Haematol (Suppl)* 31:193, 1975

77. Ljungberg O, Lange J: Skin tumours of northern pike (*Esox lucius L.*) I. Sarcoma in a Baltic pike population, *Bull Off Int Epizoot* 69:1007, 1968

78. Lucké B, Schlumberger H: Neoplasia in cold-blooded vertebrates, *Physiol Rev* 29:91, 1949

79. Lukes RJ, Collins RD: Immunological characterization of human malignant lymphoma, *Cancer* 34:1488, 1974

80. Machotka SV: Neoplasia in reptiles In *Diseases of Amphibians and Reptiles*, J Hoff, F Frye, E Jacobson (eds), Oxford, Plenum Press, pp. 519–580. 1984

81. Machotka SV, Whitney GD: Neoplasms in snakes: Report of a probable mesothelioma and a thorough tabulation of earlier cases In *The Proceedings of the Symposium on the Comparative Pathology of Zoo Animals*, R Montali, G Migaki (eds), Washington, DC, Smithsonian Institution Press, pp. 593–602. 1980

82. Mawdesley-Thomas LE: Some tumours of fish In *Diseases of Fish*, LE Mawdesley-Thomas (ed), Symposia of the Zoologi-

cal Society of London, No. 30, London, Academic Press, pp. 191–283. 1972

83. Mawdesley-Thomas LE: Neoplasia in fish In *The Pathology of Fishes*, WE Ribelin, G. Migaki (eds), Madison, Univ of Wisconsin Press, pp. 805–870. 1975

84. Moldovanu G, Moore AE, Friedman MM, Miller DG: Cellular transmission of lymphosarcoma in dogs, *Nature* 210:1342, 1965

85. Mulcahy MF: Lymphosarcoma in the pike, *Esox lucius L.* (Pisces; Esocidae) in Ireland, *Proc R Ir Acad* (D) 63:103, 1963

86. Mulcahy MF: Blood values in the pike *Esox lucius L.*, *J Fish Biol* 2:203, 1970a

87. Mulcahy MF: The thymus gland and lymphosarcoma in the pike, *Esox lucius L.*, in Ireland, Proc Int Symp Comp Leukemia Res Bibliotheca Haemat, No. 4:600, 1970b

88. Mulcahy MF: Fish blood changes associated with disease: A hematological study of pike lymphoma and salmon ulcerative dermal necrosis In *The Pathology of Fishes*, WE Pinelin, G Minaki (eds), Madison, Univ Wisconsin Press, pp. 925–944. 1975

89. Mulcahy MF, O'Leary A: Cell-free transmission of lymphosarcoma in the northern pike, *Esox lucius L.* (Pisces; Esocidae), *Experimentia* 26:891, 1970

90. Mulcahy MF, O'Rourke FJ: Lymphosarcoma in the pike (*Esox lucius L.*) in Ireland, *Life Sciences* 3:719, 1964a

91. Mulcahy MF, O'Rourke FJ: Cancerous pike in Ireland, *Ir Nature* 14:312, 1964b

92. Mulcahy MF, Winqvist G, Dawe CJ: The neoplastic cell type in lymphoreticular neoplasms of the northern pike, *Esox lucius L.*, *Cancer Res* 30:2712, 1970

93. Nigrelli RF: Spontaneous neoplasms in fishes. III. Lymphosarcoma in *Astyanax* and *Esox*, *Zoologica* 32:101, 1947

94. Ohimacher H: Several examples illustrating the comparative pathology of tumors, *Bull Ohio Hosp Epilep* 1:223, 1898

95. Penn I: Tumors arising in organ transplant recipients. *Adv Cancer Res* 28:31, 1978

96. Plehn M: *Praktikum der Fischkrankheiten* (Practical handbook of fish diseases), Stuttgart, E Schweizerbarth, pp. 301–479. 1924

97. Rappaport H: Tumors of the hematopoietic system In *Atlas of Tumor Pathology*, Sec 3, Fas 8, Washington, DC, U.S. Armed Forces Institute of Pathology. 1966

98. Rappaport H, Winter WJ, Hicks EB: Follicular lymphoma. A reevaluation of its position in the scheme of malignant lymphoma, based on a survey of 253 cases, *Cancer* 9:792, 1956

99. Rasquin P, Hafter E: Response of a fish lymphosarcoma to mammalian ACTH. *Zoologica* 36:163, 1951

100. Rasquin P, Rosenbloom L: Endocrine imbalance and tissue hyperplasia in teleosts maintained in darkness, *Bull Am Mus Nat Hist* 104:359, 1954

101. Richard CG, Barr LM, Noronha F, Dougherty E II, Post JE: C-type virus particles in spontaneous lymphocytic leukemia in a cat, *Cornell Vet* 57:302, 1967

102. Ritchie RC, cited in Schlumberger HG: Tumors characteristic for certain animal species: A review, *Cancer Res* 17:823, 1957

103. Robinson PT, von Essen CF, Benirschke K et al: Radiation therapy for treatment of an intraoral lymphoma in an Indian rock python, *J Am Vet Radiol Soc* 19:92, 1978

104. Scarpelli DG: Comparative aspects of neoplasia in fish and other laboratory animals In *Fish in Research*, OW Neuhaus, JC Halver (eds), New York, Academic Press, pp. 45–85. 1969

105. Scharrer E: The histology of the meningeal myeloid tissue in the ganoids *Ania* and *Lepisosteus*, *Anat Rec* 88:291, 1944

106. Schlumberger HG: Tumors characteristic for certain animal species. A review, *Cancer Res* 17:823, 1957

107. Schlumberger HG, Lucké B: Tumors of fishes, amphibians, and reptiles. *Cancer Res* 8:657, 1948

108. Schroeders VD: Tumors of Fishes. Dissertations. (In Russian) St Petersburg. 1900

109. Scott HH, Beattie J: Neoplasm in a porose crocodile, *J Pathol Bacteriol* 30:61, 1927

110. Smith CE: An undifferentiated hematopoietic neoplasm with histologic manifestations of leukemia in a cutthroat trout (*Salmo clarki*), *J Fish Res Bd Canada* 28:112, 1971

111. Smith GM, Coates CW, Strong LC: Neoplastic diseases in small tropical fishes, *Zoologica* 21:219, 1936

112. Snell KC: Hematopoietic neoplasms of rats and mastomys In *Comparative Morphology of Hematopoietic Neoplasms* Nat Cancer Inst Monogr 32, pp. 59–63. 1969

113. Sobel HJ, Marquet E, Kallman K, Corlay G: Melanomas in platy/swordtail hybrids In *The Pathology of Fishes*, WE Ribelin, G Migaki (eds), Madison, Univ Wisconsin Press, pp. 945–981. 1975

114. Sonstegard R: Description and spizootiological studies of infectious pancreatic necrosis virus of salmonids and lymphosarcoma of *Esox masquinongy*, Ph.D. thesis, Ontario, Univ Guelph. 1971

115. Sonstegard R: Lymphosarcoma in muskellunge (*Esox masquinongy*) In *The Pathology of Fishes*, WE Ribelin, G Migaki (eds), Madison, Univ Wisconsin Press, pp. 907–924. 1975a

116. Sonstegard RA: Studies of the etiology and epizootiology of the lymphosarcoma in *Esox* (*Esox lucius* and *Esox masquinongy*), *Progr Exp Tumor Res* 20:141, 1975b

117. Sonstegard RA, Nielsen K, McDermott LA: Epizootiological evidence for a viral etiology of lymphosarcoma in *Esox*, Int Assoc Aquatic Ani med, Ontario, Univ Guelph. 1970

118. Stevens DA: Oncogenic herpes viruses: A selective review and their possible implications for Hodgkin's Disease In *International Symposium on Hodgkin's Disease, Nat Cancer Inst Monogr* 36:55, 1973

119. Suet-Moldavsky GJ, Trubchoninova L, Ravina L: Pathoganicity of the chicken sarcoma virus (Schmidt–Ruppin) for amphibians and reptiles, *Nature* 214:300, 1967

120. Swaen GJV: Development of thymic neoplasms in rats inoculated with a murine leukemia virus (Rauscher), *J Nat Cancer Inst* 36:1027, 1966

121. Takahashi K: Studie über die Fischgeschwülste, *Z Krebsforsch* 29:1, 1929

122. Trubcheninova LP, Knutoryansky A, Svet-Moldvasky G, Kuznetsova L, Sokolov P, Belianchykova N: Body temperature and tumor virus infection. I. Tumorigenicity of Rous-sarcoma virus for reptiles, *Neoplasma* 24:13, 1977

123. Upton AC: Radiation In Cancer Medicine, 2nd ed, TF Holland, E Frei III (eds), Philadelphia, Lea and Febiger, Chap 1–6, pp. 96–109. 1982

124. Veskova TK, Trubeninova L, Dook L: Tumors in reptiles inoculated with chicken Rous sarcoma material, *Folia Biologica (Praka)* 16:353, 1970

125. Watson LJ, Schechmeister IL, Jackson LL: The hematology of goldfish, *Crassius auratus*, *Cytologia* 28:118, 1963

126. Weinberg SR, Siegal CD, Nigrelli RF, Gordon AS: The hematological parameters and blood cell morphology of the brown bullhead catfish, *Ictalurus nebulosus* (*Lesueur*), *Zoologica* 57:71, 1972

127. Weinreb EL: Studies on the fine structure of teleost blood cells. I. Peripheral blood, *Anat Rec* 147:219, 1963

128. Wellings SR: Neoplasia and primitive vertebrate phylogeny: echinoderms, prevertebrates, and fishes – a review In Neoplasms and related disorders of invertebrates and lower vertebrate animals, *Nat Inst Monogr* 31:59, 1969

129. Wessing A, von Bargen G: Untersuchungen uber einem virusbedingten tumor bei fischen (studies on a tumor caused by a virus in fish), *Arch ges Virusforsch* 9:521, 1959

130. Williams G: On various fish tumors, *Proc Trans Lpool Biol Soc* 45:98, 1931

131. Willis RA: Pathology of Tumors, 4th ed, London, Butter-

worth, p. 1019. 1967

132. Winqvist G, Ljungberg O, Hellstroem B: Skin tumors of northern pike (*Esox lucius L.*) II. Viral particles in epidermal proliferations, *Bull Off Int Epizoot* 69:1023, 1968

133. Winqvist G, Ljungberg O, Ivarsson B: Electron microscopy of sarcoma of the northern pike (*Esox lucius L.*) In Unifying Concepts of Leukemia, Bibl haemat No. 39, RM Dutcher, L Chieco-Bianchi (eds), Basel, Karger, pp. 26–30. 1973

134. Wolke RE, Wyand DS: Ocular lymphosarcoma of an Atlantic cod, *Bull Wildl Dis Ass* 5:401, 1969

135. Wright DH, Bell TM, Williams MC: Burkitt's tumor: a review of clinical features, treatment, pathology, epidemiology, entomology, and virology, *East Afr Med J* 44:51, 1967

136. Yunis JJ, Oken MM, Kaplan ME, Ensrud KM, Howe RR, Theologides A: Distinctive chromosomal abnormalities in histologic subtypes of non-Hodgkin's lymphomas. *N Engl M Jed* 307:1231, 1982

137. Zwart P, Harshbarger J: Hematopoietic neoplasms in lizards: report of a typical case in *Hydrosaurus amboiensis* and of a probable case in *Varanus salvator, Int J Cancer* 9:548, 1972

12

SPREAD AND METASTASIS OF TUMORS IN BIRDS

T.N. FREDRICKSON

Several difficulties present themselves in attempting to give
an account of how avian cancer spreads from the primary to
distant metastatic sites. Avian pathologists have concentrated most of their efforts on the virally-induced hematopoietic neoplasms which are the commercially important
diseases among chickens. Also, avian pathologists have had
only relatively young birds to examine because in commercial operations chickens are killed far short of their potential
life span of about 15 years. This may be the reason that
so few tumors of epithelial origin have been described in
chickens, with certain exceptions, although it is more
probable that it reflects a true difference in the incidence of
epithelial tumors compared to those of mammals. Thus
cases of cancer of the lungs, intestinal tract and integument,
which are not uncommon among mammals, have amounted
to only a handful of cases in the avian literature. In the face
of these difficulties this chapter attempts to: 1) cite from the
literature observations on the occurrence of epithelial
tumors among birds particularly those referring to
metastases; 2) describe certain aspects of the spread of
hematopoietic tumors in chickens; 3) describe the spread of
the two common epithelial tumors in chickens; 4) and,
finally, to point out how the bird might make an interesting
subject for work on metastatic spread of tumors.

As mentioned, the lack of substantial reports on epithelial
tumors in birds is quite apparent from a perusal of the
literature. Most reports are surveys of cases coming into
diagnostic laboratories so it is impossible to know precisely
what the general incidence of any type is among avian
populations.

In their review of the literature on avian neoplasms,
Feldman and Olson (5) cite references to two metastatic
renal carcinomas, three intestinal carcinomas, a single
pulmonary adenocarcinoma and three squamous cell
carcinomas of the skin. The very few reported cases on
record led these authors to conclude that, "In chickens the
lymphatic route of metastasis is apparently little utilized. As
a matter of fact, true metastasis as a consequence of the
conveyance of tumor cells from one situation to another by
way of vascular channels seldom occurs." There seem to
have been no reports since these words were written more
than 30 years ago to raise doubts regarding their accuracy.
Lesbouyries, writing about the same time, noted that the
lack of development of the lymphatic system in chickens did
not favour lymphatogenous spread of metastases (10). In a
description of pulmonary adenocarcinoma in birds Stewart
notes that, "Several tumors metastasized to the liver and one
to the nasal bones" (16). In their review of tumors in domestic and zoo ducks Ridgon and Leibovitz (14) cite reports of
two metastatic hepatocellular carcinomas, an osteogenic
sarcoma and a melanoma. A similar review of spontaneous
tumors in cage birds by Blackmore (1) cites 17 metastatic
tumors of a total of 168 seen in budgerigars including a
squamous cell carcinoma of skin, hepatocellular carcinoma,
two leiomyosarcomas of the spleen, two nephroblastomas
and ten testicular tumors. All those of testicular origin were
reported to have metastasized to the liver but it is not clear
if this occurred by extension, via lymphatics or hematoge-
nously. One of the few photomicrographs of obvious
pulmonary metastases of a spontaneous avian tumor is
included in a report on hepatic tumors by Wadsworth et al.
(18).

The viral aspect considerably hampers studies on
metastatic spread since one cannot be sure if tumors arising
at sites distant from the primary resulted from cellular
spread or from infection of cells at the distant sites by virus.
This dilemma casts considerable doubt on the experimental
investigation of the spread of tumors induced by Rous
sarcoma virus (RSV), a point considered in a report of such
a study (3). On the other hand, there are avian tumor viruses
with a restricted range in target cells, unlike RSV which
transforms fibroblasts anywhere in the body. These more
selective oncogenic viruses mainly transform cells of the
hematopoietic system. For myeloid and erythroid cells
transformed by avian myeloblastosis (AMV) or erythroblastosis (AEV) viruses, respectively, it is clear that foci of
transformed blast cells appear first in the bone marrow (8).
From there the leukemic cells enter the blood with stasis
occurring almost exclusively in the spleen and liver. In the
case of B cell lymphomas, induced with avian leukosis viruses (ALV), transformation occurs within follicles of the
bursa of Fabricius from where they disseminate in the
blood, mainly to the liver, spleen, kidney and gonads. It is
clear from ablation studies that the bursa, not the bone
marrow, is the site of tranformation (13). It remains unclear
if the thymus is required for transformation of T lymphocytes by Marek's disease virus (12) in which neoplastic
cells are widespread in liver, spleen, kidney, gonads, dermis,
the nervous system and skeletal muscles. Destructive lesions
are seen in the nervous system and within feather follicles so
localization of lymphoid cells at these sites may be reactive
rather than infiltrative (2). Neither T nor B lymphomas are
uniformly characterized by a leukemic phase as are myeloblastosis and erythroblastosis. In an unusual type of virally-
induced leukemia, myelocytomatosis, solid tumors, composed of myelocytes or metamyelocytes, form on the surface

H. E. Kaiser (ed.), Comparative aspects of tumor development.
© 1989, Kluwer Academic Publishers, Dordrecht. ISBN-13:978-0-89838-994-4

bones as well as the infiltrates commonly seen around the portal triads of the liver (8).

There are two exceptions to the general rule that cancer originating from epithelial tissue occurs at a very low rate in birds. These exceptions are adenocarcinomas of the oviduct and ovary, both of which are highly malignant and probably occur in all species of birds. The incidence of these genital cancers can be up to 25% in chickens by the time they have reached 5 years of age (7). The mode of spread is by abdominal seeding onto serosal surfaces of particularly the mesentery, bowel wall, ovary and oviduct. Even in cases which are not advanced, extensive seeding can have occurred. Since almost all oviductal adenocarcinomas originate from albumin secreting glands, seeding follows only after penetration of the muscularis of the oviduct. The ovary in birds is attached to the lumbar vertebrae which may facilitate abdominal seeding. Particularly striking in these cases is the aggressive infiltration of tumor tissue into the mesentery and bowel wall, causing a reactive growth of fibrous connective tissue and smooth muscle resulting in thickening of the bowel wall and shortening of the mesentery. In advanced cases the entire intestinal tract may be drawn up into a compact ball so that affected chickens die of starvation. Despite this extensive spread hematogenous or lymphatic spread occurs rarely, if at all, although there is one reference to lung metastases in a flamingo with ovarian adenocarcinoma (17).

Another exception to the low incidence of epithelial tumors is the relatively large number of renal tumors seen in budgerigars. A report on these and other budgerigar tumors (11) indicated that a relatively high proportion of renal adenocarcinomas spread to the liver but it is not clear whether this is by metastases or simply by peritoneal implantation.

The conclusion one faces is that there is relatively little that can be added to the understanding of tumor metastases through the study of avian cancer. However, this probably reflects neglect of the subject rather than a failure in its potential to give some interesting insights. Two aspects would seem to make exploitation of this model system worthwhile. The first concerns the differences between the mammalian and avian lymphoid systems. Lack of avian lymph nodes, with the duck being somewhat of an exception, presents a chance to assess the importance of these organs in metastatic spread of cancer. Avian model systems present a sort of negative control in such an assessment. Secondly, there are avian retroviruses which do induce epithelial tumors, most notably MC29 which gives about 30% hepatocellular carcinomas in chickens (9). These do metastasize to the lungs, apparently by the hematogenous route. The ease and speed with which they can be induced would seem to make them ideal for a model system.

Another experimental approach in the study of metastatic spread of tumor cells in chickens has employed transplantation of Marek's disease lymphoma cells in either syngeneic (6) or histoincompatible (4) recipients. Similar studies have been carried out using a transmissible lymphoid tumor originally induced with ALV (15). These experiments have explored factors associated with the spread of virally-induced lymphoid neoplasms and they do point to the possibility of using transplant systems in birds for other types of studies.

References

1. Blackmore DK: The clinical approach to tumors in cage birds. I. The pathology and incidence of neoplasia in cage birds. *J Small Anim Pract.* 7:217, 1966
2. Calnek BW, Witter RL: Marek's Disease. In *Diseases of Poultry*, Hofstad MS (ed.), 8th ed., p. 325, Iowa State University Press, Ames, Iowa, 1984
3. Collins WM, Brown DW, Ward PH, Dunlop WR, Briles WE: MHC and non-MHC genetic influences on Rous sarcoma metastasis in chickens. *Immunogenetics* 22:315, 1985
4. Fabricant J, Clanek BW, Schat KA, Murthy KK: Marek's disease virus-induced tumor transplants: Development and rejection in various genetic strains of chickens. *Avian Dis.* 22:646, 1978
5. Feldman WH, Olson C: *Neoplastic diseases in chickens*. In Diseases of Poultry, Biester HE and Schwarte LH (eds.), 3rd ed., p. 711, Iowa State College Press, Ames, Iowa, 1952
6. Fletcher OJ, Schierman LW: Variation in histology and growth characteristics of transplantable Marek's disease lymphomas. *Cancer Res.* 45:1762, 1985
7. Fredrickson TN, Hemlboldt CF: Tumors of Unknown Etiology. In *Diseases of Poultry*, Hofstad MS (ed.), 8th ed., p. 420, Iowa State University Press, Ames, Iowa, 1984
8. Helmboldt CF, Fredrickson TN: The pathology of avian leukemia. In *Experimental Leukemia*, Rich MA (ed.), p. 233, Appleton-Century-Crofts, New York, 1968
9. Lapis K: Histology and ultrastructural aspects of virus-induced primary liver cancer and transplantable hepatomas of viral origin in chickens. *J. Toxicol. Environ. Health* 5:469, 1979
10. Lesbouyries G: In *La Pathologie des Oiseaux*, p. 143, Vigot Freres, Paris, France, 1941
11. Neumann U, Kummerfeld N: Neoplasms in budgerigars (*Melopsittacus undulatus*): Clinical, pathomorphological and serological findings with special considerations of kidney tumors. *Avian Pathol.* 12:353, 1983
12. Payne LN, Frazier JA, Powell PC: Pathogenesis of Marek's disease. *Int Rev Exp Pathol.* 16:59, 1976
13. Peterson RD, Burmester BR, Fredrickson TN, Good RA: Prevention of lymphatic leukemia in the chicken by the surgical removal of the bursa of Fabricius. *J Lab Clin Med.* 62:1000, 1963
14. Rigdon RH, Leibovitz L: Spontaneous-occurring tumors in the duck. Review of the literature and report of three cases. *Avian Dis.* 14:431, 1970
15. Spencer JL, Gavora JS, Grunder AA, Robertson A, Speckman GW: Studies on genetic and vaccination-induced resistance of chickens to lymphoid tumor transplants. 2. Transmissible lymphoid tumors of Olson. *Avian Dis.* 20:286, 1976
16. Stewart HL: Pulmonary cancer and adenomatosis in captive wild mammals and birds from the Philadelphia zoo. *J Nat'l. Cancer Inst.* 36:117, 1966
17. Wadsworth PF, Jones DM: An ovarian adenocarcinoma in a greater flamingo (*Phoenicopterus ruber roseus*). *Avian Pathol.* 10:91, 1981
18. Wadsworth PF, Majeed SK, Brancker WM, Jones DM: Some hepatic neoplasms in non-domesticated birds. *Avian Path.* 7:551, 1978

13

PROGRESSION OF AVIAN LYMPHOID LEUKOSIS

H. GRAHAM PURCHASE

ABSTRACT

The leukosis/sarcoma viruses, members of the avian oncornavirus or oncovirus group, cause a wide spectrum of tumors in chickens. The most common under field conditions is lymphoid leukosis, a B-cell lymphoma. In susceptible chickens infected at an early age, cells of the cortex of the bursa of Fabricius of 6- to 8-week-old chickens transform and proliferate until the whole follicle is filled with transformed lymphoblasts. At about sexual maturity (18 to 20 weeks) the cells in some bursa follicles burst into the blood vessels and metastasize to other organs causing death. In other follicles the incipient tumors regress. Regression is likely enhanced by testosterone, and inhibited by the immunosuppressive effect of the virus and the tumor. Immune response genes may play a role. Resistance to tumor development in chickens susceptible to infection but genetically resistant to tumor formation could be mediated through regression of *in situ* tumors.

INTRODUCTION

There are four groups of viruses that cause tumors in avians. The herpesvirus of *Marek's disease* is likely the most common. This DNA-containing virus produces T-cell lymphomas in chickens and is the cause of severe economic loss worldwide.

The remaining 3 groups are members of the avian type C oncoviruses or retroviruses. *Turkey lymphoproliferative disease* is an RNA tumor virus of this group because it resembles these viruses morphologically and contains an RNA-dependent DNA polymerase. To date, Koch's postulates have not been fulfilled, and the virus has not yet been cultivated *in vitro*.

Reticuloendotheliosis viruses cause acute reticulum cell neoplasia, runting and chronic neoplasia of lymphoid and other tissues of chickens, turkeys, ducks, and quails. The virus can cause B-cell neoplasms in chickens.

The *leukosis/sarcoma* viruses belong to the same family as lymphoproliferative disease and reticuloendotheliosis; namely, the retroviridae. This group of viruses causes a broad spectrum of tumors as illustrated in Figure 1.

The types of tumor induced are dependent on the virus strain, the host, and the dose and route of administration of the virus. The tumor or tissue from which the virus was obtained and the passage history of the virus are important in determining the virus strain. Thus, virus preparations

Embryonic layer	Prototype strains[1] and characterizing neoplasms					
	RPL 12	BAI A	MC 29	R	MH2	RSV, OCS VII
Mesoderm						
Mesenchyme						
Sarcoma	■	■	■	■	■	■
Chondroma			■			■
Osteochondrosarcoma						■
Osteopetrosis						
Endothelioma			■		■	■
Mesothelioma[2]			■			
Meningioma[3]						
Hemangioma	■		■	■	■	■
Hemopoietic tissue						
Erythroblastosis	■		■	■	■	
Myeloblastosis		■				
Myelocytomatosis			■			
Monocytosis (?)[4]					■	
Lymphomatosis	■					■
Kidney						
Nephroblastoma[5]		■				
Adenocarcinoma[6]			■		■	
Ovary						
Thecoma		■				
Granulosa cell		■				
Testis						
Carcinoma			■			
Endoderm						
Liver						
Hepatocytoma[7]			■		■	
Pancreas					■	
Ectoderm						
Epithelioma[8]	■		■		■	
Glioma[9]						

Figure 1. Oncogenic spectrum of selected avian leukosis viruses. Black bars represent a response of that type. (Modified from Beard 1980, Raven Press.)

[1] RPL 12: Regional Poultry Laboratory strain 12, BAI A: Bureau of Animal Industry strain A, Myeloblastosis; MC29: myelocytomatosis; R: erythroblastosis; MH2: Mill Hill strain 2, Murray-Beg virus; RSV: Rous sarcoma virus; OCS VII: osteochondrosarcoma (Tyler).

[2] Metaplastic epithelial and chondromal derivatives of peritoneal, pericardial, and epicardial squamous mesothelium.

[3] Growths of meninges of mesodermal derivation induced in chickens by intracerebral inoculation of RSV and other sarcoma strains. Neurogenic growths of ectodermal origin are not produced in the chicken.

[4] Leukemia of not fully identified cells associated with MH2 strain infection.

[5] Highly complex spectrum of adenoma and carcinoma of glomerular and tubular structures, mesenchymoma, osteoma, chondroma, keratosis, and spindle cell sarcoma.

[6] Spectrum includes cystadenoma and tubular and glomerular adenocarcinoma and carcinoma, with occasional chondroma.

[7] Hepatic growths of multiple variety, trabecular carcinoma, adenocarcinoma, mosaic type growths, hepatobiliary tumors, hemorrhagic carcinoma, rifted hepatoma, chondroma, and sarcoma derived by transformation of hepatic cells in birds infected with strain MC29 virus. Adenocarcinomas and solid carcinomas of hepatocyte derivation were induced by the MH2 agent.

[8] Squamous-cell carcinoma of skin.

[9] Astrocytoma, ependymoma, oligodendroglioma, ganglioglioma.

H. E. Kaiser (ed.), Comparative aspects of tumor development.

from one type of tumor are more likely to cause that type of tumor in recipients than other types of tumors. High doses of virus tend to cause erythroblastosis, sarcomas and hemangiomas and low doses tend to cause lymphoid leukosis (LL). Subcutaneous injection causes sarcomas and intravenous injection erythroblastosis and hemangiomas. The genetic background, age, and sex of the host influence the types of tumors greatly. Thus, chickens may be genetically resistant to virus infection or to tumor development. Genetically susceptible chickens are most likely to develop tumors if they are infected in the first few days after hatching. Resistance to LL tumor development is almost complete if they are not infected till they are 3 weeks old. Thus, age resistance develops more rapidly with natural routes of infection (oral, nasal, or ocular) than with artificial routes (intravascular or intravenous). Females are more susceptible to LL than males. Under natural conditions chicks are likely infected with a low dose of virus by a natural route several days after hatching. Therefore, under natural conditions, avian leukosis/sarcoma viruses induce mainly LL.

The leukosis/sarcoma viruses are divided into subgroups A through F based on envelope glycoproteins as determined by neutralization of the virus, ability of the virus to infect genetically susceptible or resistant cells and the ability of one virus to interfere with infection by a virus of the same subgroup. These subgroup classifications, with the exception of subgroup E endogenous viruses, have no relationship to the pathogenicity of the viruses (16). Endogenous viruses have little, if any, oncogenic potential.

Epizootology of avian leukosis virus infections

Most chicken flocks worldwide are infected with the virus (usually of subgroup A or B). The virus is spread vertically from parent to offspring through the egg. This is the main means of persistence of the virus in nature and is the basis for the widespread attempt of poultry breeders to reduce or eliminate exogenous ALV. The virus is poorly contagious but does spread horizontally, particularly in young chicks when crowded together. Infection of genetically susceptible chicks with sufficient virus at an early age results in death from LL at any time after 14 weeks of age. The incidence is usually highest at about sexual maturity (20 weeks of age).

Even though infection with the virus is widespread, most susceptible chickens do not succumb to LL. Some chickens are genetically resistant to infection with avian leukosis viruses. The level of genetic resistance varies from one line of chicken to another. Sometimes chickens may be infected but the virus may not integrate into the bursal DNA. The target cell for transformation may have been destroyed by artificial (chemical or surgical bursectomy) or natural (infectious bursal disease virus infection) means. It is also possible that in some lines of chickens bursa cells are less capable of transformation (17). If transformation does occur, it is possible that the tumors regress rather than progress (7).

Target cells for transformation

It is clear that the target cell for transformation is a bursa-dependent lymphoid cell because removal of the bursa prevents LL, and reimplantation of viable cells from genetically susceptible chickens but not from genetically resistant chickens reconstitutes the ability to develop LL (15, 17). Also, surgical bursectomy between 1 day and 5 months of age (13), treatment of embryos or hatched chicks with androgens (6) or androgen analogs (11), chemical bursectomy (15) and infection with infectious bursal disease virus (14) eliminates LL. Cells of LL tumors have B cell markers and IgM on their surface (8, 12). The target cells for LL transformation are not B stem cells because the target cells for LL can be eliminated by chemical treatment without affecting the ability of the chicken to produce immunoglobulin or antibody (15). Therefore, the target cells must be B-cells that have differentiated to some extent but have not left the bursa of Fabricius.

Regression of LL tumors

Transformation of cells in the follicles of the bursa of Fabricius is a prerequisite to development of LL. Thus bursectomy eliminates LL, transformed cells can be seen on microscopic examination of bursa follicles from infected chickens but not from control chickens, transformed cells only occur in organs where the primary lymphoid tumor is found, all tumors outside the bursa are of B cells and therefore must have originated from the bursa, and cells from these tumors have the same morphology as transformed follicles in the bursa. The first transformation of cells in the follicles occurs as early as 8 weeks after infection of susceptible 1-day old chickens (7). On histologic examination, tumors appear to originate in the follicular cortex (see Figures 2 and 3). It is highly unlikely that the focal areas of transformed cells seen in the cortex are a result of metastasis because these are the first lesions seen, and because metastasis to other organs does not occur until very much later (7). These focal areas enlarge and invade the medulla. Eventually the entire follicle is composed of masses of highly uniform, transformed lymphoblasts.

At about the time of sexual maturity (18 to 20 weeks of age), the transformed cells are assumed to metastasize by bursting out of the bursa follicles into the circulation. Maximum regression of the bursa also occurs at sexual maturity so it is also possible that transformed cells accompany stem cells and B cells emigrating from the bursa. In birds that die from LL some time after sexual maturity it is sometimes difficult to find a tumor in the bursa and sometimes even the bursal remnant cannot be found. Further studies of the dynamics and mechanism of metastasis are needed.

When groups of infected chickens were examined for the presence of transformed follicles at different ages, a higher proportion of birds had transformed follicles at 16 weeks of age than had transformed follicles at 32 weeks of age and more birds had transformed follicles at 16 weeks of age than subsequently died of LL (7). Thus there was focal transformation in 70 percent of the birds yet only 40 percent died or had evidence of tumors when killed. Thus many birds must have had tumors that regressed. Commercial chickens which are susceptible to virus infection often do not develop LL and it is likely that the same regression mechanism is responsible for the low incidence of LL in commercial flocks. It is also possible that in genetically resistant com-

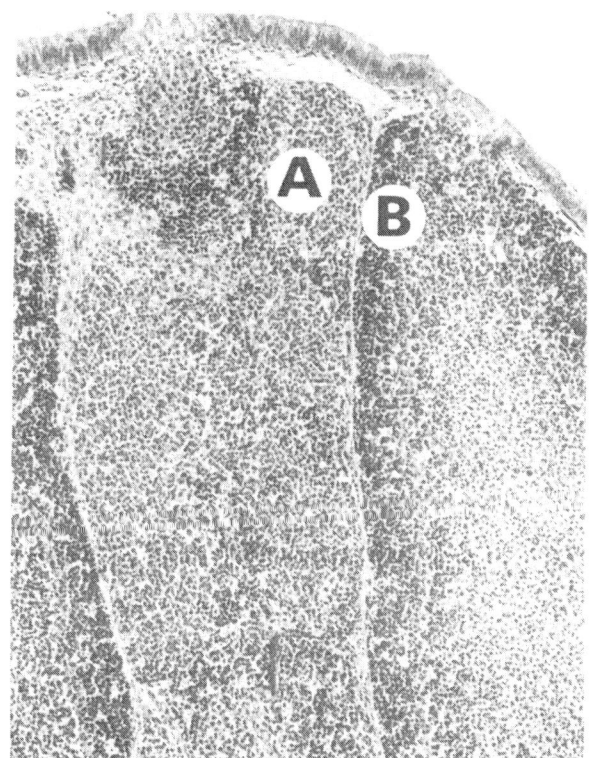

Figure 2. Low power photomicrograph of bursa of Fabricius with normal follicles at left and right and a follicle with about 6 foci of cortical transformation in the center. Neoplastic follicle (A) can easily be distinguished from normal cortex (B) by size of cells, uniformity of cells and intensity of staining. (Photograph is 900 μm wide.).

mercial flocks, fewer follicles transform. Thus transformation was detected in 82 percent of susceptible but only 11 percent of resistant commercial chickens (2). A reduction in metastasis could also be responsible (1).

The mechanism by which regression of LL tumors is induced has not been studied. Regression occurs more frequently in males than females. Thus, even though transformation occurred as frequently in males as in females, death occurred more frequently in females (7). Also, regression of the bursa occurred 1 week earlier in males than females. It is possible that this could be due to the direct effect of testosterone on the tumor cells or, more likely, the effect of testosterone on B cells in general.

Because LL tumors originate from B cells, it is possible that interference with humoral immunity may result in progression whereas a normal immune response results in regression. This hypothesis is unlikely because it has been very difficult to demonstrate any depression in humoral immune response except in those chickens that are in very advanced stages of disease (8, 10). Thus tumor cells have detectable surface IgM and variable amounts of cytoplasmic IgM. In some birds, there are high levels of IgM in the serum and the IgM is electrophoretically heterogeneous indicating that the tumors are polyclonal. The humoral response to red blood cells is increased (8) but to *Brucella* abortus, bovine serum albumin and keyhole limpit hemocyanin is depressed (10).

Some birds develop multiple foci of transformation in the bursa. It is likely that in at least some of them, the tumors that develop are clonal, i.e., only one tumor progresses per animal (1). In these animals, it is likely that all the tumors except one regress. The more transformed follicles there are within a bursa, the greater the probability that one of them will progress to neoplasia.

It is likely that, in a manner similar to homograft rejection, the cell-mediated immune response is accountable for tumor regression. The thymus alloantigen locus, Th-1 has

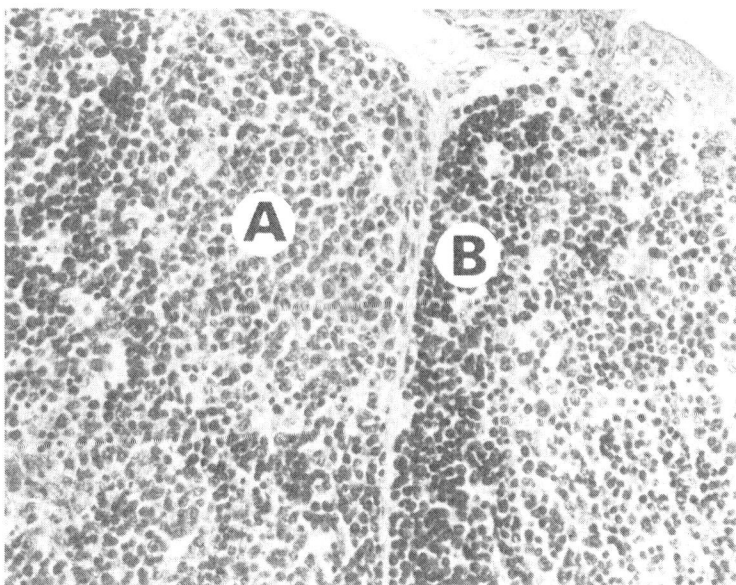

Figure 3. Higher magnification of the same bursa as in Figure 2, showing focus of transformed cells (A), and normal cortex in cells (B). (Photograph is 450 μm wide.).

been shown to influence the onset of lymphoma, and there are indications that only one subset of T lymphocytes, possibly suppressor T cells affecting immune function or B cell lymphomagenesis, is responsible (3). The major histocompatibility complex (*B*) haplotype also appears to influence the development of tumors induced by ALV, particularly erythroblastosis and to a lesser extent LL (4). This aspect needs further study.

CONCLUSION

Two levels of genetic resistance to development of LL tumors have been described. At the first level, all the cells of the chicken are resistant to infection with the virus. Thus, the chicken does not become infected, does not develop tumors, and may not even develop antibody. The frequencies of the alleles for resistance to infection vary greatly among commercial lines of chickens.

At the second level of resistance, the cells of the chicken are susceptible to infection, but tumors do not develop. This resistance is conferred by the bursa cells and not by thymic or thymus-derived cells or non-lymphocytes (17). The resistance could be mediated by resistance of the bursa cell to integration of viral DNA, to resistance of the bursa cell to transformation by integrated virus or to regression of tumors. Of these alternatives, only regression has been demonstrated though this does not preclude the other alternatives. The ability of commercial chickens to regress LL tumors may be economically exceedingly important.

REFERENCES

1. Baba TW, Humphries EH: Avian leukosis viral infection: analysis of viremia and DNA integration in susceptible and resistant chicken lines, *J Virol* 51:123, 1984
2. Baba TW, Humphries EH: Formation of a transformed follicle is necessary but not sufficient for development of an avian leukosis virus-induced lymphoma, *Proc Nat Acad Sci USA* 82:213, 1985
3. Bacon LD, Fredericksen TL, Gilmour DG, Fadly AM, Crittenden LB: Tests of Association of Lymphocyte Alloantigen Genotypes with Resistance to Viral Oncogenesis in Chickens 2. Rous Sarcoma and Lymphoid Leukosis in Progeny Derived from $6_3 \times 15_1$ and $100 \times 6_3$ Crosses[1], *Poultry Science* 64:39, 1984
4. Bacon LD, Witter RL, Crittenden LB, Fadly A, Motta J: *B*-Haplotype Influence on Marek's Disease, Rous Sarcoma, and Lymphoid Leukosis Virus-Induced Tumors in Chickens, *Poultry Science* 60:1132, 1981
5. Beard JW: Biology of Avian Oncornaviruses. In Klein G, (Ed.), *Viral Oncology* pp. 55–87, Raven Press, New York, NY, 1980
6. Burmester BR: The prevention of lymphoid leukosis with androgens, *Poultry Science* 48:401, 1969
7. Cooper MD, Payne LN, Dent PB, Burmester BR, Good, RA: Pathogenesis of avian lymphoid leukosis. I Histogenesis, *J Nat Cancer Inst* 41:373, 1968
8. Cooper MD, Purchase HG, Bockman DE, Gathings WE: Studies on the nature of the abnormality of B cell differentiation in avian lymphoid leukosis: production of heterogeneous IgM by tumor cells, *J Immunology* 113:1210, 1974
9. Crittenden LB: Two levels of genetic resistance to lymphoid leukosis, *Avian Dis* 19:281, 1975
10. Dent PB, Cooper MD, Payne LN, Solomon JJ, Burmester BR, Good RA: Pathogenesis of avian lymphoid leukosis. II Immunologic reactivity during lymphomagenesis, *J Nat Cancer Inst* 41:391, 1968
11. Kakuk TJ, Frank FR, Weddon TE, Burmester BR, Purchase HG, Romero CH: Avian lymphoid leukosis prophylaxis with mibolerone, *Avian Dis* 21:280, 1977
12. Payne LN, Rennie M: B cell markers on avian lymphoid leukosis tumor cells, *Vet Record* 96:454, 1975
13. Peterson RDA, Purchase HG, Burmester BR, Cooper MD, Good RA: Relationships among lymphomatosis, bursa of Fabricius, and bursa-dependent lymphoid tissue of the chicken, *J Nat Cancer Inst* 36:585, 1966
14. Purchase HG, Cheville NF: Infectious bursal agent of chickens reduces the incidence of lymphoid leukosis, *Avian Pathol* 4:239, 1975
15. Purchase HG, Gilmour DG: Lymphoid leukosis in chickens chemically bursectomized and subsequently inoculated with bursa cells, *J Natl Cancer Inst* 55:851, 1975
16. Purchase HG, Payne LN: Leukosis/sarcoma group In: *Diseases of Poultry*, 8th edition, 360–405, Iowa State University Press, Ames, Iowa, 1984
17. Purchase HG, Gilmour DG, Romero CH, Okazaki W: Postinfection genetic resistance to avian lymphoid leukosis resides in B target cell, *Nature* 270:61, 1977

14

IMMUNOLOGIC ASPECTS OF NEOPLASTIC PROGRESSION IN MAREK'S DISEASE

J.M. SHARMA

INTRODUCTION

A naturally occurring herpesvirus is ubiquitous among chickens and causes a progressive neoplastic disease. This disease, termed Marek's disease (MD) after its discoverer, Joseph Marek (49), is a neurologic disorder characterized by accumulation of proliferated lymphoid cells in peripheral nerves and other organs. Initially, the disease was considered a polyneuritis, although later studies established that in addition to being an inflammatory condition, the disease also has a neoplastic component. In susceptible chickens, solid lymphoid tumors are a common lesion associated with this disease.

Although MD was first recognized at the turn of the century, it appeared only sporadically for over 50 years. In the 1960s, when intensive poultry rearing practices became common, the incidence of MD increased, quickly reaching epidemic proportions. Increased disease incidence and associated economic losses to the poultry industry stimulated a great deal of research interest in this disease. The discovery in 1967–68 of the etiologic agent of MD ushered in an era of extensive research on all aspects of this disease. The labors of research were rapidly rewarded by the development of highly successful commercial vaccines that dramatically reduced the incidence of this disease in the chicken population. To date, MD remains the only naturally occurring viral neoplastic disease of any animal species against which there is a highly effective prophylactic vaccine. Despite vaccine control, MD continues to be widely studied for two main reasons. First, sporadic but significant economic losses due to MD continue to occur, ableit at much lower levels than in the pre-vaccine era, and there is a need for improved control. Second, MD is an interesting naturally occurring herpesvirus tumor model that can be readily reproduced experimentally and there is hope that the information obtained in MD will be of value in understanding and control of other viral neoplasms.

As is typical of herpes viruses, exposure to MDV leads to persistent infection of the host with the virus. In genetically resistant or vaccinated chickens, infection may not result in clinical disease although the chickens become permanent carriers of the virus. Exposure of susceptible chickens to virulent MDV results in a rapid series of events that leads to

progressive neoplastic lesions and death. For instance, if the exposure occurs at hatch, the infected chickens develop widespread lymphoid cell proliferation and solid tumors, and death usually occurs within 4–6 weeks of age. In this relatively short course of the disease, the chickens respond immunologically by generating both cellular and humoral immune responses. In the susceptible host, the immune responses are generally unable to avert the progression of the neoplastic process, but in resistant chickens the immune defense mechanisms keep the disease process under control and progressive neoplastic lesions do not develop. In this presentation, which is not intended to be a comprehensive review on any aspect of MD, I will briefly describe the pathogenesis of MD, the nature of immunity that accompanies infection with MDV and the role this immunity may play in mediating resistance to the disease. The discussion will be limited to the chicken because the chicken is the principal natural host of MDV and immunologic parameters of the disease have been studied most extensively in this animal. Certain other avian species such as turkeys, quails, ducks, etc., may either be infected experimentally or have natural antibodies to MDV.

PATHOGENESIS OF MAREK'S DISEASE IN SUSCEPTIBLE CHICKENS

Under natural conditions, chickens acquire infection with MDV via the respiratory tract. There is conclusive evidence that vertical transmission of the virus from infected parents to the progeny does not occur (102). The infectious virus suspended in the environmental air is inhaled and is presumably first deposited in the lungs. The virus then spreads to other organs without replicating to any great extent in the respiratory tract (1) Data are lacking on virus-cell interactions in the respiratory tract and on the mechanism of subsequent spread of the virus to locations outside the respiratory tract. Alveolar phagocytes and lymphoid cells may be involved in transporting the virus out of the respiratory tract.

Infection with MDV initiates a series of rapidly developing events in the host. The first evidence of viral activity is detected in the major lymphoid organs. Within 3–7 days of infection, extensive lymphoid cell destruction occurs in the bursa, thymus and spleen (31, 32, 59). Accompanying cellular lysis is the appearance of abundant amounts of viral antigens that can be readily detected by immune precipitation or immunofluorescence (1, 59). Naked virions can also

H. E. Kaiser (ed.), Comparative aspects of tumor development.
© 1989, Kluwer Academic Publishers, Dordrecht. ISBN-13:978-0-89838-994-4

be detected in infected cells (13, 22), although infectious enveloped virions are not produced. This cytolytic infection of lymphocytes without production of infectious virions has been termed as productive-restrictive infection (9). MDV is a highly cell-associated virus and all through the infectious cycle, enveloped infectious virions are produced only in the skin epithelium from where the virus is shed into the environment with dander (12). Infected chickens continue for long periods to shed infectious virus in the dander and, thus, the premises where such chickens are raised continue to be seeded with the virus.

Histologically, early lytic infection is characterized by loss of cortical lymphocytes in thymus and follicular lymphocytes in the bursa (61). Lymphocytic lysis is accompanied by hyperplasia of the reticulum type cells and other inflammatory changes. In spleen, excessive cellular destruction does not occur, although reticulum cell hyperplasia does and spleen becomes enlarged.

The target cell in the early lytic phase appears to be the B lymphocyte (96). Surgical removal of bursa or lysis of bursa cell with infectious bursal disease virus prior to MDV infection abrogates the lytic phase (79; Sharma, unpublished).

The initial cytolytic phase is transient and after 7–8 days of infection, this lytic phase subsides and the virus becomes latent in T lymphocytes. Within a few days, extensive lymphoproliferation ensues and some of the T cells undergo neoplastic transformation and lymphomas develop. Viral antigens and virions cannot be readily detected in the latent phase of infection. Solid tumors may develop in any organ or tissue, although in natural cases, nerves, gonads, liver, spleen, kidney, lung and heart are most frequently involved. Nodular tumors in the skin, generally associated with feather follicles along the major feather tracts, are most common in commercial broiler populations.

MD lymphomas are characterized by the presence of a heterogeneous population of lymphocytes that may include small, medium, or large blast-type cells, reticulum cells, macrophages and occasionally plasma cells and heterophils (61). Usually, a small proportion of tumor cells express a new antigen designated Marek's disease tumor associated surface antigen (MATSA) (71, 103). This antigen appears to be associated with MDV-induced neoplastic transformation, although data suggest that MATSA may be a differentiation or modified histocompatibility antigen (Rennie and Powell, 1979 (73); McColl, K.A., et al. In press). MATSA on different MD line cells are related but not identical (75, 94, 99).

Tumor cells can be propagated *in vitro* and numerous continuously propagating MD tumor cell lines have been developed within the last few years. Chicken MD lymphoblastoid cell lines have several important characteristics: they are Ia-bearing T lymphocytes, they express MATSA on the surface and they contain the MDV genome. Recent evidence indicates that MD may have the potential of transforming cells other than T cells. Tumor cell lines developed from experimentally induced MD lymphomas in turkeys may be of T or B origin (17, 53, 67).

IMMUNOLOGICAL RESPONSES OF THE HOST

All isolates of MDV appear to be highly antigenic and

induce persistently detectable immunity. However, infection of chickens with certain pathogenic isolates may result in rapidly progressing disease accompanied by severe immunodepression, thus preventing the host from developing lasting humoral or cellular responses (85). The immunodepression may be caused by extensive damage to lymphoid organs resulting from cytolytic infection and extensive destruction of immunologically competent lymphoid cells or from induction of suppressor cells (44). Generally, virulent strains that induce a well pronounced cytolytic phase cause a longer lasting immunodepression than the strains of low virulence that do not cause extensive lympholysis.

Humoral Immunity. Humoral antibodies in response to natural or experimental infection with MDV are directed against virus-associated antigens. Such antigens include viral envelope antigens, viral internal antigens, or membrane antigens expressed on some lytically-infected nonlymphoid cells (9, 54). Most of these antibodies appear within 1 to 2 weeks of infection and remain detectable for as long as the birds remain actively infected with the virus which, in most cases, may be for life. Numerous serologic assays have been used for assaying antibodies. These include immune precipitation tests, viral neutralization tests, immunofluorescence, indirect hemagglutination, complement fixation and, more recently, the enzyme-linked immunosorbent assay (15). The initial antibodies, detectable within a week of infection, are of IgM type, followed later by the IgG type. Humoral antibodies that participate in antibody-dependent cellular cytotoxicity reactions can also be detected in convalescent serum (39, 45). Detectable levels of anti-MATSA antibodies are not produced, even in lymphoma-bearing chickens, although chickens may be hyper-immunized against MATSA by repeated injections of MD lymphoblastoid line cells that express MATSA on their surface (98).

Besides antibodies, other humoral factors may also develop following infection of MDV. Circulating interferon, presumably of β type, has been reported to be induced by MDV (30, 34, 35). Involvement of α and γ interferons in MD has not as yet been investigated.

Cellular Immunity. Several cell-mediated immune responses have been detected in MD, both by *in vivo* and by *in vitro* systems. Tumor-bearing chickens develop a delayed type hypersensitivity reaction at the site of intradermal challenge with antigens prepared from MDV-infected cell cultures (8, 19). Antiviral cellular responses have also been detected by several *in vitro* assays. An earlier study reported on a migration inhibition test in which a partially purified antigen from MDV-infected cell cultures caused inhibition of radial migration of lymphocytes obtained from MDV-infected chickens (19). The specificity of this reaction and the mechanism of migration inhibition remain to be determined. Because of the need for a purified antigen and perhaps the complexity of test procedures, the migration inhibition assay has not been adequately studied in MD.

The most popular *in vitro* assays for measuring cell-mediated immunity have involved cytotoxic reactions. Ross (74) described a T-cell-mediated plaque reduction assay in which effector cells obtained from immunized chickens lysed virus-infected target cells and reduced their plaque-inducing potential. Several authors have used short-term ^{51}Cr-release assay to test virus-infected chickens for effector cells of cell-mediated immunity (2, 14, 16, 39, 66, 77, 84, 87, 95). In most of these studies ^{51}Cr-labelled MD lymphoblastoid line cells were used as target cells. Detectable cytotoxic effector cells appear transiently within 1–2 weeks of infection with MDV, a time period that roughly coincides with the appearance of first lymphoproliferative lesions (87) and MAT-SA-bearing cells (51). The nature of the target cell antigens recognized by the cytotoxic effector T-cells has not been clearly defined. The evidence is not clear if MATSA is the target antigen involved. Removal of surface MATSA on target cells by papain digestion or blocking MATSA by anti-MATSA antibody did not alter cytotoxicity of the effector cells (78). Further, the cytotoxic reactions were more pronounced if the effector cells were allogeneic to target cells than if the combination was syngeneic (68, 80). Because some, albeit, low, cytotoxic activity can be detected in some syngeneic target-effector combinations, MATSA may constitute a relevant target antigen for immune T-cells, although improved recognition of this antigen may be dependent upon interaction with, and possibly modification of, alloantigens on cell surfaces, as discussed by Powell *et al.*, (68).

Infection with MDV also influences NK cell activity. As in mammals, the NK cell system seems well developed in chickens (21, 41, 42, 46, 88). The avian NK cell cytotoxic activity is associated with a non-T, non-B lymphoid cell population detected in peripheral blood and spleen. The short-term ^{51}Cr-release assay is used routinely to detect this activity and, of the target cells tested thus far, cells of a retrovirus-transformed line, namely LSCC-RP9, appear most susceptible to *in vitro* lysis by avian NK cells (89). There is evidence that inoculation of chickens with MDV results in elevated NK cell activity in spleen effector cells (86). This elevation was particularly marked in line N chickens that are genetically resistant to progressive MD. Conversely, in a highly susceptible genetic line of chickens (line P), progressive MD was associated with depression in normal NK levels. Antibody-dependent cellular cytotoxic activity may also be elevated in MD (39, 45).

RESISTANCE TO MAREK'S DISEASE

Upon exposure to MDV, all chickens become infected with the virus. In susceptible chickens infection leads to progressive clinical disease that is usually fatal, whereas in resistant chickens either progressive proliferative lesions do not develop or lesion regression occurs and chickens overcome clinical MD. Resistance is expressed under several circumstances: (1) Certain chickens are resistant due to genetic background. The histocompatibility complex plays a role and several workers have shown that birds possessing the B^{21} allele show marked resistance to MD (6, 28, 48), although other alleles and minor genetic loci such as the Ly-4 locus that encodes for T-cell antigens may also determine susceptibility or resistance (23, 62). (2) Natural resistance of MD is also expressed with age, thus chickens that are fully susceptible to progressive MD if exposure to MDV is at hatch become progressively more resistant if the exposure is delayed until after 2 to 4 weeks of age (4, 81, 93,

101). There is evidence that genetic background may also to a certain extent control acquisition of age resistance so that chickens of certain genetically resistant lines express stronger age resistance than those of genetically susceptible lines (11). (3) Vaccination with the turkey herpesvirus or non-pathogenic isolates of MDV immunizes chickens against virulent MDV. Prophylactic vaccination is widely used in commercial chicken populations to keep MD under control.

MECHANISMS OF RESISTANCE

Available data indicate that the three models of resistance listed above may be mediated via common mechanisms which appear to be complex and may involve a multitude of factors. The fact that infection and early cytolytic lesions occur in most chickens but the lesions fail to progress in resistant chickens indicated that resistance is dependent primarily on host defense rather than on the inability of cells of resistant chickens to allow virus entry and replication (90, 97). There is ample evidence that the immune response of the host constitutes an important part of host defense.

An example of lesion regression is most clearly demonstrated in the age resistance model (3, 57, 93). In one study (93) chickens of two age groups, 1-day and 12-weeks, were simultaneously infected with pathogenic MDV and chronologic observations were made on the lesion responses in the two groups. Gross lesions consisting primarily of peripheral nerve enlargements were detected in both age groups at approximately 4 weeks after infection. In the 1-day group, lesions persisted and a high proportion of the chickens died during the observation period of 20 weeks, whereas in the 12-week age group, the incidence of gross lesions was 50% at 4 weeks, but these lesions apparently became resolved because chickens did not die and those examined at 8, 12, 16 and 20 weeks lacked detectable gross lesions. The initial appearance and subsequent disappearance suggested that gross lesions had regressed in the older groups. A similar pattern of regression of microscopic lesions was also observed in the two age groups of chickens.

This and other evidence on lesion regression (57, 101) prompted studies in which resistant chickens were immunosuppressed prior to infection with MDV. Immunosuppression of 8-week-old chickens prior to infection with MDV resulted in progressive lesions, whereas intact hatchmates were resistant to progressive lesions after simultaneous infection (92). Further, selective immunosuppression in the T or B-cell system revealed that resistance was more dependent on cellular immunity than on humoral immunity (83, 91, 92). Thymectomy also reduces vaccine protection (26), whereas bursectomy does not (18).

The influence of the major histocompatibility complex on resistance to MD may also be mediated through a control of this locus on immune reactions to MDV. Experimental studies have shown that the *B*-complex in chickens affects immune reactions to natural and synthetic antigens (5, 36, 63). In the mouse and in man, the genetic effects on immune response have been attributed to Ir genes that map within the major histocompatibility complex (25, 38, 50, 100). The Ir gene codes for cell surface structures on B- and T-cells and regulates cellular and humoral responses to specific antigens. Similar genetic influences may be regulated by the chicken major histocompatibility complex and in resistant chickens, a highly effective protective immunity may develop in response to infection with MDV (64).

Role of cellular immunity. As noted above, immuno-suppression studies indicated that cellular immunity mediates resistance to MD. Extensive efforts have been directed in pursuit of the antigen(s) against which the protective immunity is targeted.

Because substantial protection against challenge with virulent MDV can be obtained by immunizing chickens with non-replicating soluble or non-soluble viral antigens (33, 47, 52) or glutaraldehyde-fixed MATSA-bearing MD tumor lymphoblastoid cells (52, 65), both viral and tumor antigens appear to be involved in protective immunity (47, 52, 56, 65, 70). Thus, infected chickens must develop cellular responses against viral and tumor antigens.

The antiviral cellular immunity has been associated with T-cells or other effector cells. The T-cell-mediated antiviral activity can be assayed by plaque reduction tests or cytolytic tests in which lytically infected non-lymphoid cells are reacted *in vitro* with effector cells obtained from immune chickens (39, 74). MDV induces a multitude of antigens in infected cells and the identity of the antigen(s) against which the effector T-cell function is directed is not known.

The cellular immune reactions against the tumor antigen have not been clearly identified. If the *in vitro* cytotoxic activity of T-cells against MD tumor line cells is also directed against MATSA-bearing cells *in vivo*, the chronology of the appearance of effector cells in infected chickens does not seem to have an apparent correlation with overall resistance to clinical disease. The *in vitro* cytotoxic activity is transient and is best expressed in highly susceptible chickens or in chickens that have progressive gross lymphomas (16, 87).

Macrophages, in addition to playing an important supportive role in regulating responses of other immune cells, may in themselves engage in destruction of MDV infected target cells and thus may reduce virus levels in infected chickens (40, 43, 76). This effect is probably nonspecific and no clear differences in macrophage functions have been detected between resistant and suscep-tible chickens (27, 29, 68). Because macrophages may also act as suppressors of certain cellular immune functions in MDV infected chickens (44), the importance of these cells in resistance is doubtful.

There is evidence that regulation of NK activity by MDV in chickens may be correlated with resistance to the disease. The background NK levels present in normal chickens become elevated in resistant but not in susceptible chickens following infection with MDV (86). The specificity of NK cells seems broad because target antigens on tumor cells with diverse characteristics are involved. Because the target cells (LSCC-RP9) most sensitive to effector cell lysis *in vitro* (89) were derived from a retrovirus-induced tumor and lack viral or tumor antigens of MDV (55), and because NK cell levels may be influenced by many unrelated agents or sub-stances, the specificity of NK cells to MD is not known. Further studies to understand the NK cell regulation in chickens are needed to better appreciate the involvement of this activity in MD resistance. Similarly, antibody-depen-dent cellular cytotoxic activity that has been related with resistance needs further study (39, 45).

Role of humoral immunity. Experimentally induced immuno-deficiency in the B-cell system often leading to agamma-globulinemia does not compromise resistance to MD (18, 20, 58, 83, 91). Thus B-cell function alone is not critical for resistance. Nevertheless, anti-MDV antibodies may play an important role in modifying genesis of MD. Antibodies present at the time of infection with MDV may neutralize some or all of the inoculum. Cell-free, as well as cell-asso-ciated MDV may be neutralized (7). It is not clear whether some of the cell-associated virus is accessible for neutraliza-tion by antibody or, other mechanisms, such as antibody-dependent cellular cytotoxicity, are involved. Passively ac-quired antibodies in progeny chicks of immunized dams limit virus spread and prevent early cytolytic infection (10, 59). Partial neutralization of viral inoculum may reduce the magnitude of initial challenge and may enable the host to mount a more effective immune response than would be possible if the challenge were massive, resulting in early immunodepression.

Role of other factors. Although immunity appears to be critical for resistance, other non-immune mechanisms may also play a role. For instance, several authors have shown that certain lines of genetically resistant chickens may have fewer available lymphoid cells that may serve as targets for virus infection and transformation than do age-matched susceptible chickens (24, 45, 72). Fewer target cells may produce proportionately less virus and fewer transforming events that may be better controlled by host defense mecha-nisms than in susceptible chickens where high levels of virus are likely to initiate an overwhelming number of transform-ing events.

INTRATUMORAL IMMUNITY

Tumor progression or regression may be regulated by in-teraction of tumor cells with host defense cells at the site of the tumor, thus functional capabilities of immune cells present within solid tumors may provide information on tumorigenesis.

MD tumors consist of heterogeneous lymphoid cells with only a small fraction of the cells (1–20%) that express sur-face MATSA (71, 103). Thus the majority of the cells con-stituting a tumor are non-transformed and presumably re-present immunologically reactive host cells. Indeed, Payne and Roszkowski (60) noted that immunologically com-petent T- and B-cells could be recovered from MD lym-phomas. Recently an attempt was made to study functional diversity of intratumoral immune cells recovered by enzymatic digestion of MDV-induced progressive tumors and an MDV-derived regressive transplantable tumor (82). Cytotoxic macrophage-like cells and NK cells were recovered from both types of tumors but there were important differences between cytotoxic cells of progressive and regressive tumors. Macrophage-like cells present in progressive tumors were inactivated by treatment with carbonyl iron and carrageenan, whereas similar cells present in regressive tumors were refractory to these treatments. More importantly, the incidence and level of NK cells reac-tivity was greater in the regressive tumors than in the progressive tumors. Further, in regressive tumor-bearing animals, the NK cell activity was higher in the tumors than in the spleen. This result indicated that the cytotoxic activity was concentrated at the site of the tumor. Qualitative and quantitative differences in immune reactive cells between regressive and progressive tumors indicate that the intratumoral immunity may regulate tumor progression. Additional studies are needed to further evaluate intratumoral immunity in MD lymphomas. Such studies may facilitate modulation of local cellular immunity to promote tumor regression.

SUMMARY

Marek's disease virus, a herpesvirus, is ubiquitous among chicken populations raised under natural conditions. Although all chickens are susceptible to infection with MDV, the chickens differ in their susceptibility to the pathogenic effect of MDV. Genetic background, age at exposure and prior vaccination have a marked influence on outcome of infection with virulent MDV. Exposure to virulent MDV of unvaccinated, genetically susceptible chickens at a young age results in a rapidly progressing lymphoproliferative disease that is usually fatal. In resistant chickens, however, the virus exposure either does not result in clinical disease or virus-induced lesions are overcome by the host and recovery from clinical disease occurs.

There is extensive evidence that immunity plays an important role in regulating resistance. Selective immunosuppression studies have shown that cell-mediated immunity is more important in resistance than humoral immunity although the presence of antibody at the time of infection may reduce the severity of disease and delay tumor formation. Extensive efforts have been made in understanding cell-mediated mechanisms involved in resistance of MD. Several *in vitro* cellular immune assays have been developed that utilize effector cells from chickens infected with MDV. These effector cells seem to react against viral and possibly tumor target antigens. It is as yet not clear, however, how the immune activities detected by *in vitro* assays are related with mediating *in vivo* resistance to progressive disease.

REFERENCES

1. Aldinger HK, Calnek BW: Pathogenesis of Marek's disease: Early distribution of virus and viral antigens in infected chickens. *J Natl Cancer Inst* 50:1287, 1973
2. Aldinger HK, Confer AW: Cytotoxic in vitro reaction of chicken lymphoid cells against Marek's disease virus-infected target cells. Presented at the 3rd International Symposium on Oncogenesis and Herpesviruses, July 25–29, Harvard University, Cambridge, MA. U.S.A., 1977
3. Aigster FG: M.S. Thesis, University of Georgia, 1968
4. Anderson DP, Eidson CS, Richey DM: Age susceptibility of chickens to Marek's disease. *Am J Vet Res* 32:935, 1971
5. Benedict AA, Pollard LW, Morrow PR, Abplanalp HA, Maurer PH, Briles WE: Genetic control of immune responses in chickens. I. Responses to a terpolymer of poly (Glu^{60}Ala^{30}-Tyr^{10}) associated with the major histocompatibility complex. *Immunogenetics* 2:313, 1975
6. Briles WE, Stone HA, Cole RK: Marek's disease: Effects of B histocompatibility alloalleles in resistant and susceptible chicken lines. *Science* 195:193, 1977
7. Burgoyne GH, Witter RL: Effect of passively transferred immunoglobulins on Marek's disease. *Avian Dis* 17:824, 1973
8. Byerly JL, Dawe DL: Delayed hypersensitivity reactions in Marek's disease. *Amer J Vet Res* 33:2267, 1972
9. Calnek BW: Marek's disease virus and lymphoma. In: *Oncogenic Herpesvirus* (Rapp F, ed.), Vol. 1, pp. 103–144. Boca Raton, FL. CRC Press, 1980
10. Calnek BW: Effects of passive antibody on early pathogenesis of Marek's disease. *Infect Immun* 6:193, 1972
11. Calnek BW: Influence of age at exposure on the pathogenesis of Marek's disease. *J Natl Cancer Inst* 51:929, 1973
12. Calnek BW, Aldinger HK, Kahn DE: Feather follicle epithelium: a source of enveloped and infectious cell-free herpesvirus from Marek's disease. *Avian Dis* 14:219, 1970a
13. Calnek BW, Ubertini T, Aldinger HK: Viral antigen, virus particles, and infectivity of tissues from chickens with Marek's disease. *J Natl Cancer Inst* 45:341, 1970b
14. Calnek BW, Carlisle JC, Fabricant J, Murthy KK, Schat KA: Comparative pathogenesis studies with oncogenic and nononcogenic Marek's disease viruses and turkey herpesviruses. *Am J Vet Res* 40:541, 1979
15. Cheng YQ, Lee LF, Smith EJ, Witter RL. An enzyme-linked immunosorbent assay (ELISA) for the detection of antibodies to Marek's disease virus. *Avian Dis* 28:900, 1984
16. Dambrine G, Coudert F, Cauchy L: Cell-mediated cytotoxicity in chickens infected with Marek's disease virus and the herpes-virus of turkeys. In: *Resistance and Immunity to Marek's Disease* (Bigg PM, ed.), p. 320–337. EUR 6470 EN EEC Brussels, Luxembourg. CEC Publ., 1980
17. Elmubarak AK, Sharma JM, Witter RL, Nazerian K, Sanger VL: Induction of lymphomas and tumor antigen by Marek's disease virus in turkeys. *Avian Dis* 25:911, 1981
18. Else RW: Vaccinal immunity to Marek's disease in bursectomised chickens. *Vet Rec* 95:182, 1974
19. Fauser IS, Purchase HG, Long PA, Velicer LF, Mallmann VH, Fauser HT, Winegar GO: Delayed hypersensitivity and leucocyte migration inhibition in chickens with BCG or Marek's disease. *Avian Pathol* 2:55, 1973
20. Fernando WWD, Calnek BW: Influence of bursa of Fabricius on infection and pathological response of chickens exposed to Marek's disease herpesvirus. *Avian Dis* 15:467, 1971
21. Fleischer B: Effector cells in avian spontaneous and antibody-dependent cell-mediated cytotoxicity. *J Immunol* 125:1161, 1980
22. Frazier JA, Biggs PM: Marek's disease herpesvirus particles in tissues from chickens free of precipitating antibodies. *J Natl Cancer Inst* 48:1519, 1972
23. Fredericksen TL, Longenecker BM, Pazderka F, Gilmour DG, Ruth RF: A T-cell antigen system of chickens: Ly-4 and Marek's disease. *Immunogenetics* 5:535, 1977
24. Gallatin WM, Longenecker BM: Genetic resistance to herpesvirus-induced lymphoma at the level of the target cell determined by the thymic microenvironment. *Intl J Cancer* 27:373, 1981
25. Green I: Genetic control of immune responses. *Immunogenetics* 1:4, 1974
26. Gupta SK, Kharole MU, Kalra DS: Role of thymus-dependent immune system in HVT protection against Marek's disease. *Avian Dis* 26:7, 1982
27. Haffer K, Sevoian M, Wilder M: The role of macrophage in Marek's disease: *In vitro* and *in vivo* studies. *Intl J Cancer* 23:648, 1979
28. Hansen HP, van Zandt JN, Law GRJ: Differences in susceptibility to Marek's disease in chickens carrying two different B locus blood group alleles. *Poultry Sci* 46:1268, 1967
29. Higgins DA, Calnek BW: Some effects of silica treatment on Marek's disease. *Infect Immun* 13:1050, 1976
30. Hong CC, Sevoian M: Comparison of indirect hemagglutination and immunodiffusion tests for detecting type II leukosis

(Marek's) infection in S- and K-line chickens. *Appl Microbiol* 23:449, 1972

31. Jakowski RM, Fredrickson TN, Luginbuhl RE, Helmboldt CF: Early changes in bursa of Fabricius from Marek's disease. *Avian Dis* 13: 215, 1969

32. Jakowski RM, Fredrickson TN, Chomiak TW, Luginbuhl RE: Hematopoietic destruction in Marek's disease. *Avian Dis* 14:374, 1970

33. Kaaden OR, Dietzschold B, Ueberschar S: Vaccination against Marek's disease: Immunizing effect of purified turkey herpesvirus and cellular membranes from infected cells. *Med Microbiol Immunol* 159:261, 1974

34. Kaleta EF, Bankowski RA: Production of circulating and cell-bound interferon in chickens by type 1 and type 2 plaque-producing agents of the Cal-1 strain of Marek's disease herpesvirus and herpesvirus of turkeys. *Am J Vet Res* 33:573, 1972a

35. Kaleta, EF, Bankowski RA: Production of interferon by the Cal-1 and turkey herpesvirus strain associated with Marek's disease. *Am J Vet Res* 33:567, 1972b

36. Karakoz I, Krejci J, Hala K, Blaszczyk B, Hraba T, Pekarek J: Genetic determination of tuberculin hypersensitivity in chicken inbred lines. *Eur J Immunol* 4:545, 1974

37. Kermani-Arab V, Moll T, Cho BR, Davis WC, Lu Y-S: Effect of cyclophosphamide on the response of chickens to a virulent strain of Marek's disease virus. *Infect Immun* 12:1058, 1975

38. Klein J: *Biology of the mouse histocompatibility-2 complex*. p. 192–219. New York, NY. Springer-Verlag, 1975

39. Kodama H, Sugimoto C, Inage F, Mikami T: Anti-viral immunity against Marek's disease virus infected chicken kidney cells. *Avian Pathol* 8:33, 1979a

40. Kodama H, Mikami T, Inoue M, Izawa H: Inhibitory effects of macrophages against Marek's disease virus plaque formation in chicken kidney cell cultures. *J Natl Cancer Inst* 63:1267, 1979b

41. Lam KM, Linna TJ: Protection of newly-hatched chickens from Marek's disease (JMV) by normal spleen cells from older animals. In: *Advances in Comparative Leukemia Research* 1977 (Bentzvelzen P, Hilgers J, Yohn DS, eds.), p. 111–113. Amsterdam. Elsevier/North Holland Biomedical Press, 1978

42. Lam KM, Linna TJ: Transfer of natural resistance to Marek's disease (JMV) with non-immune spleen cells. I. Studies of cell population transferring resistance. *Intl J Cancer* 24:662, 1979

43. Lee LF: Macrophage restriction of Marek's disease virus replication and lymphoma cell proliferation. *J Immunol* 123:1088, 1979

44. Lee LF, Sharma JM, Nazerian K, Witter RL: Suppression of mitogen-induced proliferation of normal spleen cells by macrophages from chickens inoculated with Marek's disease virus. *J Immunol* 120:1554, 1978

45. Lee LF, Powell PC, Rennie M, Ross LJN, Payne LN: Nature of genetic resistance to Marek's disease. *J Natl Cancer Inst* 66:789, 1981

46. Leibold W, Janotte G, Peter HH: Spontaneous cell mediated cytotoxicity (SCMC) in various mammalian species and chickens: Selective reaction pattern and different mechanisms. *Scand J Immunol* 11:203, 1980

47. Lesnik F, Ross LJN: Immunization against Marek's disease using Marek's disease virus-specific antigens free from infectious virus. *Intl J Cancer* 16:153, 1975

48. Longenecker BM, Pazderka F, Gavora JS, Spencer JL, Ruth RF: Lymphoma induced by herpesvirus: Resistance associated with a major histocompatibility gene. *Immunogenetics* 3:401, 1976

49. Marek J: Multiple Nervenentzundung (Poly-6 neuritis) bei Huhnern (Polyneuritis of chickens). *Dtsch Tierarztl Wschr* 15:417, 1907

50. Mozes E: Expression of immune response (Ir) genes in T and B cells. *Immunogenetics* 2:397, 1975

51. Murthy KK, Calnek BW: Marek's disease tumor-associated surface antigen (MATSA) in resistant versus susceptible chickens. *Avian Dis* 23:831, 1979a

52. Murthy KK, Calnek BW: Pathogenesis of Marek's disease: Effects of immunization with inactivated viral and tumor antigens. *Infect Immun* 26:547, 1979b

53. Nazerian K, Elmubarak AK, Sharma JM: Establishment of B-lymphoblastoid cell lines from Marek's disease virus-induced tumors in turkeys. *Intl J Cancer* 29:63, 1982

54. Nazerian K, Lee LF, Sharma JM: The role of herpes-viruses in Marek's disease lymphoma of chickens. *Progr Med Virol* 22:123, 1976

55. Okazaki W, Witter RL, Romero C, Nazerian K, Sharma JM, Fadly A, Ewert D: Induction of lymphoid leukosis transplantable tumour and the establishment of lymphoblastoid cell lines. *Avian Pathol* 9:311, 1980

56. Payne LN: Pathogenesis of Marek's disease – A review. In: Oncogenesis and Herpesviruses (Biggs PM, de The G, Payne LH, eds.), p. 21–37. Lyon, France, IARC, 1972

57. Payne LN, Biggs PM: Studies on Marek's disease II. Pathogenesis. *J Natl Cancer Inst* 39:281, 1967

58. Payne LN, Rennie M: Lack of effect of bursectomy on Marek's disease. *J Natl Cancer Inst* 45:387, 1970

59. Payne LN, Rennie M: Pathogenesis of Marek's disease in chicks with and without maternal antibody. *J Natl Cancer Inst* 51:1559, 1973

60. Payne LN, Roszkowski J: The presence of immunologically uncommitted bursa and thymus dependent lymphoid cells in the lymphomas of Marek's disease. *Avian Pathol* 1:27, 1972

61. Payne LN, Frazier JA, Powell PC: Pathogenesis of Marek's disease. *Intl Rev Exp Pathol* 16:59, 1976

62. Pazderka F, Longenecker BM, Law GRJ, Stone HA, Ruth RF: Histocompatibility to chicken populations selected for resistance to Marek's disease. *Immunogenetics* 2:93, 1975

63. Pevzner I, Nordskog AW, Kaeberle ML: Immune response and the B blood group locus in chickens. *Genetics* 80:753, 1975

64. Pevzner IY, Kujdych I, Nordskog AW: Immune response and disease resistance in chickens. II. Marek's disease and immune response to GAT. *Poultry Sci* 60:927, 1981

65. Powell PC: Immunity to Marek's disease induced by glutaraldehyde-treated cells of Marek's disease lymphoblastoid cell lines. *Nature* 257:684, 1975

66. Powell PC: Studies on Marek's disease lymphoma-derived cell lines. *Bibl Haemat* 43:348, 1976

67. Powell PC, Howes K, Lawn AM, Mustill BM, Payne LN, Rennie M, Thompson MA: Marek's disease in turkeys: The induction of lesions and the establishment of lymphoid cell lines. *Avian Pathol* 13:201, 1984

68. Powell PC, Mustill BM, Rennie M: The role of histocompatibility antigens in cell-mediated cytotoxicity against Marek's disease tumor-derived lymphoblastoid cell lines. *Avian Pathol* 12:461, 1983

69. Powell PC, Rennie M, Hartley KJ, Mustill BM: Macrophage activity following Marek's disease virus infection. In: *Leukemia Review International* (Rich M, ed.), p. 123–124. Marcel Dekker, Inc. New York/Basel, 1983

70. Powell PC, Rowell JG: Dissociation of antiviral and antitumor immunity in resistance to Marek's disease. *J Natl Cancer Inst* 59:919, 1977

71. Powell PC, Payne LN, Frazier JA, Rennie M: T lymphoblastoid cell lines from Marek's disease lymphomas. *Nature* (Lond) 251:79, 1974

72. Powell PC, Lee LF, Mustill BM, Rennie M: The mechanism of genetic resistance to Marek's disease in chickens. *Intl J Cancer* 29:169, 1982

73. Rennie M, Powell PC: Serological characterization of Marek's disease tumour-associated surface antigens on Marek's disease lymphoma cells and on cell lines derived from Marek's disease lymphomas. *Avian Pathol* 8:173, 1979

74. Ross LJN: Antiviral T cell-mediated immunity in Marek's disease. *Nature* (Lond) 266:644, 1977

75. Ross LJN: Characterization of an antigen associated with the Marek's disease lymphoblastoid cell line MSB-1. *J Gen Virol* 60:375, 1982

76. Schat KA, Calnek BW: *In vitro* inactivation of cell-free Marek's disease herpesvirus by immune peripheral blood lymphocytes. *Avian Dis* 22:693, 1978

77. Schat KA, Calnek BW: *In vitro* cytotoxicity of spleen lymphocytes against Marek's disease tumor cells: Induction by SB-1, an apparently non-oncogenic Marek's disease virus. In: *Resistance and Immunity to Marek's Disease* (Biggs PM, ed.), p. 301–316. EUR 6470 EN, EEC Brussels, Luxembourg, CEC Publ., 1980

78. Schat KA, Murthy KK: In vitro cytotoxicity against Marek's disease lymphoblastoid cell lines after enzymatic removal of Marek's disease tumor-associated surface antigen. *J Virol* 34·130, 1980

79. Schat KA, Calnek BW, Fabricant J: Influence of the bursa of Fabricius on the pathogenesis of Marek's disease. *Infect Immun* 31:199, 1980

80. Schat KA, Shek WR, Calnek BW, Abplanalp H: Syngeneic and allogeneic cell-mediated cytotoxicity against Marek's disease lymphoblastoid tumor cell lines. *Intl J Cancer* 29:187, 1982

81. Sevoian M, Chamberlain DM, Larose RN: Avian lymphomatosis. V. Air-borne transmission. *Avian Dis* 7:102, 1963

82. Sharma JM: Presence of adherent cytotoxic cells and nonadherent natural killer cells in progressive and regressive Marek's disease tumors. *Vet Immunol Immunolpathol* 5:125, 1983

83. Sharma JM: Resistance of Marek's disease in immunologically deficient chickens. *Nature* 247:117, 1974

84. Sharma JM: Cell-mediated immunity to tumor antigen in Marek's disease: susceptibility of effector cells to antilymphocyte serum and enhancement of cytotoxic activity by *Vibrio cholerae* neuraminidase. *Infect Immun* 18:46, 1977

85. Sharma JM: Immunosuppressive effects of lymphoproliferative neoplasms of chickens. *Avian Dis* 23:315, 1979

86. Sharma JM: Natural killer cell activity in chickens exposed to Marek's disease virus: Inhibition of activity in susceptible chickens and enhancement of activity in resistant and vaccinated chickens. *Avian Dis* 25:882, 1981

87. Sharma JM, Coulson BD: Cell-mediated cytotoxic response to cells bearing Marek's disease tumor-associated surface antigen in chickens infected with Marek's disease. *J Natl Cancer Inst* 58:1647, 1977

88. Sharma JM, Coulson BD: Presence of natural killer cells in specific pathogen-free chickens. *J Natl Cancer Inst* 63:527, 1979

89. Sharma JM, Okazaki W: Natural killer cell activity in chickens: Target cell analysis and effect of antilymphocyte serum on effector cells. *Infect Immun* 31:1078, 1981

90. Sharma JM, Purchase HG: Replication of Marek's disease virus in cell cultures derived from genetically resistant chickens. *Infect Immun* 9:1092, 1974

91. Sharma JM, Witter RL: The effect of B-cell immunosuppression on age-related resistance of chickens to Marek's disease. *Cancer Res* 35:711, 1975

92. Sharma JM, Witter RL, Purchase HG: Absence of age-resistance in neonatally thymectomized chickens as evidence for cell-mediated immune surveillance in Marek's disease. *Nature* 253:477, 1975

93. Sharma JM, Witter RL, Burmester BR: Pathogenesis of Marek's disease in old chickens: Lesion regression as the basis for age-related resistance. *Infect Immun* 8:715, 1973

94. Sharma JM, Nazerian K, Stephens EA, Witter RL: Lack of serologic identity of Marek's disease associated tumor surface antigen (MATSA) in various Marek's disease cell lines. In: *Adv. Comp. Leuk Res.* (Bentvelzen P., Hilgers J, Yohn DS, eds.), p. 191–192. Elsevier/North-Holland Biomedical Press. Amsterdam/New York, 1977

95. Sharma JM, Witter RL, Coulson BD: Development of cell-mediated immunity to Marek's disease tumor cells in chickens inoculated with Marek's disease vaccines. *J Natl Cancer Inst* 61:1273, 1978

96. Shek WR, Calnek BW, Schat KA, Chen CH: Characterization of Marek's disease virus-infected lymphocytes: Discrimination between cytolytically and latently infected cells. *J Natl Cancer Inst* 70:485, 1983

97. Spencer JL: Marek's disease herpesvirus: *In vivo* and *in vitro* infection of kidney cells of different genetic strains of chickens. *Avian Dis* 13:753, 1969

98. Stephens EA, Witter RL, Nazerian K, Sharma JM: Development and characterization of a Marek's disease transplantable tumor in inbred line 7_2 chickens homzygous at the major (B) histocompatibility locus. *Avian Dis* 24:358, 1980

99. Sugimoto C, Mikami T, Susuki K: Antigenic dissimilarity of cell surface antigens of two Marek's disease lymphoma-derived cell lines (MSB-1 and RPL-1). *Avian Dis* 23:357, 1979

100. Vladutiu AO, Rose NR: HL-A antigens: Association with disease. *Immunogenetics* 1:305, 1974

101. Witter RL, Sharma JM, Solomon JJ, Champion LR: An age-related resistance of chickens to Marek's disease: Some preliminary observations. *Avian Pathol* 2:43, 1973

102. Witter RL, Solomon JJ: Prospects for the control of Marek's disease through isolation rearing. *Progr Immunobiol Standard* 5:163, 1972

103. Witter RL, Stephens EA, Sharma JM, Nazerian K: Demonstration of a tumor-associated surface antigen in Marek's disease. *J Immunol* 115:177, 1975

15

FEATHER-PULP LESIONS DURING THE COURSE OF MAREK'S DISEASE VIRUS-INDUCED LYMPHOMA FORMATION IN CHICKENS

R. MORIGUCHI

Marek's disease (MD) is a highly contagious lympho-proliferative and neuropathic disease of domestic fowls caused by a cell-associated herpesvirus (Marek's disease virus: MDV). The latent period prior to development of clinical disease is relatively long, and virus infection persists, even in the presence of antibody, for the life of most chickens. It is notable that MD is effectively controlled by vaccination with herpesvirus of turkeys or apathogenic MDV, which has certain antigenic similarities with virulent MDV. Lymphoma in MD may occur in one or more of a variety of organs. The liver, spleen, kidney, heart, lung, gonad and proventriculus are most often affected, but the lymphomatous lesions can also be found in the mesentery, adrenal gland, pancreas, intestine, thymus, iris, skeletal muscle and skin. Affected organs show enlargement and a diffuse grayish discoloration. In some birds nodular tumor-like growths are found within and extending from the parenchyma of the organs. The histopathology of MD has been described by many workers, who were in agreement about the type of lesions and the cell type involved. However, the significance and interpretation of some of the histological changes have not been so universally agreed upon.

MD lymphoma has the following characteristics: 1) the lymphoma consists of proliferated lymphocytes of various sizes (small, medium and large), reticulum cells, pyknotic lymphoid cells, referred to as "MD" cells and rarely plasma cells (6, 18, 22); 2) the lymphoma is composed mainly of thymus-dependent (T) cells, with a minor component of bursa-dependent (B) cells (8, 19, 20); 3) not all of the T cells constituting the tumor seem to be malignantly transformed by MDV, because only a small number appear to have tumor-associated surface antigens, and the rest of the T cells present in the tumor may be reactive cells mediated by the host immune response (24); 4) some of the lymphomatous lesions may regress to a more inflammatory one (18).

Cutaneous involvement in MD was first described by Helmboldt *et al.*, (7), who observed tumor-like aggregates of lymphoid cells in the skin. Other workers (9, 10) studied subsequently the pathology and pathogenesis of the lymphoid lesions in the skin. The most noticeable discoveries of skin involvement in MD were the presence of immunofluorescent (IF) antigen associated with MD and a large number of naked and enveloped herpesvirus particles in the feather-follicle epithelium (FFE) (2, 3, 4, 17). By light microscopy, cytoplasmic and nuclear-inclusion bodies (NI) formation in the FFE and associated lymphoid cell response in the perifollicular dermis are characteristically seen in MDV-infected chickens (Figure 1). We recently reported

feather pulp lesions (FPLs) of MD and revealed a close correlation among the FPLs, NI formation in the FFE and incidence of MD in chickens experimentally inoculated with MDV (12, 13). These studies shed some light on the pathogenesis of MD in chickens. To examine the chronological

Figures 1–8. All micrographs were taken from skin specimens collected by biopsy from birds of various ages that were post-inoculated (PI) with MDV at 2 days old.

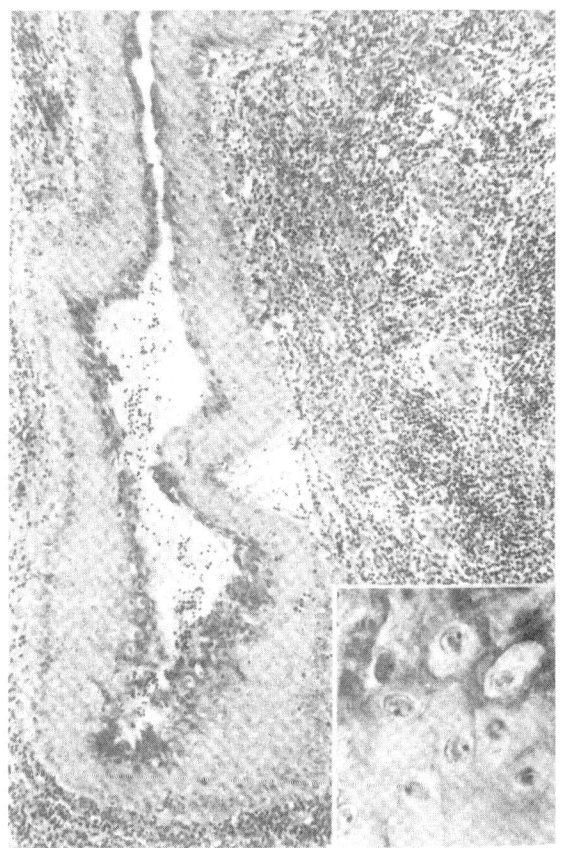

Figure 1. Severe nuclear-inclusion (NI) formation in the superficial layers of the feather-follicle epithelium (FFE) and associated lymphoid lesions in the perifollicular dermis. Inset shows higher magnification of NI-positive cells with vacuolated cytoplasm in the FFE. Skin biopsy at 21 days PI. × 126, Inset × 570.

H. E. Kaiser (ed.), Comparative aspects of tumor development.

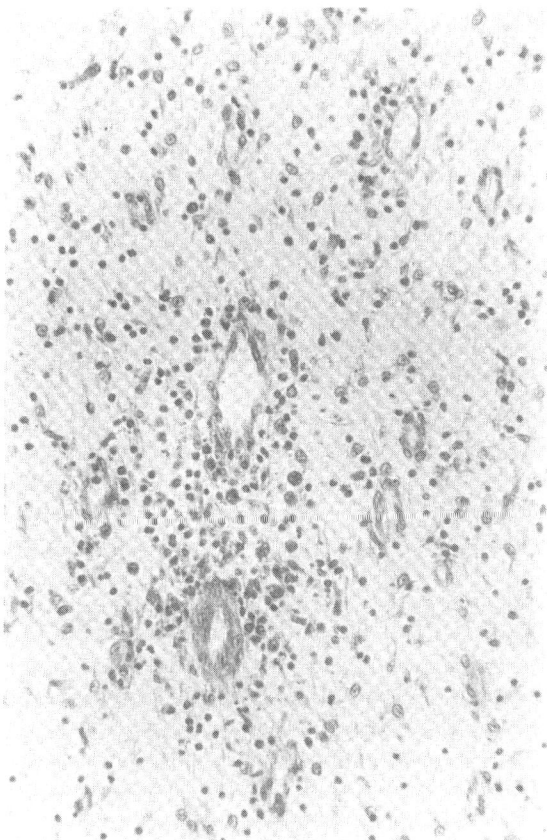

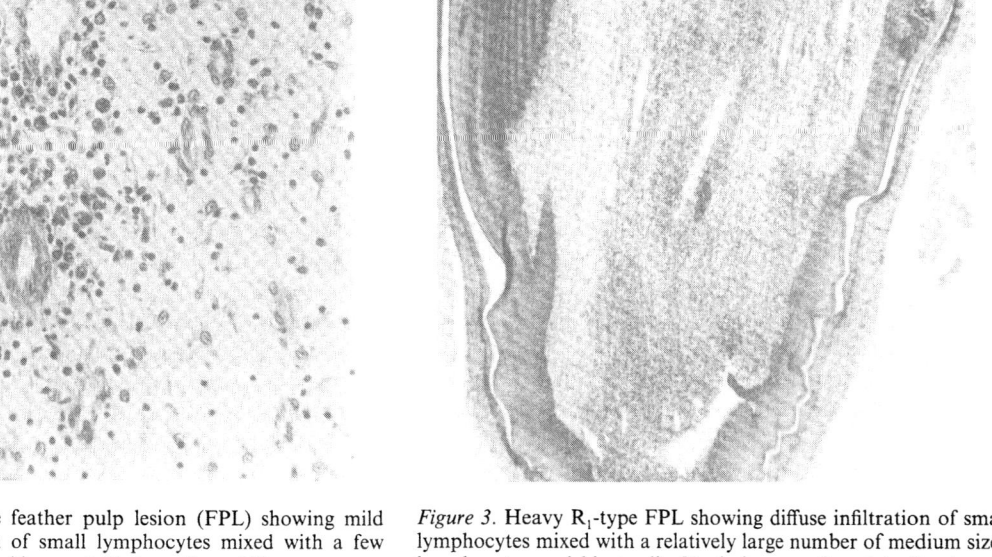

Figure 2. Mild R_1-type feather pulp lesion (FPL) showing mild perivascular infiltration of small lymphocytes mixed with a few large lymphocytes. Skin biopsy at 28 days PI. × 280.

Figure 3. Heavy R_1-type FPL showing diffuse infiltration of small lymphocytes mixed with a relatively large number of medium sized lymphocytes and blast cells. No lesions are found in the dermis. Skin sample taken from a bird that was killed at 123 days PI due to MD; necropsy showed nontumorous MD-associated lymphoid lesions in the viscera and peripheral nerves. × 72.

changes of FPLs or NI formation in the FFE, skin specimens including five growing feathers were taken at intervals from the ventral feather tracts of individual birds and examined by light microscopy. In chickens inoculated with MDV at 1 day or 3 weeks of age, 60–90% of the birds developed MD by 17–20 weeks of age.

The FPLs found in MDV-infected chickens were classified into 3 types, based on a previously described classification of MD lesions in the peripheral nerves (6), i.e., R_1-type: from minimal perivascular to diffuse infiltration of small lymphocytes mixed with a few medium lymphocytes or blast cells, and activation and proliferation of mesenchymal cells mainly in the periphery of blood vessels (Figures 2, 3); R_2-type: edema, infiltration of plasma cells or heterophils and perivascular germinal center formation (Figures 3, 4); T-type: tumorous proliferation of lymphoid cells predominantly composed of large lymphocytes or blast cells. Mitotic figures were common (Figures 6, 7, 8).

Chronological observations of feather pulp samples from birds infected with MDV revealed that the earliest observable changes in the pulp were the occurrence of constantly mild R_1-type lesions (Figure 2) and that certain patterns of lesion progression were present, i.e., R_1-type → T-type and R_1-type → R_2-type. Noticeable evidences were that the FPL patterns were related to the incidence of MD or NI forma-

tion in the FFE. The former pattern, R_1-type → T-type, was seen exclusively in the chickens showing evidences of both persistent NI formation in the FFE and development of lymphoma in the viscera, and the latter pattern, R_1-type → R_2-type, was seen exclusively in the chickens that showed transient or no evidence of NI formation in the FFE and failed to develop lymphoma in the viscera. Within the feather pulp samples from MD-affected chickens, occurrence of R_1-type lesion usually persisted, and in samples from these birds taken prior to development of clinical disease, marked R_1-type lesion (Figure 3), mixed R_1 + T-type lesion or mild to severe T-type lesion were commonly seen. Within the limits of examining five feathers per chicken FPL was not necessarily found in every chicken, however, occurrence of T-type lesions in the feather pulp was found in 74.1% of the birds that developed lymphoma in the viscera. In chickens that had fully developed lymphoma in the viscera, there were T-type lesions present throughout the feather pulp (Figures 7, 8c, 8d).

The diversity of the nerve lesion of MD is reflected in the lack of agreement on their pathogenesis and nature. Chronological observations of nerve lesions of MD de-

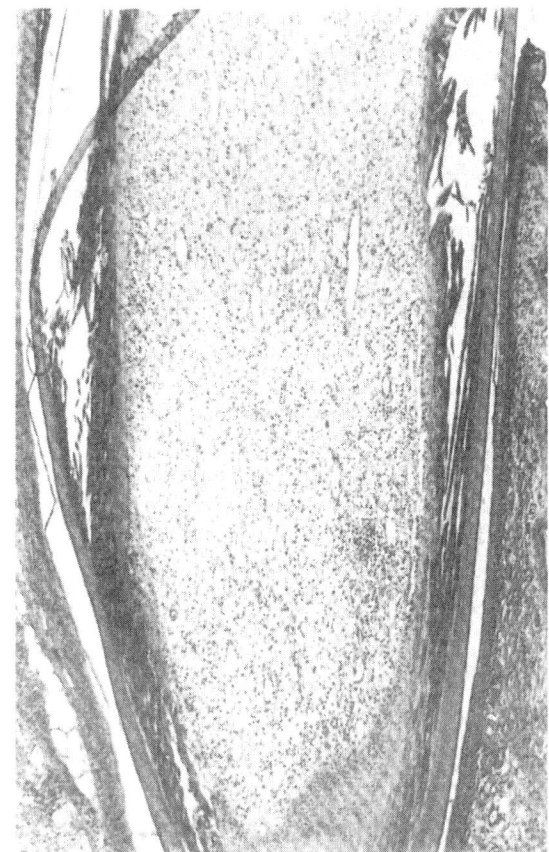

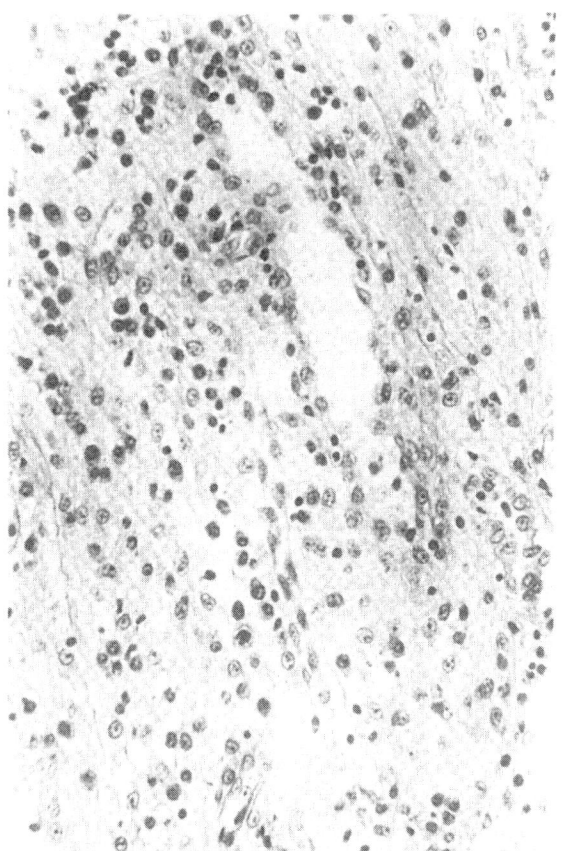

Figure 4. R$_2$-type FPL showing edema and infiltration of plasma cells and small lymphocytes. Skin biopsy at 28 days PI. The chicken survived in a healthy state up to 170 days old. × 72.

Figure 5. R$_2$-type FPL showing perivenous plasma cellular infiltration. Skin biopsy at 84 days PI. The chicken was killed 12 days later due to MD; necropsy showed absence of lymphoma in the viscera and development of peripheral nerve lesions. × 470.

scribed by Payne & Biggs (18) and Lawn & Payne (11) resembled those of the FPLs described herein. The inflammatory nature of the R$_2$-type lesion and the neoplastic nature of the T-type lesion have been confirmed, but the nature of the R$_1$-type lesion is unclear.

Perivascular lymphoid aggregates were commonly seen in the perifollicular skin dermis adjacent to the NI-positive FFE. Lapen *et al.* (10) suggested from their chronological observations that gross cutaneous lymphoid lesions of MD arose from aggregates which developed initially in response to MDV activity in the FFE. In our experimental studies, however, tumorous proliferation of lymphoid cells in the dermis was rare, in spite of frequent occurrences of T-type lesion in the feather pulp. It appeared that the MD lesion response in the feather pulp of chickens infected with MDV was different, to some extent, from that observed in the skin dermis. The distinct differences of NI formation in the FFE between MD-affected and healthy birds supported and advanced previous studies indicating that incidence of MD is closely related to virus multiplication, especially at an early stage after infection, and to persistence of infection (1, 5, 21, 23). We proposed that the information on NI formation in the FFE and the presence of FPLs in feather samples may be useful for further study of the pathogenesis of MD, and

that these lesions are useful measures to predict the fate of MDV-induced lymphoma formation in chickens.

We studied subsequently MD-associated FPLs in field chickens (14–16); unpublished data. In the field MD tended to occur in chickens aged over about 16–20 weeks of age. Table 1 shows the incidences of FPLs and NI formation in the FFE of 79 chickens aged 18–35 weeks that developed MD-associated lymphoma in the viscera. Most of the chickens with generalized and severe lymphoma had severe T-type FPL, the chickens with moderate lymphoma had mild to severe T-type FPL occasionally with concomitant R$_2$-type FPL, and the chickens with mild and localized lymphoma had occasionally T-type FPL and frequently R$_2$-type FPL. To investigate the chronological changes of FPLs and their association with NI formation in the FFE during the course of MD lymphoma formation in chickens, 15 chickens that developed lymphoma in the viscera and a number of birds that failed to develop lymphoma were sampled, five feathers per chicken at intervals during their life. In chickens that developed lymphoma in the viscera, occurrence of T-type FPL persisted from 4 to 11 weeks prior to death. The extent of T-type FPL varied due to the course of a period after the initial occurrence of tumorous lesion. The chronological

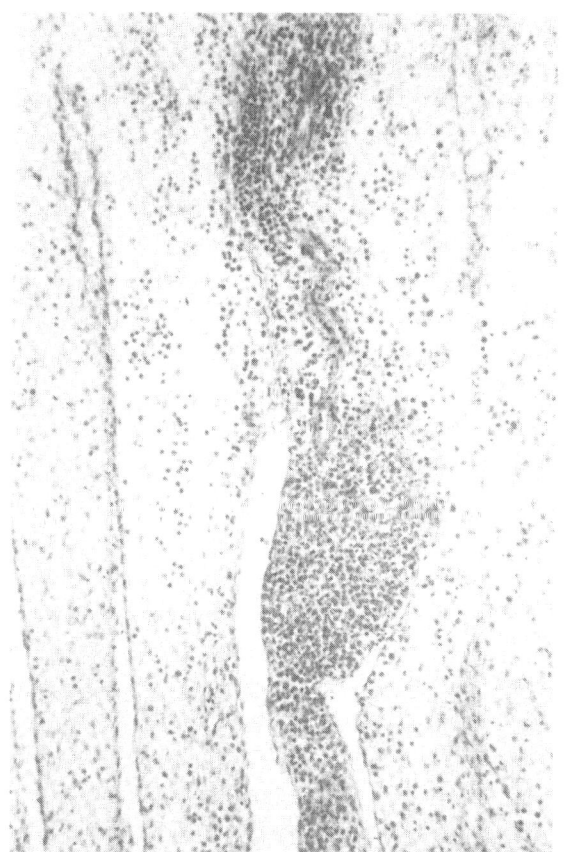

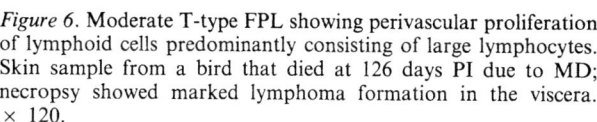

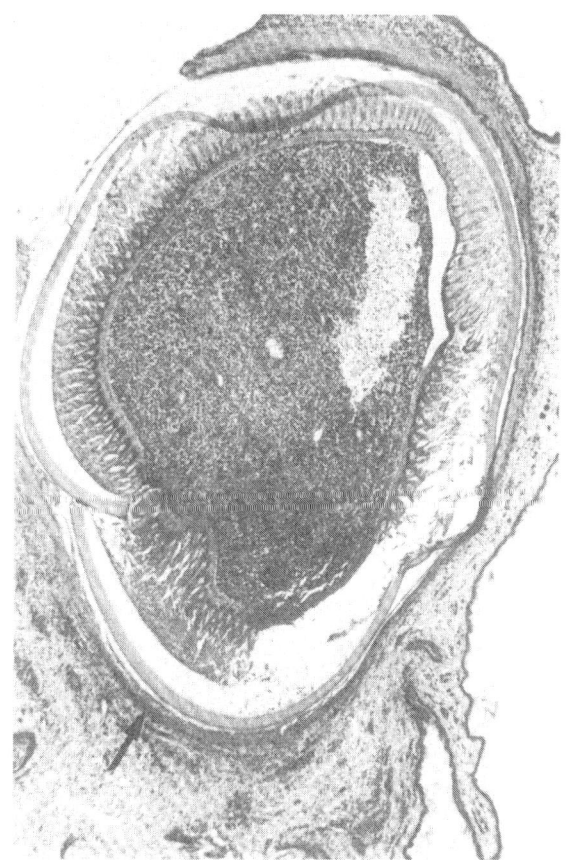

Figure 6. Moderate T-type FPL showing perivascular proliferation of lymphoid cells predominantly consisting of large lymphocytes. Skin sample from a bird that died at 126 days PI due to MD; necropsy showed marked lymphoma formation in the viscera. × 120.

Figure 7. Heavy T-type feather pulp lesion showing diffuse proliferation of lymphoid cells, which completely replaced the feather pulp. NI formation in the FFE is seen (arrow). In the skin dermis no evidence of T-type lesion is seen. Skin biopsy at 84 days PI. The bird died of MD 12 days later; necropsy showed marked lymphoma formation in the viscera. × 50.

changes of FPLs during the course of MD lymphoma formation in chickens were classified into three patterns, i e , pattern A: development of severe T-type FPL within a period of several weeks followed by outbreak of heavy clinical MD (Figure 9); pattern B: definite fluctuation in the extent of T-type FPL during a relatively long time period (8–12 weeks) up to the outbreak of heavy clinical MD, indicating progressive stage, regressive stage and recurrent stage of T-type FPL (Figure 10); pattern C: inconsistent occurrences of T-type FPL and occasional occurrences of R$_2$-type FPL during a relatively long period (up to 15 weeks), with or without outbreak of clinical MD. Noticeable evidences were that above-mentioned FPL patterns correlated well with the dynamics of NI formation in the FFE and pathologic pictures of lymphoma in the viscera, i.e., pattern A was found in chickens that had persistent NI incidence and developed severe, generalized lymphoma; pattern B was observed in chickens that had persistent (in some birds transiently disappeared) NI incidence and developed moderate to severe, generalized lymphoma with R$_2$-type lesion (plasma cellular infiltration, fibrous proliferation, hypertrophy of the parenchymal tissues) in the lesion sites; pattern C appeared in chickens that had persistent NI in-

cidence that subsequently disappeared and developed mild, localized and nodular lymphoma with R$_2$-type lesion. On the other hand, almost all of the birds that failed to develop lymphoma in the viscera showed lesion progression, R$_1$-type → R$_2$-type FPL. It was also evidenced that a small proportion of the birds transiently developed mild to severe T-type FPL and that regression of T-type lesion not only

Table 1. Incidence of feather-pulp lesions(FPLs) and nuclear-inclusion (NI) formation in the feather-follicle epithelium(FFE) of 79 birds, aged 18–35 weeks that developed MD lymphoma in the viscera.

Severity of lymphoma	No. birds	Incidence (%) of FPLs		Incidence of NI in the FFE
		T-type	R$_2$-type	
Severe	26	100	7.7	76.9
Moderate	45	91.1	28.9	86.7
Mild	8	25	87.5	37.5

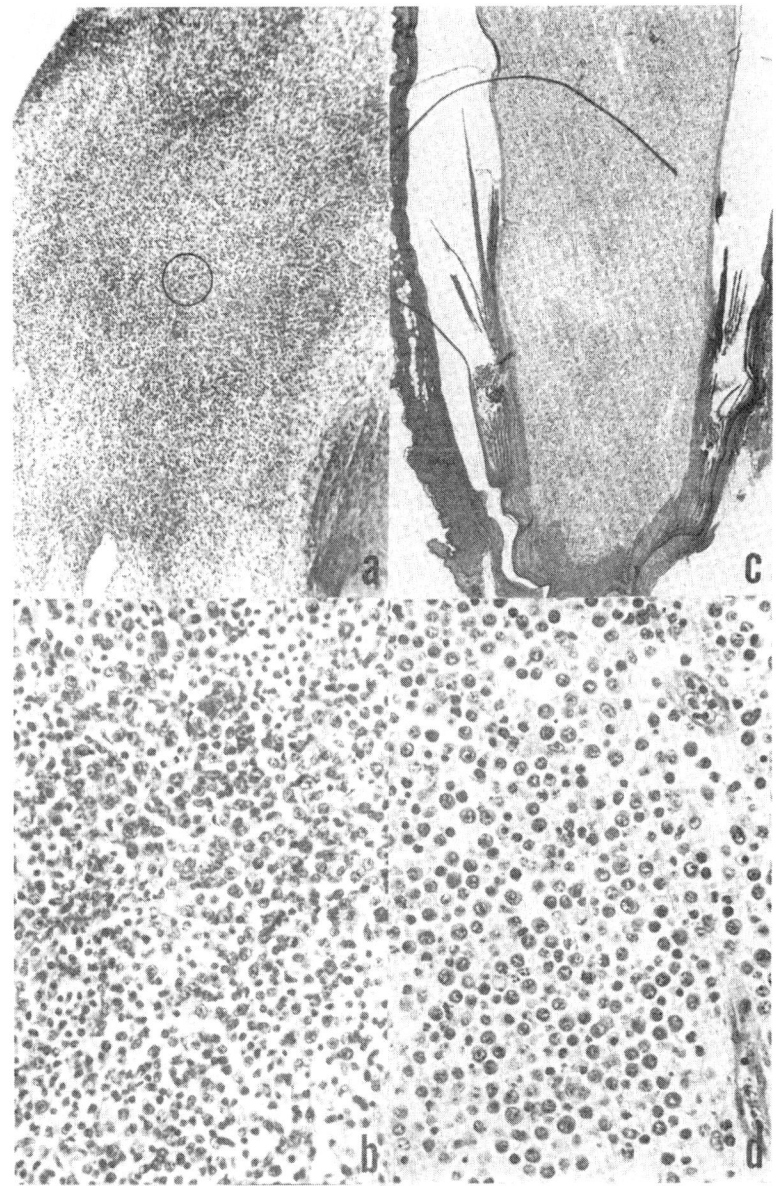

Figure 8a-d. Progression of T-type FPL in a chicken. *a* and *b* = mixed R_1 + T-type lesions in the skin sample at 126 days PI. *a*: low power view, × 120. *b*: high power view of the boundary portion (demarcated by circle in Figure 8*a*) of both type lesions. × 455. *c* and *d* = advanced T-type FPL in skin sample taken at 137 days PI when the chicken was killed due to MD. *c*: low power view, × 56. *d*: high power view, × 540.

occurred in the feather pulp but also occurred in the viscera (Figure 11).

Low power views of figures 9–11 are showing chronological changes of FPLs during the proceeding of MD lymphoma formation in field chickens. Only the T-type lesion is visible within these feather pulp samples. Numbers of upper left corner indicate age (weeks) of birds when feather samples were obtained.

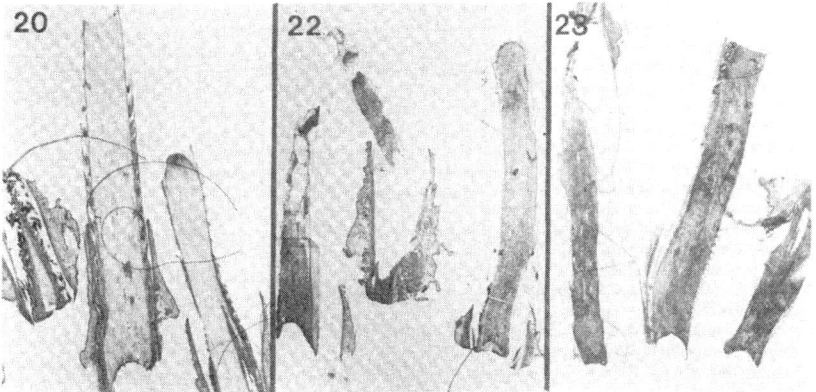

Figure 9. FPL pattern A. Rapid increase reaching to peak level in the extent of T-type FPL between 20–23 weeks of age. The bird died of MD at 23 weeks of age; necropsy showed severe, generalized lymphoma in the viscera.

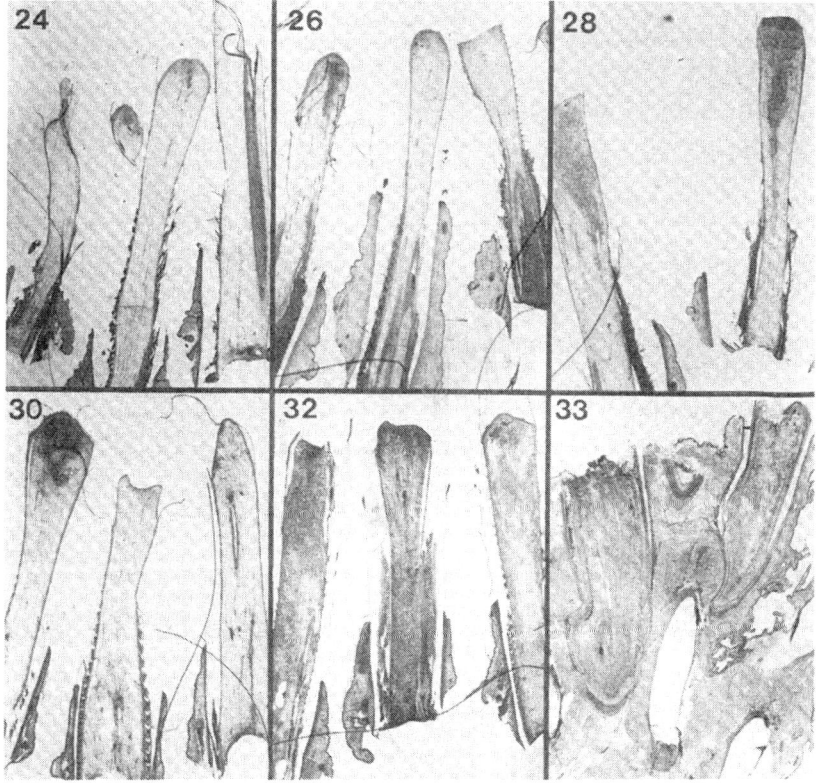

Figure 10. FPL pattern B. Definite fluctuation in the extent of T-type FPL during 24–33 weeks of age, indicating progressive lesion (24–28 weeks of age), regressive lesion (30 weeks of age) and recurrent lesion (32 and 33 weeks of age). The bird was killed at 33 weeks of age; necropsy showed severe, generalized lymphoma with R_2-type lesions (plasma cellular infiltration, fibrous proliferation, etc.) in the viscera.

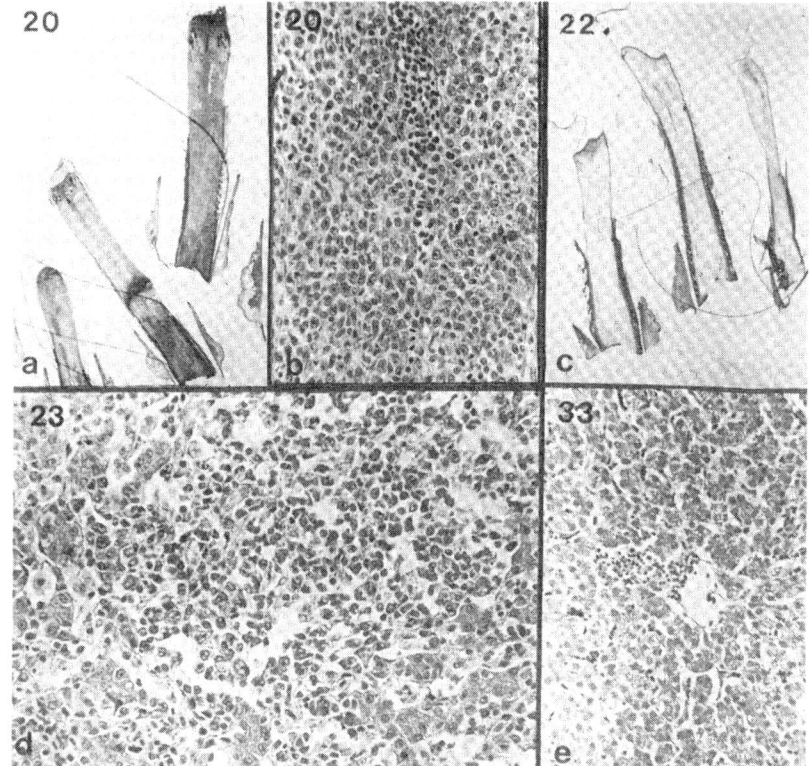

Figure 11a–e. Transient occurrence of severe T-type FPL at 20 weeks old (a, b; low and high power view) in chicken that survived in a healthy state up to 33 weeks old. The T-type FPL disappeared in samples biopsied at (and after) 22 weeks of age (c). Regression of the T-type lesion was also found in the viscera, i.e., heavy T-type lesion was found in the liver biopsy samples obtained at 23 weeks old (d), but no lesions were found in the liver examined at 10 weeks later (e).

REFERENCES

1. Biggs PM, Powell DG, Churchill AE, Chubb RC: The epizootiology of Marek's disease 1. Incidence of antibody, viraemia and Marek's disease in six flocks. *Avian Pathol* 1:5, 1972
2. Calnek BW, Hitchner SB: Localization of viral antigen in chickens infected with Marek's disease herpesvirus. *J Natl Cancer Inst* 43:935, 1969
3. Calnek BW, Aldinger HK, Kahn DE: Feather follicle epithelium: a source of enveloped and infectious cell-free herpesvirus from Marek's disease. *Avian Dis* 14: 219, 1970
4. Calnek BW, Ubertini T, Aldinger HK: Viral antigen, virus particles, and infectivity of tissues from chickens with Marek's disease. *J Natl Cancer Inst* 45:341, 1970
5. Fabricant J, Ianconescu M, Calnek BW: Comparative effects of host and viral factors on early pathogenesis of Marek's disease. *Infect Immun* 16:136, 1977
6. Fujimoto Y, Nakagawa M, Okada K, Okada M, Matsukawa K: Pathological studies of Marek's disease I. The histopathology on field cases in Japan. *Jpn J Vet Res* 19:7, 1971
7. Helmboldt CF, Wills FK, Frazier MN: Field observations of the pathology of skin leukosis in *Gallus gallus*. *Avian Dis* 7:402, 1963
8. Hudson L, Payne LN: An analysis of Marek's disease lymphomas of the chicken. *Nature New Biol* 241:52, 1973
9. Lapen RF, Piper RC, Kenzy SG: Cutaneous changes associated with Marek's disease of chickens. *J Natl Cancer Inst* 45:941, 1970
10. Lapen RF, Kenzy SG, Piper RC, Sharma JM: Pathogenesis of cutaneous Marek's disease in chickens. *J Natl Cancer Inst* 47:389, 1971
11. Lawn AM, Payne LN: Chronological study of ultrastructural changes in the peripheral nerves in Marek's disease. *Neuropathology and Applied Neurobiology* 5:485, 1979
12. Moriguchi R, Izawa H: Marek's disease in chickens: correlation of Marek's disease with nuclear-infusion formation in feather-follicle epithelium. *Avian Dis* 23:547, 1979
13. Moriguchi R, Fujimoto Y, Izawa H: Chronological observations of feather pulp lesions in chickens inoculated with Marek's disease virus. *Avian Dis* 26:375, 1982
14. Moriguchi R, Fujimoto Y, Izawa H: Marek's disease in field chickens: correlation between incidence of Marek's disease and nuclear-inclusion formation in the feather-follicle epithelium. *Avian Dis* 28:331, 1984
15. Moriguchi R, Fujimoto Y, Mori F, Izawa H: Chronological observations of Marek's disease-associated feather pulp lesions in field chickens. *Avian Dis* 30:284, 1985
16. Moriguchi R, Yoshida H, Okada H, Izawa H, Fujimoto Y: Feather pulp lesions in chickens with naturally occurring Marek's disease lymphoma. *Avian Dis* 31:156, 1987
17. Nazerian K, Witter RL: Cell-free transmission and *in vivo* replication of Marek's disease virus. *J Virol* 5:388, 1970
18. Payne LN, Biggs PM: Studies on Marek's disease. II. Pathogenesis. *J Natl Cancer Inst* 39:281, 1967
19. Payne LN, Powell PC, Rennie M: Response of B and T lymphocytes and other blood leukocytes in chickens with

Marek's disease. *Cold Spr Harb Symp Quant Biol* 39:817, 1974

20. Rouse BT, Wells RJH, Warner NL: Proportion of T and B lymphocytes in lesions of Marek's disease: theoretical implications for pathogenesis. *J Immunol* 110:534, 1973
21. Steck F, Haberstich HU: Marek's disease in chickens: development of viral antigen in feather follicles and of circulating antibodies. *Infect Immun* 13:1037, 1976
22. Wight PAL: Variation in peripheral nerve histopathology in fowl paralysis. *J Comp Pathol Ther* 72:40, 1962

23. Witter RL, Solomon JJ, Champion LR, Nazerian K: Long-term studies of Marek's disease infection in individual chickens. *Avian Dis* 15:346, 1971
24. Witter RL, Stephens EA, Sharma JM, Nazerian K: Demonstration of a tumor cell-associated surface antigen in Marek's disease. *J Immunol* 115:177, 1975

16

TESTICULAR TUMORS: SPECIES AND STRAIN VARIATIONS

HOWARD M. HAYES, Jr. and BERNARD SASS

The testis is a complex organ fundamentally composed of two components producing germ cells and sex hormone. The germ cell component consists of the seminiferous tubules lined with spermatogenic cells in various stages of maturation. The sex hormone component consists of interstitial (Leydig) cells and Sertoli (sustentacular) cells. Testis development bears a similarity among mammalian species. Among mammals with scrotal testis, the descent of the testes is also often similar, particularly between man, dog, horse, cow, and the pig (46).

The epidemiologic features of testis neoplasia are likewise similar between many species, based on a cell-type to cell-type comparison. Etiologically, testis neoplasms may be the product of genetic influence, induction by chemical carcinogens, or spontaneous occurrence. It may be presumptuous to regard any tumor, occurring in any animal species, as "spontaneous" (113). However for the purpose of this report, a "spontaneous" testis tumor is one reported in an animal not known to have been exposed to any carcinogenic agent related to the induction of testis tumors.

As a general rule, spontaneous testis tumors rarely occur in mammals. But when they do, particularly in man, they are often highly malignant and pose a threat to life. In man, testicular cancer accounts for only 0.4% of all cancer deaths among those living in the United States. Yet among 15–34 year old men, this is the most common primary cancer and causes 12% of their cancer-related deaths (163).

Worldwide, human testicular cancer is not common in any geographic region, despite the wide variations that exist in incidence rates. Highest rates occur in Denmark and West Germany, lowest rates are in African blacks (79). Blacks in the United States likewise have a lower risk than whites for the malignancy (14). Internationally, the incidence and mortality rate has been rising (98). In the United States, a pronounced increase over time has been noted, particularly for white men aged 15–44 years (14).

Approximately 93% of primary human testis tumors originate from germ cells. In boys under 15 years, about 75% of these tumors are either infantile embryonal carcinoma or teratoma, or a mixture of both cell-types. Choriocarcinoma is not seen in childhood. Seminoma is the predominate testis tumor in middle-aged men, particularly among those over 50 years of age (25).

Among the known causes of testicular tumors, the most reliable determinant is cryptorchism, the presence of which increases man's (27, 95) and dog's (59) risk about 9 fold versus that in non-cryptorchids. Other factors possibly involved in the human disease include prenatal exposures, such as maternal use of exogenous estrogens (27), radiography (13), and genetic predisposition (44). Postnatal factors may involve low birth weight independent of cryptorchism (13), inguinal hernia (27), living in rural areas (83, 148), or urban areas (19), or near incinerators, and/or sewage disposal plants (33), participating in certain recreational sport activities, such as cycling (22), and employment as a professional (e.g., medical, clergy) or in certain skilled occupations (e.g., saw mill, crude oil, and natural gas extraction workers) (94).

The histologic classification of testis tumors has suffered some confusion over the years. The source may have been the attempt of some to classify on the basis of cell origin, when such was not completely understood. Also, there was a failure to appreciate the necessity for definitive identification of the individual components of mixed tumors. At times, investigators from one country seem to have used only their own classification scheme. For example, while there has been no particular dispute regarding what constitutes a seminoma or choriocarcinoma, British investigators often referred to embryonal carcinoma, teratoma, and teratocarcinoma as simply teratomas. French investigators, on the other hand, used other terminology (7).

The array of testicular tumors, by cell-type, occur with considerable variety. Presented is the available information on the occurrence of germ cell tumors (seminoma, embryonal carcinoma, infantile embryonal carcinoma, teratoma, and choriocarcinoma), gonadal stromal tumors, and tumors of the collecting duct system (rete testis) to serve as a reference guide. Because of the voluminous amount of literature published, no attempt has been made to present a complete bibliography. Rather, a representative example is offered in situations where there have been more than one report of a particular cell-type with similar presenting characteristics in the same animal species or laboratory animal strain.

Reports of testis tumors are uncommon-to-rare in domesticated animals (132) (Table 1). Farm animals, in particular, are most often castrated at a young age thereby removing them from the "at-risk" population. Old bulls are reported to develop interstitial cell tumors (91) as do Angora goats (73). Only a few testis tumors have been recorded in sheep (129); the same is true for swine although Steiner and Bengston (137) reported observing a "few" teratomas in their extensive abbatoir survey. In horses, about 200 testis tumors have been reported. Teratomas and seminomas appear to occur with about equal frequency (55); rarely have interstitial cell or Sertoli cell tumors been diagnosed in the horse.

H. E. Kaiser (ed.), Comparative aspects of tumor development.
© 1989, Kluwer Academic Publishers, Dordrecht. ISBN-13:978-0-89838-994-4

Table 1. Spontaneous testicular tumors reported in domestic animal species.

Species	Testis tumor cell type*	Comments	Reference
Bovine	ICT	Adult animal	(100)
Bovine	SEM	2 cases	
Bovine	ICT	3 month old calf	(70)
Bovine	ICT	12% prevalence in old bulls (7 1/2 years+)	(91)
Bovine	SCT	1 case	(9)
Bovine	SCT	10+ year old; Simmental breed	(55)
Bovine	Teratocarc.	3 cases	(132)
Canine	ICT	See TABLE 2	
Canine	SCT	See TABLE 2	
Canine	SEM	See TABLE 2	
Caprine	ICT	29% incidence in Angora breed	(73)
Caprine	SEM	1 case; both testes	(103)
Equine	Embryoma (teratoma?)	2 cases; right intra-abdominal testis; 2 and 3 year old Shires; very rare	(60)
Equine	ICT	Cryptorchid; rare	(131)
Equine	SCT	Tumor in scrotal left testis; right testis undescended; rare	(107)
Equine	SEM	Common equine testis tumor	(12)
Equine	SEM	One case; left scrotal testis and right inguinal testis; both malignant	(154)
Equine	Teratoma	Common equine testis tumor; may occur in undescended testes and be bilateral; usually seen in colts 1–3 years of age	(159, 160)
Feline	Embryonal carc.	13 years old; left testis	(76)
Feline	ICT	3 year old cryptorchid American domestic shorthair cat	(55)
Feline	ICT	10+ year old mixed breed cat	(55)
Feline	SCT, SEM	SCT and SEM in scrotal testis of mixed breed cat; SCT in bilateral cryptorchid mixed breed cat	(92)
Feline	Teratoma	Mixed breed	Peyron and Cocu, 1938; cited by (92)
Ovine	SCT	1 case; Romney ram	
Ovine	SEM	2 cases; Romney Marsh rams 4 and 5 years of age	(128, 129)
Ovine	SEM	5/78; abattoir survey; 1 Columbia breed 4 years of age; 1 Hampshire breed 5 years of age; 3 Hampshire and Suffolk crossbreds 6–8 years of age, 2 of which had bilateral involvement	(72)
Ovine	Adenocarc. rete testis	Merino ram; right testis	(125)

Table 1. Continued

Species	Testis tumor cell type*	Comments	Reference
Porcine	SCT	1 case; seen at Iowa State Veterinary University	(108)
Porcine	SEM	7 year old large white English race	(62)
Porcine	Teratoma	Several cases seen in abattoir survey	(137)

* SCT = Sertoli cell tumor
  SEM = Seminoma
  ICT = Interstitial cell tumor

The domestic cat is another species about which only a few reports of testis tumors exist. The citations in Table 1 represent all of the available literature.

The "pet dog" is the exception to the typical "castration" practice of domestic animals. He is often permitted to live his life sexually intact. Because of this, or possibly due to a species' characteristic, canine testicular tumors are a common recognized occurrence.

The largest case series of canine testicular tumors presented with a referent hospital population at-risk involved 410 dogs (56) collectively seen at collaborating colleges of veterinary medicine in North America (58). A current review of the data from North American veterinary colleges (1500

cases; (57)) indicates Sertoli cell tumor, seminoma, and interstitial cell tumor represent almost all of the primary cell-types and occur with equal frequency. This cell-type distribution, however, is altered in the cryptorchid dog which more often develops a Sertoli cell tumor and to a lesser extent, the seminoma (59). Other relative information on the dog is presented in Table 2. There were reports 50 years ago citing canine testicular teratomas (124); none recently have been described. There has been one report of a canine gonadoblastoma (151).

There is a paucity of reports of spontaneous testis tumors in wildlife and zoo animals (Table 3). Interstitial cell tumor, seminoma, and Sertoli cell tumors have been reported in non-human primates. Considering the few opportunities to observe testis tumors in jungle cats and other "big" cats, the three cases reported (32, 121, 157) suggest that these ani-

Table 2. Spontaneous and genetically influenced testicular tumors in canines.

Characteristic	Sertoli cell tumor	Seminoma	Interstitial cell tumor	Reference
Hospital prevalence in 1,242 cases with only one testis tumor cell type	32%	34%	34%	(57)
Mean age (years) at diagnosis	9.8 (N = 399)	11.0 (N = 425)	11.6 (N = 418)	(57)
Percentage reported as malignant	28%	26%	14%	(57)
Familial association	Yes	Yes	Yes	(56)
Associated with cryptorchism	Yes	Yes	No	(59)
Occurrence in abdominal or inguinal testes	> 50%	38%	5%	(82)
Clinical signs of feminization	24%	6%	1.5%	(82)
Clinical signs of prostatic disease other than neoplasia	19%	14%	17%	(57)
Prevalence when seen with adrenocortical neoplasms	10%	14%	76%	(57)
Prevalence when seen with chemodectoma	8%	31%	61%	(57)
Prevalence when seen with perianal gland neoplasms	13%	22%	65%	(161)
Prevalence when seen with prostatic carcinoma	15%	39%	46%	(57)

Table 3. Spontaneous testicular tumors reported in wildlife and zoo animal species.

Order/species/strain	Testis tumor cell type*	Comments	Reference
ARTIODACTYLA			
Cervus canadensis (Elk)	SEM	10 years old	(126)
CARNIVORA			
Felis chaus (Jungle cat)	SCT	Washington DC zoo; 23 years; right testis	(121)
Neofelis nebulosa (Clouded leopard)	SCT	San Diego zoo	(32)
Neofelis nebulosa (Clouded leopard)	SEM	San Diego zoo	(157)
Thalarctos maritimus (Polar bear)	SEM	London zoo; 22 years; possibly malignant	(3)
Vulpes vulpes (Red fox)	SEM	10 years old; right inguinal testis; cyst in right testis	(45)
MARSUPIALIA			
Megalela rufa (Red kangaroo)	SCT	San Diego zoo; aged animal	(157)
PERISSODACTYLA			
Equus zebra x Equus caballus (Zebra cross)	SEM	Naples Zoo; 22 years; monorchid; left scrotal testis malignant	(104)
PRIMATE			
Gorilla gorilla (Lowland gorilla)	ICT	Regent's Park Zoo, London; 33 years old; left testis	(75)
Pongo pygmaeus (Orangutan	SEM		(156)
Alouatta caraya (Howler monkey)	SEM	1/174; tumor weighed 5 kg	(88)
Macaca mulatta (Rhesus monkey)	SEM	Left testis	(90)
Aotus trivirgatus (Owl monkey)	SCT	Right scrotal testis	(36)

* SCT = Sertoli cell tumor
SEM = Seminoma
ICT = Interstitial cell tumor

Table 4. Spontaneous and genetically influenced testicular tumors reported in laboratory animal species.

Species/strain	Testis tumor cell type*	Comments	Reference
Gerbil (Mongolian)	SEM	1/50; right testis; 24 months old	(5)
Gerbil (Mongolian)	Teratoma	15 months old; left testis	(155)
Guinea pig	Embryonal carc.	1 in 25 surviving over age 3 years	(115)
Hamster, Syrian	SEM	1/7,200	(77)
Mastomys	Adenocarc. rete testis	2.7% incidence in those > 18 months of age	(134)
	SEM	2.1% incidence in those > 18 months of age	(134)
Woodchuck	ICT	1 case from the Penrose colony	(135)
Rabbit strains			
Chinchilla	SEM (?)	4 year old	(61)

Table 4. Spontaneous and genetically influenced testicular tumors reported in laboratory animal species.

Species/strain	Testis tumor cell type*	Comments	Reference
Domestic	SEM	7–9 years old, malignant	(55)
Dutch	ICT,	1/14	(67)
	SEM	1/14; bilateral	(67)
New Zealand	ICT	5 1/2 year old monorchid	(16)
New Zealand	ICT	5 year old; bilateral in scrotal testes	(37)
"Stock"	ICT		(26)
Strain III	Teratoma		(93)
Mouse strains			
A, hybrids	ICT		(41)
AxC	ICT		Hare and Stewart, 1953; cited by (35)
A/HeJ	Teratocarc.	2 weeks old; right testis	(93)
Alderley Park (strain 1)	ICT	5.9% incidence per 100 testes	(66)
BALB/c	Choriocarc.		(96)
BALB/c	ICT	Small tumor; < 1% incidence	(2)
BALB/c	ICT	Cryptorchid	(68)
BALB/cJ	ICT	Transplantable	(85)
BALB/cCr	ICT,	6/2088; 18 months old	(87)
	SEM	1/2088; 18 months old	
B6C3 (F_1)	Embryonal carc.	2 cases	(1)
B6C3 (F_1)	ICT	3 cases	
B6C3 (F_1)	SEM	1 case	
C	ICT	Transplantable	(64)
C3H/A	SCT		(97)
C3H Heston	ICT, SCT	Both in same testis	(38)
C57BL	SCT		(97)
C57BL/Ka	ICT	13% incidence; mean life span was 23 months	(165)
C57BL/6	ICT	3 cases; 0.75% incidence	(1)
DB	ICT	When transplanted, causes greatest increase in plasma volume	(158)
DBAxCE hybrid	ICT	3% incidence	(30)
(DBA/2x4BR) F_1	ICT	AFIP files	(96)
DBA/2J	Teratocarc.	Left testis; 4 months old	(93)
DBA/2J	SCT	Right testis; 7 months old; incomplete undifferentiated form	(93)
H	ICT	25% incidence; associated with mammary tumors	(39)
Icr:Ha (ICR)	ICT	1/166	(31)
JCLxICR	Adenocarc. of rete testis	1 case; 0.4% incidence	(162)
Nude-BALB/c	ICT	< 1% incidence	(146)
Nude-CBA/H	ICT	1/33	(146)
Nude-CBA/H-A^{vy}	ICT	1/40	(146)
RF	ICT	Transplantable; may be hormonally inactive, secrete estrogen or androgen	(20)
(Y/B2xAKR) F_1	ICT	AFIP files	(96)

Table 4. Continued

Species/strain	Testis tumor cell type*	Comments	Reference
129	Embryonal carc.	16 day old fetus	(141)
129	Teratoma	1% incidence; 3:1 left side differential	(144)
129/Dr	Teratoma	1.1% incidence	(145)
129/J	Teratoma	1.7% incidence	(145)
129/Re	Teratoma	0.3% incidence	(145)
129/Rr	Teratoma	0.6% incidence	(145)
129/Sv	Teratoma	1.6% incidence	(145)
129/Sv-Sl	Teratoma	Same incidence in 15–19 day fetuses as in older mice	(138)
129/Sv-SlCP	Teratoma	10% incidence	(145)
129/Sv-Sl^{d}CP	Teratoma	16.5% incidence; left side differential	(143)
129/Sv-Sl^{j}CP	Teratoma	18% incidence; left side differential	(143)
129/Sv-W^{v}CP	Teratoma	5–10% incidence	(143)
129/ter-Sv	Teratoma	32% incidence; left side differential	(142)
129/ter-Sv	Teratoma	Familial predisposition possibly due to single gene	(102)
"Stock mouse"	ICT	28/9500	(130); classification by Horn and Stewart, (65)
"White mouse"	SEM	0.09% incidence	(96)
Rat strains			
ACI	ICT	20% incidence in older animals	(136)
ACI/N	ICT	20% incidence in 12–18 months old; 85% incidence in > 18 months of age	(133)
BDX	ICT	1/37	(164)
Fischer	ICT	68% incidence; 3/4ths were bilateral	(71)
Fischer 344	ICT	86% incidence	(122)
Fischer 344	ICT	Frequently bilateral	(21)
Fischer 344	ICT	Malignant; 2.5% incidence in combined reports of those aged 24+ months	(1)
Fischer 344	SEM	Very rare; 0.6% incidence	(122)
Fischer 344/N	ICT	70% incidence in < 18 month old virgins; 30% incidence in same age breeders	(136)
King-Holtzman hybrids	ICT	Testes had morphologic characteristics of steroid-producing cells	(18)
M520/N	ICT	35% incidence in virgin males > 18 months of age	(53)
MRC	SEM	1% incidence	(150)
MRC(WI)BR	ICT	18% incidence	(119)
Oregon	ICT	3.7% incidence	(86)
Osborne-Mendel (Yale)	Embryonal carc., ICT	1 case each	(123)
Osborne-Mendel (Yale)	ICT	4/975	(49)
Sprague Dawley	ICT	5-fold increase between ages 18–24 and > 24 months	(1)

Table 4. Spontaneous and genetically influenced testicular tumors reported in laboratory animal species.

Species/strain	Testis tumor cell type*	Comments	Reference
(WAGxBN) F₁	ICT	6% incidence	(15)
WAG/Rij	ICT	3% incidence	(15)
Wistar/Copenhagen	ICT	8% incidence	(47)
Wistar/GG	ICT	18% incidence	(47)
Wistar/Johannesburg	ICT	19% incidence 13–32 months of age; 84% had pheochromocytoma	(48)
Wistar/PVG	ICT	60% incidence by 2 years of age	(23)
Wistar/Rochester	ICT	20% incidence at age 18–24 months	(24)
Wistar/Utrecht	ICT	5% incidence	(47)
Wistar/Furth	SEM	1 case	(147)

* SCT = Sertoli cell tumor
 SEM = Seminoma
 ICT = Interstitial cell tumor

Table 5. Experimentally induced or environmentally influenced testicular tumors reported in laboratory animal species.

Species/strain	Testis tumor cell type*	Comments	Reference
Rhesus monkey	SEM	Exposed to irradiation; 18 years old	(90)
Hamster strains			
Syrian golden	Embryonal carc.	Induced with zinc chloride (intratesticular); 2/49	(52)
Syrian golden	Embryonal carc.	Induced with ethylurea sodium nitrite; 1/28	(118)
Syrian golden	ICT	5 of 50 induced with subcutaneous implant of diethylstilbestrol	(110)
Syrian golden	SCT	1 case; induced with estradiol	(4)
Syrian golden	SEM	1 case; induced with 2-aminoacetophenone	(54)
Syrian golden	SEM	1 case; induced with diethylstilbestrol	(112)
European (strain MHH:EPH)	ICT	27 of 50 induced with subcutaneous implant of diethylstilbestrol	(110)
Rabbit strains			
Dutch	ICT,	1/20 receiving neutron irradiation	(67)
	SCT,	4/20 – neutron irradiation; 3/15 – gamma irradiation	
	SEM	1/20 – neutron irradiation; 1/15 – gamma irradiation	
Mouse strains			
A	ICT	Estrogen induced	(11)
A	ICT	Estradiol benzoate and stilbestrol	(63)
A	ICT	Pregnant mare serum injections	(105)
(AxA.SW) F₁ hybrids	ICT	3/70 induced with flank implant of diethylstilbestrol; transplantable	(78)

Table 5. Continued

Species/strain	Testis tumor cell type*	Comments	Reference
(A/HexC57L) F₁	ICT	Radiation induced	(153)
BLAC/c	ICT	Occurred after being made cryptorchid by surgery	(69)
BLAC/c & F₁ hybrid	ICT	Induced with tri-p-anisylchloroethylene given subcutaneously	(106)
BALB/c & hybrids	ICT	Estrogen induced; 80% incidence	(2)
C	ICT	Induced with subcutaneous implant of stilbestrol-cholesterol pellets	(127)
CBA	ICT	Estrogen induced	(40)
CD-1 outbred	Adenocarc. rete testis	4.7% incidence in prenatal exposure to diethylstilbestrol	(101)
C_3H	ICT	Estrogen induced	(40)
C57	ICT	Chlorotrianisene	(42)
C57BL	ICT	Estrogen induced; 3% incidence	(2)
C57BLxCBA	ICT	Chlorotrianisene	(43)
DBA/2	ICT	Estrogen induced; 10% incidence; 16 months average age	(2)
DBA/2eB	ICT	1/60 induced with flank implant of diethylstilbestrol	(28)
DD	ICT	Cyclophosphamide	(149)
IFS	ICT	Estrogen induced; ingested 3 mg. in oil weekly for 20–99 weeks	(10)
JCLxICR	Adenoma of rete testis	Fed chlorpromazine in food; 1 case; 0.4% incidence	(162)
JK	ICT	Estrogen induced; 7 of 13, all developed unilateral tumors	(40)
Nude-BLAC/c	ICT	Estrogen induced; 56%+ incidence	(146)
R III	ICT	Estrogen induced	(10)
(YBRxAKR) F₁	ICT	22% incidence with (aa) and 5% with lethal yellow gene (A^4a)	(29)
WLL	ICT	Estrogen induced	(10)
129/Sv	Teratoma	Transplanted tubal ova to adult testes	(140)
129/Sv-S1	Teratoma	2.4% incidence increasing to 5.6% after 1st litter when gene Steel (Sl) introduced	(145)
129/Sv-Sl	Teratoma	Transplanted 12.5 day-old genital ridges from male fetuses to adult testes; 82% developed tumors	(139)
"Albino mouse" Charles River cesarean-derived strain	ICT	Cadmium chloride	(50)
Rat strains			
Chester Beatty	ICT	Cadmium sulfate	(114)
Fischer	ICT	5-azacytidine	(17)
Fischer	Gonadal stromal	68% incidence with N-nitrosobis (2-oxopropyl)amine	(109)

Table 5. Continued

Species/strain	Testis tumor cell type*	Comments	Reference
Long-Evans	ICT	Localized irradiation; 40/74 that received 500 rad	(81)
MRC outbred	Adenocarc.	Fed carrageenan for 110 days	(120)
MRC(WI)BR	ICT	47% incidence with 0.6% metronidazole	(119)
R	ICT	Transplanted testis tissue to anterior eye chamber in gonadectomized males and females	(80)
Sherman	Granulosa-theca like	Transplant infantile testis in spleen of castrated adults	(8)
Sprague-Dawley	Embryonal carc., ICT, SEM, Teratocarc.	Whole body radiation; 11/19 were affected; all were 15–18 months post-irradiation at death	(6)
Sprague-Dawley	ICT	1/42 induced with 430 rad of x radiation; concomitant with adrenocortical adenoma, pheochromocytoma, pituitary adenoma and islet cell tumor	(116)
Sprague-Dawley	ICT	1/74 induced with 320 rads of neutrons; concomitant with thyroid and islet cell tumor	(117)
Wistar	ICT	Cadmium chloride	(50)
Wistar	ICT	Flank injection of 4′-fluoro-4-Aminodiphenyl	(89)
Wistar	ICT	Ligation of spermatic vessels ligation plus zinc	(51)
Wistar	ICT	Transplanted testis tissue under splenic capsule	(74)
Wistar IC	ICT, SEM ICT, Teratoma	Induced with zinc chloride at 28 months; zinc chloride plus gonadotropic hormone at 20 months	(111)
Wistar/Twombly	ICT	Transplanted testis tissue to spleen of gonadectomized males and females	(152)
"White rat"	SEM	Injection of methylcholanthrene	(84)
"Stock rat"	ICT	Induced by ligation of the internal spermatic & deferential arteries with the vas deferens	(34)

* SCT = Sertoli cell tumor
  SEM = Seminoma
  ICT = Interstitial cell tumor

Table 6. Summary of testicular tumors reported in animals.

Species	Embryonal carcinoma	Interstitial cell tumor	Seminoma	Sertoli cell tumor	Teratoma
Bull	−	+	+	+	+
Boar	−	−	+	+	+
Cat	+	+	+	+	+
Dog	−	+	+	+	−
Elk	−	−	+	−	−
Gerbil	−	−	+	−	+
Goat	−	+	+	−	−
Guinea pig	+	−	−	−	−
Hamster	+	+	+	+	−
Marsupial	−	−	−	+	−
Mastomys	−	−	+	−	−
Mouse	+	+	+	+	+
Primates	−	+	+	+	−
Rabbit	−	+	+	+	+
Rat	+	+	+	−	+
Ram	−	−	+	+	−
Stallion	−	+	+	+	+
Woodchuck	−	+	−	−	−

mals, as a group, may have a higher frequency of the disease than their domesticated relatives.

Laboratory animals have provided a wealth of information on testicular neoplasia. The experimental work of Stevens and Little (144) established a milestone as it served to confirm the germ cell origin of teratomas. A wide range of testis tumor cell-types have been reported, particularly in outbred and inbred rats, mice, and rabbits (Table 4). Within these species exists a wide variation of "strain" differences in frequency and cell-type specificity of spontaneous tumor occurrence.

Experimentally induced testis tumors usually have been interstitial cell tumors, particularly in laboratory mice and rats (Table 5). Agents such as exogenous estrogen (40), irradiation (153), zinc (111), and cadmium (114) have been proven in the laboratory to be testis carcinogens. Although strikingly, a combination of zinc and cadmium did not induce interstitial cell tumors in mice and rats in one study (50). Note that the strain designation presented in Tables 4 and 5 is that cited by the investigator. These designations may differ from the nomenclature employed today.

An abbreviated overall summary of this review is presented in Table 6.

ACKNOWLEDGMENTS

We thank Drs. H.L. Stewart and A.G. Liebelt for critique and helpful suggestions.

REFERENCES

1. Altman PL: (ed.): Pathology of Laboratory Mice and Rats. Elmsford, NY, Pergamon Press, 246, 1985
2. Andervont HB, Shimkin MB and Canter HY: Susceptibility of seven inbred strains and the F_1 hybrids to estrogen-induced testicular tumors and occurrence of spontaneous testicular tumors in strain BALB/c mice. *J Natl Cancer Inst* 25:1069, 1960
3. Appleby EC: Tumours in captive wild animals: some observations and comparisons. *Acta Zool Path Antverpiensia* 48:77, 1969
4. Bacon RL and Kirkman H: The response of the testis of the hamster to chronic treatment with different estrogens. *Endocrinol* 57:255, 1955
5. Benitz K-F and Kramer AW Jr: Spontaneous tumors in the Mongolian gerbil. *Lab Anim Care* 15:281–294, 1965
6. Berdjis CC: Protracted effects of repeated doses of x-ray irradiation in rats. *Exp Molec Pathol* 2:157–172, 1963
7. Berdjis CC: Testicular tumors in infants and children: a comparative study of similar tumors in animals. *In*: Tumours of Early Life in Man and Animals. Severi, L. (ed.), Perugia, Perugia University, pp. 1111–1129, 1978
8. Biskin MS and Biskind GR: Tumor of rat testis produced by heterotransplantation of infantile testis to spleen of adult castrate. *Proc Soc Exp Biol Med* 59:4–8, 1945
9. Blom E and Christensen NO: Sertoli cell tumour combined with lack of epididymis in a bull. *Acta Pathol Microbiol Immun Scand* 90A(4):283–288, 1982
10. Bonser GM: Mammary and testicular tumours in male mice of various strains following oestrogen treatment. *J Path Bact* 56:15–26, 1944
11. Bonser GM and Robson JM: The effects of prolonged oestrogen administration upon male mice of various strains: development of testicular tumours in the Strong A strain. *J Path Bact* 51:9–22, 1940
12. Bourgoin JJ: Les cancers spontanes des animaux. *Bull Soc Sci et Med comparée* (Lyon) 74:307 314, 1972
13. Brown LM, Pottern LM and Hoover RN: Prenatal and perinatal risk factors for testicular cancer. Submitted for consideration, *Cancer Res* 46, 1812–1816, 1986
14. Brown LM, Pottern LM, Hoover RN, Devesa SS, Aselton P and Flannery JT: Testicular cancer in the United States: trends in incidence and mortality. *Int J Epid* 5:164–170, 1986
15. Burek JD: Pathology of Aging Rats. West Palm Beach, FL, CRC Press, p. 136, 1978
16. Byoung IY: Interstitial cell tumor in a monorchid rabbit. (Abstract) *Lab Anim Sci* 35:538, 1985
17. Carr BI, Reilly JG, Smith SS, Winberg C and Riggs A: The tumorigenicity of 5-azacytidine in the male Fischer rat. *Carcinogenesis* 5:1583–1590, 1984
18. Chung KW, Allison JE and Stanley AJ: Structural and functional factors related to testicular neoplasia in feminized rats. *J Natl Cancer Inst* 65:161–168, 1980

19. Clemmesen J: A doubling of morbidity from testis carcinoma in Copenhagen. 1943–1962. *Acta Pathol Microbiol Scand* 72:348–349, 1968

20. Clifton KH, Bloch E, Upton AC and Furth J: Transplantable Leydig-cell tumors in mice. *Arch Path* 62:354–368, 1956

21. Cockrell BY and Garner FM: Interstitial cell tumor of the testis in rats. *Comp Pathol Bull* 8:2–4, 1976

22. Coldman AJ, Elwood JM and Gallagher RP: Sports activities and risk of testicular cancer. *Br J Cancer* 46:749–756, 1982

23. Cotchin E and Roe FJC: Pathology of Laboratory Rats and Mice. Oxford, Blackwell Scientific Publications, p. 423, 1967

24. Crain RC: Spontaneous tumors in the Rochester strain of the Wistar rat. *Amer J Pathol* 34:311–335, 1958

25. Culp DA, Boatman DL and Wilson VB: Testicular tumors: 40 years' experience. *J Urol* 110:548–553, 1973

26. De Faria JF: Tumor de celulas intersticiais do testiculo em coelho. *Arch Inst Biol Anim* (Rio de Janeiro) 4:127–131, 1961

27. Depue RH, Pike MC and Henderson BE: Estrogen exposure during gestation and risk of cancer of the testis. *J Natl Cancer Inst* 71:1151–1155, 1983

28. Deringer MK: Development of tumors, especially mammary tumors, in agent-free strain DBA/2eB mice. *J Natl Cancer Inst* 28:203–210, 1962

29. Deringer MK: Influence of the lethal yellow (A^y) gene on development of reticular neoplasms. *J Natl Cancer Inst* 45:1205–1210, 1970

30. Dickie MM: The use of F₁ hybrid and backcross generations to reveal new and/or uncommon tumor types. *J Natl Cancer Inst* 15:791–799, 1954

31. Eaton GJ, Johnson FN, Custer RP and Crane AR: The Icr:Ha(ICR) mouse: a current account of breeding, mutations, diseases and mortality. *Lab Animals* 14:17–24, 1980

32. Effron M, Griner L and Bernirschke K: Nature and rate of neoplasia found in captive wild mammals, birds, and reptiles at necropsy. *J Natl Cancer Inst* 59:185–198, 1977

33. Feldman PS, Howards SS, Harris C and Harris C: A geographic cluster of testicular seminomas. *J Urol* 129:839–840, 1983

34. Fels E and Bur GE: Modification du testicule du rat par ligature du pedicule vasculaire. *Comptes Rendus Soc Biol* (Paris) 152:1395–1396, 1958

35. Firminger HI: Testicular tumors. *In*: The physiopathology of Cancer. Homburger F and Fishman WH (eds.), New York, Paul B. Hoeber, Inc., pp. 149–164, 1953

36. Fiske RA, Woodard JC and Moreland AF: Sertoli cell tumor in an owl monkey. *J Amer Vet Med Assoc* 163:1206–1207, 1973

37. Flatt RE and Weisbroth SH: Interstitial cell tumor of the testicle in rabbits: a report of two cases. *Lab Anim Sci* 24:682–685, 1974

38. Franks LM: Spontaneous interstitial and Sertoli cell tumors of a testis in a C3H mouse. *Cancer Res* 28:125–127, 1968

39. Furtado-Dias MT: Spontaneous testicular tumours in mice of the H strain. *In*: II. International Symposium on Mammary Cancer. Severi,L. (ed.), Perugia, Univ. Perugia, pp. 505–512, 1958

40. Gardner WU: Testicular tumors in mice of several strains receiving triphenylethylene. *Cancer Res* 3:92–99, 1943a

41. Gardner WU: Spontaneous testicular tumors in mice. *Cancer Res* 3:757–761, 1943b

42. Gardner WU: Testicular tumorigenesis. *Ciba Found Colloq Endocrinol* [*Proc.*] 12:239–249, 1958

43. Gardner WU and Boddaert J: Testicular interstitial cell tumors in hybrid mice given tri-p-anisyl-chloro ethylene. *Arch Pathol* 50:750–764, 1950

44. Gedde-dahl T Jr, Hannisdal E, Klepp OH, Grottum KA, Waksvik H, Fossa SD, Stenwig AE and Brogger A: Testicular neoplasms occurring in four brothers. *Cancer* 55:2005–2009, 1985

45. Gelberg HB and McEntee K: Cystic rete testis in a cat and fox. *Vet Pathol* 20:634–636, 1983

46. Gier HT and Marion GB: Development of mammalian testes and genital ducts. *Biol Reprod* (*Suppl.*) 1:1–23, 1969

47. Gilbert C, Gillman J, Loustalot P and Lutz W: The modifying influence of diet and the physical environment on spontaneous tumour frequency in rats. *Br J Cancer* 12:565–593, 1958

48. Gillman J, Gilbert C and Spence I: Phaeochromocytoma in the rat. *Cancer* 6:494–511, 1953

49. Goodman DG, Ward JM, Squire RA, Paxton MB, Reichardt WD, Chu KC and Linhart MS: Neoplastic and nonneoplastic lesions in aging Osborne-Mendel rats. *Tox Appl Pharm* 55:433–447, 1980

50. Gunn SA, Gould TC and Anderson WAD: Cadmium-induced interstitial cell tumors in rats and mice and their prevention by zinc. *J Natl Cancer Inst.* 31:745–759, 1963

51. Gunn SA, Gould TC and Anderson WAD: Comparative study of interstitial cell tumors of rat testis induced by cadmium injection and vascular ligation. *J Natl Cancer Inst.* 35:329–337, 1965

52. Guthrie J and Guthrie OA: Embryonal carcinomas in Syrian hamsters after intratesticular inoculation of zinc chloride during seasonal testicular growth. *Cancer Res.* 34:2612–2614, 1974

53. Hansen CT, Potkay S, Watson WT and Whitney RA Jr: NIH Rodents 1980 Catalogue. Bethesda, MD, NIH Pub. No. 83–606, 1982

54. Harkovskaja NA: [Carcinogentic action of 2-aminoacetophenone in Syrian hamsters]. *Vop Onkol* 25:81–84, 1979

55. Hayes HM Jr: Unpublished observations from the Veterinary Medical Data program, 1986

56. Hayes HM Jr and Pendergrass TW: Canine testicular tumors: epidemiologic features of 410 dogs. *Int J Cancer* 18:482–487, 1976

57. Hayes HM Jr, Sass B and Wilson GP: Testis tumors: a report on 1,500 cases. In preparation, 1986.

58. Hayes HM Jr, Wilson GP and Moraff H: The Veterinary Medical Data Program (VMDP): Past, Present, and Future. *In*: Proceedings of International Symposium on Animal Health and Disease Data Banks, December 4–6, 1978, Washington, D.C., USDA, APHIS, Misc. Pub. # 1381, pp. 127–132, 1979

59. Hayes HM Jr, Wilson GP, Pendergrass TW and Cox VS: Canine cryptorchidism and subsequent testicular neoplasia: case-control study with epidemiologic update. *Teratology* 32:51–56, 1985

60. Hobday F: Cryptorchidism in animals and man. *Proc Roy Soc Med* (Oct. 24, 1923) 17:3–17, 1924

61. Hoffmann JA: Hodenkrebs bei einem Kaninchen. *Berl Münch Tierarztl Ztschr* 67:350–353, 1954

62. Holst SJ: Sterility in boars. *Nord Vet Med* 1:87–120, 1949

63. Hooker CW and Pfeiffer CA: The morphology and development of testicular tumours in mice of the A strain receiving estrogens. *Cancer Res* 2:759–769, 1942

64. Hooker CW, Strong LC and Pfeiffer CA: A spontaneous transplantable testicular tumor in a mouse. (Abstract) *Cancer Res* 6:503, 1946

65. Horn HA and Stewart HL: A review of some spontaneous tumors in noninbred mice *J Natl Cancer Inst* 13:591, 1952

66. Hulse EV: Can radiation induce interstitial-cell (Leydig-cell) tumours of the testes? *Int J Radiat Biol* 32:185–190, 1977

67. Hulse EV: Tumour incidence and longevity in neutron and gamma-irradiated rabbits, with an assessment of r.b.e. *Int J Radiat Biol* 337:633–652, 1980

68. Huseby RA: Interstitial cell tumours of the mouse testis. Studies of tumorigenesis, dependency and hormone production. *In*: Hormone Production in Endocrine Tumors. *Ciba Foundation Colloquia on Endocrinology* 12:216–230, 1958

69. Huseby RA and Bittner JJ: The development of interstitial-

cell tumors of the testes in experimentally cryptorchid Bagg albino C mice bearing grafted ovaries. (Abstract) *Sc Proc Amer Assoc Cancer Res Cancer Res* 12:271, 1952

70. Innes JRM: Neoplatic diseases of the testis in animals. *J Path Bact* 54: 485–498, 1942

71. Jacobs BB and Huseby RA: Neoplasms occurring in aged Fischer rats, with special reference to testicular, uterine, and thyroid tumors. *J Natl Cancer Inst* 39:303–309, 1967

72. Jensen R and Flint JC: Intratubular seminomas in testes of sheep. *J Comp Path* 73:146–149, 1963

73. Johns DE, Street CS, Terner JY and Berdjis CC: Incidence of cryptorchidism and tumors in the goat testes. EASP 100-38, Research Laboratories, Edgewood Arsenal, MD, 1968.

74. Jones A: Experimental production of interstitial cell tumours. *Br J Cancer* 9:640–645, 1955

75. Jones DM, Dixson AF and Wadsworth PF: Interstitial cell tumor of the testis in a western lowland gorilla (*Gorilla gorilla gorilla*). *J Med Primatol* 9:319–322, 1980

76. Joshua JO: The Clinical Aspects of Some Diseases of Cats. Philadelphia, J.B. Lippincott, pp. 119–140, 1965

77. Kirkman H: A preliminary report concerning tumors observed in Syrian hamsters. *Stanford Med Bull* 20:163–166, 1962

78. Klein G and Hellstrom KE: Transplantation studies on estrogen-induced interstitial-cell tumors of testis in mice. *J Natl Cancer Inst* 28:99–115, 1962

79. Kolonel LN, Ross RK, Thomas DB and Thompson DJ: Epidemiology of testicular cancer in the Pacific basin. *Natl Cancer Inst Monogr* 62:157–160, 1982

80. Kullander S: On tumor formation in gonadal and hypophyseal transplants into the anterior eye chambers of gonadectomized rats. *Cancer Res* 20:1079–1082, 1960

81. Lindsay S, Nichols CW Jr, Sheline GE and Chaikoff IL: Leydig-cell tumors in rat testes subjected to low-dose x-irradiation. *Rad Res* 40:366–378, 1969

82. Lipowitz A, Schwartz A, Wilson GP and Ebert JW: Testicular neoplasms and concomitant clinical changes in the dog. *J Amer Vet Med Assoc* 163:1364–1368, 1973

83. Lipworth L and Dayan AD: Rural preponderance of seminoma of the testis. *Cancer* 23:1119–1122, 1969

84. Llombart A and Sansano-pena V: La production experimental de tumores testiculare por el metil-colantreno. *Cir Ginecol Urol* 11:81–92, 1957

85. Lucis OJ and Lucis R: Metabolism of steroids by transplantable mouse interstitial cell tumor. *Cancer Res* 29:1647–1652, 1969

86. MacKenzie WF and Garner FM: Comparison of neoplasms in six sources of rats. *J Natl Cancer Inst* 50:1243–1257, 1973

87. Madison RM, Rabstein LS and Bryan WR: Mortality rate and spontaneous lesions found in 2,928 untreated BALB/cCr mice. *J Natl Cancer Inst* 40:683–685, 1968

88. Maruffo CA: Spontaneous tumours in Howler monkeys. *Nature* 213:521, 1967

89. Matthews JJ and Walpole AL: Tumours of the liver and kidney induced in Wistar rats with 4'-fluoro-4-Aminodiphenyl. *Br J Cancer* 12:234–241, 1958

90. McClure HM: Neoplasia in Rhesus monkeys. *In*: The Rhesus Monkey. Volume II., Bourne, G.H. (Ed.), New York, Academic Press, pp. 369–398, 1975

91. McEntee K: Pathological conditions in old bulls with impaired fertility. *J Amer Vet Med Assoc* 132:328–331, 1958

92. Meier H: Sertoli-cell tumor in the cat. Report of two cases. *North Amer Vet* 37:979–981, 1956

93. Meier H, Myers DD, Fox RR and Laird CW: Occurrence, pathological features, and propagation of gonadal teratomas in inbred mice and in rabbits. *Cancer Res* 30:30–34, 1970

94. Mills PK, Newell GR and Johnson DE: Testicular cancer associated with employment in agriculture and oil and natural gas extraction. *Lancet* (#8370) 1:207–210, 1984

95. Morrison AS: Cryptorchidism, hernia, and cancer of the testis. *J Natl Cancer Inst* 56:731–733, 1976

96. Mostofi FK and Bresler VM: Tumours of the testis. *In*: Pathology of Tumours in Laboratory Animals. Volume II. – Tumours of the Mouse. Turusov, V.S. (ed.), Lyon, Internatiional Agency for Research on Cancer, pp. 325–350, 1979

97. Mostofi FK and Sesterhenn I: Neoplasms of the male reproductive tract. *In*: The Mouse in Biomedical Research. Volume IV. Experimental Biology and Oncology. Foster, H.L., Small, J.D. and Fox, J.G. (eds.), New York, Academic Press, pp. 413–438, 1982

98. Muir CS and Nectoux J: Epidemiology of cancer of the testis and penis. *Natl Cancer Inst Monogr* 53:157–164, 1979

99. Mustacchi P and Millmore D: Racial and occupational variations in cancer of the testis: San Francisco, 1956–65. *J Natl Cancer Inst* 56:717–720, 1976

100. Nascimento EF, Chquiloff MA and Maia PCC: Alteracoes testiculares e epididimarias em bovinos. IV. Neoplasias. *Arquivo Brasil Med Vet Zootecnia* 35:515–521, 1983

101. Newbold RR, Bullock BC and McLachlan JA: Lesions of the rete testis in mice exposed prenatally to diethylstilbestrol. *Cancer Res* 45:5145–5150, 1985

102. Noguchi T and Stevens LC: Primordial germ cell proliferation in fetal testes in mouse strains with high and low incidences of congenital testicular teratomas. *J Natl Cancer Inst* 69:907–913, 1982

103. Pamukcu AM: Seminoma of the testicles in an Ankara goat. *Vet Fak Derg* 1:42–46, 1954

104. Pandolfi F and Roperto F: Seminoma with multiple metastases in a zebra (*Equus zebra*) × mare (*Equus caballus*). *Eq vet J* 15:70–72, 1983

105. Pfeiffer CA and Hooker CW: Testicular changes resembling early stages in the development of interstitial cell tumors in mice of the A strain after long-continued injections of pregnant mare serum. *Cancer Res* 3:762–766, 1943

106. Pourreau-Schneider N: Cytoplasmic inclusions in estrogen-induced testicular interstitial-cell tumors in mice. *J Natl Cancer Inst* 39:67–74, 1967

107. Rahaley RS, Gordon BJ, Leipold HW and Peter JE: Sertoli cell tumour in a horse. *Eq vet J* 15:68–70, 1983

108. Ramsey FK and Migaki G: Tumors, intestinal emphysema, and fat necrosis. *In*: Diseases of Swine. Dunne, H.W. (ed.), Ames, IO, Iowa State University Press, pp. 956–970, 1970

109. Rao MS, Subbarao V and Scarpelli DG: Carcinogenic effect of N-nitrosobis(2-oxopropyl)amine in newborn rats. *Carcinogenesis* 6:1395–1397, 1985

110. Reznik-Schuller H: Carcinogenic effects of diethylstilbestrol in male Syrian golden hamsters and European hamsters. *J Natl Cancer Inst* 62:1083–1088, 1979

111. Riviere MR, Chouroulinkov I and Guerin M: Production de tumeurs par injections intratesticulaires de chlorure de zinc chez le rat. *Bull assoc Fr Étude Cancer* 47:55–87, 1960

112. Riviere MR, Chouroulinkov I and Guerin M: Contribution a la carcinogenese hormonale chez le hamster. *Acta UICC* 20:1509–1511, 1964

113. Roe FJC: Spontaneous tumours in rats and mice. *Fd Cosmet Toxicol* 3:707–720, 1965

114. Roe FJC, Dukes CE, Cameron KM, Pugh RCB and Mitchley BCV: Cadmium neoplasia: testicular atrophy and Leydig cell hyperplasia and neoplasia in rats and mice following subcutaneous injection of cadmium salts. *Br J Cancer* 18:674–681, 1964

115. Rogers JB and Blumenthal HT: Studies of Guinea pig tumors. I. Report of fourteen spontaneous Guinea pig tumors, with a review of the literature. *Cancer Res* 20:191–197, 1960

116. Rosen VJ Jr, Castanera TJ, Jones DC and Kimeldorf DJ: Islet-cell tumors of the pancreas in the irradiated and nonirradiated rat. *Lab Invest* 10:608–616, 1961

117. Rosen VJ Jr, Castanera TJ, Kimeldorf DJ and Jones DC:

Pancreatic islet cell tumors and renal tumors in the male rat following neutron exposure. *Lab Invest* 11:204–210, 1962

118. Rustia M: Multiple carcinogenic effects of the ethylnitrosourea precursors ethylurea and sodium nitrite in hamsters. *Cancer Res* 34:3232–3244, 1974

119. Rustia M and Shubik P: Experimental induction of hepatomas, mammary tumors, and other tumors with metronidazole in noninbred Sas:MRC(WI)BR rats. *J Natl Cancer Inst* 63:863–868, 1979

120. Rustia M, Shubik P and Patil K: Lifespan carcinogenicity tests with native carrageenan in rats and hamsters. *Cancer Ltr* 11:1–10, 1980

121. Sagartz JW, Garner FW and Sauer RM: Multiple neoplasia in a captive jungle cat (*Felis chaus*) – thyroid adenocarcinoma, gastric adenocarcinoma, renal adenoma, and Sertoli cell tumor. *J Wildlife Dis* 8:375–380, 1972

122. Sass B, Rabstein LS, Madison R, Nims RM, Peters RL and Kelloff GJ: Incidence of spontaneous neoplasms in F344 rats throughout the natural life-span. *J Natl Cancer Inst* 54:1449–1456, 1975

123. Saxton JA Jr, Sperling GA, Barnes LL and McCay CM: The influence of nutrition upon the incidence of spontaneous tumors of the albino rat. *Acta UICC* 6:423–431, 1948

124. Schlotthauer CF, McDonald JR and Bollman JL: Testicular tumors in dogs. *J Urol* 40:539–550, 1938

125. Searson JE: Testicular adenocarcinoma in a ram. *Vet Pathol* 17:391–393, 1980

126. Seefeldt S and Helfer D: Seminoma in an elk (*Cervus canadensis*). *Vet Pathol* 17:248–249, 1980

127. Shimkin MB, Grady HG and Andervont HB: Induction of testicular tumors and other effects of stilbestrol-cholesterol pellets in strain C mice. *J Natl Cancer Inst* 2:65–80, 1942

128. Shortridge EH: Lesions of the testicle and epididymis of rams. *NZ Vet J* 10:23–26, 1962

129. Shortridge EH and Cordes DO: Seminoma in sheep. *J Comp Path* 79:229–232, 1969

130. Slye M, Holmes HF and Wells HG: Primary spontaneous tumors of the testicle and seminal vesicle in mice and other animals. *J Cancer Res* 4:207–228, 1919

131. Smith HA: Interstitial cell tumor of the equine testis. *J Amer Vet Med Assoc* 124:356–359, 1954

132. Smith HA and Jones TC: Veterinary Pathology. Philadelphia, Lea & Febiger, p. 228, 1957

133. Snell KC: Spontaneous lesions of the rat. *In*: The Pathology of Laboratory Animals. Ribelin, W.E., Jr. and McCoy, J.R. (eds.), Springfield, Charles C. Thomas, pp. 241–302, 1965

134. Snell KC and Hollander CF: Tumors of the testes and seminal vesicle in *Praomys* (*Mastomys*) *natalensis*. *J Natl Cancer Inst* 49:1381–1393, 1972

135. Snyder RL: The laboratory woodchuck. *Lab Anim* 14(1):20–32, 1985

136. Squire RA, Goodman DG, Valerio MG, Fredrickson T, Strandberg JD, Levitt MH, Lingeman CH, Harshbarger JC and Dawe CJ: Tumors. *In*: Pathology of Laboratory Animals. Volume II., Benirschke K, Garner FM and Jones TC (eds.), New York, Springer-Verlag, pp. 1051–1283, 1978

137. Steiner PE and Bengston JS: Research and economic aspects of tumors in food-producing animals. *Cancer* 4:1113–1124, 1951

138. Stevens LC: Testicular teratomas in fetal mice. *J Natl Cancer Inst* 28:247–267, 1962

139. Stevens LC: Experimental production of testicular teratomas in mice. *Proc Natl Acad Sci* (*Wash.*) 52:654–661, 1964

140. Stevens LC: The development of teratomas from intratesticular grafts of tubal mouse eggs. *J Embryo exp Morph* 20:329–341, 1968

141. Stevens LC: Embryonal carcinoma in mouse. *In*: Tumors of the Male Genital System. Mostofi, F.K. and Price, E.B., Jr. (eds.), Washington, D.C., Armed Forces Institute of Pathology, pp. 14–14a, 1973a

142. Stevens LC: A new inbred subline of mice (129/terSv) with a high incidence of spontaneous congenital testicular teratomas. *J Natl Cancer Inst* 50:235–242, 1973b

143. Stevens LC: Spontaneous testicular teratomas: mouse. *In*: Inbred and Genetically Defined Strains of Laboratory Animals. Part 1. Mouse and Rat. Altman, P.L. and Katz, D.D. (eds.), Bethesda, MD, *Fed Amer Soc Exper Biol* pp. 207–208, 1979

144. Stevens LC and Little CC: Spontaneous testicular teratomas in an inbred strain of mice. *Proc Natl Acad Sci* USA 40:1080–1087, 1954

145. Stevens LC and Mackensen JA: Genetic and environmental influences on teratocarcinogenesis in mice. *J Natl Cancer Inst* 27:443–453, 1961

146. Stutman O: Spontaneous, viral, and chemically induced tumors in the nude mouse. *In*: The Nude Mouse in Experimental and Clinical Research. Fogh, J. and Giovanella, B.C. (eds.), New York, Academic Press, pp. 411–435, 1978

147. Takizawa S and Miyamoto M: Observations on spontaneous tumors in Wistar Furth strain rats. *Hiroshima J Med Sci* 25:89–98, 1976

148. Talerman A, Kaalen JG and Fokkens W: Rural preponderance of testicular neoplasms. *Br J Cancer* 29:176–178, 1974

149. Tokuoka S: Induction of tumor in mice with N,N-bis(2-chloroethyl)-N′, O-propylenephosphoric acid ester diamide (cyclophosphamide). *Gann* 56:537–541, 1965

150. Toth B and Toth T: Investigation on the tumor producing effect of isonicotinic acid hydrazide in ASW/Sn mice and MRC rats. *Tumori* 56:315–324, 1970

151. Turk JR, Turk MAM and Gallina AM: A canine testicular tumor resembling gonadoblastoma. *Vet Pathol* 18:201–207, 1981

152. Twombly GH, Meisel D and Stout AP: Leydig-cell tumors induced experimentally in the rat. *Cancer* 2:884–892, 1949

153. Upton AC, Kimball AW, Furth J, Christenberry KW and Benedict WH: Some delayed effects of atom-bomb radiations in mice. *Cancer Res* 20 (Suppl No 8, Part 2):1–60, 1960

154. Vaillancourt D, Fretz P and Orr JP: Seminoma in the horse: report of two cases. *J Eq Med Surg* 3:213–218, 1979

155. Vincent AL and Ash LR: Further observations on spontaneous neoplasms in the Mongolian gerbil, *Meriones unguiculatus*. *Lab Anim Sci* 28:297–300, 1978

156. Voronoff S: Tumeurs spontanées chez les singes; in groupes sanguins chez les singes; la greffe du cancer humain aux singes. Paris, Doin, pp. 63–129, 1949

157. Wallach JD and Boever WJ: Diseases of Exotic Animals. Philadelphia, W.B. Sanders, pp. 386, 600, 1983

158. Wilhelmina JPR, Tengbergen E and Muhlbock O: Disorders of the blood in mice bearing spontaneous or transplanted tumours. *Br J Cancer* 12:81–98, 1958

159. Willis RA: Pathology of Tumours. 4th edition, London, Butterworths, pp. 992–993, 1967

160. Willis RA and Rudduck HB: Testicular teratomas in horses. *J Path Bact* 55:165–171, 1943

161. Wilson GP and Hayes HM Jr: Castration for treatment of perianal gland neoplasms in the dog. *J Amer Vet Med Assoc* 174:1301–1303, 1979

162. Yoshitomi K and Morii S: Benign and malignant epithelial tumors of the rete testis in mice. *Vet Pathol* 21:300–303, 1984

163. Young JL, Percy CL and Asire AJ: Surveillance, Epidemiology, and End Results: Incidence and Mortality Data, 1973–1977. *Natl Cancer Inst Monogr* 57, 1981

164. Zoller M, Matzku S and Goerttler K: High incidence of spontaneous transplantable tumours in BDX rats. *Br J Cancer* 37:61–66, 1978

165. Zurcher C, Nooteboom AL and Hollander CF: Neoplastic and non-neoplastic lesions in ageing C57BL/Ka mice. Rijswijk, *Ann Rep Org for Hlth Res TNO* pp. 252–254, 1975

SPECIES SPECIFIC INTERACTION OF THE BREAST AND THE LYMPHATIC SYSTEM (LYMPH NODES) IN MAMMALIAN TUMORIGENESIS

H.E. KAISER

The mammary glands and the lymphatic system of the body at its highest phylogenetic stage are both characteristics of the mammalian body. Both structures exhibit primary and secondary neoplasms. Primary neoplasms derive from both groups (see chaps 12/I, 20/V) and secondary neoplasms develop from the respective neoplasms of both units or enter from other structures to find a soil in the mammary glands or the structures of the lymphatic system in the mammal. This chapter deals only with the secondary neoplasms of both types of structures, especially of those which build secondary deposits from other primary sources (see chapters 9 + 10/Vol VII and 13/Vol VIII).

The breast gland as a soil for secondary neoplasms belongs to the rare sundry locations (7). More common is the spreading of breast tumors from one side to the others.

The interaction of the mammary glands which organs give the mammals the name, with the lymphatic system, the most potential transmitter of neoplastic distribution may offer some new insight into the development of cancer in man. Breast cancer comprises a group of neoplasms which disseminate most widely and unpredictably. This is especially true in the female but mammary (breast) occurs also to a lesser degree in the male. In comparison to the lymphatic structures we deal with the following separable units of the breast: the alveolus, the ducts, and the nipple in man. In the lymphatic system we deal with the following structures: (1) lymph vessels: capillaries, small and medium-sized lymph vessels, large lymph vessels, and collecting ducts (e.g., thoracic duct); (2) lymphatic tissue: diffuse lymphatic tissues, lymph nodules, tonsils; (3) lymphatic organs, thymus, lymph nodes, hemolymph-nodes, spleen.

Mammary glands and abundant lymphatic system are two mammalian characteristics (the one circumscribed, the other widely disseminated)

The topic of our interest is well circumscribed because it is only common in the mammal, as is the case with both organs under concern. This is a particular advantage for research and resulting understanding. The mammary gland is a circumscribed organ in man, and certain domestic animals as in form of the udder in such animals as cow and goat, but less so in dog, cat, pig or laboratory rodents. Contrastingly, the lymphatic system is widely distributed in the mammal's body and intensively connected with the hematogenic system as the other part of the circulatory system. Only in the central nervous system of the mammal the lymphatic system is missing. From the topographic condition of both systems it is self-explanatory that the dissemination from the circumscribed breast to the other organs via the lymphatic system will dominate the picture in some species as man but not in others as in cattle; contrary to the widely distributed lymphatic system to the circumscribed mammary glands as in man.

The interaction of both systems, a phylogenetic young development

As stated in chapter 3, it can be assumed that the culmination of neoplastic development took place in the mammal, perhaps especially in man. That it happened in man in particular is due to the fact that man is a mammal, and to man's special position as a highly specialized mammal (particular brain development, erect position) and the resulting introduction of unnatural cancer causing factors into man's life such as unhealthy nutrition, analgesics, chemical waste, and following pollution, behavioral habits, smoking. One remarkable peak of development is the interaction of the mammary glands with the lymphatic system in man's body. Kaiser stated elsewhere that the phylogenetic age of tissues and their width of distribution are unmistakenly connected. The development of both systems in the mammalian body according to the fossil contents of the earth's crust must have come into existence not before the upper triassic period (160 million years ago) concerning the mammals; but regarding man not earlier than at the upper border of the Pliocene and therefore the lower border of the Plistocene (lower border of the Quaternary). The wide distribution of breast cancer metastasis gives a hint to my statement of man as being one of the culmination points of neoplastic development, at least in these aspects. This new development is reflected in two ways: (1) free-ranging mammals and certain mammals of domestic species mentioned before have a very low occurrence of spontaneous development of mammary cancers; (2) the fluctuation in man is seen as we find in this species the highest occurrence of breast cancer in women of the United States and Western Europe in contrast to the lowest occurrence in such countries as Japan, Singapore and Algeria. How much the different types of the female breast in women of the Caucasian, yellow (oriental) and black populations may indicate, perhaps also biochemically variations or other distinguishing factors of the various neoplastic differentiation potential is not known. These less often considered ideas of possible variabilities are connected with

H. E. Kaiser (ed.), Comparative aspects of tumor development.

those of the species and lower taxonomic differences of the lymphatic system. The lymphatic system of the mammal characterized by the abundant lymph nodes is a system widely distributed in the body. In contrast, the system in the mammary glands is especially in the woman restricted where only two mammae exist to the cat with four, in the dog with six. We can state that in man, *Homo sapiens*, the extreme reaches a peak. It can also be said that the secondary spreading, especially metastasis, from the breast, as direct spread from the breast reaches frequently the lymphatic system, especially the lymph nodes. The breast as a host for secondary tumor spreading is in contrast very restricted in size, so the breast as location for metastasis can be considered an organ of sundry location.

SUMMARY AND CONCLUSION

The potential for secondary neoplastic spreading of the lymphatic system and the metastatic potential of breast neoplasms, at least in certain populations and certain strains of laboratory animals can be seen as a peak development of neoplastic growth in the mammal. Species-specific interaction of the breast and the lymphatic system (lymph nodes) in mammalian tumorigenesis indicates that

1. Breast and abundant lymphatic system are two mammalian characteristics: one circumscribed, the other widely distributed in the body.
2. This development is phylogenetically young.
3. Differences exist among species, in human population groups, in races, strains, and breeds.

4. Spreading of lymphatic or other neoplasms to human breasts are rare. In the human female spreading from one breast to the other is the most commonly observed.
5. Spreading of breast neoplasms to and via the lymphatic system occur in abundancy to nearly all regions of the body, with exception of the central nervous system because lymphatics are lacking there.

REFERENCES

1. Ashley DJB: Evans' Histological Appearances of Tumours. (3rd edition), vols. 1 and 2. Edinburgh–London–New York: Churchill Livingstone 1978
2. DeVita VT Jr, Hellman S, Rosenberg SA: Cancer Principles & Practice of Oncology. (2nd edition). Philadelphia – Toronto: J.B. Lippincott Co 1985
3. Holland JF, Frei E III (eds): Cancer Medicine. (2nd edition). Philadelphia: Lea & Febiger 1982
4. Kaiser HE (ed.): Neoplasms – Comparative Pathology of Growth in Animals, Plants, and Man. Baltimore: Williams & Wilkins, 1981
5. Kampmeier OF: Evolution and Comparative Morphology of the Lymphatic System. Springfield, Ill.: Charles C. Thomas 1969
6. Nowak RM, Paradiso JL: Walker's Mammals of the World. (4th edition). Baltimore and London: The Johns Hopkins University Press 1983.
7. Von Albertini A: Histologische Geschwulstdiagnostik. Stuttgart: Georg Thieme Verlag 1974
8. Willis RA: The Spread of Tumours in the Human Body. (3rd edition) London: Butterworths 1973

MULTIPLE ENDOCRINE SYNDROME IN SHN MICE: MAMMARY TUMORS AND UTERINE ADENOMYOSIS

TAKAO MORI and HIROSHI NAGASAWA

INTRODUCTION

It is recognized that in laboratory rodents normal and neoplastic mammary gland growth is dependent upon prolactin and the ovarian steroid hormones (estrogen and progesterone) (2, 37, 41). Normal and abnormal proliferation of the uterus is also under the control of similar hormones (6, 8, 14, 25), although the mechanism is not always well understood.

Recently, it has been found that the SHN strain of mice, which was established as a high mammary tumor strain from Swiss albino mice independently of any other mammary tumor susceptible strains (49), frequently develops adenomyosis after 4 months of age (30, 32, 33, 45). This strain may be a good animal model for study of the endocrine regulation of multiple lesions, mammary tumors and adenomyosis.

In this chapter, we shall review general features of mammary tumors and uterine adenomyosis of the SHN strain of mice and the control of these lesions by hormones, with special reference to prolactin, and discuss the value of these systems as animal models for human cases.

GENERAL FEATURES OF SPONTANEOUS MAMMARY TUMORIGENESIS IN SHN MICE

Mammary tumor incidence

Mammary tumor incidence in SHN mice finally reaches 100 % in both breeders and virgins. Unlike most other high mammary tumor strains, the pattern of mammary tumor incidence is similar in breeders and virgins of the SHN strain; about 50 % of mice develop before 7 months of age and additionally more than 90 % of mice have tumors by 10 months of age (Figure 1). This small difference in age at onset of mammary tumors is one of the characteristics of this strain (49). As shown in Figure 2, nearly 60 % of the mice have only one tumor in their life span; however, four or five tumors develop in about 5 % of the mice (49).

Mammary hyperplastic alveolar nodules (HAN), one preneoplastic state in high mammary tumor strains of mice appear after three or four months of age, and 100 % of the mice have HAN by seven months. The number of HAN per gland increases with age (49).

Lung metastases

One of the marked differences between human breast cancer and experimental mammary tumors is the evidence of metastases. The low incidence of metastases in experimental animals is a serious disadvantage for an animal model. However, the incidence of metastases of mammary tumors to lung could be increased by frequent surgical removal of tumors soon after appearance (Table 1) and by lengthening the survival time of the animals (Mori and Nagasawa, submitted for publication). Thus the low incidence of metastases of spontaneous mammary tumors of this strain should not be ascribed to the intrinsic characteristics of the tumors, but to early death of the host animals.

Hormonal control of mammary tumors

As seen in other strains of mice (67), the formation and growth of HAN and the development of mammary tumors in SHN mice are also highly dependent upon prolactin. Pituitary grafting at weaning (20–23 days of age) resulted in a marked decline in the age of mammary tumor onset (47). Moreover, it has recently been demonstrated that even this type of mammary tumor, which is hormone-independent and, therefore, autonomous during progression, is still largely dependent upon prolactin at the initial phase of progression (39).

Meanwhile, little difference was found in serum prolactin levels in various reproductive states between SHN and SLN which was established as a low mammary tumor strain from the same basal stock as SHN (42, 49). On the other hand, the former shows a higher mammary gland response to prolactin than the latter (44), indicating that mammary gland susceptibility is much more important than the circulating level for manifestation of the effects of the hormone (42). Sinha (59) claimed that level estimated by radioimmunoassay represents only a fraction of the total prolactin circulating in blood. Therefore, it is not surprising that most of the studies conducted so far have failed to find a strong, clinically useful correlation between plasma prolactin and the incidence of breast cancer in experimental animals and humans.

Another hormone-related characteristic of the SHN strain is the continued estrous/metestrous vaginal smears

H. E. Kaiser (ed.), Comparative aspects of tumor development.

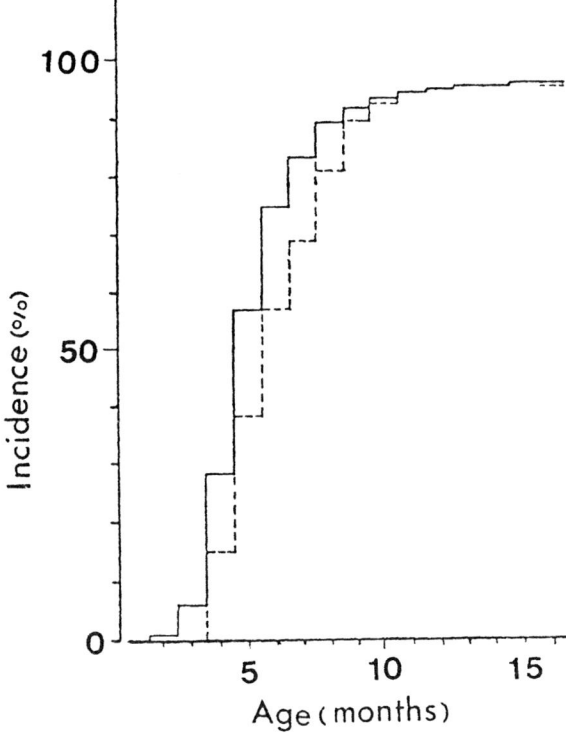

Figure 1. Spontaneous mammary tumor incidence (%) in virgin (----: No. of mice = 94) and breeding (——: No. of mice = 300) SHN mice.

after six months of age (Nagasawa and Fujii, unpublished). This is of great interest in relation to the premise that one of the major causes of human breast cancer is the non-cyclic and constant exposure of normal and malignant mammary foci to estrogen after menopause. This further suggests the value of the SHN to study the genesis of postmenopausal breast cancer.

GENERAL FEATURES OF UTERINE ADENOMYOSIS IN SHN MICE

Hormonal control of the development of adenomyosis

Adenomyosis is a benign pathological state of endometrial tissues, aberrant endometrial glands or stroma, or both, within the myometrium. It occurs spontaneously in many animal species: cats, dogs, guinea pigs, mice, rabbits, etc. (60).

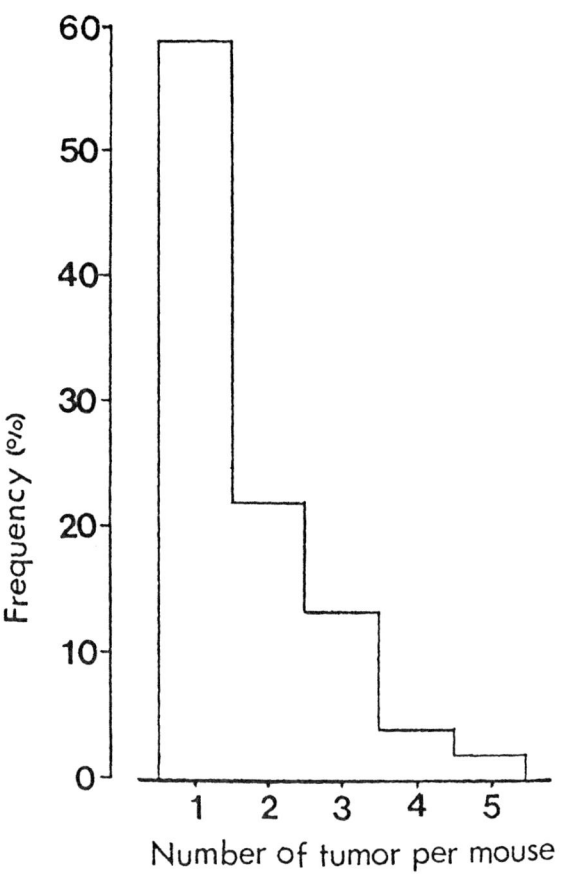

Figure 2. Number of mammary tumors per tumor bearing SHN virgin mouse (No. of mice = 151).

It was found that SHN mice given pituitary isografts into the mammary fat pad for the induction of mammary tumors showed cystic dilatation of the endometrial glands and the presence of aberrant tissues within the myometrium (29). This raised the question as to whether the direct implantation of pituitary tissue into the uterine lumen can induce such abnormal changes. Fifty-day-old female mice of SHN strain were each given a single anterior pituitary in the lumen of the right uterine horn. Control mice were each given a piece of submaxillary gland at the same site. All grafts were obtained from age-matched male mice. Intrauterine pituitary implantation produced adenomyosis in 100 % of the mice by 5 months after grafting, while spontaneous development of adenomyosis was observed in only 20 % of the control mice without the pituitary graft; a

Table 1. Relationship between the rate of lung metastases and the survival time in tumorous SHN mice.

Months after the first mammary tumor appearance	0–1	1.1–2	2.1–3	3.1–4
Rate of lung metastases (%)	0 (0/43)*	6.2 (6/97)	28.8 (17/59)	35.3 (6/17)

*Number of mice with lung metastases/total number of mice with mammary tumors examined.

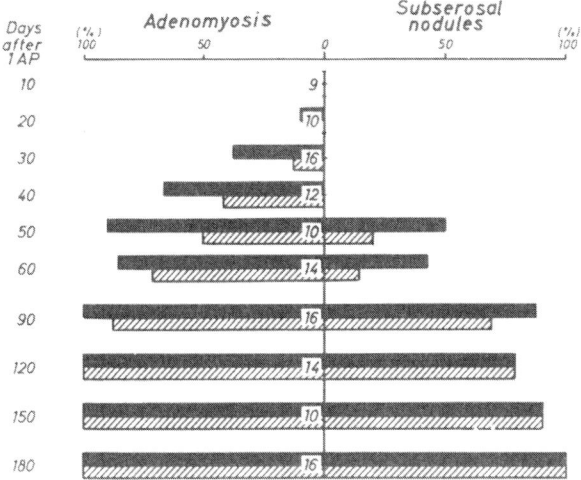

Figure 3. Changes with age in the incidence (%) of adenomyosis and subserosal nodules in SHN mice given an isograft of an anterior pituitary (1 AP) each in the right horn at 50 days of age. ■: right horn, ▨: left horn. The number of samples is indicated at the bottom of each column. (From T. Mori, H. Nagasawa, *Acta Anat* 116:46, 1983).

statistically significant difference (32, 33). Ectopic transplantation of an anterior pituitary results in hyperprolactinemia. Apparently the elevation of the circulating levels of prolactin by intrauterine pituitary grafting is favorable for the rapid induction of adenomyosis in SHN mice (30, 32). The induction of adenomyosis by ectopic pituitary grafting has been reported by some other workers (10, 11).

Adenomyosis has also been experimentally induced by continuous treatment with estrogen for a relatively long time (usually over a year); thus in mice (19, 21, 22, 55), in guinea pigs (52), in rabbits (27) and in monkeys (5). These studies suggest that the development of adenomyosis is attributable

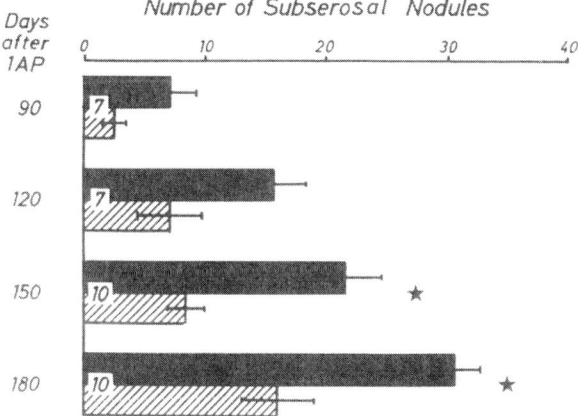

Figure 4. Number of subserosal nodules in uteri of SHN mice given an isograft of an anterior pituitary (1 AP) each in the right horn at 50 days of age. ■: right horn, ▨: left horn. The number of samples is indicated at the bottom of each column. Standard errors are represented by the transverse lines on each column. *Significantly different between the right and left horns at 0.05 level. (From T. Mori, H. Nagasawa, *Acta Anat* 116:46, 1983).

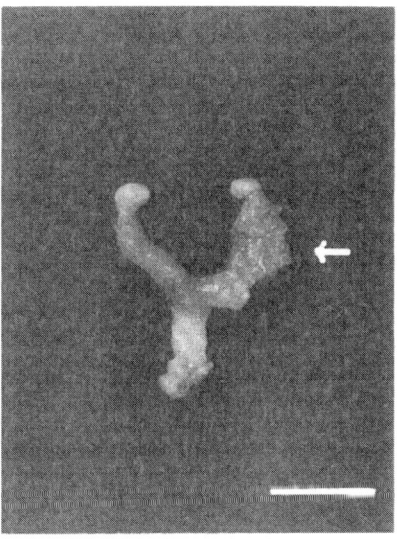

Figure 5. The uterus of a SHN mouse given an isograft of an anterior pituitary in the right horn at 50 days of age and killed 150 days after the grafting. Note the large numbers of the subserosal nodules in the right horn (arrow). Line = 1 cm. (From T. Mori et al., *Life Sci* 29:1277, 1981).

to a chronic hormonal imbalance, since continuous supplement with estrogen leads to an increase of prolactin release by the pituitary. In addition, prenatal exposure to estrogens also leads to adenomyosis in mice in old age (7, 10, 26). Nagasawa et al. (50, 51) have reported that neonatal exposure to estrogen results in hyperprolactinemia at advanced age. Further, Kalland, Forsberg and Sinha (13) have stated that neonatal treatment with diethylstilbestrol enhances the pituitary release of prolactin in response to estrogen induction later in life. Thus, all the results clearly indicate the importance of prolactin for the development of adenomyosis. We have found that continuous treatment with estradiol benzoate induced an early appearance and high incidence of adenomyosis in intact SHN mice associated with the elevated levels of plasma prolactin and decreased levels of plasma progesterone compared to the control (30). Therefore, such hormonal milieu as increased circulating levels of prolactin and estrogen, and decreased levels of progesterone would be responsible for the genesis of adenomyosis. In our experimental system of pituitary grafting into the right uterine horn, adenomyosis appears earlier in the right horn than in the left one (Figure 3) and the incidence of subserosal nodules, an advanced state of adenomyosis, is higher in the right than in the left (Figures 4 and 5) (30, 32). On the other hand, pituitary transplantation under the renal capsule, which is also favorable for the induction of adenomyosis, does not lead to any difference in the time of onset and incidence of adenomyosis between the two uterine horns (30). These results strongly suggest that prolactin plays a direct primary role in the formation of adenomyosis. However, Ostrander, Mills and Bern (54) claim that the production of adenomyosis is accounted for by a hormonal imbalance involving high levels of circulating progesterone.

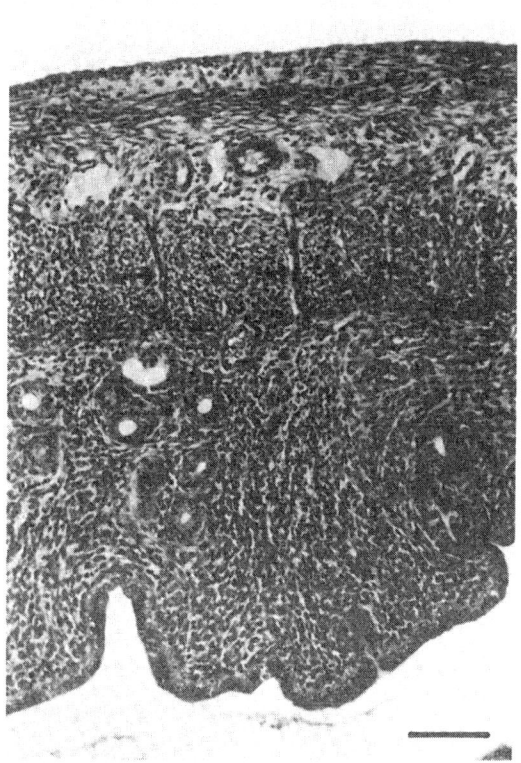

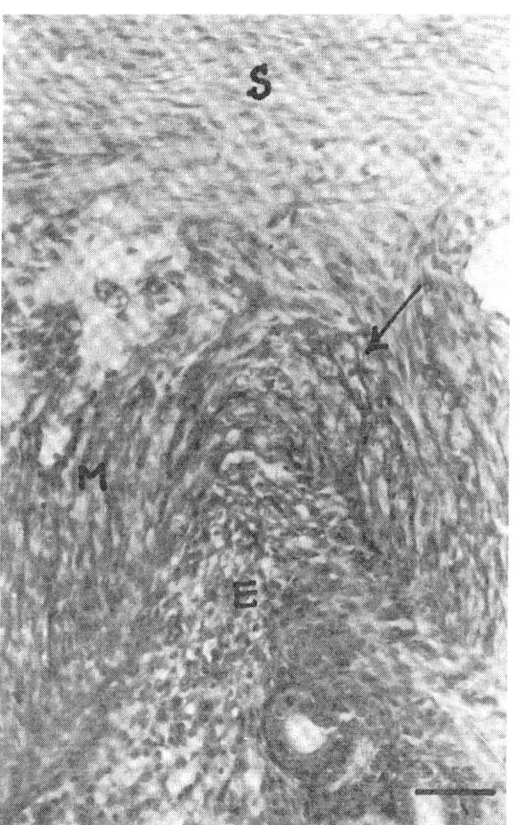

Figure 6. The section of uterus of a SHN mouse given an isograft of an anterior pituitary in the right horn at 50 days of age and killed 20 days after the grafting. Note conspicuous blood vessels with the endometrial stromal cells (arrows). Line = 100 μm. Hematoxylin and eosin. (From T. Mori, H. Nagasawa, *Acta Anat* 116:46, 1983).

Figure 7. The section of uterus of a SHN mouse given an isograft of an anterior pituitary in the right horn at 50 days of age and killed 30 days after the grafting. Note invasion of a large amount of the endometrial stromal cells into the myometrium (arrow). E = endometrium, M = myometrium, S = subserosa, Line = 25 μm. Hematoxylin and eosin.

Ovariectomy immediately after pituitary grafting eliminates the development of adenomyosis, and continuous treatment with estrogen in combination with progesterone restores the pathological state in ovariectomized mice bearing pituitary isografts (32). The presence of ovarian hormones is important for manifestation of the prolactin effect.

Histogenesis and morphology

The presence of endometrial glands or stroma or both in abnormal locations has been termed endometriosis. The disorder showing the presence of endometrial tissues in ectopic sites outside the uterus was called external endometriosis. When the aberrant tissues were contained within the myometrium, the condition was termed as internal endometriosis or adenomyosis (16). At present, however, it is generally accepted that external endometriosis is simply referred to as endometriosis and the internal case as adenomyosis (53). Adenomyosis occurs in a wide variety of animal species, but endometriosis occurs only in those species that menstruate, namely primates (15)

Adenomyosis induced in SHN mice differs little histologically from that developing spontaneously (30, 32, 33, 45).

Morphological disorders appear 20 days after the pituitary is grafted into the uterine lumen (Figure 3). The early sign of the development of adenomyosis is the invasion of a small amount of endometrial stromal tissue into the myometrium along the branches of the blood vessels (Figure 6), followed by a large amount of stromal tissue which displaces the muscle layer (Figure 7) (Grade 1). Thereafter, uterine glands invade the myometrium through the invaded stromal tissue (Figures 8 and 9) (Grades 2 and 3, respectively). Associated with these changes, the myometrium as a whole becomes loose (30, 34). At the advanced stages, a large amount of endometrial tissue invades the myometrium and breaks up the circular arrangement of the layer of smooth muscle bundles. The aberrant endometrial tissues continue to invade through the myometrium and reach the subserosa, forming subserosal nodules which are easily recognized at laparotomy (Figures 5 and 10) (Grade 4). The nodules consist of endometrial glands surrounded by stromal cells, smooth muscle cells and serosa, or when highly cystic, by serosa only. The progression of adenomyosis is accompanied by glandular proliferation. The glands vary in size and shape, and many show cystic hyperplasia, resulting in a Swiss cheese type of endometrium. The surface of the en-

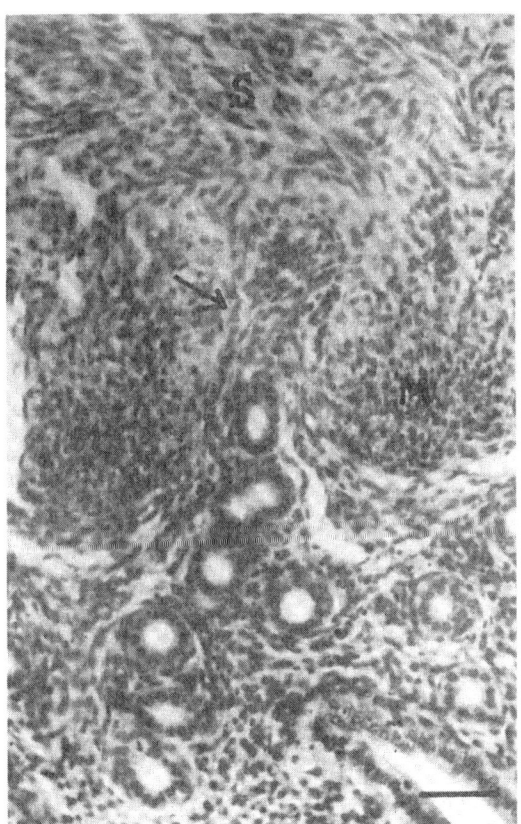

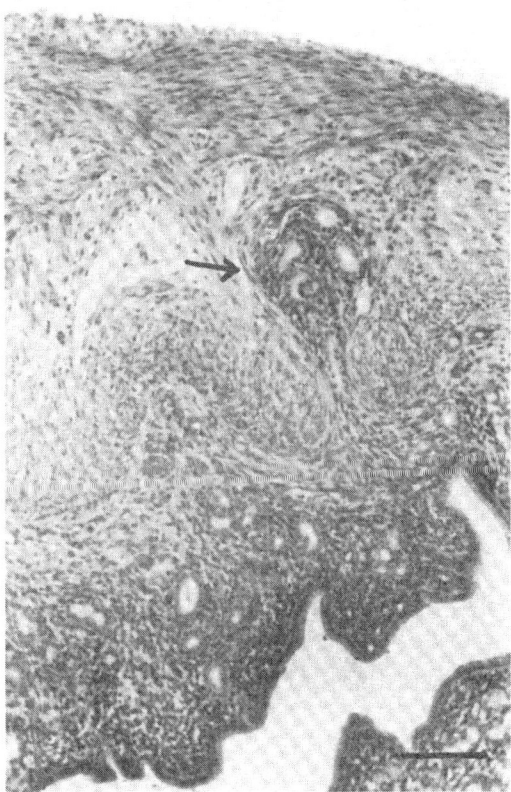

Figure 8. The section of uterus of a SHN mouse given an isograft of an anterior pituitary in the right horn at 50 days of age and killed 30 days after the grafting. Note invasion of the endometrial glands into the myometrium (arrow). M = myometrium, S = subserosa, Line = 25 μm. Hematoxylin and eosin. (From T. Mori, H. Nagasawa, *Acta Anat* 116:46, 1983).

Figure 9. The section of uterus of a SHN mouse given an isograft of an anterior pituitary in the right horn at 50 days of age and killed 50 days after the grafting. Note invasion of the endometrial tissues into the subserosa (arrow). Line = 100 μm. Hematoxylin and eosin. (From T. Mori et al., *Experientia* 40: 1385, 1984).

dometrium is irregular and contains small polyps (Figure 11) (Grade 5). Classification of progression of adenomyosis is presented in Table 2. Direct connection between the endometrial surface and the lumen of the subserosal nodule is frequently observed (Figure 12). The subserosal nodules appear bilaterally on the part of the uterine horn adjacent to the fallopian tubes, although both appearance and progression of the nodules are earlier in the right horns bearing the pituitary grafts than in the left ones without the grafts (Figures 4 and 5). Once the lesion becomes this advanced, it may be irreversible since the lesion does not disappear following ovariectomy (30).

On the other hand, it has been reported that prolactin enhances the response of the rodent uterus to trauma or formation of decidua (1, 12, 61). Prolactin caused an acceleration of estrogen binding to uterine explants (20) and enhanced the ability of uterine homogenates to metabolize progesterone (1), although there are some conflicting results showing no alteration of estrogen receptor levels by prolactin (57, 62). Prolactin binding has been found in the uterus of rabbits and sheep (56) and rats (68). Prolactin exerts a marked inhibitory effect on oxytocin-induced myometrial contraction both in rats primed with estrogen and progesterone (9) and in pregnant rabbits (24). These results suggest

that prolactin may alter the responsiveness of the uterus to other hormones. When endometrial tissues penetrated through the myometrium in our experimental system, the myometrium became loose as observed histologically. Thus, it is possible that the changes in the myometrium may be ascribed to the effect of prolactin. Immunohistochemical studies by the unlabeled antibody peroxidase-antiperoxidase method to search for immunoreactive prolactin (30) showed that endometrial gland cells contained the immunoreactive material and myometrial cells also had slight immunoreactivity (Figure 13). However, stromal cells did not contain the immunoreactive material. In uterus, there is no distinct barrier such as basement membrane between endometrium and myometrium. Extension of endometrial tissues under normal physiological condition is protected by the barrier of the circular layer of smooth muscle bundles. However, the looseness of the myometrium induced by prolactin may not allow resistance to the pressure of aggressive extension of endometrial tissues. Moreover, it is plausible that the areas where blood vessels penetrate the endometrial stroma from the myometrium are the weakest sites of the muscle barrier; blood vessels may act as a part for the invasion of endometrial tissues into the myometrium. It has already been pointed out that hypertrophy and hyperplasia of uterine vessels may play an im-

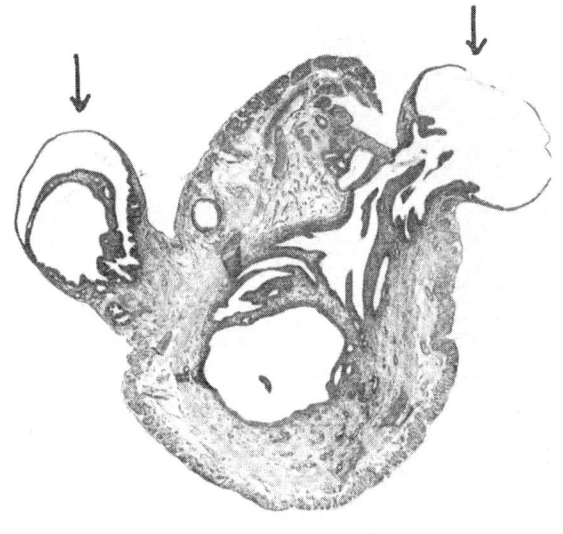

Figure 10. The vertical section of uterus of a SHN mouse given an isograft of an anterior pituitary in the right horn at 50 days of age and killed 150 days after the grafting. Note protrusion of two subserosal nodules (arrows). Line = 1 mm. Hematoxylin and eosin. (From T. Mori et al., *Lab Anim Sci* 32:40, 1982).

portant role in the development of human adenomyosis (58).

Strain difference on the development of adenomyosis

We have found strain differences in the induction of adenomyosis by pituitary grafting (33): a high incidence of

Table 2. Criteria for classification of progression of adenomyosis in SHN mice.

Degree	No. of figure in the text	Histological features
Grade 1	Fig. 7	Endometrial stromal cells are present in the inner layer of myometrium.
Grade 2	Fig. 8	Endometrial glands are present in the inner layer of myometrium.
Grade 3	Fig. 9	Endometrial glands are present between the inner layer and the outer layer of myometrium.
Grade 4	Fig. 10	Endometrial glands reach subserosa and protrude outside uterus as subserosal nodules.
Grade 5	Fig. 11	Uterus contains cystic hyperplasia of endometrial glands (Swiss cheese endometrium) and subserosal nodules, and lose circular arrangement of myometrium.

adenomyosis is observed in the three mammary tumor virus (MTV)-expressed strains, SHN, SLN and C3H, and a low incidence in MTV-unexpressed C57BL strain of mice by 10 months after grafting. In a previous study (29), adenomyotic changes did not occur in MTV-expressed BALB/cfC3H mice 12 months after pituitary grafting. In contrast, Huseby and Thurlow (10) have reported that adenomyosis can be induced by prenatal exposure to diethylstilbestrol or by pituitary grafting in both BALB/c and C3H × BALB/c hybrid mice, and incidence also being lower in the MTV-unexpressed strain than in the MTV-expressed strain. However, it is unlikely that MTV plays a role in this process, since spontaneous development of adenomyosis is found in MTV-unexpressed virgin IF mice (28). There are two plausible explanations for the strain differences in the induction of adenomyosis by pituitary grafting: (1) different sensitivity

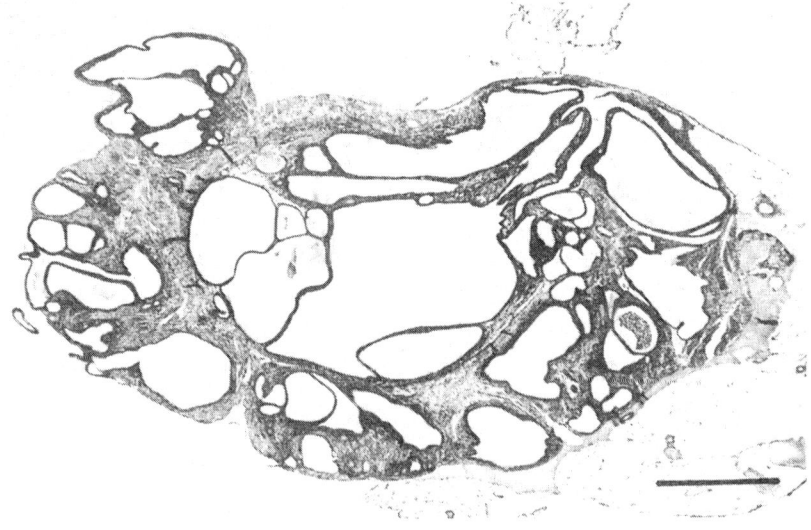

Figure 11. The vertical section of uterus of a SHN mouse given an isograft of an anterior pituitary in the right horn at 50 days of age and killed 150 days after the grafting. Note cystic hyperplasia of the endometrial glands, polyps of the endometrial surface and protrusion of the subserosal nodules. Line = 1 mm. Hematoxylin and eosin. (From T. Mori et al., *Life Sci.,* 29:1277, 1981).

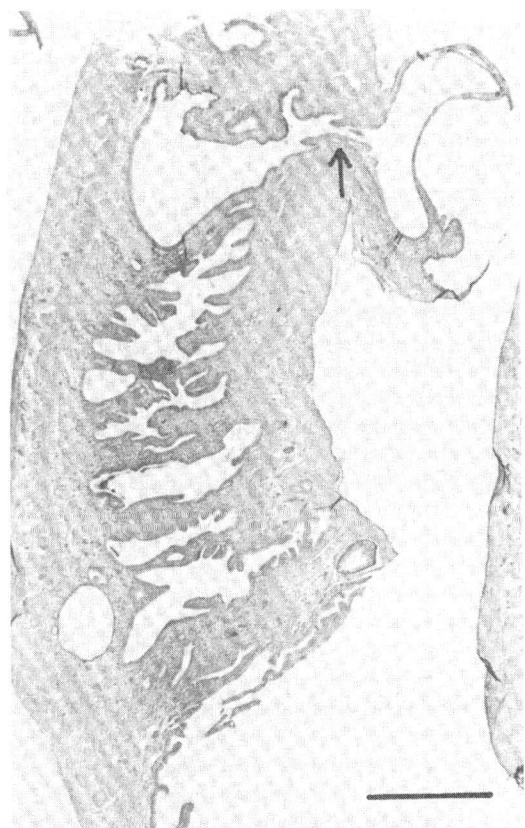

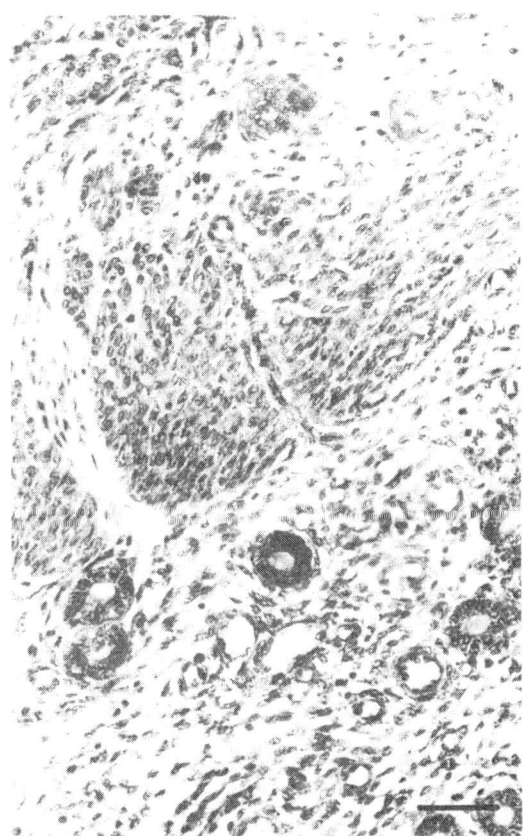

Figure 12. The horizontal section of uterus of a SHN mouse given an isograft of an anterior pituitary in the right horn at 50 days of age and killed 150 days after the grafting. Note direct connection between the endometrial surface and the lumen of subserosal nodule (arrow). Line = 1 mm. Hematoxylin and eosin.

Figure 13. The section of uterus of a SHN mouse given an isograft of an anterior pituitary in the right horn at 50 days of age and killed 60 days after the grafting. The section was stained immunohistochemically for mouse prolactin and lightly counterstained with hematoxylin. Endometrial glands and myometrium contain the immunoreactive material. Line = 25 μm.

of the uterine endometrium to the synergistic effect of prolactin with ovarian sex steroids, and (2) different sensitivity of the hypothalamo-pituitary-ovarian axes to prolactin.

Effect of carcinogen on adenomyosis

Fifty-day-old female SHN mice were each given two isologous anterior pituitary grafts under the right renal capsule and implanted simultaneously with a small amount of 7, 12-dimethylbenz (a) anthracene (DMBA) and 3-methylcholanthrene (MC) in the right and left uterine horns, respectively. However, neither DMBA nor MC induced uterine adenocarcinomas, squamous cell carcinomas, fibromas or leiomyomas by 150 days after the treatment.

Implication for human cases

The general features of human adenomyosis are not intrinsically different from that of SHN mice. Human adenomyosis is not a congenital malformation, since adenomyosis is not seen in children and is much less common in young women. The peak incidence occurs at the fourth and fifth

decades (16, 53). The generally accepted origin of adenomyosis is that it is derived from penetration of endometrial glands and stroma into the myometrium, because the glands within the myometrium are often continuous with the endometrium. This concept was confirmed by our experiments dealing with the histogenesis of adenomyosis in mice (30).

In the human, one of the factors responsible for initiating the glandular penetration into the myometrium has been considered to be uterine trauma generally occurring at the time of delivery, but adenomyosis also occurs in nulliparous women who do not have a prior history of curettage or myomectomy. Therefore, it is thought that some adenomyosis develops as a metaplastic process from uncommitted stromal cells in the myometrium. These cells are located adjacent to blood vessels lying between the smooth muscle bundles (18). In SHN mice, the early step of adenomyotic changes commences with the invasion of endometrial stromal cells into the myometrium along the blood vessels, although metaplasia of stromal cells preexisting around blood vessels, if present, cannot be excluded.

However, adenomyosis does seem to occur more frequently in women with endometrial hyperplasia or carcinoma (3, 4, 17, 23, 53). In such cases the foci of adenomyosis may occasionally also appear hyperplastic or neoplastic in step with the endometrial lesion.

EFFECTS OF TEMPORARY INHIBITION OF PROLACTIN ON THE DEVELOPMENT OF MAMMARY TUMORS AND ADENOMYOSIS IN SHN MICE

Mammary gland DNA synthesis is a limiting factor for mammary tumorigenesis (35, 38) and is primarily controlled, in part, by prolactin (36, 37). In rats, mammary gland DNA synthesis is high only during youth with a peak around 7 weeks of age and decreases thereafter with increasing age (40, 48). Therefore, prolactin suppression by ergot alkaloids, a potent suppressor of pituitary prolactin secretion, during youth (4–11 weeks of age) markedly protects against spontaneous development of mammary tumor, but suppression during older age (11–18 weeks of age) beyond the active phase of DNA synthesis had little effect (43, 46). On the other hand, mammary gland DNA synthesis in SHN mice is not age-related and is much higher than that in rats (36). While ergot-induced prolactin suppression throughout the experiment is found markedly to inhibit spontaneous mammary tumor development in C3H mice (65, 66, 69), treatment with an ergot alkaloid, bromocriptine-mesilate (CB-154), during youth (4–11 weeks of age) enhanced the development of both HAN and tumors (31, 45). CB-154 treatment during –18 weeks of age also accelerated the development of su n mammary lesions (31). Thus, temporary treatment wit CB-154 is not effective in preventing against mammary tumorigenesis in species in which mammary gland DNA synthesis continues at a high rate throughout the lifetime.

On the other hand, in uterus of the intact SHN mice, CB-154 treatment during 4–11 weeks of age completely inhibits spontaneous adenomyosis later in life (31, 45). The uterus of SHN mice shows rapid growth and reaches maturity between 4 and 8 weeks of age (31). CB-154 treatment administered during 11–18 weeks of age, beyond maturation of the uterus, does not show any inhibitory effects on the development of adenomyosis (31). These results strongly suggest that there is a critical period for forming favorable characteristics for the abnormal growth of endometrial tissues. In addition, the inhibitory effect of CB-154 on the development of adenomyosis cannot be nullified by pituitary grafting (31). Therefore, the inhibitory effect by prolactin suppression during youth would be strong enough to cancel the influence of a later increase of the circulating prolactin levels.

FUTURE PROSPECTS

Endocrine mechanisms in the development and progression of either breast cancer (63, 64) and/or uterine adenomyosis (16, 18, 53) in human are still obscure.

In most high mammary tumor strains of mice currently available, breeders generally develop mammary tumors earlier and have a higher incidence than virgins, and the difference between the age of tumor onset is large. These findings make it very difficult and impractical to use the mouse system as an animal model for human breast cancer,

despite its value in presenting spontaneous tumors comparable to human cancers. On the other hand, both breeders and virgins develop mammary tumors early with high incidence and small variations in onset in our SHN strain. Moreover, the survival time of tumorous individuals can be lengthened by frequent surgical removal of tumors which resulted in the increased lung metastases. Similar advantages are also found with respect to another lesion, adenomyosis. Up to the present time, more than a year is usually needed for the induction of adenomyosis in experimental animals. In the SHN-strain this lesion can be induced in only 20 days by our technique of intrauterine pituitary grafting in young mice; furthermore, several characteristics of this lesion appear to be similar to human adenomyosis. Thus, extensive use of these animal systems having the above advantages would give valuable information on the etiology, diagnosis, therapy, and finally prophylaxis of human breast cancer and adenomyosis.

SUMMARY

General features and hormonal control of mammary tumors and adenomyosis in SHN mice were summarized. All data collected herein strongly suggest that hyperprolactinemia may be a primarily important etiological factor in the development of this endocrine syndrome. While both lesions are largely dependent upon prolactin, adenomyosis, but not mammary tumors, has a critical period for development. Finally, the usefulness of these systems as an animal model for human cases was discussed.

References

1. Armstrong DT, King ER: Uterine progesterone metabolism and progestational response: effects of estrogens and prolactin. *Endocrinology* 89:191, 1971
2. Beuving LT, Bern HA: Hormonal influence upon normal, preneoplastic, and neoplastic mammary gland. In: *Estrogen: Target Tissues and Neoplasia.* Dao TL ed., p. 257, Chicago & London, Univ. Chicago Press 1972
3. Colman HI, Rosenthal AH: Carcinoma developing in areas of adenomyosis. *Obstet Gynecol* 14:342, 1959
4. Cope E: Adenocarcinoma of the endometrium with malignant stromatosis. *J Obstet Gynecol Brit Emp* 65:58, 1958
5. Crossen RJ, Suntzeff V: Endometrial polyps and hyperplasia produced in an aged monkey with estrogen plus progesterone. *Arch Pathol* 50: 721, 1950
6. Drill VA: Relationship of estrogens and oral contraceptives to endometrial cancer in animals and women. *J Reprod Med* 24:5, 1980
7. Güttner J: Adenomyosis in mice. *Z Versuchstierk* 22:249, 1980
8. Heywood R, Wadsworth PF: The experimental toxicology of estrogens. *Pharmac Ther* 8:125, 1980
9. Horrobin DF, Lipton A, Muiruri KL, Manku MS, Bramley PS, Burstyn PG: An inhibitory effect of prolactin on the response of rat myometrium to oxytosin. *Experientia* 29:109, 1973
10. Huseby RA, Thurlow S: Effects of prenatal exposure of mice to "low-dose" diethylstilbestrol and the development of adenomyosis associated with evidence of hyperprolactinemia. *Am J Obstet Gynecol* 144:939, 1982
11. Huseby RA, Soares MJ, Talamantes F: Ectopic pituitary grafts in mice: hormone levels, effects on fertility, and the

development of adenomyosis uteri, prolactinomas, and mammary carcinoma. *Endocrinology* 116:1440, 1985

12. Joseph MM, Mubako HB: Extraovarian effect of prolactin on the traumatized uterus in the rat. *J Reprod Fert* 45:413, 1975
13. Kallad T, Forsberg J. -G, Sinha YN: Long-term effects of neonatal DES treatment on plasma prolactin in female mice. *Endocrinol Res Commun* 7:157, 1980
14. Kimura J, Okada H: Uterine tumors and hormone dependency. In *Hormone Related Tumors*. Nagasawa H, Abe K. eds., p. 201. Tokyo & Berlin, Japan Sci. Soc. Press/Springer-Verlag, 1981
15. King NW: The reproductive tract. In: *Pathology of Laboratory Animals*. Benirschke K, Garner FM, Jones TC. eds., vol. 1, chapter 7. p. 510, New York, Heidelberg & Berlin, Springer-Verlag, 1978
16. Kraus FT: Female genitalia. In: *Pathology*. Anderson W.A.D. Kissane JM. eds., vol. 2, 7th ed., chapter 40, p. 1680, Saint Louis, The CV Mosby Comp, 1977
17. Kumar D, Anderson W: Malignancy in endometriosis interna. *J Obstet Gynecol Brit Emp* 65:435, 1958
18. Kurman RJ: Benign diseases of the endometrium. In: *Pathology of the Female Genital Tract*. Blaustein A. ed., 2nd ed., chapter 12. p. 279, New York, Heidelberg & Berlin, Springer-Verlag, 1982
19. Lacassagne A: Modifications progressives de l'utérus de la souris sous l'action prolongée de l'oestrone. *C. r. Séanc Soc Biol* 120:1156, 1935
20. Leung BS, Sasaki GH: Prolactin and progesterone effect on specific estradiol binding in uterine and mammary tissues *in vitro*. *Biochem biophys Res Commun* 55:1180, 1973
21. Lipschütz A, Iglesias R, Panasevich VI, Salinas S: Pathological changes induced in the uterus of mice with the prolonged administration of progesterone and 19-nor-contraceptives. *Brit J Cancer* 21:160, 1967
22. Loeb L, Burns EL, Suntzeff V, Moskop M: Carcinoma-like proliferation in vagina, cervix and uterus of mouse treated with estrogenic hormones. *Proc Soc exp Biol Med* 35:320, 1936
23. Marcus CC: Relationship of adenomyosis uteri to endometrial hyperplasia and endometrial carcinoma. *Am J Obstet Gynecol* 82:408, 1961
24. Mati JKG, Mugambi M, Muriuki PL, Thairu K: Effect of prolactin on isolated rabbit myometrium. *J Endocrinol* 60:379, 1974
25. McKay DG: A review of the status of endometrial cancer. *Cancer Res* 25:1182, 1965
26. McLachlan JA, Newbold RR, Bullock BC: Long-term effects on the female mouse genital tract associated with prenatal exposure to diethylstilbestrol. *Cancer Res* 40:3988, 1980
27. Meissner WA, Sommers SC, Sherman G: Endometrial hyperplasia, endometrial carcinoma, and endometriosis produced experimentally by estrogen. *Cancer* 10:500, 1957
28. Mody JK: Structural changes in the ovaries of IF mice due to age and various other states: Demonstration of spontaneous pseudopregnancy in grouped virgins. *Anat Rec* 145:439, 1963
29. Mori T, Bern HA: Longterm effects of neonatal anterior hypophysial isografts on the mammary gland of mammary tumor virus-expressed mice. *Proc Soc exp Biol Med* 161:48, 1979
30. Mori T, Nagasawa H: Mechanisms of development of prolactin-induced adenomyosis in mice. *Acta Anat* 116:46, 1983
31. Mori T, Nagasawa H: Alteration of the development of mammary hyperplastic alveolar nodules and uterine adenomyosis in SHN mice by different schedules of treatment with CB-154. *Acta Endocrinol* 107:245, 1984
32. Mori T, Nagasawa H, Takahashi S: The induction of adenomyosis in mice by intrauterine pituitary isografts. *Life Sci* 29:1277, 1981
33. Mori T, Nagasawa H, Nakajima Y: Strain-difference in the induction of adenomyosis by intrauterine pituitary grafting in mice. *Lab Anim Sci* 32:40, 1982

34. Mori T, Ohta Y, Nagasawa H: Ultrastructural changes in uterine myometrium of mice with experimentally-induced adenomyosis. *Experientia* 40:1385, 1984
35. Nagasawa H: Mammary gland DNA synthesis as a limiting factor for mammary tumorigenesis. *Forum. IRCS Med Sci* 5:405, 1977
36. Nagasawa H: Prolactin: Its role in the development of mammary tumours. *Med Hypoth* 5:1117, 1979
37. Nagasawa H: Hormones and experimental mammary tumorigenesis. In: *Hormone Related Tumors*. Nagasawa H, Abe K. eds. p. 137, Tokyo, Berlin, Japan Sci. Soc. Press/Springer-Verlag, 1981
38. Nagasawa H: Causes of age-dependency of mammary tumour induction by carcinogens in rats. *Biomedicine* 34:9, 1981
39. Nagasawa H: Prolactin as a promoter of initial progression of spontaneous mammary tumors in mice and lack of relationship to age. *Life Sci* 33:1451, 1983
40. Nagasawa H, Yanai R: Frequency of mammary cell division in relation to age: Its significance in the induction of mammary tumors by carcinogen in rats. *J Nat Cancer Inst* 52:609, 1974.
41. Nagasawa H, Yanai R: Normal and abnormal growth of mammary glands. In: *Physiology of Mammary Glands*. Yokoyama A, Mizuno H, Nagasawa H. eds., p. 121, Baltimore, Univ. Park Press, 1978
42. Nagasawa H, Yanai R: Mammary gland prolactin receptor and pituitary prolactin secretion in lactating mice with different lactational performance. *Acta Endocrinal* 88:94, 1978
43. Nagasawa H, Morii S: Prophylaxis of spontaneous mammary tumorigenesis by temporal inhibition of prolactin secretion in rats at young ages. *Cancer Res* 41:1935, 1981.
44. Nagasawa H, Yanai R: The *in vitro* mammary gland response to mammotropic hormones in mice with different mammary tumorigenesis. *Europ J Cancer* 17:503, 1981
45. Nagasawa H, Mori T: Stimulation of mammary tumorigenesis and suppression of uterine adenomyosis by temporary inhibition of pituitary prolactin secretion during youth in mice. *Proc Soc exp Biol Med* 171:164, 1982
46. Nagasawa H, Morii S: Inhibition by early treatment with CB-154 (bromocriptine) of spontaneous mammary tumor development in rats with no side-effects. *Acta Endocrinol* 101:51, 1982
47. Nagasawa H, Yanai R, Taniguchi H: Reduction by pituitary grafts of mammary tumor age. Its variability in a high mammary tumor strain of mice: Effects on mammary DNA synthesis. *Europ J Cancer* 12:1017, 1976
48. Nagasawa H, Yanai R, Taniguchi H: Importance of mammary gland DNA synthesis on carcinogen-induced mammary tumorigenesis in rats. *Cancer Res* 36:2223, 1976
49. Nagasawa H, Yanai R, Taniguchi H, Tokuzen R, Nakahara W: Two-way selection of a stock of Swiss albino mice for mammary tumorigenesis: Establishment of two new strains (SHN and SLN). *J Natl Cancer Inst* 57:425, 1976
50. Nagasawa H, Mori T, Yanai R, Bern HA, Mills KT: Long-term effects of neonatal hormonal treatments on plasma prolactin levels in female BALB/cfC3H and BALB/c mice. *Cancer Res* 38:942, 1978
51. Nagasawa H, Yanai R, Jones LA, Bern HA, Mills KT: Ovarian dependence of the stimulatory effect of neonatal hormone treatment on plasma levels of prolactin in female mice. *J Endocrinol* 79:391, 1978.
52. Nelson WO: Endometrial and myometrial changes, including fibromatus nodules, induced in the uterus of guinea pig by prolonged administration of oestrogenic hormone. *Anat Rec* 68:99, 1937
53. Novak ER, Woodruff JD: Adenomyosis (adenomyoma) uteri. In: Novak's *Gynecologic and Obstetric Pathology with Clinical and Endocrine Relations*. Novak ER, Woodruff JD (eds.), 8th ed. ch. 12, p. 280. Philadelphia, London, Toronto, W.B. Saunders Company, 1979
54. Ostrander PL, Mills KT, Bern HA: Long-term responses of

the mouse uterus to neonatal diethylstilbestrol treatment and to later sex hormone exposure. *J Natl Cancer Inst* 74:121, 1985

55. Pan SC, Gardner WU: Carcinomas of uterine cervix and vagina in estrogen- and androgen-treated hybrid mice. *Cancer Res* 8:337, 1948

56. Posner BI, Kelly PA, Shiu RPC, Friesen HG: Studies of insulin, growth hormone and prolactin binding: tissue distribution, species variation and characterization. *Endocrinology* 95:521, 1974

57. Saiduddin S, Zassenhaus HP: Effect of prolactin on specific oestradiol receptors in the rat uterus. *J Endocrinol* 72:101, 1977

58. Schwarz OH, Sherman A: Hyperplasia of the endometrium, its relationship to hypertrophy and hyperplasia of the uterine vessels. *Am J Obstet Gynecol* 59:1330, 1950

59. Sinha YN: Plasma prolactin analysis as a potential predictor of murine mammary tumorigenesis. In Banbury Report 8: *Hormones and Breast Cancer*. Dike MC, Siiteri PK, Welsch CW. eds., p. 377, New York, Cold Spring Harbor Lab, 1981

60. Squire RA, Goodman DG, Valerio MG, Fredrickson T, Strandberg JD, Levitt MH, Lingeman CH, Harschbarger JC, Dawe CJ: Female reproductive system. In: *Pathology of Laboratory Animals*. Benirschke K, Garner FM, Jones TC eds., vol. 2. chapter 12, p. 1172, New York, Heidelberg, Berlin, Springer-Verlag, 1978

61. Terranova PF, Kent GC: Uterine trauma: Its anabolic effect and influence on uterine sensitivity to prolactin in ovariecto-mized hamsters. *Endocrinology* 94:1484, 1974

62. Vignon F, Rochefort H: Regulation of estrogen receptors in ovarian-dependent rat mammary tumors. I. Effects of castration and prolactin. *Endocrinology* 98:722, 1976

63. Vorherr H: Breast cancer. Epidemiology, Endocrinology, Biochemistry and Pharmacology, Baltimore, Munich, Urban, Schwarzenberg, 1980

64. Vorherr H: Hormones and prostaglandins in relation to breast cancer. In: *Hormone Related Tumors*. Nagasawa H, Abe K. eds., p. 137. Tokyo, Berlin, Japan Sci. Soc. Press/Springer-Verlag, 1981

65. Welsch CW, Gribler C: Prophylaxis of spontaneous mammary carcinoma in C3H/HeJ female mice by suppression of prolactin. *Cancer Res* 33:2939, 1973

66. Welsch CW; Gribler C, Clemens JA: 6-methyl-8-β-ergolineacetonitrile (MEA)-induced suppression of mammary tumorigenesis in C3H/HeJ female mice. *Europ J Cancer* 10:595, 1974

67. Welsch CW, Nagasawa H: Prolactin and murine mammary tumorigenesis: a review. *Cancer Res* 37:951, 1977

68. Williams GH; Hammond JM; Weisz J, Mortel R: Binding sites for lactogenic hormone in the rat uterus. *Biol Reprod* 18:697, 1978

69. Yanai R, Nagasawa H: Inhibition of mammary tumorigenesis by ergot alkaloids and promotion of mammary tumorigenesis by pituitary isografts in adreno-ovariectomized mice. *J Nat Cancer Inst* 48:715, 1972

ETIOLOGY, MORPHOLOGY AND PATHOGENESIS OF PROLIFERATIVE AND HYPERPLASTIC LESIONS AND NEOPLASMS OF MOUSE MAMMARY GLAND

BERNARD SASS

INTRODUCTION

Apolant, in 1906 (3) described focal hypertrophic lesions of the mouse mammary gland which he felt resembled adenomas and which were later classified as hyperplastic alveolar lesions. Haaland, in 1911 (36) reported the existence of hyperplastic changes which preceded neoplasia and also showed that increased frequency of hyperplastic mammary gland lesions in mice was related to both increasing age and the subsequent occurrence of cancer. Murray, in 1911 (75) discovered a hereditary factor in the etiology of mouse mammary tumors.

Fekete (27) examined persistently growing areas of mammary gland epithelium in mouse strains with high and low tumor incidence and demonstrated that these areas eventually transformed to cancer. Gardner et al. (35) described hyperplastic ductal and alveolar lesions and suggested that the lesion progressed to neoplasia.

Foulds (29, 31) used the term tumor progression for the sequence of events that determine the behavior of mouse mammary tumors and of neoplasms in general. The development of carcinomas from preneoplastic lesions such as plaques were considered by Foulds (32) under the heading of "group B lesions". Among the characteristics cited for group B lesions was that: "conditional tumors that grow only whilst they are stimulated by extrinsic factors, regress when these factors are withdrawn and reoccur from a persistent focus of residual neoplasia when the stimulus is restored". This characteristic was the only one which would apply to mouse mammary tumor progression, the other six characteristics named by Foulds applied specifically to skin papillomas. Specific fates theorized for type B lesions were as follows: 1) progression to another type B lesion of higher neoplastic capacity or to carcinoma, 2) progressive growth without qualitative change, 3) regression. The concept that development of neoplasms is a multistage phenomenon became widely accepted based on the work in experimental skin carcinogenesis by Mottram (72), Berenblum (7–9), Rous and Kidd (88), and others (33, 34). Intermediate stages of neoplasia in skin are difficult to visualize, especially when one agent is the initiator and a second agent is the promoter.

The mouse mammary gland and liver are the two major systems in which intermediate cell populations exist. Using transplantation, fat pad clearing, and more recently cell organ culture techniques, investigators could study precursor lesions in detail in mouse mammary tumor model systems.

Morphology

Hyperplastic alveolar nodules (HAN) were described by numerous authors (20, 39, 74, 80, 83, 101, 104, 105, 108). Medina (57) defined HAN as foci of hyperplastic lobuloalveolar development in an area of nonstimulated mammary gland. Using a dissecting microscope at 8–12 magnifications, Muhlbock and Tengbergen (74) described HAN as yellow nodules, owing to their hemosiderin content. Because it is difficult to visualize HAN in this manner, the preferred method is to subcutaneously inject the animals on each of 3 successive days with a combination of the hormones somatotrophin, 125 mcg., luteotrophin, 125 mcg., and hydrocortisone acetate, 250, mcg. (11). By this method, HAN, if present, appear grossly as alveolar foci of milky white material.

Whole mounts of mammary gland tissue are widely used to study the morphology of mouse mammary gland lesions, especially HAN and other precursor lesions. Briefly, the method (57) consists of killing the animal by cervical dislocation, and then removing the skin to which the mammary glands remain attached. The skin is pinned to a cork board which is suspended in 12% formalin for 24 hours. The five pairs of mammary glands are carefully peeled off as a unit and placed in a nylon staining basket and defatted with two changes of acetone. Next, the tissues are rinsed twice with alcohol, and stained with hematoxylin. The vessels, nerves, and hair follicles are removed under a dissecting microscope. The glands are then stored in methyl salicylate and examined by the dissecting microscope for the presence of lesions.

Histologically, HAN consist of alveoli lined by a single row of cuboidal cells surrounding a small lumen, and unless they have progressed, are histologically indistinguishable from normal prelactating mammary gland epithelium, but differ from normal mammary tissue by their biological properties (82). The most common variations in the histomorphology of HAN are the size of the lumen and the degree of secretory activity. (45, 22, 23).

HAN also showed diffuse progression and were classified (47, 48) as type A, B, and adenoacanthoma using the classification of Dunn 1959 (25). Huseby and Bittner (44) classified HAN with progression as inflammatory, ductal and noninflammatory types. Sass and Vlahakis (93) examined histologically, described and illustrated HAN with inflammation, with secretion, keratinization and malignant foci. However, Bittner (14) considered HAN as early ade-

H. E. Kaiser (ed.), Comparative aspects of tumor development.

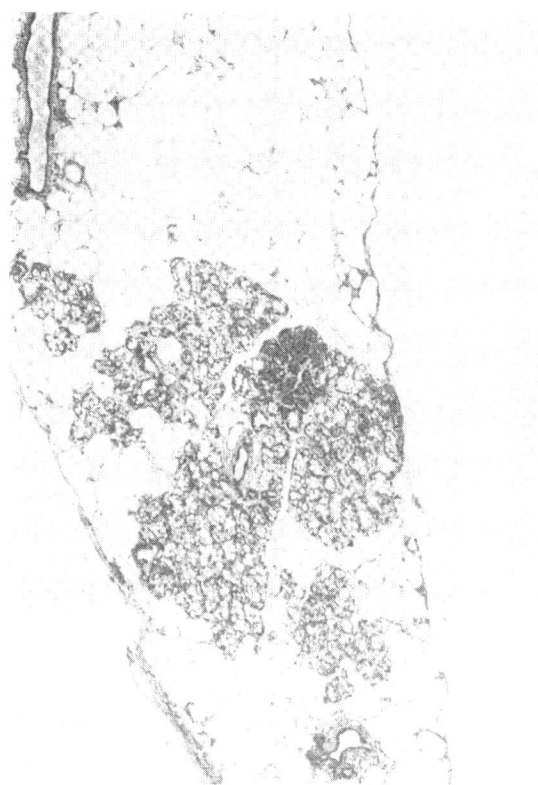

Figure 1. HAN = multiple, some confluent. Deeply stained area center is a neoplastic focus. Strain C3H/A^{vyf}BfDD 12 mos. Hematoxylin and eosin 55X.

mas, if there was necrosis of the epithelium, acidophilic secretion and escape of the contents into the surrounding tissue. Sass and Vlahakis (93) classified the above lesions as HAN with inflammatory reaction, providing inflammatory cells, usually lymphocytes were present. Another common feature of HAN, which also is occasionally found in normal mammary glands, is the presence of mineral concretions known as corpora amylacea (93).

HAN with malignant foci are composed of groups of acini lined by multiple layers of cells which stain more deeply than the cells lining the normal acini, and thus show histologic evidence of malignant progression (93) (Figure 1). Often, HAN show progression throughout the lesions and are thus microcarcinomas.

Foulds (29, 30) described mammary tumors in certain hybrid mice: RIIIxC57BL, C57BLXRIII and inbred strains BR6 and RIII. More recently, tumors arising in strains GR (100, 109, 117), DD (40) and RIII (100) were described. Unlike the mammary tumors in other strains of mice, some of Fould's mice developed tumors originating from lesions termed plaques which were responsive to reproductive activity, since such tumors grew during pregnancy and regressed partially or completely after parturition. Tumors which were unaffected by pregnancy were termed unresponsive.

At autopsy, plaques that were palpable measured 0.5–1.0 cm. in diameter and 0.1 to 0.2 cm. in thickness. Smaller non-palpable plaques could however, be visualized grossly at post mortem (30).

Plaques have been subclassified as perfect, imperfect, incomplete and complex. The latter type is further subclassified as multilobular, giant, irregular and as plaques with epidermal reaction (30).

Histologically, plaques are elliptical or disc-shaped circumscribed and unencapsulated; perfect plaques have a myxomatous core of loosely arranged connective tissue (Figure 2). The epithelial elements exhibit radial symmetry, and the cortex enlarges during pregnancy. After parturition, plaques regress and exhibit cortical atrophy. Malignant foci, however, persist and enlarge (Figure 3).

Imperfect plaques lack the radial symmetry of perfect plaques, have an incomplete cortex and are triangular in shape, with the base toward the skin surface and the apex related to a mammary duct (Figure 4).

Complex multilobular plaques involve several lobes of mammary tissue in which the medullary zones communicate and each individual lobe resembles a single simple plaque.

Certain plaques called giant plaques by Foulds can be very large growths which histologically resemble simple plaques and may include multilobular areas of hyperplasia. Irregular complex plaques lack orderly internal structure; the branching tubules often lack radial symmetry. Large and complex plaques represent further progression of plaques and are difficult to distinguish from carcinomas. Regressing plaques contain epithelial cells undergoing necrosis and have a hyalin stroma, which often becomes sclerotic.

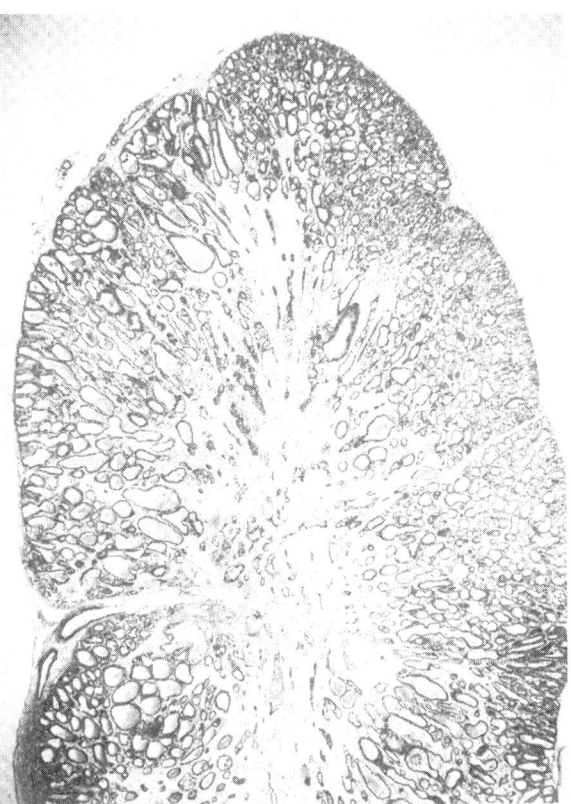

Figure 2. Plaque – the lesion consists of tubules which appear to radiate from a central point which is myxomatous. Strain GRS, 9 mos. Hematoxylin and eosin 25X.

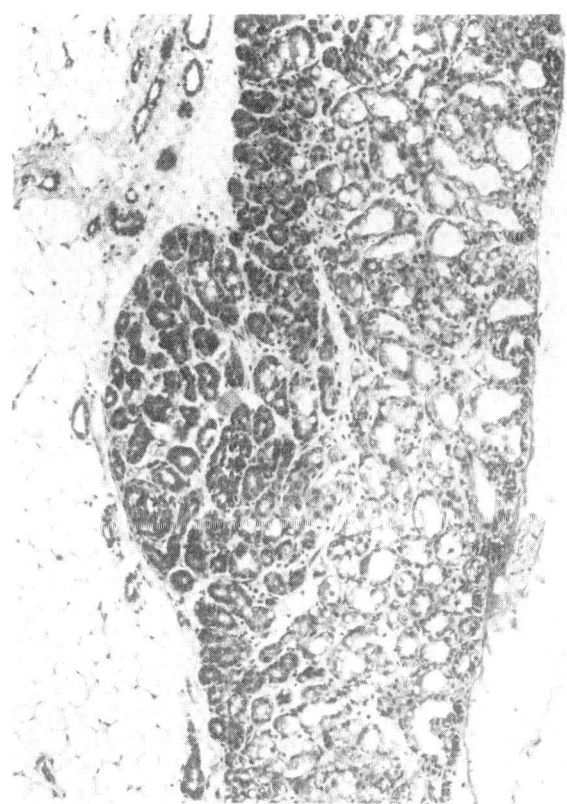

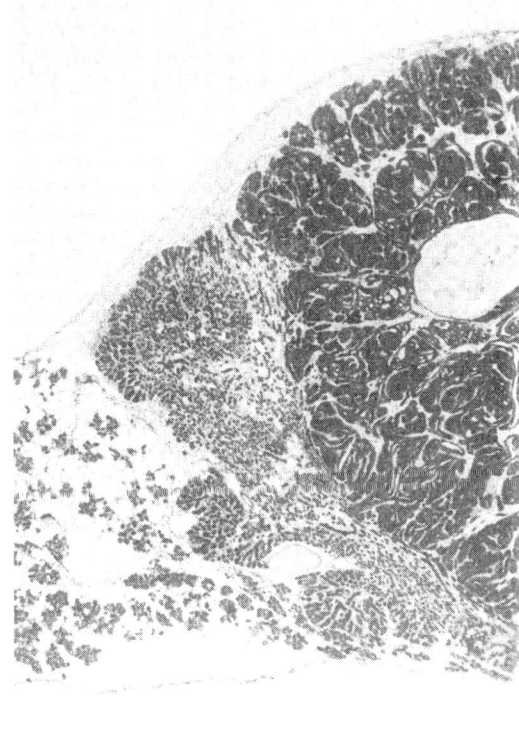

Figure 4. Imperfect plaque adjacent to adenocarcinoma type B, right. Strain GRS 7 mos. Hematoxylin and eosin 28X.

Figure 3. Plaque with malignant area, left center; cells are deeply stained. Strain C3H/A^vyfBfDD, 17 mos. Hematoxylin and eosin 130X.

Plaques with epidermal reaction were reported by Foulds (30). Such lesions are characterized by the presence of plaques with hyperplasia of the overlying epidermis. Tumors of mammary gland with participation of skin and adnexae have also been reported (30). Such tumors are characterized by domed elevation of the skin with acanthosis, proliferation of the basal cell layer and of the adnexal epithelium and, in particular, of hair follicles. Underlying the adnexal derived neoplasms are mammary tumors resembling imperfect plaques with secretion (93) (Figure 5).

Mammary adenocarcinomas containing sebaceous cells are occasionally found (93) (Figure 6). Such sebaceous cells are present within the tumor tissue, are surrounded by mammary tumor cells and may occur singly or as nests. In humans (52) and possibly in rodents, the mammary gland is derived from sweat glands. It is not known if the neoplastic epithelial elements in such tumors could be derived entirely from sebaceous cells, however, the presence of both cell types suggests parallel modes of development of mammary gland and sebaceous glands.

The term organoid tumor (30) is applied to plaques which become enlarged, do not regress after parturition and histologically maintain neoplastic tubular structures showing radial symmetry (Figure 7). Hormone-responsive tumors occurring in strain GRS mice are composed of acini lined by basophilic stellate shaped cells arranged in multiple layers which do not regress, resemble the giant plaques and organoid tumors of Foulds, but were termed type P tumors by

vanNie (109). HAN were also found in strain GRS.

The term adenocarcinoma type P (92) is used to designate similar tumors in strain GRS. These tumors were distinguished from plaques on the basis of increased cell atypia and basophilia, lobular areas of ingrowth into tubular structures lined by multiple layers of neoplastic epithelial cells and a more irregularly distributed abundant stroma than occurs in plaques (Figure 8).

Adenocarcinomas type P often contain plaques and areas

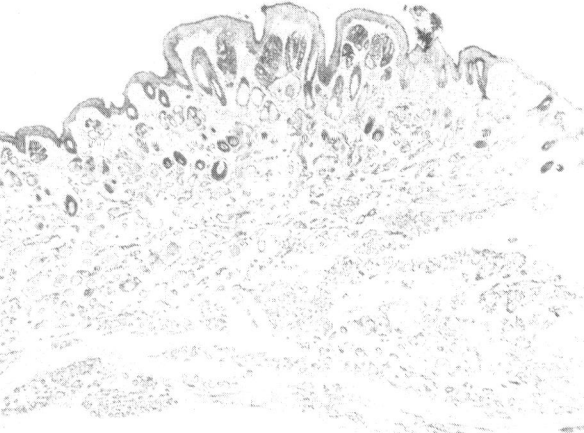

Figure 5. Dome shaped neoplasm of epidermis with papillary elements, beneath which lies imperfect plaque. Strain DD female, 10 mos. Hematoxylin and eosin 38X.

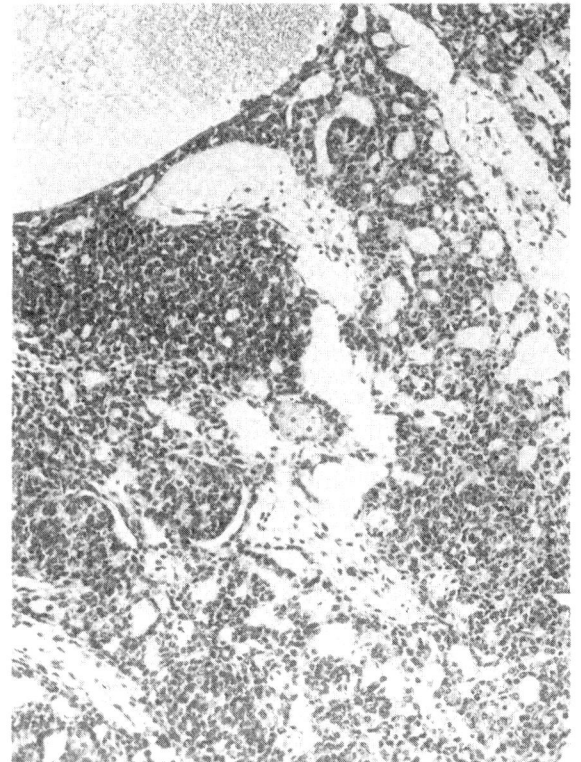

Figure 6. Adenocarcinoma type B. There is a nest of normal sebaceous glands in the center. Strain (C3HXVob)F₁, 12 mos. Hematoxylin and eosin 130X.

of adenocarcinoma type B which may progress (93) thus attesting to their transitional nature and providing a link between reversibility and nonreversibility of hormone dependent tumors.

Pale cell carcinomas are tumors of strain GRS mice (106, 92, 93), RIII (100) or BALB/Cf RIII (101) which often assume the shape of plaques or are intimately associated with plaques (Figure 9), and contain areas of squamous differentiation characterized by the presence of individual cell keratinization and intercellular bridges. The pale cells which exhibit this differentiation usually surround cells bordering cystic spaces. In some sections, dark cells surround cords of pale cells separated by intervening stroma (Figure 10). Pale cell carcinomas can arise in three different precursor lesions (93):
1) Plaques – such tumors often have the shape of plaques, or contain plaques.
2) Adenocarcinomas type P – transplants of adenocarcinomas type P give rise to pale cell carcinomas (109).
3) Adenocarcinoma type B (25) – tumors with cystic and papillary architecture having large areas of blood-filled spaces and necrosis occur with some frequency in mice of strain GRS.
   Foci of pale cell carcinoma were observed in a number of such tumors (93). The areas of adenocarcinoma type P possibly arise in plaques.

Strum (102) studied the ultrastructure of the pale and dark cells in pale cell carcinomas of strain GRS/S. The pale cells had electron lucent or clear cytoplasm. Some of the pale

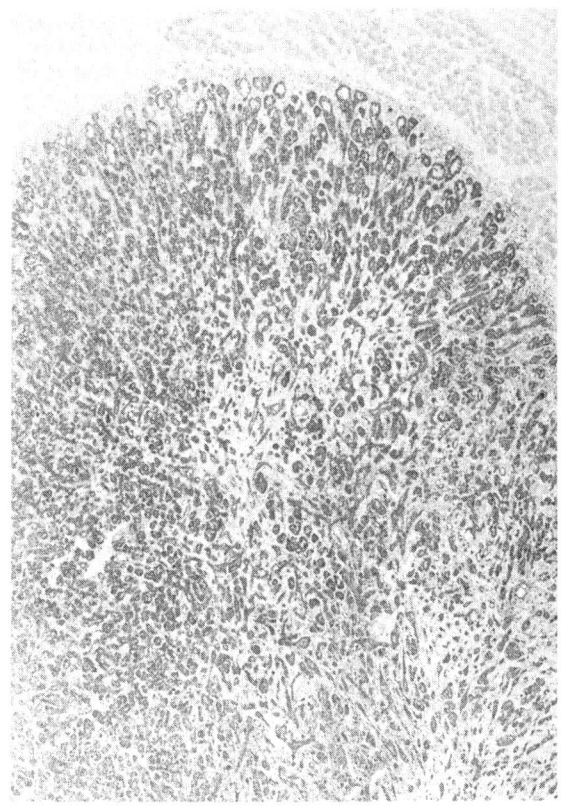

Figure 7. Organoid tumor showing radiate tubular pattern. Strain GRS, 11 mos. Hematoxylin and eosin 38X.

cells contained intracytoplasmic keratin. Others had evidence of squamous differentiation.

The dark cells were considered to be either active or inactive. Ultrastructurally, the active dark cells sometimes contained microglandular lumens with viral particles. Many of the inactive cells were interpreted as "apoptotic cells", that is, they were programmed to die. The pale cells were aligned along vascular channels, whereas the dark cells often surrounded lumens. On the basis of morphometric examinations, Strum postulated that the pale cells underwent degeneration and cytoplasmic swelling and then become keratinized. The cystic spaces lined by basophilic cells as described by Sass and Dunn (92) were identified ultrastructurally. They were considerd to be intracellular alveoli containing fluid and mammary tumor virus.

Slemmer (97) studied the interactions of different cell types using two different genotypes from normal and neoplastic mammary glands. Mosaic tissues were produced by associating mammary cells from two different mouse strains *in vitro* and then subjecting them to serial transplantation by the mammary fat pad technique (20) to F₁ hybrids of the parent strains, and to the original strains. Cells from one strain produced only alveolar cells and from another strain only ducts. Three different cell types were identified using this technique: alveolar, ductal, and myoepithelial. The findings suggest existence of cells with the capacity of self renewal and the capability of producing the same cell type on serial transplantation (97). Thus, alveolar epithelial cells

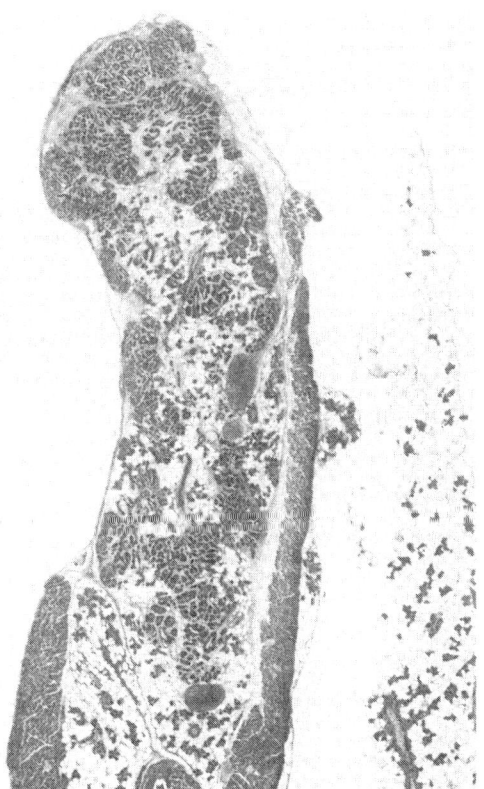

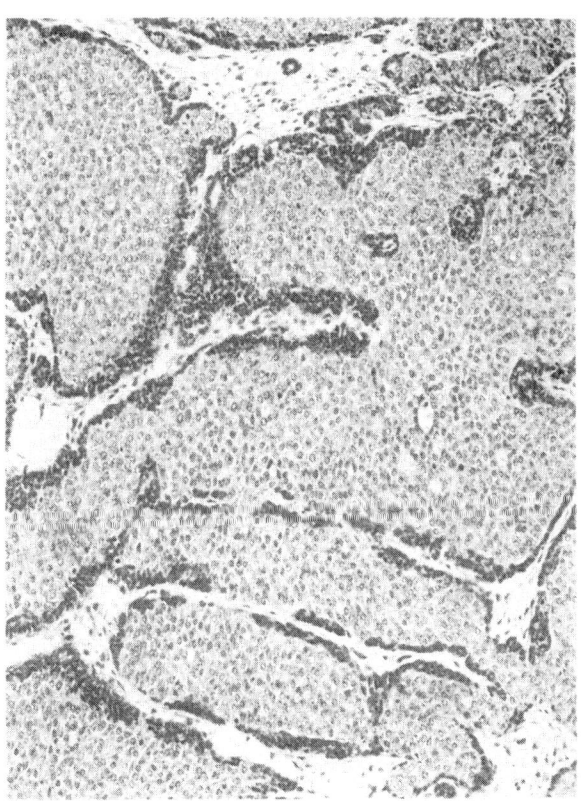

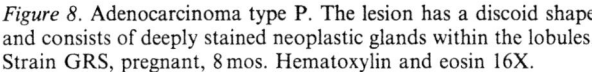

Figure 8. Adenocarcinoma type P. The lesion has a discoid shape and consists of deeply stained neoplastic glands within the lobules. Strain GRS, pregnant, 8 mos. Hematoxylin and eosin 16X.

Figure 9. Pale cell carcinoma. The pale cells are arranged in sheets. Dark cells line cystic spaces. Strain GRS, 10 mos. Hematoxylin and eosin 130X.

produce alveolar preneoplasia and duct epithelial cells produce ductal hyperplasia. The cell lines consisting of only myoepithelium gave rise to epidermoid-mesenchymal neoplasms and adenoacanthomas which arise late in BALB/c mice. Myoepithelial cells were shown to regulate the space between ducts and that normal myoepithelial cells cannot survive in the absence of epithelium (97).

Etiologic factors

1. Viruses

HAN are histologically indistinguishable from the normal mammary gland in the prelactating state and their recognition requires the use of non-pregnant, non-lactating mice (20, 21, 39, 44). Pitelka (84) examined HAN ultrastructurally and found that the major difference between prelactating mammary gland alveoli and HAN was the presence of large numbers of particles characteristic of MMTV (mouse mammary tumor virus).

According to Bernhard and Granboulan (12) four different virus particles can be found in thin sections of mammary gland. They are as follows:

1) Intracisternal A particles – are crescent-shaped or doughnut-shaped incomplete particles with 30 mu shells located in the cisternae of endoplasmic reticulum (12, 84). They can be found in a variety of mouse tumors (84) and in the mammary gland (17, 18, 19, 24). The biological signifi-

cance of intracisternal A particles is unknown.

2) Intracytoplasmic A particles are doughnut shaped and contain two concentric rings approximately 30 mu to 85 mu in diameter. They often form inclusion bodies (12).

3) B particles are characteristic of MMTV and appear to bud off the apical cell membrane, or appear as mature, extracellular particles with four shells, an eccentric electron dense nucleoid and spikes on the outer shell (91).

4) C particles are similar to B particles, but contain three shells, a central electron dense nucleoid, and lack spikes on the outer membrane.

Virus particles of type A and B are frequent (100% of cells) in HAN, but are infrequent (25% of cells) in normal mammary epithelial cells (84, 86); they may also be found in the male reproductive system.

More recently, MMTV has been classified by Medina (62) into the following variants: MMTV-S, the Bittner virus, which is transmitted through the milk; 2) MMTV-L, the nodule inducing virus which is weakly oncogenic and is transmitted through germ cells; 3) MMTV-P is found in strains GR, RIII, DDD, DD, and BR6. This virus is transmitted thorough both the germ cells and milk in GR mice, but is only milk transmitted in RIII and DD mice (73); 4) MMTV-O is the putative endogenous virus present in the genome of all mice (73). Activation and transmission patterns of this agent are not yet established (71).

In strain C3HA^{vy} the agent was shown to be transmitted by either parent and/or through the milk (110). This agent,

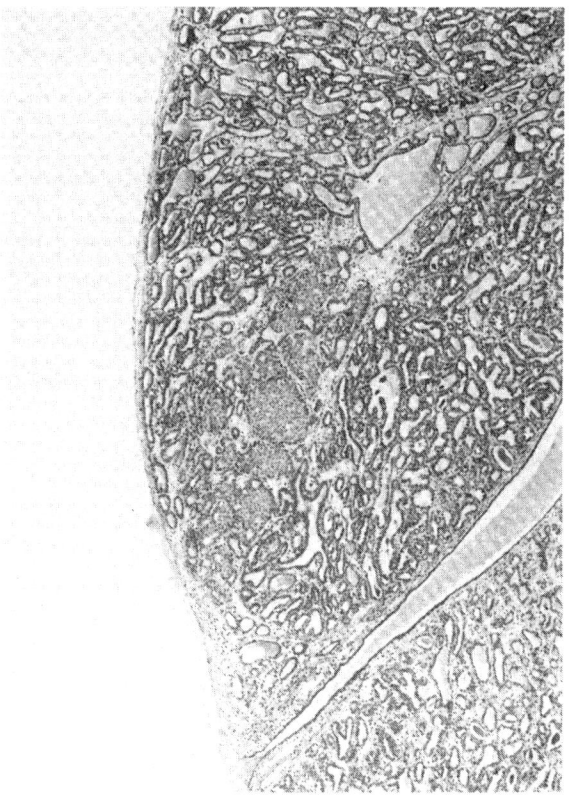

Figure 10. Plaque with areas of early pale cell carcinoma Strain GRS, 11 mos. Hematoxylin and eosin 55X.

though originating from strain C3H mice, thus seems to be different from MMTV-S as defined by Medina (62).

Recently, a new MMTV from Mus cervicolor was characterized (95). This agent is immunologically related to MMTV from MUS musculus.

MMTV-S and MMTV-L induce HAN and adenocarcinomas (80), whereas MMTV-P induces plaques and adenocarcinomas type P (99), respectively.

According to Hilgers and Bentvelzen (42) MTV can replicate in different tissues, but transforms only mammary tissues efficiently. MMTV from C3H mice induces transformation of only alveolar cells, whereas, MMTV of strain GR transforms duct-alveolar cells (42).

2. The role of hormones

Lathrop and Loeb, in 1916, (51) recorded a decrease in the incidence of mammary tumors in spayed females as compared to controls, thus demonstrating the role played by hormonal factors. Bittner (14) showed that the difference in mammary tumor or incidence in strains A and C3H was attributable to what he termed "inherited hormonal influence." Bern and Nandi (10) suggested that the inherited hormonal influence in virgin C3H mice reflected responsiveness to growth hormone when it was administered as a mixture of hormones. Strain A mice, which have few HAN and mammary tumors if they remain virgins have a higher incidence of mammary tumors if prolactin is included in the mixture of hormones. Other workers (96), using *in vitro*

assays, could not establish a correlation between growth hormone sensitivity for lobuloalveolar development and tumor incidence in virgins.

Hormones have the capability of influencing MMTV infection of mammary tissue (56, 67). The use of pituitary isografts enhances infection and replication of MMTV-S and MMTV-L in normal and HAN containing mammary gland (63, 64, 68, 82). The use of hormone antagonists is a useful method for establishing the role of hormones in mammary carcinogenesis. Several workers (114, 115, 116) have established that ergocarnine, an inhibitor of prolactin synthesis, when given to animals which were MMTV-S positive, inhibited both HAN and tumor formation.

Neonatal mice of strain SHN that were positive for MMTV-S, when treated with B-dihydrotestosterone (118), or strain C3H/HeJ female mice (41) which were fed diethylstilbesterol, and castrated male (C3HXRIII)F₁ mice given estrone or estradiol by injection (89) had an increased incidence of mammary tumors. However, mice of strain C3HeB/FeJ, which are negative for MMTV-S when fed diethylstilbestrol did not have increased incidence of mammary tumors. The effect of estrogen and progesterone on mammary gland is mediated by prolactin, since the number of pituitary mammotroph cells in mice neonatally treated with steroids is correlated with the effect of treatment (49).

Insulin and glucocorticoids enhance replication of MMTV-S in tumor cells *in vitro* (56). Parks et al. (81) used the synthetic glucocorticoid dexamethasone to stimulate expression of MMTV *in vitro*. Harbell and Medina (37) developed a model *in vitro* system for the study of strain GRS mammary tumor phenotype regulation using insulin, prolactin and progesterone, and both Aidells and Daniel (1) and vanNie and Dux (109) showed that *in vivo*, estrogen and progesterone promote the expression of the tumor phenotype.

Systems such as those mentioned above should provide the basis for careful detailed quantitative studies on the regulation of tumor expression and growth by hormones.

The most frequently used technique of determining the role of hormones in the development of preneoplastic lesions and mammary tumors is the fat pad transplantation technique (20, 21). Weanling (3 week old) mice are anesthetized, an abdominal midline skin incision made and the inguinal (no. 4) fat pads are exposed. Then the nipples and large vessels from the level of the inguinal node to the inguinal fat pads caudal to the no. 5 mammary gland are cauterized. The exposed pads are excised and removed. The resulting space is then available as a transplantation site. Small (.5 mm³) samples of mammary gland tissue from young untreated mice are inserted into this space. The effects of MMTV, pituitary isografts and hormones on transplanted mammary fat pads have been studied using this technique (57, 62, 63).

It should be mentioned in passing, that induction of so called "nodules" by a putative nodule inducing virus (NIV) constitutes a useful biological test for MMTV (77, 78). However, convincing evidence for the spontaneous occurrence of this entity in mice is lacking; rather, nodules occurred only upon transplantation of mammary tissue with MMTV or as a result of administering MMTV in tissue suspensions. Furthermore, no difference in histomorphology between the so-called nodules and HAN were described

(77, 78, 79). Cancer chemotherapeutic agents can be tested in nodule outgrowth lines (65).

The development of nodule outgrowth lines that can be serially transplanted by use of the fat pad transplantation technique is considered equivalent to *in vitro* cell lines. Using these outgrowth lines, morphology, tumor induction and heterogeneity, growth kinetics, response to viruses, and physical agents can be studied.

In vitro studies comparing normal and mouse mammary epithelial cells transformed *in vitro* indicate that *in vitro* transformed neoplastic cells but not *in vivo* grown neoplastic cells have altered morphology, absence of microfilament and microtubule networks, increased agglutination with plant lectins and cell surface topography (5, 70). Other *in vitro* studies with neoplastic mouse mammary epithelium indicate stimulation of DNA synthesis by insulin (111) altered the sensitivity to mitotic regulation by lipids (43) or by serum (28). Mammary tumor cell lines have also proven useful for the study of hormonal regulation of MMTV production (4, 76, 81, 116, 119).

Chemical and physical carcinogenesis

Mammary tumors can be induced by a variety of chemical carcinogens: 3-methylcholanthrene (2, 13, 15, 26, 38, 53, 87); urethane (58, 60) and 9, 10, Dimethyl-1,2-benzanthracene (DMBA) are the most widely used; the latter is the most potent carcinogen inducing a 40–70% mammary tumor incidence within 10–14 months in virgin mice (16, 53, 69). The disadvantage of using DMBA, however, is that leukemias, pulmonary and gastric tumors and ovarian tumors are also increased up to an incidence of 25% (62).

To overcome this disadvantage, Medina (69) treated (C57BLXDBA/2f)F₁ females with DMBA and obtained a 70% incidence of mammary tumors in 9 months, and also a few leukemias. In strain BALB/c which carries little or no MMTV, hormone stimulation by pituitary isografts is obligatory for the rapid induction of carcinogen altered cells into neoplastic cells (59).

In addition to HAN, Faulkin (26) using the whole mount technique, described other lesions induced by methylcholanthrene alone or in combination with hormones. These were as follows: 1) fibrous nodules, 2) area nodules, 3) noduloids, and 4) alveoli along ducts. HAN from chemically treated animals, when transplanted into syngeneic hosts, give rise to adenocarcinomas; the other lesions were not transplanted. However, fibroadenomas believed to develop from fibrous nodules arise frequently in chemically treated mice. Medina and Warner (66) using the whole mount technique and histological examination observed what they termed terminal ductal hyperplasia in 50% of pituitary isograft DMBA or urethane treated virgin BALB/C mice. From the illustrations in their paper, the ductal lesions appear as tubules or cords and could be derived from alveoli or ductules or from a combination of the two.

Medina (58, 59) and Medina and Warner (66) administered DMBA to strain BALB/c, C57/B1, (C57BLxDBA/2f)F₁ and C3H/StWi (MMTV-S free) mice. The tumor incidence varied from 50–80%. Duct hyperplasias subclassified as simple, lobular and papillary, and end bud types were described. The first three types, simple, lobular and papillary, when transplanted into mammary gland fat pads of syngeneic mice gave rise to mammary carcinomas. In their illustrations depicting ductal lesions, they appear as tubules, glands, and duct-like structures (60, 61). Smith et al. (98) distinguish the virus-induced transformation of alveolar cells from chemically induced transformation of only ductal cells and Slemmer (97) has shown outgrowth of ductal cells from transplants of the mammary tissue derived from donors treated with methylcholanthrene. Wellings and Jensen (112) developed, a quantitative 3 dimensional whole mount technique correlated with histology, to examine sixty whole human breasts with and without coincident infiltrating duct carcinomas. On the basis of these studies, the hypothesis developed was that since the smallest solitary independent foci of ductal carcinoma observed were located in terminal ductal lobular units, then ductal carcinomas arise in these units rather than larger ducts.

In a later study, Wellings et al. (113) examined 196 human breasts and 16 biopsy specimens with a variety of dysplastic, metaplastic and neoplastic lesions including adenosis, fibroadenoma, fibrocystic, metaplastic disease and various cancers, including ductal and lobular carcinoma in situ. All lesions were examined as previously by a modification of the whole mount method used in mice, confirmed and correlated histologically. Morphologic evidence was given which indicated that most of the lesions arose in terminal ductal lobular units and that with progression, the unfolded lobule resembled a duct and gave the impression of a ductal lesion. Further, lesions classified as atypical lobules gave rise to both duct carcinoma in situ and lobular carcinoma in situ. Wellings further stated that the mouse mammary tumor is a valid model for the study of the above mentioned human breast lesions. Since several authors claim that chemically induced tumors of the mouse mammary gland originate in ducts, cytochemical markers could be developed to test the hypothesis that chemically induced mouse mammary tumors arise in glandular epithelial cells or in the epithelial cells of the terminal ductuloalveolar units rather than in duct epithelium. The organoid tumor of Foulds would serve as an excellent model to test this hypothesis.

Although the mechanism of chemical induction of mammary tumors is not fully understood, it has been shown that chemical carcinogens can alter the host's immune and endocrine status (50, 103). Ruppert et al. (90) using BALB/c mice bearing transplanted nodule outgrowth lines showed that immunogenicity of tumors derived from HAN exposed to DMBA depends on events occurring during the transformation of HAN to neoplasms. Ovarian and adrenal function is affected by carcinogens (90), but no correlation between appearance of mammary tumors and a decrease in progesterone and prolactin levels has been shown. In BALB/c mice (58, 59) the addition of hormones is essential to rapid induction of carcinogen altered cells and subsequent conversion into neoplastic cells. Pituitary isografts were not considered to act as a classic promoter in this system. The use of organ cultures should allow investigation of direct effect of various carcinogens (6, 54, 106).

Possible interactions of MMTV and chemical carcinogens are being studied intensively. Chemically induced mammary tumors in strains C3H/StWi (98), BALB/cCrgl, BALB/cfC3H (104), (C57BlxDBA/2f)F₁ (69), BALB/cAn, 020, and C3Hf (71) had the same levels of MTV-DNA, RNA and protein (gp 52) as homologous normal mammary gland. The spontaneous mammary tumor incidence ranged from 1% for strains C3H/StWi, BALB/cCrgl, (C57BLxDBA/2f)F$_1$ to 35% for C3Hf/He and 020, and to 90% for (BALB/cfC3H)F$_1$. Thus, persistent high levels of MTV-RNA and viral protein synthesis are not necessary for maintenance of the neoplastic phenotype and suggests that chemical carcinogens do not act by activating the MTV genome (61).

Reports of induction of mammary tumors by irradiation are few in number. Long-term gamma irradiation of strain LAF$_1$ and C3H hybrids using exposure levels of 8.8, 4.4, 2.2, and 1.1. R per day resulted in an increased incidence of both sarcomas and carcinomas (55). No mammary tumors occurred in the controls.

Strain BALB/c female mice receiving 200 R of gamma irradiation or neutron irradiation given as 1R/day induced 45% incidence of mammary tumors (107). In another study (57), administration of 400 R of whole body irradiation to BALB/c mice bearing nodule outgrowth lines, enhancement of tumor-producing capabilities was demonstrated.

Iyer and Banerjee (46) showed *in vitro* transformation of gland free strain BALB/c mouse mammary fat pads using 7.8 uM dimethylbenzanthracene (DMBA). The authors monitored transformation by enzymatically dissociating the cells, and inoculating them into syngeneic mice. HAN resulted from 26/48 such transplants and tumors from 8. Twelve serial transplant lines produced hyperplastic alveolar outgrowths and mammary tumors in a sequential manner for up to 20 generations.

Schaefer et al. (94) repeated these experiments using 3.9, 1.95, .40 and .004 uM concentrations of DMBA. The resultant HAN, when transplanted into young female syngeneic did not result in the development of HAN or tumors. The authors postulated that the reason for the transplantation failure was the occurrence of cytotoxicity in the organ cultures treated with high concentrations of DMBA. This cytotoxicity could lead to a multistep process of transformation in the surviving cells, but with less cytotoxicity more cells survived and less transformation occurred.

REFERENCES

1. Aidells BD, Daniel CW: Hormone-dependent mammary tumors in strain GR/A mice. Alternation between ductal and tumorous phases of growth during serial transplantation. *JNCI* 52:1855–1863, 1974
2. Andervont HB, Dunn TB: Response of strain, DBA/2f mice, without the mammary tumor agent, to oral administration of methylcholanthrene. *JNCI* 14:329–339, 1953
3. Apolant H: Die epithelialen Geschwülste der Maus. Arbeiten aus dem Königlichen Institut für experimentelle Therapie zu Frankfurt- a.M. 11–62, 1906
4. Arthur LO, Fine DL, Bentvelzen P: Oncogenicity of murine mammary tumor virus produced in tissue culture: Brief communication. *JNCI* 60:461–464, 1978
5. Asch BB, Medina D: Concanavalin A-induced agglutinability of normal, preoplastic and neoplastic mouse mammary cells. *JNCI* 61:1423–1430, 1978
6. Banerjee MR, Wood BG, Washburn LL: Chemical carcinogen-induced alveolar nodules in organ culture of mouse mammary gland. *JNCI* 53:1387–1393, 1974
7. Berenblum I: A speculative review: The probable nature of promoter action and its significance in the understanding of the mechanism of carcinogenesis. *Cancer Res* 14:471–477, 1954
8. Berenblum I: "Carcinogenesis; Mechanisms of Action" pp. 55–64. Edited by G.E.W. Wolstenholme and M. O'Connor Little, Brown Boston, Mass., 1958
9. Berenblum I: "Cellular Control Mechanisms and Cancer." pp. 259–267, Edited by: P. Emmelot and O. Muhlbock, Elsevier, Amsterdam, 1964
10. Bern HA, Nandi S: Recent studies of the hormonal influence in mouse mammary tumorigenesis. *Prog Exp Tumor Res* 2:91–145, 1961
11. Bern HA, Nandi S, Finster V: Induction of Lactation in precancerous hyperplastic alveolar nodules in the mammary gland of C3H HeCrgl mice. *Experientia* 15:155–157, 1959
12. Bernhard W, Granboulan N: "Tumor viruses of murine origin." pp. 6–49. Edited by: G.E.W. Wolstenholme and M. O'Connor. Churchill, London, 1962
13. Biancifiori C, Caschera F: The relation between pseudopregnancy and the chemical induction by four carcinogens of mammary and ovarian tumors in BALB/c mice. *Br J Cancer* 16:722–730, 1962
14. Bittner JJ: Some enigmas associated with the genesis of mammary cancer in mice. *Cancer Res* 8:625–639, 1948
15. Bonser GM: The evolution of mammary cancer induced in virgin female IF mice and minimal doses of locally-acting methylcholanthrene. *J Pathol Bacteriol* 68:531–546, 1954
16. Bonser GM: The mammary changes in IF female mice following a limited dose of four carcinogenic chemicals. *Int Symp Mammary Cancer Proc*, 2nd, 1957, pp. 576–584, 1958
17. Dalton AJ, Felix MD: The electron microscopy of normal and malignant cells. *Ann NY Acad Sci* 63:1117–1140, 1956
18. Dalton AJ, Potter M, Merwin RM: Some ultrastructural characteristics of a series of primary and transplanted plasma cell tumors of the mouse. *JNCI* 26:1221–1268, 1961
19. de Harven E, Friend C: Electron microscopic study of a cell free induced leukemia of the mouse. A preliminary report. *J Biophysics Biochem Cytol* 4:151–156, 1958
20. DeOme KB, Bern HA, Nandi S, Pitelka D, Faulkin CJ Jr: The precancerous nature of the hyperplastic alveolar nodules found in the mammary glands of old female. C3H/HeCrgl mice in: Genetics and Cancer. pp. 327–248. U. of Texas Press, 1959
21. DeOme KB, Faulkin LJ Jr, Bern HA, Blair PE: Development of mammary tumors from hyperplastic alveolar nodules transplanted into gland-free mammary fat pads of female C3H mice. *Cancer Res* 19:515–520, 1959
22. DeOme KB, Blair PB, Faulkin CJ Jr: Some characteristics of the preneoplastic-hyperplastic alveolar nodules of C3H/Crgl mice. *Acta Unio Contre le Cancer*. 17:973–982, 1961
23. DeOme KB, Nandi S, Bern HA, Blair PB, Pitelka DR: Morphological precursor of cancer. pp. 349–368, edited by Lucio Severi. Div of Cancer Res Perugia, 1962
24. Dmochowski L, Grey CE: Electron microscopy of known and suspected viral etiology. *Tex Repts Biol and Med* 15:704–753
25. Dunn TB: Morphology of Mammary tumors in mice. In: "The Physiopathology of Cancer" pp. 38–84. Edited by: F. Homburger. Harper (Hoeber) New York, 1957
26. Faulkin LJ Jr: Hyperplastic lesions of mouse mammary glands after treatment with 3-methylcholanthrene. *JNCI* 36:289–298, 1966
27. Fekete EA: A comparative morphological study of the mammary gland in a high and low incidence tumor strain of mice. *Am J of Pathol* 14:557–578, 1938
28. Feldman MK: Decreased serum responsiveness by primary cultures of preneoplastic and neoplastic mammary epithelial cells. *Experientia* 15:97–98, 1978
29. Foulds L: Mammary tumors in hybrid mice: Growth and

progression of spontaneous tumors. *Br J Cancer* 3:345–375, 1949

30. Foulds L: The histologic analysis of mammary tumors in mice. *JNCI* 17:701–801, 1956
31. Foulds L: In: Cellular control mechanisms and cancer. Edited by P. Emmelot and O. Muhlbock, pp. 242–258. Elsevier, Amsterdam, 1964
32. Foulds L: Neoplastic development. Vol. 1 pp. 24–81. Academic Press, London, 1969
33. Friedewald WF, Rous P: The initiating and promoting elements in tumor production. An analysis of the effect of tar, benzol and pyrene and methylcholanthrene on rabbit skin. *J Expt Med* 80:101–128, 1944
34. Friedewald WF, Rous P: Pathogenesis of deferred cancer; study of the after-effects of methylcholanthrene upon the rabbit skin. *J Exptl Med* 91:459–484, 1950
35. Gardner WU, Strong LC, Smith GM: The mammary glands of mature female mice of strains varying in susceptibility to spontaneous tumor development. *Am J Cancer* 33:510–517, 1939
36. Haaland M: "Spontaneous tumors in mice." In: Fourth Scientific Report, pp. 1–111. *Imperial Cancer Research Fund London*, 1911
37. Harbell JW, Daniel CW: Induction of the GR pregnancy-dependent mammary tumors by hormones *in vitro* (meeting abstract). *In Vitro* 14:361, 1978
38. Haran-Ghera N: The mechanism of carcinogenesis in breast tumor development in mice. *Acta Unio Contra Cancrum* 19:765–768, 1963
39. Harkness MN, Bern HA, Alfert M, Goldstein NO: Cytochemical studies of hyperplastic alveolar nodules in the mammary gland. *JNCI* 19:1023–1033, 1957
40. Heston WE, Vlahakis G, Tsubura Y: Strain DD, a new high mammary tumor strain and comparison of DD with strain C3H. *JNCI* 32:237–251, 1964
41. Highman B, Norvell MJ, Shellenberger TE: Pathological changes in female C3H mice continuously fed diets containing diethylstilbestrol or 17 B-estradiol. *J Environ Pathol Toxicol* 1:1–30, 1977
42. Hilgers J, Bentvelzen P: Interactions between viral and genetic factors in mouse mammary cancer. *Adv Cancer Res* 29:143–195, 1978
43. Hosick HL, Angello JC, Anderson ME: Stimulation of mammary epithelial growth by free fatty acids and changes in this response during neoplastic progression (meeting abstract) *Proc Am Assoc Cancer Res* 19, 178, 1978
44. Huseby RA, Bittner JJ: A comparative morphological study of the mammary glands with reference to the known factors influencing the development of mammary carcinoma in mice. *Cancer Res* 6:240–255, 1946
45. Ingraham RL: Variability of mouse mammary hyperplastic nodules maintained in organotypic culture. *JNCI* 40:1273–1286, 1968
46. Iyer AP, Banerjee MR: Sequential expression of preneoplastic and neoplastic characteristics of mouse mammary epithelial cells transformed in organ culture. *JNCI* 66:893–905, 1981
47. Jones EE: A comparative study of hyperplastic nodules in mammary glands of mice with and without the mammary inciter. *Acta Unio Contra Cancrum* 7:262–265, 1951
48. Jones EE: Studies on the mammary glands of hybrid mice theoretically free of the milk agent. *Acta Unio Contra Cancrum* 12:638–652, 1956
49. Kawashima S, Bern HA, Jones LA, Mills KT: Histometric study of the pituitary in mice treated neonatally with steroids and the relationship between prolactin cells and mammary tumorigenesis. *Endocrinol Japan* 25:341–348, 1978
50. Krarup T: Effect of 9,10-dimethyl-1,2-benzanthracene on the mouse ovary. *Br J Cancer* 24:168–186, 1970

51. Lathrop AEC, Loeb L: Further investigations on the origins of tumors in mice. On the part played by hormones in spontaneous development of tumors. *J Cancer Res* 1:1–20, 1916
52. Lennox B: Some relationships between tumours of the breast and the sweat glands. In: "The Morphological Precursor of Cancer" pp. 423–428 (Ed.) L. Severi, Division of Cancer Research, Perugia, 1962
53. Liebelt AG, Liebelt RA: Chemical factors in mammary tumorigenesis. *Annu Symp Fundam Cancer Res [Proc]* 20:315–345, 1967
54. Lin FL, Banerjee MR, Crump LR: Cell cycle related hormone carcinogen interaction during chemical carcinogen induction of nodule-like mammary lesions in organ culture. *Cancer Res* 36:1607–1614, 1976
55. Lorenz E, Jacobson LO, Heston WE, Shimkin M, Eschenbrenner AB, Deringer MK, Donniger J, Schweisthal R: In: "Biological Effects of External X and Gamma Radiation." Pt. 1, chapter 5, p. 207. Edited by Zirkel RE. McGraw-Hill, New York, 1954
56. McGrath CM: Replication of mammary tumor virus in tumor cell cultures; dependence on hormone-induced cellular organization. *JNCI* 47:455–467, 1971
57. Medina D: Preneoplastic lesions in mouse mammary tumorigenesis. *Methods Cancer Res* 7:353–414, 1973
58. Medina D: Mammary tumorigenesis in chemical carcinogen-treated mice. 1. Incidence in BALB/c and C57BL mice. *JNCI* 53:213–221, 1974
59. Medina D: Mammary tumorigenesis in chemical carcinogen-treated mice. II. Dependence on hormone stimulation for tumorigenesis. *JNCI* 53:223—226, 1974b
60. Medina D: Preneoplastic lesions in murine mammary cancer. *Cancer Res* 36:2589–2595, 1976a
61. Medina D: Mammary tumorigenesis in chemical carcinogen-treated mice. VI. Tumor-producing capabilities of mammary dysplasias in BALB/cCgl mice. *JNCI* 57:1185–1189, 1976b
62. Medina D: Mammary Tumors. In: "The Mouse in Biomedical Research." Vol. IV, pp. 373–396. Edited by Foster, M.L., Small, J.D., and Fox, J.G. Academic Press, New York, 1982
63. Medina D, DeOme KB: Influence of mammary tumor virus on the tumor-producing capabilities of nodule outgrowths free of mammary tumor virus. *JNCI* 40:1303–1308, 1968
64. Medina D, DeOme KB: Effects of various oncogenic agents on tumor-producing capabilities of D series BALB/c mammary nodule outgrowth lines. *JNCI* 45:353–363, 1970
65. Medina D, Shepherd F: Enhancement and inhibition of mammary tumor formation and growth by cytostatic drugs. *Cancer Res* 37:3571–3577, 1977
66. Medina D, Warner M: Mammary tumorigenesis in chemical carcinogen-treated mice. IV. Induction of mammary ductal hyperplasias. *JNCI* 57:331–337, 1976
67. Medina D, Bern HA, Brown D, DeOme KB: Mammary tumor virus activity in mammary tissues of hormone stimulated BALB/cfC3H, Crgl mice. *Proc Soc Exp Biol Med* 131:180–183, 1969
68. Medina D, DeOme KB, Pitelka DR, Colley VB: Appearance of virus particles in BALB/c mammary nodule outgrowth lines transplanted into BALB/cfC3H and (C3hXBALB/c)F₁ mice. *JNCI* 46:1153–1160, 1971
69. Medina D, Butel JS, Socher SH, Miller FL: Mammary tumorigenesis in 7,12 dimethylbenzanthracene treated (C57BLxDBA/2f)F₁ mice. *Cancer Res* 40, 368–373, 1980a
70. Medina D, Asch BB, Brinkley BR, Mace ML: *In vitro* and *in vivo* models for transformation of breast cells. Breast Cancer: "New Concepts in Etiology and Control." pp. 53–66. Edited by M.J. Brennan, C.M. McGrath, M.A. Rich. Academic Press, New York, 1980b
71. Michalides R, Van Deemter L, Nusse R, Ropcke G, Boot L: Involvement of mouse mammary tumor virus in spontaneous and hormone-induced mammary tumors in low mammary-

tumor mouse strains. *J Virol* 27, 551–559, 1978

72. Mottram JC: A developing factor in experimental blastogenesis. *J Pathol Bact* 56:181–187, 1944

73. Muhlbock O, Bentvelzen P: The transmission of the mouse mammary tumor viruses. *Persp in Virol* 6:75–87, 1969

74. Muhlbock O, Tengbergen EW van: Studies on the development of mammary tumors in dilute-brown DBA/s mice without the agent. *JNCI* 13:505–532, 1952

75. Murray JA: Cancerous ancestry and the incidence of cancer in mice. *Scient Rep Invest Imp Cancer Res Fund* 4:114–130, 1911

76. Nagle SC, Fine DL: Demonstration of components of serum-free culture medium effecting maximum *in vitro* expression of mouse mammary tumor virus. *In Vitro* 14 (2), 218–226, 1979

77. Nandi S: A new method for detecting mouse mammary tumor virus I Influence of foster nursing on incidence of hyperplastic mammary nodules in BALB/cCrgl mice. *JNCI* 25:753–778, 1963a

78. Nandi S: A new method for detection of mouse mammary tumor virus. II. Effect of administering lactating tissue extracts on the incidence of HAN in BALB/cCrgl mice. *JNCI* 31:75–89, 1963b

79. Nandi S: Interactions among hormonal, viral and genetic factors in mouse tumorigenesis. *Can Cancer Conf* 6:69–81

80. Nandi S, MCGrath CS: Mammary neoplasia in mice. *Adv Cancer Res* 17:353–414, 1973

81. Parks WP, Scolnick EM, Kozikowski EH: Dexamethasone stimulation of murine mammary tumor virus expression: A tissue culture source of virus. *Science* 184:158–160, 1974

82. Pauley RJ, Medina D, Socher SH: Murine mammary tumor virus expression during mammary tumorigenesis in BALB/c mice. *J Virol* 29:483–493, 1979

83. Pitelka DR, Bern HA, DeOme KB, Schooley CN, Wellings SR: Virus like particles in hyperplastic alveolar nodules of the mammary gland of the C3H/He mouse. *JNCI* 20:541–554, 1958

84. Pitelka DR, DeOme KB, Bern HA, Nandi S: On the significance of virus-like particles in mammary tissues of C3Hf mice. *JNCI* 33:867–885, 1958

85. Pitelka DR, Unemori EN, Field MF *et al*: Cell-cell and cell-stroma interactions in Metastasis. In: Understanding Breast Cancer: Clinical and Laboratory Concepts. Rich MA, Hager JC, Furmanski P (eds). New York, Marcel Dekker, pp. 99–118, 1983.

86. Pitelka DR, DeOme KB, Bern HA: Virus-like particles in precancerous hyperplastic mammary tissues of C3H and C3Hf mice. *JNCI* 25:753–778, 1960

87. Ranadive KB, Hakim SA: The chemical induction of mammary cancer in different inbred strains of mice. *Int Symp Mammary Cancer Proc*, 2nd 1957, pp. 575–584, 1958

88. Rous P, Kidd JG: Conditional Neoplasms and subthreshold states. A study of the tar tumor of rabbits. *Expt Med* 73:365–389, 1941

89. Rudali G, Julline P, Nives C, Apiou F: Dose-effect studies on estrogen induced mammary cancer in mice. *Biomedicine* 29:45–46, 1978

90. Ruppert B, Wei W, Medina D, Medina GH: Effect of chemical-carcinogen treatment on the immunogenicity of mouse mammary tumors arising from hyperplastic alveolar outgrowth lines. *JNCI* 61:1165–1169, 1978

91. Sarkar NH, Nowinski RC, Moore DH: Characteristics of structural components of the mouse mammary tumor virus. I. Morphological and Biochemical Studies. *Virol* 46:1, 1971

92. Sass B, Dunn TB: Classification of mouse mammary tumors in Dunn's miscellaneous group including recently reported types. *JNCI* 62:1287–1293, 1979

93. Sass B, Vlahakis G, Heston WE: Precursor lesions and pathogenesis of spontaneous mammary tumors in mice. *Toxicologic Path* 10:12–21, 1982

94. Schaefer FV, Tonelli QJ, Dickens MS, Custer RP, Sorof S: Nononcogenic hormone-independent alveoli produced by carcinogens in cultured mouse mammary glands. *Cancer Research* 43:3310–3315, 1983

95. Schlom J, Hand PH, Teramoto YA, Callahan R, Topdaro G, Schidlorsky G; Characterization of a new virus from MUS cervicolor immunologically related to the mouse mammary tumor virus. *JNCI* 61:1509–1519, 1978

96. Singh DV, DeOme KB, Bern HA: Strain differences in response to the mouse mammary gland to hormones *in vitro*. *JNCI* 45:657–675, 1970

97. Slemmer G: Interactions of separate types of cells during normal and neoplastic gland growth. *J Invest Dermtol* 63:27–47, 1974

98. Smith GH, Pauley RJ, Socher SH, Medina D: Chemical carcinogenesis in C3H/StWi mice. A worthwhile experimental model for breast cancer. *Cancer Res* 38:4504–4509, 1978

99. Squartini F: Mammogenesis and breast carcinogenesis in virgin female mice of BALB/c_f substrain with the milk agent. *JNCI* 23:1227–1238, 1959

100. Squartini F, Bistocchi M: Bioactivity of C3H and RIII mammary tumor viruses in virgin female BALB/c mice. *JNCI* 58:1845–1847, 1977

101. Squartini F, Bistocchi M, Buongiorno L: Development, morphology and progression of mammary tumors during and after fertile life in BALB/cfRIII mice. *JNCI* 66:311–319, 1981

102. Strum J: Pale cell carcinoma-ultrastructure of a hormone dependent mammary tumor in GR mice. *Am J Path* 103:283–291, 1981

103. Stjernsward J: Immunodepressive effect of 3-methylcholanthrene: Antibody formation at the cellular level and reaction against weak antigenic homografts. *JNCI* 35:885–892, 1965

104. Swartz-Dusing SD, Medina D, Butel JS, Socher SH: Mouse mammary tumor virus genome expression in chemical carcinogen-induced mammary tumors in a low and high tumor incidence mouse strain. *Proc Natl Acad Sci USA* 76:5360–5364, 1979

105. Taylor HC Jr, Waltman CA: Hyperplasia of mammary gland in human and in the mouse; morphological and etiological contrasts. *Arch surg* 40:733–840, 1940

106. Tonelli QJ, Custer RP, Sorof S: Transformation of cultured mouse mammary glands by aromatic amines and amides and their derivatives. *Cancer Res* 39:1784–1792, 1979

107. Ullrich RL, Jernigan MC, Storer JB: Neutron carcinogenesis: Dose and dose-rate effects in BALB/c mice. *Radiat Res* 72:487–498, 1977

108. van Gulik PJ, Korteweg R: The anatomy of mammary gland in mice in regard to the degree of its disposition for cancer. *Neth Akad Wettenschappen* 43:891–900, 1940

109. vanNie R, Dux A: Biological and morphological characteristics of mammary tumors in GR mice. *JNCI* 46:885–897, 1971

110. Vlahakis G, Heston WE, Smith GH: Strain C3H/A^{vy}fB mice: Ninety percent incidence of mammary tumors transmitted by either parent. *Science* 170:185–187, 1970

111. Voyles BA, McGrath CM: Differential responses of malignant BALB/c mammary epithelial cells to the multiplication-stimulating activity of insulin. *Cancer Res* 62:597–605, 1979

112. Wellings SR, Jensen HM: On the origin and progression of ductal carcinoma in the human breast. *JNCI* 50:1111–1118, 1973

113. Wellings SR, Jensen HM, Marcum RG: An atlas of subgross pathology of the human breast with special reference to possible precancerous lesions. *JNCI* 55:231–273, 1975

114. Welsch CW, Gribler C: Prophylaxis of spontaneously developing mammary carcinoma in C3H/HeJ female mice by suppression of prolactin. *Cancer Res* 33:2939–2946, 1973

115. Welsch CW: Prophylaxis of early preneoplastic lesion of the mammary gland. *Cancer Res* 36:2621–2625, 1976

116. Yagi MJ: Cultivation and characterization of BALB/cfC3H mammary tumor cell lines. *JNCI* 51:1849, 1973

117. Yanai R, Nagasawa H: Development and growth of pregnancy-dependent and – independent mammary tumors in GR/A strain of mice and their interrelationship. *GANN* 69:25–30, 1978

118. Yanai R, Mori T, Nagasawa H: Long-term effects of prenatal and neonatal administration of 5-beta-dihydrotestosterone on normal, and neoplastic mammary development in mice. *Cancer Res* 37:4566–4459, 1977

119. Young LJT, Cardiff RD, Ashley RL: Long-term primary culture of mouse mammary tumor cells: Production of virus. *JNCI* 54:1215–1221, 1975

COMPARATIVE ASPECTS OF MAMMARY CANCER

H.E. KAISER

INTRODUCTION

Mammary cancer is one group of neoplasms which exhibits striking human and species differences. Mammary glands characterize the class of mammals named after them. In the industrialized world of the United States and Western Europe cancers of the breast are very frequent in women and occur also in the male. Little is known about the mammary cancers which appear in wild, zoo and the majority of domestic animals. Cancers of the mammary glands are common in some species of domesticated animals such as the bitch and laboratory animals such as certain strains of mice (CH3), as well as in the human population of particular nations, such as the USA. In the population of other nations as in Singapore and in certain domestic animals, such as horse and cow and laboratory animals, such as guinea pig and rabbit mammary cancers are rare. This aspect suggests that a comparison of mammary cancers between different species and human population groups may result in new understanding useful for future therapy.

Neoplasms are generally considered as diseases of the aged but this is a misconception because only certain types of neoplasms occur in the aged and quite a number of histologic tumor types are characteristic diseases of the young. Tumors of different kind appear in all age brackets. Domestic mammalian species, such as cattle, do not outlive their life in general but dairy cows do reach the carcinogenic age and due to the fact that so many millions of cows are slaughtered makes it unprobably that the scarcity of mammary cancer in these animals is artificial. The extensive use of the udder has to be considered. It can also not be assumed that free-ranging animals, such as whales, deer and fox so often hunted, exhibit so few mammary tumors. Of course, many mammalian species have not been investigated for neoplastic diseases but from the extensive material of free-ranging, zoo, domestic and laboratory animals with their variation in the occurrence of mammary neoplasms it is necessary to assume, that we experience remarkable differences in the development of mammary cancer in the various species of mammals. This view is supported by the differences of breast cancer frequency in different human populations.

(1) Too little information is available to resolve the question if the domestication of animals, as dog and cat, and the cultural technology in women has something to do with the increase of breast cancer in these females.

The epidemiology of health experience in women is incomplete (85). Similar gaps are present concerning the pre-malignant stages of breast neoplasms of which some metastasize very fast whereas others proliferate not before 10 or 30 years. A large heterogeneity also in regard to physiological factors may exist (82). Not enough attention has been placed on genetics in these processes (56). The role of lymph nodes was investigated experimentally in regard to tumor immunity and it could be shown that nodes negative for metastasis are suggestive of tumor immunity and positive ones characterize low tumor immunity (73).

(2) Is the hormonal balance as changed by feeding of the youngster, obesity, etc. related to the high level of the disease in various human races and other species? In man such relations have been observed and in the mouse, plaque formations (pregnancy-responsive tumors) are related to such facts.

(3) Is the different form of the breast in white (bulb-like), black (like goat udder), and oriental woman (cone-like) an indication of additional metabolic variations?

(4) The extreme rarity of mammary cancer in free-ranging, terrestrial, aquatic and flying mammals should be evaluated, and correlated with conditions in women, cat and dog on a species level, and among women with high incidence of breast cancer and controls in such countries as the United States and West Germany as compared to Japan which has a low incidence of the disease.

Comparative view of the types of mammary cancer in different mammalian orders

Comparative aspects and their interpretation may offer improved insights into the nature and origin of this threatening disease group in humans. Special emphasis is put on comparison with dog and cat, the domestic animals most often experiencing breast cancer and which are generally allowed to live out their natural life even though many are killed when cancer develops. Man and these two species should be compared with species exhibiting no breast cancer.

As stated in chapter 2, the class of mammals comprises 19 orders, 134 families, 1018 genera and 4145 species (Nowak and Paradiso, 1983). Spontaneous mammary cancers are known in less than 100 species of mammals. Table 1 reviews in which orders mammary cancers have been reported. Some gaps of knowledge in various species may be due to the fact that we have not looked close enough, this means that necropsy data are not available. But the knowledge we have in form of data indicates racial, breed and species variations of mammary neoplasms.

142

Table 1. The distribution of mammary cancers in mammalian orders.

Order	Number of species	Species/mammary tumors	Comments
Monotremata	3	0	
Marsupialia	258	Tasmanian devil (*Sarcophilus harrisi*)	mammary tumor known
Insectivora	379	0	
Dermoptera	2	0	
Chiroptera	942	0	
Primata	203	several species	exhibited mammary tumors (see table 2)
Edentata	33	0	
Pholidota	7	0	
Lagomorpha	65	several species	e.g. rabbit shows mammary tumors
Rodentia	1687	several species	e.g. mouse, rat, hamster, guinea pig, *Praomys* show variable frequency of mammary tumors
Cetacea	79	0	
Carnivora	238	several species	dog and cat have frequently mammary tumors beside other species
Pinnipedia	34	0	
Tubulidentata	1	0	
Proboscidia	2	0	
Hyracoidea	7	0	
Sirenia	4	0	
Perissodactyla	17	several species	in the horse mammary neoplasms are extremely rare
Artiodactyla	192	several species	mammary tumors are rare in cattle, pig and not as rare in goat

Mammary cancer in free-ranging animals

Surprisingly, this cancer is very rare in free-ranging animals. It is worth mentioning that it is not known in animals, such as whales, which have been frequently hunted and processed just as deer.

In reviewing the cases known from the North American continent Shivaprasad (1984) described a gray squirrel (*Sciurus carolinensis*) with mammary cancer metastatic to the left axillary lymph node. Cosgrove (personal communication) dissected 1673 small rodents of 14 different species and found only two benign fibroadenomas.

Mammary cancer in zoo animals

Mammary cancer are also rare in this group of animals and some data from the San Diego Zoo are given in Table 2.

Mammary cancers in domestic animals

In domestic animals, these cancers are common in certain species such as the dog and cat, and very rare in others such as the horse. The most common cancer is that of the bitch. There are variations with breeds of dogs, with miniature

Table 2. Selected cases of mammary cancer in zoo animals*.

Order	Species	Type of mammary cancer
Marsupialia	*Sarcophilus harrisi*, Tasmanian devil	adenocarcinoma
Primates	*Tupaia bilangeri*, tree shrew	adenocarcinoma
Rodentia	*Dicrostonyx groenlandicus*, collared lemming	
	Dipodomys heermanni, kangaroo rat	adenocarcinoma
	Mus musculus, mouse	adenocarcinoma
Carnivora	*Arctictis binturong*, binturong	adenocarcinoma
Artiodactyla	*Camelus ferrus arabicus*, camel	intraductal papillary adenoma

* after Griner (36).

poodle, English setter, German shorthair pointer, and pointer having the highest prevalence (41).

In the dog (*Canis familiaris*) breast tumors are the most common neoplasms, second only to those of the skin. They are by far the most common in the bitch. Twenty five percent of breast tumors are carcinomas followed by adenomas, myoepitheliomas and malignant mixed tumors. Benign mixed tumors comprise 65% of mammary tumors in the dog. The frequency of types differs but behavior and histological origin are similar if human and dog mammary neoplasms are compared. In the dog exists no geographical variation in frequency. Mammary tumors of the dog are nearly always diseases of the female and occur in the male dog only sporadically. The frequency of benign and malignant mammary tumors increases from the most cephalad to the most caudal mammary glands. There is almost no evidence that mammary tumors of dogs may be of viral origin. It is possible to distinguish between adenoma, benign mixed tumors and carcinoma. Based on the cell type carcinoma may be classified as acinar, clear, spheroidal, mucous or squamous cells; according to tissue change as cribriform, solid, papillary, tubular or glandlike, medullary; necrosis in solid ducts as known as Comedo carcinoma, the infiltration or lack of the same, and according to stroma (scirrhous or fibrosing). Histologic classification results in the following types of carcinoma: Adenocarcinoma, papillary carcinoma, scirrhous carcinoma, lobular carcinoma, solid carcinoma, squamous cell carcinoma, and Padget's carcinoma of the nipple. Only one case is known from the last tumor of the dog (2). Other tumors are the malignant mixed tumors and myoepithelioma (68).

Malignant tumors originating from the canine mammary glands may metastasize either by the lymphatic or the hematogenous route (23). Spread to the lymph nodes is most common. If the primary mammary tumor develops in the cranial half of the mammary chains, lymphatic spread is to the axillary lymph nodes. The caudal mammary glands usually demonstrate lymphatic spread to the superficial and deep inguinal and sublumbar lymph nodes. Radiographic evaluation of the abdomen, but not with plain films, best reveals enlargements of sublumbar nodes. If hematogenous spread has occurred, metastasis appears most commonly in the lungs. Mammary carcinoma is the most common malignant neoplasm. In the bitch, the annual prevalence rate of malignancies was 453.3/100,000 and mammary cancer comprised 41.7% (63). Mammary tumors for the entire dog population make up 12% to 44% of the tumors observed (23, 67).

The risk for developing mammary cancer is much higher in the older bitch. First diagnosis of mammary tumor in bitches less than 2 years of age is very low, begins to increase slowly by 6 years of age, and obtains a median age of 10 years and 2 months (22). Over 25% of dogs with malignant mammary tumors have radiographic evidence of lung metastasis on initial presentation (29). Half of all bitches with malignant mammary cancer survive less than 8 months following surgical resection alone and 75% of all bitches operated die from their cancer within 2 years (64). Over half initially present with regional lymph node metastasis.
Hormonal influence: Bitches neutered (ovariohysterectomized) at an early age have a significantly lower risk of developing mammary cancer than intact bitches (22, 80).

Proestrus, estrus, metestrus, and anestrus comprise the estrous cycle in the bitch. The length of anestrus varies among breeds, among individuals within the breeds, and within an individual's own cycling pattern (83). Estrus the period of sexual receptivity usually occurs every 6 months in the majority of bitches, lasting 6–12 days.

Proestrus lasts for approximately 6 to 9 days, beginning with the onset of vaginal bleeding and ending with sexual receptivity. The major estrogens found in the bitch are 17 B-estradiol, 17 a-estradiol, estrone, and estriol.

Anestrus, the period of reproductive rest when the body is not influenced by elevated hormone levels, begins after the endometrium has returned to normal and may last up to 100 or 150 days.

Hormonal stimulation becomes apparent at 6 to 10 months of age.

Bitches spayed before experiencing a single estrous cycle have approximately 5% of the mammary cancer risk experienced by intact multiestrous ones (22). The cancer risk for bitches undergoing only one estrous cycle before neutering is only 8% (80). Animals spayed after two to four estrous cycles experience, as a group, 26% of the cancer risk of intact multiestrous bitches (80). Spaying after $2\frac{1}{2}$ years of age (after five estrous cycles) does not significantly reduce mammary cancer risk (80).

Oophorectomy at the time of cancer excision does not cause a significant increase in survival or an effect on mortality (15, 80). The effect of castration at the time of cancer removal on the development of new mammary cancer is unknown.

Estrogen receptors have been demonstrated in canine mammary tumors (26, 65).

Although experimental hormonal induction of mammary neoplasia has not been proven in the bitch, development of mammary cancer is definitely influenced by events associated with intense hormonal stimulation.

Anatomy, vascular supply and lymphatics of the mammary glands

The mammae of the bitch are composed of five paired glands numbered one to five from cranial to caudal.

The arterial supply to the thoracic mammary glands comes from perforating branches of the internal thoracic arteries, cutaneous branches of the intercostal arteries from T-7 caudally, and the lateral thoracic arteries. Venous drainage parallels the arterial supply.

Lymphatic drainage, comprising a series of anastomotic branches beginning in the tests, are joined by branches from the subcutis and parenchyma and empty into lymphatics that drain to adjacent glands or directly into the regional lymph nodes. The cranial and caudal thoracic and cranial abdominal glands drain to the axillary node on the ipsilateral side. The drainage of the caudal thoracic and cranial abdominal glands overlap and have multiple anastomotic branches between the two glands. The caudal abdominal and inguinal glands drain through a common network to the superficial inguinal lymph nodes on the same side.

Mammary neoplasia occurs most commonly in the most caudal glands and becomes progressively less frequent in the more cranial glands. The two most caudal glands contain almost 60% of the mammary tumors of all types (67).

Mammary tumors spread by direct invasion, hematogenous routes, and lymphatic channels. Metastases most frequently affect the regional lymph nodes and lungs (67, 68).

Mammary tumors may range from small, firm masses under the dermis to large, ulcerating tumors. Regional lymph node involvement usually indicates metastasis.

Clinical staging of mammary tumors is based upon tumor size (T), regional lymph node metastasis (n), and distant metastasis (M). After TNM classification is completed, a clinical state I-IV is determined.

A review of the literature reveals considerable controversy in the terminology used to describe mammary tumors.

Histologic type using WHO classification, shows that sarcomas have a poorer prognosis than simple carcinomas, which, in turn, have a poorer prognosis than complex carcinomas. Additionally, severely infiltrating tumors have a poorer prognosis than do moderately infiltrating ones. Extending growth patterns have the best prognosis (64). At the time of surgical removal, the smaller the size of the tumor the better the prognosis.

The location of the tumor within the mammary chains, invasion into lymphatics, and regional lymph node involvement do not affect the 2 year survival rate for dogs operated on for malignant mammary tumors.

Comparison of Human and Canine Mammary Tumors (see also Bonser (10))

Impressive similarities between breast cancer in bitches and women exist (22) including age distribution, metastatic behavior, apparent hormonal control of development and clinical staging.

The onset of mammary tumors in dogs compares well with the onset of mammary carcinomas in women (68).

Lactation disturbances, e.g. mastitis, occur frequently in both bitches and women.

Most human breast cancers but only 30 to 50% of canine mammary tumors are carcinomas, the tissue of origin in the majority of both being the ductular epithelium.

Favored metastatic sites for breast cancer in women include lymph nodes, lungs and bones, while the lymph nodes and lungs are the most frequently affected sites in the dog.

No clinical evidence exists to confirm that the canine skeletal system is significantly affected by metastatic mammary neoplasia. Such metastases do occur, but not with the same frequency as in women.

Regional lymph node involvement carries important prognostic value in human breast cancer, although it has no apparent value in dogs.

Breast cancer in the bitch has been treated by surgery alone in most cases. Although chemotherapy has been used in severely infiltrative and metastatic breast cancers, no studies have been performed to document the success of such treatment.

Hormonal therapy has had no effect in controlling metastatic mammary cancer in the bitch.

Radiotherapy, alone or in combination with surgery, has not been well evaluated, and existing accounts do not suggest good results (72).

Cat (Felis cattus)

Breast neoplasms are the most common tumors besides those of skin, and the lymphoid and hematopoietic tissues. Siamese cats have twice the risk of other breeds for mammary carcinoma, they are younger at diagnosis (40). The age specific incidence of mammary tumors of cats is the same for dogs and increases with age. Carcinomas are found in older casts, mostly 11 to 12 years old (68).

The location of mammary tumors in cats differs somewhat from dogs, most tumors in cats develop in the first two pairs of glands (67). In the majority of cats only one mammary gland is involved. It is not known if virus play a role (68).

Almost all tumors are carcinomas and behave in a very malignant manner (3, 67). Metastasis usually develops by way of lymphatics, also hematogenous spread may occur. Simple tubular adenocarcinomas occur most frequently.

Therapy seems to depend on early aggressive surgery. Although bilateral resection of the mammary chains and regional lymph nodes is recommended, no significant studies available have evaluated various surgical modes of therapy.

The content of tumor receptors showed no correlation with the stage of the estrous cycle or the fact whether the cat was intact or neutered (47).

Fibroepithelial hyperplasia (feline mammary hypertrophy) occurs rarely most often in queens under 2 years of age (68).

Other species

Lagomorpha. Rabbit (*Oroctolagus cuniculus*). Mammary neoplasms are rare. The number of reported cases can be said to be low. Carcinoma in the rabbit occurs generally in multiparous females 3 to 4 years old. The cases reported by Green belong to Belgian and English breeds. Two major types of tumors adenocarcinoma of papillary or solid type and medullary adenocarcinoma were distinguished; the first tumor resembles the same type in the dog whereas intracystic adenomata of humans were also comparable to rabbit adenocarcinoma developing from cystic disease. Metastasis involved the lungs and regional lymph nodes and in case of the English breed to thoracic and abdominal organs and regional lymph nodes (94).

Perissodactyla; *Horse (Equus caballus)*. Mammary tumors of the horse are rare. Schmahl (see 1) described a solid mammary carcinoma which produced pulmonary metastases by hematogenous spreading. Acland and Gillette (1) observed in a 19 year old thoroughbred brook mare an early abortion and an enlargement of the right mammary gland. The left supramammary and external iliac lymph nodes were also enlarged. No other metastases were seen in this case of solid carcinoma. A 10-year-old Arabian mare exhibited a mammary adenocarcinoma of papillary type metastatic to the liver a tumor histologically similar to intraductal carcinomas of women (42). The incidence of mammary tumors in a big study in Paris with 40,000 horses of a slaughterhouse was estimated 0.11% (28); see also (54, 86).

Artiodactyla: *Pig (Sus scrofa)*
Mammary carcinoma of the sow were rarely seen (e.g. 75).

Cases of breast cancer from the Bactrian camel (*Camelus bactrianus*), the camel (*Camelus dromedarus*), the Llama (*Lama glama*), the alpaca (*Lama pacas*), and the reindeer (*Rangifer tarandus*) have not come to my attention. Domestic cattle (*Bos taurus*). The incidence of mammary neoplasia is very low (67); approximately 25 cases have been recorded in the literature. The rare occurrence of mammary tumors in the cow is interesting because many dairy cows are allowed to survive to "cancer age" (50). Carcinomas, fibromas, fibrosarcomas, papillary adenomas, osteomas, and fibroadenomas have been seen. Primary carcinoma of the mammary gland are rare and involved always the duct system never the alveolar epithelium. Metastasis spread to supramammary lymph nodes and in one case to lung and liver. Primary parenchymal carcinoma is much more rare than squamous cell carcinoma of the udder invading the gland (68).

Water buffalo (Bubalus bubalis). Also in the water buffalo the mammary duct system exhibited papillomas and fibroadenomas (8, 9). Among 300 others from female buffaloes in Indian slaughterhouses an intraductal carcinoma comparable to a comedo carcinoma of man was seen in an 8 to 12-year old animal (59).

Goat (Capra hircus). Among 4000 examined female goats 10 cases of fibrocystic disease and two intraductal carcinomas were found (81).

Sheep (Ovis aries). As in the goat mammary gland tumors are extremely rare.

Mammary cancer of laboratory animals

Mammary cancer in laboratory animals in its spontaneous chapter 19/Vol V. As in other species, especially the rat, there exist pronounced strain differences. The induced mammary cancers of laboratory animals are not considered in this chapter. The taxonomic sequence is given according to the importance of the members of the orders in the laboratory.

Rodentia: *Mouse (Mus musculus).* Spontaneous mammary tumors constitute the most common tumor in mice, especially in breeding females (6). Histopathologic classification is as follows: adenocarcinoma, adenoacanthoma, carcinosarcoma, sarcoma, and miscellaneous. Viral agents have caused some mouse mammary tumors (see also chapters 18 & 19).

Rat (Rattus norwegicus). Rat mammary tumors may be malignant or benign (70). Spontaneous and induced tumors may develop, the type and behavior depending on the strain of rat. Mammary tumors account for approximately 20% of all naturally occurring tumors in mixed strains of rats. The incidence of tumors by sex is 6 to 1 with female predominance.

The most frequently occurring tumors are fibroadenomas and fibromas. Malignant spontaneous tumors, of epithelial and/or mesodermal origin, are classified respectively as adenocarcinomas, solid carcinomas, cystadenocarcinomas, papillary carcinomas, and rarely, squamous cell carcinomas. Fibrosarcomas frequently develop, and mixed tumors combining adenocarcinoma and squamous cell cancer have occurred as well.

Most frequent fibroepithelial tumors occur as spontaneous lesions in the rat mammary gland. Next in frequency are fibroadenomas. Compound tumors also are distinctive in the rat mammary gland and the most often presenting experimental tumors. Carcinosarcomas are rare (0.6%). As epithelial tumors, tubular adenomas, cystadenomas, anaplastic adenocarcinomas, and squamous cell tumors have been observed. True fibromas and fibrosarcomas appear as pure connective tissue lesions. The great histologic diversity in the same rat tumor distinguishes it from human breast tumors. In the rat occurred metastasizing compound tumors lacking nuclear pleomorphism characteristic of cancer. In both rats and humans lobular carcinomas have been found. The tumor type which resembles most its counterpart in humans is the fibroadenoma of the rat mammary gland. Some neoplasms of the rat mammary gland exhibit a similar histology to those in mice. The basic structure of mouse tumors is showing an acinar structure whereas the mammary tumors in the rat are basically tubulopapillary. Therefore only a few mammary tumors between these two species may be compared, such as simple adenomas in rats to type C tumor in mice (52). In contrast to spontaneous tumors, most induced tumors are carcinomas, having varying degree of hormone responsiveness.

Hamsters: *Common hamster (Cricetus cricetus) and Golden hamster (Mesocricetus auratus).* Spontaneous mammary tumors in hamsters are very rare, but have been reported (17). A spontaneously occurring transplantable not metastasizing tumor exhibited in the 91st transplant generation metastases in axillary and inguinal lymph nodes (31). Adenocarcinomas are the main tumor type.

Guinea pig (Cavia porcellus). Adenocarcinomas are the most frequently reported malignant mammary tumors. They are of ductal origin and occur also more often than in other species. A transplanted mammary adenocarcinoma metastasized to the inguinal lymph nodes, another one to the kidney and an inguinal lymph node. Fibroadenomas, a liposarcoma, direct spreading by tumor embolus in a pulmonary artery and a carcinosarcoma metastasizing to kidney and spleen have been observed (92). The most recent report on mammary tumors in the guinea pig, spontaneous and irradiated is this one by Hoch-Ligeti and coworkers (45). Neoplasms in 62 animals arose either as lobular acinar carcinoma or cystadenocarcinoma or as papillary carcinomas within large ducts near the mammilla. The frequency in male animals were remarkable. Two irradiated males and one female metastasis occurred. Differences between nontreated and irradiated animals were not pronounced (45).

African soft-furred rat (Praomys natalensis). Due to a lack of intensive reports dealing with mammary cancer in *Praomys* this experimental study of Hoch-Ligeti *et al.* (44) is introduced to supplement. Eight female Praomys treated with N,N-2,7-fluorenylenebisacetamide developed carcinomas of the mammary glands affecting one or all 8 glands in the animals. The animals were a mixture of adenos-

Table 3. Selected neoplasms of the mammary gland in nonhuman primates.

Species	Age	Type of neoplasm	Comments	References
Tupaia glis	adult	adenocarcinoma	pregnant	(25)
Lemur catta		mammary neoplasm		(91)
Galago crassi caudatus	13 yrs	spindle cell sarcoma	metastases to liver, lung, kidney perhaps spleen, heart, cecum, omentum	(4, 5, 6)
	15 yrs	mixed mammary t.	metastasized to local lymph nodes and kidney	
Cebus apella	42 yrs	mammary adenoca.	metastases to intercostal muscles, lungs, lymph nodes and adrenal	(61)
Macaca mulatta (rhesus)	8 yrs	carcinoma	isolation of virus, metastases	(20)
	10 yrs	adenoca.	lymph node metastases	(?)
	adult	carcinoma	adenoma of kidney, ovarian endometrial cyst	(90)
	8–10 yrs	ductal carcinoma	received oral contraseptive; metastasis to local lymph nodes, liver, lungs	(51)
	9 yrs	adenocarcinoma	received irradiation, lymph node metastases	(19)
		intraductal carcinoma		(87)
		nodular hyperplasia		(69)
Papio hamadryas		squamous cell epithelioma		(6)
Mandrillus sphinx	5 yrs	adenocarcinoma	metastasized to liver, lung, axillary lymph nodes	(6)
Cercopithecus aethiops	5 yrs	fibrosarcoma		(71)
Pongo	15 yrs	carcinoma	metastasized to lymph nodes and lung	(?)

quamous carcinoma and adenocarcinoma and myoepithelioma. Four tumors produced multiple metastases to the lungs. One untreated female 25.2-months-old exhibited a mammary gland myoepithelioma with regions of adenocarcinoma. In the male of this species mammary tumors have not been observed.

Nonhuman primates
Mammary gland neoplasms occur in female nonhuman primates and rarely in males. Reports on mammary tumors in New World monkeys are lacking. These spontaneous tumors found were histologically nearly similar to the same tumor types in women (6). Nodular hyperplasia was observed by Valerio (84) in three rhesus monkeys and resembled as reported by McDivitt (62), Hutter (46), and Dawson (21) atypical terminal duct hyperplasia, atypical lobular hyperplasia and epitheliosis in humans. Neoplasms of the female breast gland have been found with considerable frequency in nonhuman primates (60, 61).

Comparative experimental work

The types and forms of myoepithelial cells' hyperplasia in

dysplasia and benign mammary gland tumors in the dog and man were studied by indirect Coon's method, using highly purified monospecific antiserum to smooth muscle myosin and performing alkaline phosphatase test. Studying surgical materials from 75 patients and 12 dogs using the histochemical method, researchers performed a comparative analysis of immunohistochemical and histochemical MC and discovered that differences in the results of staining in 7 out of 38 observations were due to negative test for alkaline phosphatase in the presence of fluorescence. The high degree of coincidence of positive tests in immunohistochemical and histochemical methods suggests that the test for alkaline phosphatase is a sufficiently reliable marker of MC. The principal similarity of types and forms of MC hyperplasia in dogs reveals that dogs may be used as an adequate model to study diseases of this organ. In addition to the known centripetal and centrifugal types, a uniformly concentric and smooth muscle proliferation of MC was noted in parallel immunohistochemical and histochemical studies on variants of MC proliferation (78).

Researchers used protein A-positive or -negative *Staphylococcus aureus* preparations in an extracorporal system to treat dogs with spontaneously occurring cancers. Four of the seven dogs treated by reinfusion of plasma incubated with protein A-positive *S. aureus* Cowan I strain (SAC) experienced tumor regression. Therapy was associated with fever, liver enzyme abnormalities and hypocomplementia. More extensive washing of the SAC preparation could diminish tumor response and toxicity. Two of our animals experienced tumor regression. Additionally, tumors regressed in 3 of 4 dogs treated with infusions of protein A-free saline extracts from *S. aureus*. These results suggest that the release of a non-protein A bacterial product contributes to tumor regression following incubation of plasma with *S. aureus*.

Four′–epi-doxorubicin displays greater antitumor activity than doxorubicin in Lewis lung carcinoma, MS-2 sarcoma lung metastasis, and human melanoma and thymic mice. Four′-epi-DX has proven to be less toxic and less cardiotoxic than its parent compound. The hepatobiliary metabolism and excretion of 4′-epi-DX investigated in the rat indicated that the new analogue was more extensively metabolized than the parent compound.

The main pharmacokinetic characteristics of 4′-epi-DX were a high plasma clearance (0.9–1.41/min), a terminal half-life of about 30 to 40 hours and a large volume of distribution. Four′-epi-DX has shown activity in a variety of tumors, including breast carcinoma, soft tissue sarcomas, non-Hodgkin's lymphomas, leukemias, ovarian cancer, and gastric cancer. Melanoma, rectal cancer, and pancreatic cancer have displayed preliminary evidence of activity, hence suggesting a broad spectrum of activity.

Estradiol and progesterone receptors were measured in tumor cytosols from 3 intact and 4 neutered female cats with spontaneously occurring mammary adenocarcinomas. Serum from 2 of intact cats, which has experienced estrous 4 and 4 to 6 weeks before tumor excision, contained progesterone concentrations of 16.2 and 2.2 ng/ml, respectively. Serum progesterone extracted from the other cats contained less than 2 ng/ml. Whereas estradiol receptors were not detected in any cytosols, progesterone receptors existed in all cytosols in concentrations ranging from 4.0 to 11.7 (means = 7.2) fmol/ng of protein. A scatched plot analysis of tumor cytosol from an 8th cat with mammary adenocarcinoma revealed the presence of high affinity progesterone binding with a dissociation constant (Kd) of 3.47 aM. The tumor receptor content could not be correlated with the stage of the estrus cycle whether the cat was intact or neutered.

Hayden, Johnson and Ghobrial studied the ultrastructure of feline mammary hypertrophy in a 5-year old cat which had recently aborted, a 10-year old cat one month postestrus, and a 4-year old progestin treated neutered male. When the subject cats' tissues were compared to normal mammary tissue from a 1-year old cat, the hypertrophied mammary tissue contained the same cell types and spatial relationships as did the normal gland. Major differences included a more highly developed duct system composed of metabolically active cells, often arranged in multiple cell layer, and periductular stroma with increased fibroblasts and vascularization. Smooth-contoured nuclear membranes, more evenly dispersed heterodiromatin, prominent nucleoli, increased polyribosomes, and elongated mitochondria characterized the hypertrophied epithelial cells. Only the cat which had aborted recently had significantly developed sectory activity. Myoepithelial cells displayed such modifications as more evenly dispersed nuclear heterochromatin, thicker bundles of cytoplasmic filaments, straighter plasma membranes along the basal lamina, elongated hemidesmosomes, and accentuated multilayering of the basal lamina. Nuclear heterochromatin in the stromal fibroblasts were distributed similarly to that of epithelial and myoepithelial cells and increased rough endoplasmic reticulum. Myoepithelial cells did not contribute to the increased stromal cellularity. Mammary hypertrophy in young, old, and progestin-treated cats displayed no significant ultrastructural differences from one another.

By detecting and describing oncogenes via RNA tumor viruses (or retroviruses) and recognizing their location at chromosomal translocation breakpoints frequently formed in some human neoplasms, researchers have increased their understanding of molecular mechanisms underlying carcinogenesis. Oncogenes are cellular genes which can be transduced by RNA tumor viruses and can induce malignant transformation under experimental conditions *in vivo* and *in vitro*. Epidemiological observations, the isolation of retroviruses from several human T-cell leukemias and lymphomas (human T-cell leukemia/lymphoma virus of HTLV), and the biochemical association of retroviral markers with human leukemias have pointed to a role of retroviruses in human leukogenesis. A human immune deficiency syndrome (AIDS) has also suggested a role of HTLV. In view of the well known role of many factors in carcinogenesis, the concept of carcinogenesis as a multistep process, as well as the concept of cocarcinogenesis and the role of cofactors other than viruses (e.g., radiation and chemicals, aging, hormones, graft vs. host reaction, environmental factors, etc.) must be carefully considered.

Mammary cancer in human types

As indicated above, human breast cancer, especially those in the female, vary in their appearance in different geographic regions, population groups and races. In the United States and western Europe, including Great Britain, the frequency of breast cancer is very high. Within the United States, Washington, DC, for example, exhibits a very high risk and this in the various racial groups. This fact may be explainable on the basis that breast cancer dependent also on two environmental factors, the socioeconomic status and diet. Other factors are surely involved but we do not know how they work. In India were breast cancer is less common. Comparisons of the frequency of breast cancer and cancer of the female genital organs have been undertaken but exhibit variable tumor frequency. Columbia and Yugoslavia are countries with a medial frequency of breast cancer in their female population. Countries with the lowest incidence of breast cancer are Japan, Singapore, and Nigeria. As we see there are many variations. But new comparative studies based on epidemiologic investigations in humans are essential and have to be interrelated to results concerning other species.

Suggestions for clinical implications from the field of veterinary and human medicine

The clinical implications rest on two facts: (1) through the comparative variations our knowledge about the mechanisms of neoplasms of the mammary glands may be promoted; (2) clinically, these tumors are highly important and we possess an extensive material.

Details of importance are: (1) Mammary glands occur only in mammals and present therefore species-wise a well circumscribed basis for comparison; (2) mammary glands are phylogenetically young organs, which developed since the Triassic; (3) the large variations in frequency and secondary development in the various mammalian species offer the comparative background for this model of experimental and clinical tumor investigations; (4) species variations can not be attributed to small numbers of animals investigated, because several species such as dogs, cats, mice, rats, cattle (especially the dairy cow, which reaches a tumor prone age), whales slaughtered in the thousands have been routinely examined by veterinarians; (5) the metastatic distribution is very incompletely investigated, even in such species as dog and cat but exhibits a pronounced departure from the metastatic path in women and mice; (6) the majority of species seems to have an infrequent appearance of mammary cancer which is also the case in certain human population as in the Japanese (but changes in tumor pattern have been observed recently); (7) the variation in incidence in human races is also based on an extensive clinical and pathological experience.

CONCLUSIONS

This topic offers a new avenue of research if the reasons for this variation are blended into cancer causing aspects. The chance to investigate why these differences in races, breeds, strains, and individual mammals exist, have never been exploited in a satisfying way. The normal situation seems to be a scarcity of mammary cancer in the mammals as illustrated by findings of free-ranging mammals, zoo-, domestic and laboratory animals and certain human populations. The question still remains: What are the reasons which are responsible for the variation in frequency, histologic and other aspects of mammary tumors contrasting similarities among species?

REFERENCES

1. Acland HM, Gillette DM: Mammary Carcinoma in a Mare. *Vet Path* 19:93, 1982
2. Ajello A: Il considdetto morbo di Paget della mammella nella cagna. *Annal Fac Med Vet* Messina 13:201, 1976
3. Anderson LJ, Jarrett WFH: Mammary neoplasia in the dog and cat. II. Clinico-pathologic aspects of mammary tumors in the dog and cat. *J Small Anim Pract* 7:697, 1966
4. Appleby EC: Tumors in captive wild animals: Some observations and comparisons. *Acta Zool Pathol Antverpiensia* 48:77, 1969
5. Appleby EC, Keymer IF: Some tumors in captive wild mammals and birds: A brief report. Verhandlungsbericht des X. Internationalen Symposiums über die Erkrankungen der Zootiere, Salzburg 10:199, 1968
6. Appleby EC, Keymer LF, Hime JM: Three cases of suspected mammary neoplasia in nonhuman primates. *J Comp Pathol* 84:351, 1974
7. Banks WC, Morris E: Results of radiation treatment of naturally occurring animal tumors. *JAVMA* 166(1):1063, 1975
8. Bhowmik MK: A note on mammary fibroadenoma in a buffalo (*Bubalus bubalis*). *Indian J Anim Sci* 49:147, 1979
9. Bhowmik MK, Iyer PKR: Studies on the pathology of chronic lesions in the mammary glands of buffaloes (*Bubalus bubalis*). *Indian Vet J* 55:418, 1978
10. Bonser GM, Dossett JA, Jull JW: Mammary carcinogenesis in experimental animals, chapter 7. In: Human and Experimental Breast Cancer. London: Pitman Medical Publishing Co., p. 130, 1961
11. Brack M: Carcinoma solidum simplex mammae bei einem Orang utan (*Pongo pygmaeus*). *Zentralbl Allg Pathol* 109:474, 1966
12. Bradley RL: Selected oral, pharyngeal, and upper respiratory conditions in the cat. Oral tumors, nasopharyngeal and middle ear polyps, and chronic rhinitis and sinusitis. *Vet Clin North Am* (*Small Anim Pract*) 14(6):1173, 1984
13. Bradley RL, MacEven EG, Loar AS: Mandibular resection for removal of oral tumors in 30 dogs and 6 cats. *J Am Vet Med Assoc* 184(4):460, 1984
14. Brewer WG, Turrel JM: Radiotherapy and hyperthermia in the treatment of fibrosarcomas in the dog. *JAVMA* 181(2):146, 1982
15. Brodey RS, Fidler IJ, Howson AE: The relationship of estrous irregularity, pseudopregnancy, and pregnancy to canine mammary neoplasms. *J Am Vet Med Assoc* 149:1047, 1966
16. Cameron AM, Faulkin LJ: Hyperplastic and inflammatory nodules in the canine mammary gland. *J Natl Cancer Inst* 47:1277, 1971
17. Cardesa A, Handler AH, Kelman AD: Tumours of the mammary gland. In: Pathology of Tumours in Laboratory Animals, vol. III, edited by Turusov VS Lyon: International Agency for Research on Cancer, p. 33, 1982
18. Chapman WL: Neoplasia in nonhuman primates. *J Am Vet Med Assoc* 153:872, 1968
19. Chapman WL, Allen JR: Multiple neoplasia in a rhesus monkey. *Pathol Vet* 5:342, 1968a
20. Chopra HC, Mason MM: A new virus in a spontaneous mammary tumor of a rhesus monkey. *Cancer Res* 30:2081, 1970
21. Dawson EK: Carcinoma in the mammary lobule and in origin. *Edinb Med J* 40:57, 1933
22. Dorn CR, Taylor DON, Frye FL, Hibbard HH: Survey of animal neoplasms in Alameda and Contra Costa counties, California. I. Methodology and description of cases. *J Natl Cancer Inst* 40:295, 1968
23. Dorn CR, Taylor DON, Schneider R et al: Survey of animal neoplasms in Alameda and Contra costa counties, California. II. Cancer morbidity in dogs and cats from Alameda county. *J Natl Cancer Inst* 40:307, 1968a
24. Dubielzig RR: Proliferative dental and gingival diseases of dogs and cats. *JAAHA* 18(4):577, 1982
25. Elliot OS, Elliot MW, Lisco H: Breast cancer in a tree shrew (*Tupaia glis*). *Nature* 211:1105, 1966
26. Evans CR, Pierrepoint CG: Tissue steroid interaction in canine hormone dependent tumor. *Vet Res* 79:464, 1975
27. Feldman DG, Gross L: Electron microscopic study of spontaneous mammary carcinomas in cats and dogs: virus-like particles in cat mammary carcinomas. *Cancer Res* 31:161, 1971
28. Feldmann WH: Malignant growths in domestic animals. *J Am Vet Med Assoc* 75:192, 1929
29. Fidler IJ, Abt DA, Brodey RS: The biological behavior of canine mammary neoplasms. *J Am Vet Med Assoc* 151:1311, 1967
30. Floid MFA: Bibliography of Camelids. Damaskus, Syria: Arab Center for Studies of Arid Zones, 1981
31. Fortner JG, Mahy AG, Cotran RS: Transplantable tumors of the Syrian (golden) hamster. II. Tumors of the hematopoietic tissues, genitourinary organs, mammary glands and sarcomas.

Cancer chemotherapy screening data X. *Cancer Res* 21:199, 1961

32. Ganzina F: 4′-epi-doxorubicin, a new analogue of doxorubicin: a preliminary overview of preclinical and clinical data. *Cancer Treat Rev* 10(1):1, 1983

33. Gillette EL: Indications and selection of patients for radiation therapy. *Vet Clin North Am* 4(4):889, 1974

34. Gordon BR, Matus RE, Saal SD et al: Protein A-independent tumoricidal responses in dogs after extracorporeal perfusion of plasma over *Staphylococcus aureus*. *JNCI* 70(6):1127, 1983

35. Grier RI *et al*: Regression of cutaneous melanosarcoma following intralesional *Mycobacterium bovis* BCC injection: A case report. *JAAHA* 14(1):76, 1978

36. Griner LA: Pathology of Zoo Animals. San Diego: Zoological Society of San Diego, 1983

37. Hargis AM: A review of solar induced lesions in domestic animals. *Compend Contin Educ Pract Vet* 3(4):287, 1981

38. Harvey HJ *et al*: Prognostic criteria for dogs with oral melanoma. *JAVMA* 178(6):580, 1981

39. Hayden DW, Johnson KH, Ghobrial HK: Ultrastructure of feline mammary hypertrophy. *Vet Pathol* 20(3):254, 1983

40. Hayes HM, Milne KL, Mandell CP: Epidemiological features of feline mammary carcinoma. *Vet Rec* 108:476–9, 1981

41. Hayes HM: Epidemiology of selected aspects of dog and cat neoplasms and comparison with man. In: Neoplasms – Comparative Pathology of Growth in Animals, Plants, and Man, edited by Kaiser HE. Baltimore: Williams & Wilkins, p. 499, 1981

42. Hayes HM: (personal communication)

43. Hehlmann R, Schatters R, Kreeb G *et al*: RNA-tumoriviruses, oncogenes, and their possible role in human carcinogenesis. *Klin Wochenschr* 61(24):1217, 1983

44. Hoch-Ligeti C, Wagner BP, Deringer MK, Stewart HL: Tumor induction in *Praomys (Mastomys) natalensis* by N, N′-2,7-fluorenylenebisacetamide. *JNCI* 74(4):909, 1985

45. Hoch-Ligeti C, Liebelt AG, Congdon CC, Stewart HL: Mammary gland tumors in irradiated and untreated guinea pigs. *Toxicol Path* 14:289, 1986

46. Hutter RV: The pathologist's role in minimal breast cancer. *Cancer* 28:1527, 1971

47. Johnston SD, Hayden DW, Kiang DT *et al*: Progesterone receptors in feline mammary adenocarcinomas. *Am J Vet Res* 45(2):379, 1984

48. Karelina TV, Rukosuev VS, Golubeva VA, Ermilova VD: Types of myoepithelial cell proliferation in dyshormonal breast dysplasias and benign breast tumors. *Arkh Patol* 45(8):27, 1983

49. Kazantseva IA, Karelina TV: Role of myoepithelial cells in the histogenesis of lobular breast cancer. *Arkh Patol* 46(5):32, 1984

50. Kenny JE: Primary adenocarcinoma of the udder of a milk cow. *Vet Res* 54:240, 1942

51. Kirschstein RL, Rabson AS, Rusten GW: Infiltrating duct carcinoma of the mammary gland of a rhesus monkey after administration of an oral contraceptive: a preliminary report. *J Natl Cancer Inst* 48:551, 1972

52. Komitowski D, Sass B, Laub W: Rat mammary tumor classification: notes on comparative aspects. *JNCI* 68(1):147, 1982

53. Levene A: Upper digestive tract neoplasia in the cat in comparative study. *J Laryngol Otol* 98(12):1221, 1984

54. Lombard and Tagand: Carcinome encephaloide de la mammelle chez une jument. *Rev Vet* (Toulouse) 75:725, 1923

55. Lowenstine L: (unpublished data)

56. Lynch HT, Albano WA, Hsieck JJ *et al*: Genetics, biomarkers, and control of breast cancer: a review. *Cancer Genet Cytogenet* 13(1):43, 1984

57. MacEwen EG: Melanoma. Proc 9th Annu Vet Surg Forum, Chicago, IL, p. 198, 1981

58. Maclean U: Women and health in Europe: the scope and limits of epidemiology. *Int J Health Serv* 15(4):665, 1985

59. Mandal PC, Iyer PKR: Mammary intraductal carcinoma in a buffalo (*Bubalus bubalis*). *Vet Path* 6:534, 1969

60. McClure HM: Neoplasia in rhesus monkeys, I. Tumors of the genital organs and mammary glands, p. 381. In: The Rhesus Monkey, vol. II, Management, Reproduction, and Pathology. New York-San Francisco-London: Academic Press, 1975

61. McClure HM: Neoplastic diseases in nonhuman primates: Literature review and observations in an autopsy series of 2,176 animals, p. 549. In: The Comparative Pathology of Zoo Animals, edited by Montali RJ, Migaki G. Washington, DC: Smithsonian Institution Press, 1980

62. McDivitt RW, Stewart FW, Berg JW: Tumors of the Breast. Atlas of Tumor Pathology, 2nd series, Fascicle 2, Washington, DC: Armed Forces Institute of Pathology, 1968

63. Miller ME, Christensen GC, Evans HE: Anatomy of the Dog. Philadelphia: WB Saunders, 1964

64. Misdorp W, Hart AAM: Prognostic factors in canine mammary cancer. *J Natl Cancer Inst* 56:779, 1976

65. Monson KR, Malbirn JO, Hubber K: Determination of estrogen receptors in canine mammary tumors. *Am J Vet Res* 38:1937, 1977

66. Moulton JE: Tumors of the alimentary tract. In: Tumors in Domestic Animals, 2nd edition, edited by JE Moulton. Berkeley: University of California Press, p. 240, 1961

67. Moulton JE: Tumors of the mammary glands. In: Tumors of Domestic Animals, edited by Moulton JE. Berkeley: University of California Press, chapter 11, 1978

68. Moulton JE: Tumors of the mammary gland. In: Tumors in Domestic Animals (3rd edition), edited by Moulton JE. Berkeley-Los Angeles-London: University of California Press, 1987

69. Nelson LW, Shott LD: Mammary nodular hyperplasia in intact rhesus monkeys. *Vet Pathol* 10:130, 1973

70. Noble RL, Cutts JH: Mammary tumors of the rat: a review. *Cancer Res* 19:125, 1959

71. O'Connor P: Occurrence of tumors in zoo animals. *Animaland* 14:2, 1947

72. Owen LN: Mammary neoplasia in the dog and cat III. Prognosis and treatment of mammary tumours in the bitch. *J Small Anim Pract* 7:703, 1966

73. Papaioannou A: The contribution of regional lymph nodes in the resistance against breast cancer: practical implications. *J Surg Oncol* 25(4):232, 1984

74. Priester WA, McKay FW: The occurrence of tumors in domestic animals. *Natl Cancer Inst Monogr* 54, 1980

75. Rao AT, Iyer PKR, Chaudary C, Nayak BC: Mammary intraductal carcinoma in a pig. *Indian Vet J* 53:892, 1976

76. Reil JS, Cohen D: The environmental distribution of canine respiratory tract neoplasms. *Arch Environ Health* 22(1)136, 1971

77. Richardson RC: Mammary tumors in animals. In: Breast Cancer, edited by Hoogstraten B, McDivitt RW. Boca Raton, FL: CRC Press. Chapter 2, p. 27, 1981

78. Richardson RC: Spontaneous canine and feline neoplasms as models for cancer in man. Kal Kan Forum Fall 1983, p. 88, 1983

79. Ruch TC: Diseases of Laboratory Primates. Philadelphia: Saunders contents citation of Griffith, 1959

80. Schneider R, Dorn CR, Taylor DON: Factors influencing canine mammary cancer development and post-surgical survival. *J Natl Cancer Inst* 43:1249, 1969

81. Shivaprasad HL, Sundberg, JP, Ely R: Malignant mixed (carcinosarcoma) mammary tumor in a gray squirrel. *Vet Pathol* 21:115, 1984

82. Smith HS, Wolman SR, Hackett AJ: The biology of breast cancer at the cellular level. *Biochim Biophys Acta* 738(3):103, 1984

83. Sokolowski JH: Reproduction patterns in the bitch. *Vet Clin North Am* 7:651, 1977

84. Squire RA, Goodman DG, Valerio MG *et al*: Mammary

gland. In: Pathology of Laboratory Animals, edited by Benirschke K, Farner FM, Jones TC, chapter 12, p. 1194. New York-Heidelberg-Berlin: Springer Verlag, 1978

85. Stannard AA, Pulley LT: Tumors of the skin and soft tissues. In: Tumors in Domestic Animals, edited by Moulton JF (2nd edition). Berkeley: University of California Press, p. 17, 1961

86. Surmont J: L'epitheliome mammaire de la jument et ses metastases pulmonaires. *Bull Ass franc Etude Cancer* 15:98, 1926

87. Tekeli MM, Ford: Carcinoma, intraductal. *Vet Pat* 17(4):502, 1980

88. Thrall DE: Orthovoltage radiotherapy of oral fibrosarcomas in dogs. *JAVMA* 179(2):159, 1981

89. Todoroff RJ *et al*: Oral and pharyngeal neoplasia in the dog. Retrospective survey of 361 cases. *JAVMA* 175(6):567, 1979

90. Vadova AV, Gel'shtein VI: Spontaneous tumors in catarrhine monkeys according to the data obtained in the monkey colony of the Sukhumi Medico-Biological station. Utkin Theoretical and Practical Questions of Medicine and Biology in Experiments on Monkeys. New York: Pergamon Press, p. 137, 1960

91. Wadsworth JR: Mammary neoplasms – *Lemur catta*. *Vet Pathol* 17:386, 1980

92. Wagner JE, Manning PJ: Tumors of the mammary glands. In: The Biology of the Guinea Pig, edited by Wagner JE, Manning PJ. New York-San Francisco-London: Academic Press, p. 217, 1979

93. Wallach JD, Boever WJ: Diseases of Exotic Animals. p. 110. Philadelphia-London-Toronto; WB Saunders, 1983

94. Weisbroth SH, Flatt RE, Kraus AL (eds): Tumors of the mammary gland. In: The Biology of the Laboratory Rabbit. New York-London: Academic Press, p. 345, 1974

95. Withrow SJ: Oral and pharyngeal tumors. Proc. 9th Annu Vet Surg Forum, Chicago, IL, p. 186, 1981

96. World Health Organization (WHO): Histological Classification of Tumors. No. 2. Histological Typing of Breast Tumors (2d ed). Geneva: WHO, 1981

CARDIAC TUMORS IN LABORATORY RODENTS –
COMPARATIVE PATHOLOGY

CORNELIA HOCH-LIGETI* and HAROLD L. STEWART

This survey of spontaneous and induced cardiac tumors of rats, mice, guinea pigs and hamsters is based on a critical review of the literature and the hitherto unpublished data of a study of the material accessed of the NCI Registry of Experimental Cancers. The frequency of cardiac tumors in laboratory rodents, the location within the heart, the histologic classification and heredity aspect are compared with these features in humans with cardiac tumors.

In her review of spontaneous tumors in small laboratory mammals, Tamaschke (122) refers to the only report she could find up to the date of her publication of a cardiac tumor in a rodent, a sarcoma of the heart of a guinea pig (7). Comprehensive reviews of cardiac tumors in several rodent species have appeared: on the guinea pig (82), on the rat (1, 57), on the mouse (116), and on rodents and other animal species (111).

Foremost among the reviews of cardiac tumors in man are those by Mahaim (81), Prichard (91), Heath (47), Sytman and MacAlpin (120), and McAllister and Fenoglio (73).

CARDIAC TUMORS IN RATS

Tumors of the endocardium and myocardium

The first cardiac tumor reported in a rat (87) arose in an animal, 8.2 months of age, which had ingested a diet to which 2-FAA, dissolved in warm corn oil solution, had been added. Subsequently, cardiac tumors were induced in rats by a number of other carcinogenic agents, in particular by derivatives of nitrosourea and nitrosamine, the names, abbreviations and chemical formulae of which are listed in Table 1. Table 2 lists in chronological order reports of cardiac tumors induced in rats. The carcinogenic chemicals were administered by various routes (intravenous, intraperitoneal, subcutaneous or transplacental) to rats of different strains and of various ages, the details of which are given in the original publications.

Cardiac tumors have also been reported in "untreated rats" which had either been used as controls in different experiments or been treated with agents considered to be non-tumorigenic. In 1973, Boorman and associates (12), under the title "Naturally occurring endocardial disease," described this lesion in the heart of rats of three different strains from the Institute for Experimental Gerontology, Rijswijk, The Netherlands. The lesion consisted of proliferation of fibroblast-like cells within the endocardium. Out of

the total of 40 rats with the "endocardial disease," 9 were untreated controls, and it is unlikely that the experimental procedures to which the other rats had been subjected, had exerted any decisive influence on the initiation of cardiac lesions. In 6 rats large tumor-like masses were found in the heart. Prior to this publication, no cardiac tumors had been reported in untreated rats. Ivankovic and associates (58) stated that among approximately 15,000 untreated BD rats, which had been necropsied, tumors of the heart were not observed. Following 1973, cardiac lesions in untreated rats of several strains were found in increasing numbers. We now believe that these lesions, reported under a variety of diagnoses, represent different stages of neoplastic development and progression. In Table 3, data pertaining to these cardiac lesions in untreated rats are tabulated chronologically in order of their publication and with the authors' designations of them. Cardiac tumors of histologic types, other than the endocardial tumor, but observed in untreated rats, are appended to Table 3.

Studying Tables 2 and 3, one is impressed by the diversity of the diagnoses applied to the lesions which we regard as endocardial tumor. Owing to this diversity, clarification is rendered difficult by the disparate sources of the material collected. Several of the cardiac tumors are excerpted from publications dealing with the overall occurrence of tumors of different sites in a given strain of rat (40, 41, 75–77). In these publications only the occurrence and the diagnosis of the cardiac tumor are stated without any indication of its exact location within the heart or description of its morphology. In some other publications, the histology of the cardiac tumor is carefully described, but its exact location within the heart is not specified.

Photomicrographs of cardiac lesions published by different authors and designated by different terms are reproduced in Figures 1–8. The viewer will appreciate that the morphology of the lesions illustrated is identical, both in the early or advanced stage of development, irrespective of whether the rat had or had not been treated. The lesion develops in the subendothelial layer of the endocardium by an increase of the size and number of elongated cells and the formation of two or more cell layers. The endothelium overlying the lesion remains intact and no thrombi form (Figures 1 and 2). There may be a single focus or several foci of proliferating subendothelial cells. Although foci may appear to be separated by normal-appearing subendocardial tissue, nonetheless, since serial sections were not examined, the presence of these skip areas may be accounted for by the

---

*Deceased May 17th, 1986.

H. E. Kaiser (ed.), Comparative aspects of tumor development.
© 1989, Kluwer Academic Publishers, Dordrecht. ISBN-13:978-0-89838-994-4

Table 1. Abbreviations for the cardiac carcinogens used.

AMMN	acetoxymethyl-methyl-nitrosamine		ENBU	N,N ethylnitrosobiuret	
CD	carbamate derivatives 1,1 diphenyl 2 propynyl N ethylcarbamate 1(4 chlorophenyl)-1 phenyl 2 propynylcarbamate				
CHC	cyclohexylcarbamate		2 FAA	N 2 fluorenylacetamide	
DMN	dimethylnitrosamine		2,7 FAA	N,N' 2,7 fluorenylene bisacetamide	
DMNU	N,N' dimethylnitrosourea		2,7 FAA F$_6$	N,N' 2,7 fluorenylenebis 2,2,2 trifluoroacetamide	
DPP	3,3-diphenyl-3 (pyrrolicin-carbonyloxy)-1 propyne		MCA	20 methylcholanthrene	
DSF	disulfiram		MNU	N,N-methylnitrosourea	
EC	ethylcarbamate urethane		PDET	1 pyridyl 3,3 diethyl triazene	
EMS	ethylmethane sulfonate		PhDMT	1 phenyl 3,3 dimethyl triazene	
ENU	N,N ethylnitrosourea		PS	1,3 propane sulton	

Table 2. Cardiac tumors induced in rats.

Compound	Administration	Strain	Rats with cardiac tu. total nr. M	F	Age*, months (Range)	Tumor designation	Reference
2-FAA	oral	Buffalo	1/18	–	8	Anitschkow cell	(87)
PhDMT	s.c.	BDIX	2/21		8, 13	Sarcoma NOS	(27)
EC	i.p.	MRC	3/80	2/80	(10–17)	Anitschkow cell sarcoma	(129)
2,7-FAA	oral	Sprague-Dawley	1/12	–	8	Adenoma**	(124)
MNU		Hooded	38/591	–	8	Sarcoma NOS	(102)+
	i.v., i.p.	Wistar	–	6/148			
DMNU		Hooded	1/60		–	Sarcoma NOS	(102)
MNU	oral	Wistar	–	1/156	10	Sarcoma	(123)
PS	i.v.	BD	1/32		15	Fibrosarcoma	(26)
ENU	oral	BDIX	4/145		(10, 12)	Malignant neurinoma	(29)
	i.v.		5/64		16		
EC	i.p.	MRC	13/542		12	Anitschkow cell sarcoma	(65)
ENBU	i.g. to mother	BD	2/34		5, 6	Malignant neurinoma	(28)
		Hooded	66				
MNU	i.v., i.p., i.g.		368 74		7	Fibroma, fibro-sarcoma	(103)
		Wistar	6/148	–			
PDET	oral	BD	11/27	5/17	(12–23)	Neurinoma, neurofibro-ma, neurosarcoma	(58)
EMS			2 6 118				
DMN	i.p.	Wistar	1/34	–	(8–22)	Neurinoma, neurosarcoma	(42)
DMN + EMS			2 3 109				
MNU	i.v.	Sprague-Dawley	1/52		(4–9)	Anaplastic neurinoma	(118, 119)
MNU	i.v., i.p., t.p.	BDIX	60/278		(4–27)	Fibroma, fibrosarcoma, undifferentiated sarcoma	(104)
ENU	s.c.		8/312				
AMMN	s.c.	Sprague-Dawley	1/35	–	6		
AMMN	i.v.		30/62	–	(5–9)	Rhabdomyo-sarcoma	(43)
AMMN	i.v. newborn	Sprague-Dawley	10/31	–	–	Schwannoma	(8)
AMMN	i.v.	Sprague-Dawley	1/18	–	5		
DSF + AMNN	i.v., oral		4/36	–	(7–12)	Fibrosarcoma	(44)
DSF	oral		0/36	–	–		
2,7-FAA	oral	Buffalo	1/18	–	23		
2,7-FAA-F$_6$	oral	Buffalo	–	1/18	11		
2,7-FAA + 2OMCA	oral	ACI	1/20	–	11	Endocardial mesen-chymal tumor	(50)
CHC	oral or topical		10/90	3/25			
CD	oral	Wistar	2/45	–	(8–21)		
DPP	oral		3/23	–			
fibrous	intrathoracic	Osborne-Mendel	–	8/135		Endocardial mesen-chymal tumor	(51)
material	i.v.		–	1/15			
ENU	oral	F344/DuCrj	1/52	–	(15–38)	Myxoma?	(78)

*If the age of death of the tumor-bearing rat(s) is not given, the range for the whole treated group is quoted.
*The histologic description is that of myogenic lesion. + The data are quoted in the 1972 report, which is on the same MNU-treated rats, with some additional observations.

Table 3. Cardiac tumors in untreated rats.

Strain	Rats with cardiac tu. total nr. M	F	Age, months (Range)	Designation by the author(s)	Reference
CIVO (Wistar)	17 $\overline{1990}$	2	(16–25)	Endocardial disease. (fibroblast-like cell	
WAG/Rij (Wistar)	2 $\overline{344}$	12	(21–39)	proliferation within the endocardium*)	(12)
BN/Rij		7/95	(21–39)		
Sprague-Dawley		1/217		Fibroma	
Osborne-Mendel		1/131		Fibrosarcoma	(75)
Oregon		1/673		Fibroma	
ACI/N	1/55	3/209	26, 25	Fibroma	(77)
Sprague-Dawley	1/–	–	12	Fibromatous proliferation	(34)
BN/Bi	1/74	–	13	Fibrosarcoma	(13)
F344	1/1794	1/1754	25	Adenoca. [+], fibroma, sarcoma, Anitschkow cell sarcoma.	(10)
CFHB (Wistar)	3 $\overline{1224}$	2	(20–24)	Sub-endocardial fibrosis	(70)
Sprague-Dawley	–	1/99	20	Undifferentiated sarcoma	(8)
Osborne-Mendel	4/975	1/970	(24–27)	Fibroma Sarcoma NOS	(41)
–	1/–	–	–	Schwannoma	(11)
Osborne-Mendel		1/252			
F344	1/–		(25–26)	Neurilemmoma	(95)
Sprague-Dawley	–	6/480	(6–25)	Endocardial thickening	(143)
F344/DuCrj	1/296	2/297		Fibroma or myxoma	(76)
Wistar	2/–	–	17, 22		
Buffalo	–	1/–	15	Endocardial mesenchymal tumor	(50)
Osborne-Mendel	–	1/–	19		
F344/DuCrj	–	1/52	(15–38)	myxoma?	(78)
Sprague-Dawley	–	1/3397	15	Endothelioma	(101)
Wistar	1/1342		(26–28)	Paraganglioma	(36)
Albino	1/–	–	36	Aortic body tumor	(127)
Wag/Rij	–	14/484	(22–47)		
Sprague-Dawley	–	1/–	23	Aortic body tumor	(130)
NZR/Gd	12/100	4/100	> 24	Atriocaval mesothelioma	(38, 39)
COBS Charles River	1/–	–	18	Mesothelioma	(105)

* Gross tumor in the heart of 4M and 1F CIVO rats, and of 1F WAG/Rij rat.
+ Dr. Goodman now considers this tumor as an atrio-caval mesothelioma (personal communication).

plane of the section, and cannot be accepted as proof that the initial lesion arose multifocally. With most lesions studied, the subendothelial neoplastic proliferative cells cover ribbon-like the entire myocardial surface (Figures 3 and 4). In lesions consisting of more than 10 rows of cells, two layers can be distinguished (Figures 5 and 6). In the more cellular, superficial layer, the cells are rounded, ovoid or polygonal with large hyperchromic nuclei and prominent nucleoli; occasionally, mitotic figures are present. The cytoplasm of many cells in this layer exhibit fine vacuolization resembling honeycombing. The deeper layer is formed by fibroblast-like cells, which are elongated with elongated nuclei and are arranged in a herringbone pattern. Bands of collagen fibers of different thicknesses and fibroglia are present among and between the cells. Elastic fibers could not be found in the lesions, although a few fibers have been demonstrated in the endocardium of normal rats, mostly in the endocardium of

the right atrium. Cells with Anitschkow nuclear morphology are present in the majority of the lesions and in some, the Anitschkow cells are so numerous that they form the prevalent cell type (Figure 9). None of the cells show cross or longitudinal striations and, although a herring-bone pattern is often discernable in the subendocardial proliferative cell layers, palisading, Verocay bodies and other features pathognomonic of schwannoma are absent.

The proliferating endocardial cell layers are initially sharply separated from myocardium; in some areas the thickened endocardial layers come into contact with each other and form confluent masses. Later, however, the proliferating cells, lying against the myocardium extend along the perimysium and compress the myocardial fibers, particularly those of the papillary and trabecular muscles, resulting in atrophy of these. With the lesion advanced, the tumor in areas has lost its subendothelial character and has become

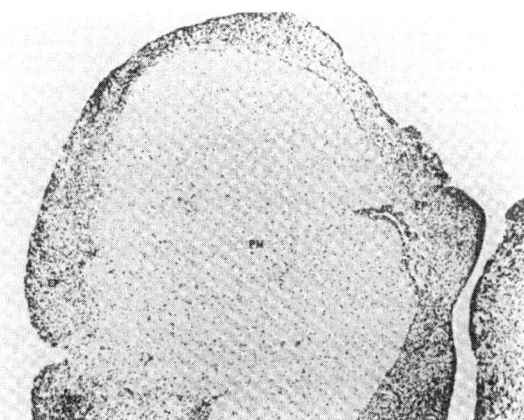

Figure 1. Marked subendocardial proliferation of papillary muscle. H & E × 50. Reproduction of Figure 1 and its legend from Lewis, (70). Author's diagnosis: Subendocardial fibrosis.

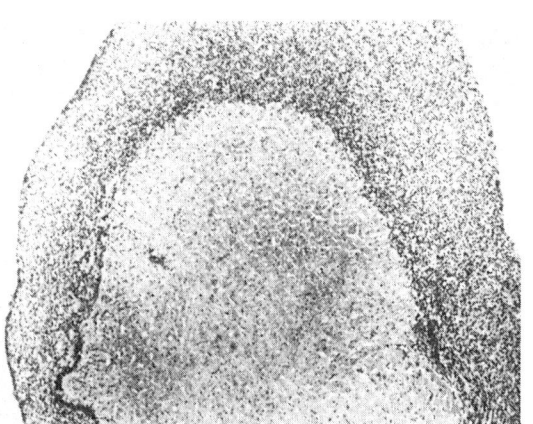

Figure 2. Rat No. 1227. Time of latency 192 days, D. 31.3 mg MNU intravenous. A spindle-shaped cell cardiac tumor covering hood-like the papillary muscle. HE, magnification 75. Reproduction of Figure 2 and translation of its legend from Schreiber et al., (103). Authors' diagnosis: Fibrosarcoma.

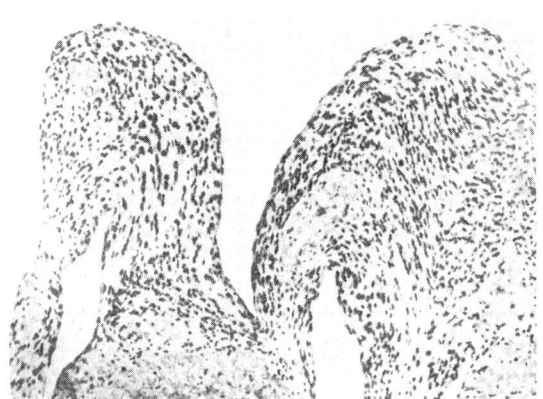

Figure 3. Papillary aspect of lesion seen in WAG/Rij. (Hematoxylin-phloxin-safran). Original magnification × 210. Reproduction of Figure 6 and its legend from Boorman et al., (12). Authors' diagnosis: Endocardial disease (Proliferation of fibroblast-like cells within the endocardium).

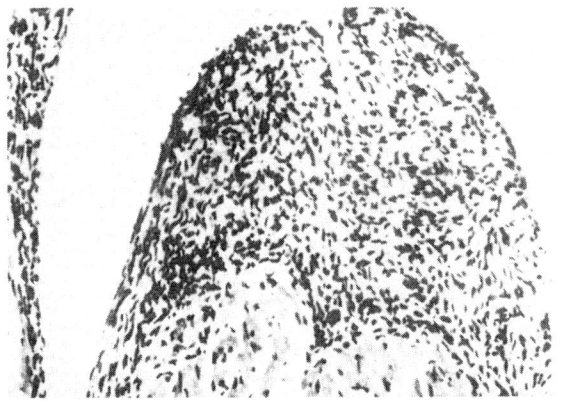

Figure 4. Neurinoma (Antoni type A) in which there are sharply defined boundaries between the tumor and the heart tissue. There is little infiltration of the heart muscle. H & E × 100.

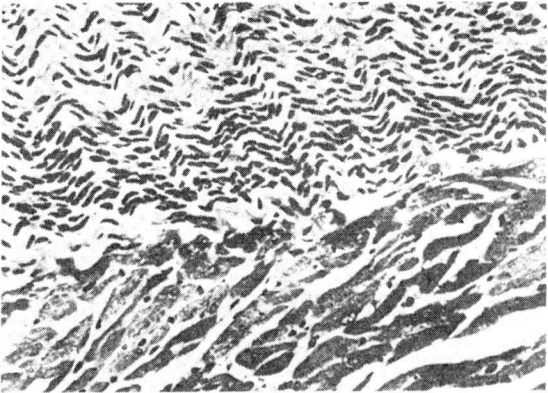

Figure 5. Coronary neurofibroma. The spindle-shaped cells of the tumor are arranged in a distinctly wave-like pattern. Male; survived 77 weeks; treated with 30 mg DMN + 100 mg EMS/kg.b.w.; H & E. Reproduction of Figure 1 and translation of its legend from Haas et al., (42).

exophytic, or anaplastic cells with numerous mitoses have infiltrated the myocardium, forming a large neoplastic mass. The exophytic tumor may fill the cardiac chamber (Figures 7, 8). Even at this stage, the subendocardial character of the tumor is retained in other areas of the same heart. Endocardial tumors develop at an earlier age in the carcinogen-treated rats than in untreated rats, are more frequent in males than in females, are preferentially localized within the left ventricle and commonly involve the interventricular septum. Several, however, have involved the right ventricle or both ventricles and the atria. While exophytic, space-occupying, growths were described by several previous authors who reported on this lesion, its neoplastic nature remained questionable, and proliferative growth was taken into consideration. The demonstration that an endocardial tumor had metastasized to the lung (50), provided evidence of its neoplastic nature (Figures 10–12). Since a progressively increasing cell dedifferentiation has been demonstrated in the morphologic characteristics of the small endocardial lesions as they evolve in the direction of the large infiltrating lesions (50, 104), the identical neoplastic nature of all such

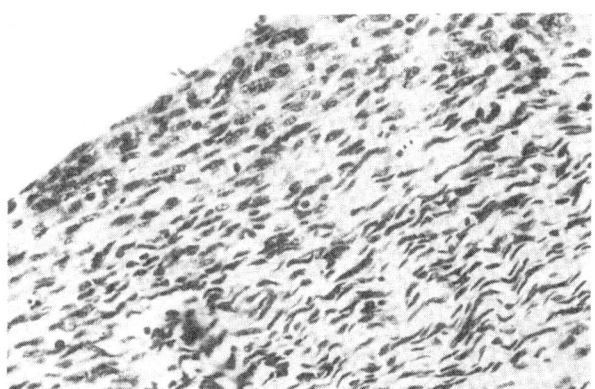

Figure 6. Endocardial tumor. Intact endothelial lining covers the cellular upper layer of rounded cells with hyperchromic nuclei. The sparse elongated cells in the lower layers are separated by interstitial collagen fibers. Male Wistar rat, 25 weeks of age, treated with 3,3-diphenyl-3-(pyrrolidine-carbonyloxy)-1-propane. H & E × 330. Reproduction of Figure 1 and its legend from Hoch-Ligeti et al., (50).

endocardial lesions can be postulated. Hence the lesions designated by different authors as endocardial or subendocardial fibrosis or endocardial fibromatous proliferation can with justification be tabulated as endocardial tumor (Table 3). Cellular atypia, numerous, often multipolar mitoses and infiltration of the myocardium attest to the malignant neoplastic nature of the lesion from an early stage.

It may be relevant to compare on the one hand the evolution of the space-occupying cardiac tumor from the preceding endocardial fibrous proliferation to, on the other hand,

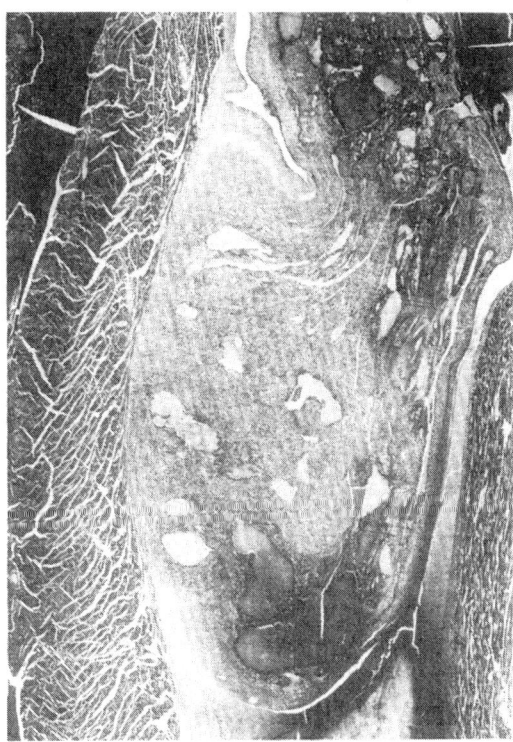

Figure 8. Endocardial tumor filling the left ventricle and extending into the lumen of the aorta. Female Osborne-Mendel 75-weeks-old rat treated with i.v. injection of 0.05 ml air particulates of urban atmosphere extracted with hexafluorotetrachlorobutane. H & E × 14. Enlarged photograph of endocardial tumor shown in Figure 2 of Hoch-Ligeti et al., (50).

the progression of the lesion of the trigeminal nerve induced by ENU. This neural lesion progresses from the early proliferative cell change to the stage of genuine schwannoma. The early manifestation of the lesion proved to be

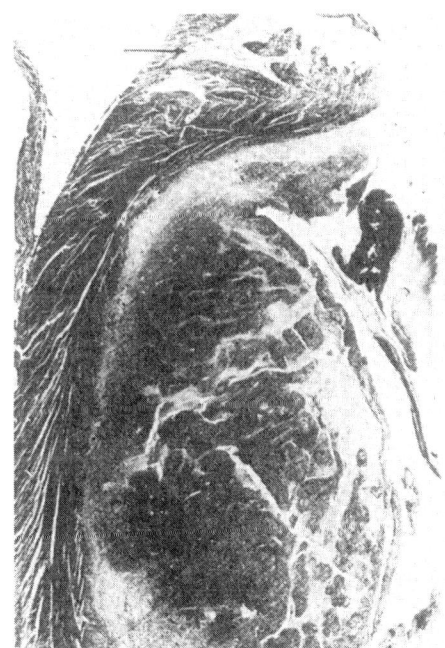

Figure 7. Tumor mass filling left ventricle of CIVO rat. Note also endocardial disease in left atrium (arrow) (H & E, original magnification × 11). Reproduction of Figure 7 and its legend from Boorman et al., (12).

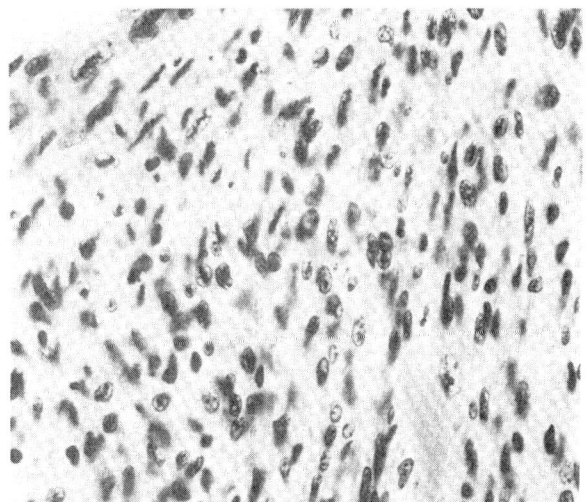

Figure 9. Endocardial tumor. Numerous tumor cells exhibit Anitschkow cell nuclear morphology. Male BUF rat, 58 weeks of age, treated with 2-FAA. H & E × 220.

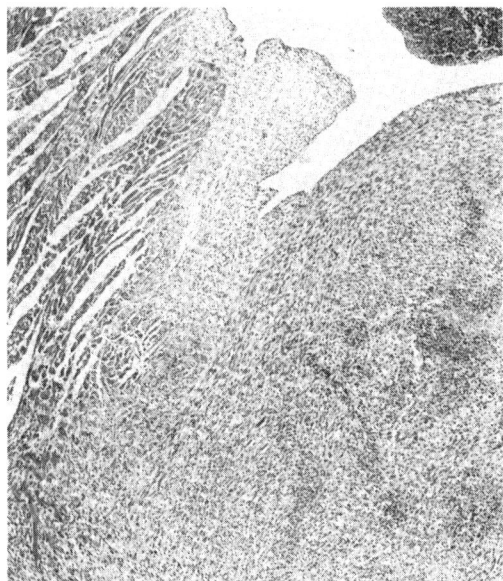

Figure 10. Myocardium, left ventricle, showing invasion with resulting destruction of myofibers by tumor. Note the continuity of the tumor with the endocardial lesion at its margin. Male BUF rat 99 weeks of age, treated with injections of 2,7-FAA. H & E × 54.

transplantable at a stage when only a minimal increase of the cellularity of the nerve had developed (118). Based on the success of their transplantation experiments with this lesion, the authors concluded that the preceding changes

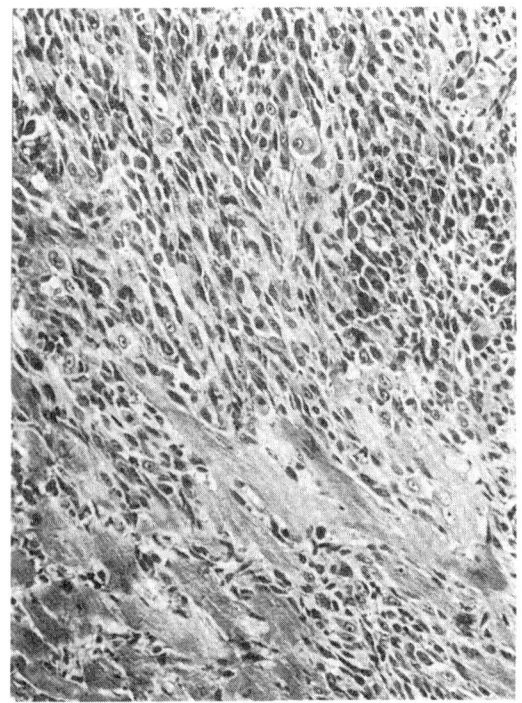

Figure 11. Cellular details of the tumor shown in Figure 10. The tumor cells are of varying size and shape with large hyperchromic nuclei. H & E × 220.

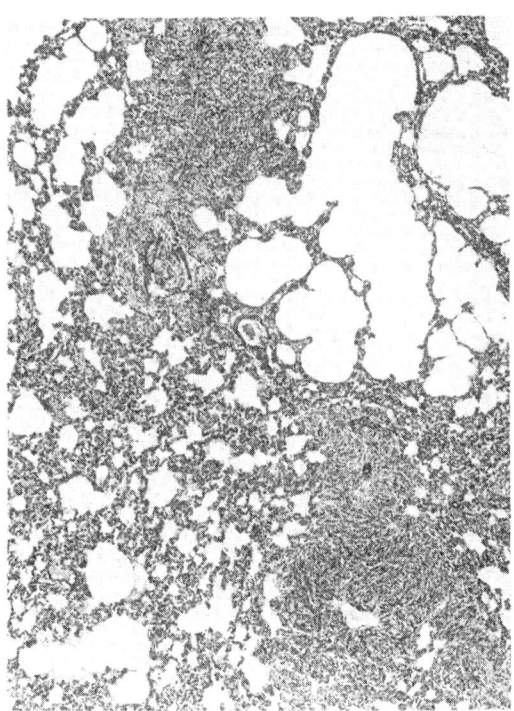

Figure 12. Lung. Numerous metastatic nodules from tumor shown in Figures 10 and 11. H & E × 54.

represent a genuine neoplastic transformation rather than a preneoplastic process. Transplantation of endocardial tumors has not as yet been attempted at any stage of their development. This should encourage investigators to attempt transplantation of the early cardiac *in situ* lesion which we believe does in time progress to the exophytic and infiltrating and metastasizing neoplasms.

Most rats with induced cardiac tumors also had tumors at other primary sites; most of these were diagnosed as neurogenic, hepatic, gastro-intestinal or mammary tumors.

The cytogenesis of the endocardial tumors is not yet unequivocally established. On the basis of the overwhelming numbers of cells with the typical Anitschkow cell nuclear morphology, Morris and associates (87), Vesselinovitch and Mihailovich (129), and Kommineni and associates (65) reported their cardiac tumors under the designation of Anitschkow cell sarcoma. Druckrey and associates, in their early work (26, 27) and Schreiber and associates (102–104) reported their cardiac tumors as sarcoma, not otherwise specified, or as fibrosarcoma. Only later did Druckrey and associates (29) classify the cardiac tumors, that they had induced by a single administration of ENU, as neuromas or neurosarcomas. These diagnoses were based in part on the morphology of the tumor and in part were influenced by analogy to the proven neurotropic property of ENU. Of the ENU-induced tumors at various sites in 296 rats, 144 were primary in brain, 70 in spinal cord, 89 in cranial nerves, and 140 in peripheral nerves. Ivankovic and associates (58) and Berman and associates (8) also classified the cardiac tumors they found in rats as neurogenic in type. Mennel, (84), studied by light-microscopy 17 cardiac tumors, provided by Druckrey, that had been induced by administration by different routes of the neurotropic carcinogens ENU (11 cases), ENB (2 cases), triazene derivatives (2 cases), methyl-benzyl-hydrazine (transplacental, 1 case), and DEN (transplacental, 1 case). He divided the tumors into 2 groups: In one, "the morphologic properties of neurinoma were still detectable," the other consisted of sarcomas "which could arise by extensive de-differentiation from neurinomas, or they could as well be of primarily connective tissue nature."

Hoch-Ligeti and associates (50) reported that one of the histologic patterns, duplicated repeatedly in endocardial tumors induced by carbamate derivatives, is a herringbone arrangement of the cells in the deeper layer of the lesion. This pattern might be misinterpreted as the parallel bundles and fibers designated the Antoni type A tissue, which is the most constant but least significant diagnostic feature of schwannoma. Absent, however, from these endocardial tumors were features that are pathognomonic of schwannoma, including palisading of nuclei, Verocay bodies, Antoni type B tissue, pigmented regions, foci of degeneration which progress to the formation of small cysts, and neoplastic lipoid-containing pseudo-xanthomatous cells. From comparison of the endocardial tumors of rats and mice with schwannomas primary in cranial and spinal nerves at various sites, we have concluded that the cardiac tumors are not schwannomas but instead mesenchymal type tumors.

Holzhausen and Schreiber (53) studied by electron-microscopy incipient cardiac tumors induced by MNU, and confirmed the subendocardial location of the lesion. They concluded that the tumors "probably developed from neoplastic Schwann cells, but an additional mesenchymal component seems to be engaged." Also on the basis of EM studies, Berman and associates (8) concluded without reservation that the cells composing the cardiac tumors induced by AMMN in Sprague-Dawley rats are of Schwann cell origin. On the other hand Lewis (70), from his EM examination of cardiac tumors in untreated Wistar rats concluded that the neoplastic cells are of the fibroblast type. Berman and associates (8) based their diagnosis on the EM observation of basal membranes on the surface of the tumor cells and of "convoluted plasma membranes." Basal membranes are, however, observed also on fibroblastic cells, endothelial cells and smooth muscle cells (35).

There is thus lack of unanimity as to the cell of origin of the cardiac tumor. This result is not unexpected, since even by extensive light- and electron-microscopic investigations of the cells of tumors classified as peripheral neurinomas induced in rats by the administration of MNU, the origin of the neoplastic cells from Schwann cells could, in the opinion of Jänisch and associates (59), be demonstrated in only 3 tumors. Russell and Rubinstein (98) in their discussion of the cytohistogenesis of tumors diagnosed as neurinoma in the human "placed the debate firmly between the Schwann cell and the perineural cell, both of which possess a distinctive basal membrane. In conclusion, regarding the peripheral neurinomas, the debate remains open." Based on their electron-microscopic studies of tissue culture cells derived from malignant nerve sheath tumors induced in rats by transplacental administration of ENU, Conley and associates (20) advanced the concept that "Schwann cells and perineural fibroblasts are functional variants of the same cell type."

A soluble protein, S-100, characteristic for the nervous tissue, was described by Moore in 1965. This protein was demonstrated by a microcomplement fixation method in 21 of 22 tumors of the peripheral nervous system induced in the rat by MNU or ENU (135). The technique might be applied to a study of the endocardial tumors in order to investigate further the possibility of their origin from Schwann cells. Recently, however, Weiss and associates (136), in an evaluation of the accuracy of S-100 protein in the diagnosis of soft tissue tumors, concluded that, although S-100 protein is characteristic of neural crest-derived tumors, it is not restricted to them, since occasionally several types of mesenchymal tumor may show cells immunoreactive to S-100 protein.

The endocardial tumor of the rat considered in this publication appears to be a unique and characteristic tumor of this species. The question arises whether all induced cardiac tumors in the rat are endocardial or whether some might arise from tissues in other locations within the heart.

Several publications lack details in regard to the anatomical location and histologic characteristics of the cardiac tumors which arose spontaneously or were induced. The location of the majority of spontaneous cardiac tumors in the endocardium is suggested by their designation as endocardial disease, endocardial fibrosis, endocardial thickening, endocardial fibromatous proliferation. An exception is the report by Robertson and Associates (95), who located within the myocardium the tumors they designated as schwannoma.

A description of the condition of the endocardium is lacking in several reports of induced cardiac tumors. Thus Vesselinovitch and Mikhailovich (129) did not describe the endocardium in their report while they state that "careful inspection of the heart muscle revealed in several instances the presence of greyish 2–3 mm nodules." Similarly, the endocardium was not described by Mennel (84) in his detailed light-microscopic study of the morphology of the cardiac tumors that Druckrey and associates had induced by a variety of mostly neurogenic carcinogens.

In 1976, Schreiber and associates reported a careful anatomical and light-microscopic study of cardiac tumors that had been induced by intravenous, intraperitoneal, subcutaneous or transplacental administration of MNU and ENU to 590 BDIX rats, whose average age at death was 287 days. After excluding the animals with inflammatory changes in the endo-, myo- or pericardium, 66 rats remained with cardiac tumors, of which 22 were of considerable size. The less advanced tumors were confined exclusively to the subendocardium; none originated in the myocardium. A study of the advanced tumors revealed their progression from the endocardium to involve the myocardium. Only 4 tumors "exhibited an unusual localisation; 3 infiltrated the mural and septal myocardium without involvement of the endocardium, and one infiltrated diffusely the myocardium."

Of the 50 cardiac tumors of the rat that we have examined, in all but 5 the direct evolution of the tumor from a proliferative lesion of the endocardium was clearly evident. With these 5 exceptions we could not determine whether the tumor originated in the endocardial lesion or whether the endocardial lesion was independent of the myocardial tumor or whether the latter had infiltrated the endocardium secondarily. All 5 hearts exhibited endocardial proliferation

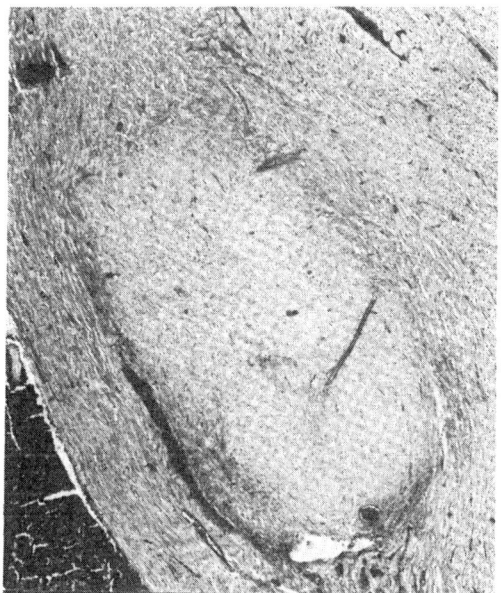

Figure 13. Wall, left ventricle with moderately well circumscribed tumor. Male Wistar rat, 25 weeks of age, had ingested a diet containing 3,3-diphenyl-3-pyrrolidine-carbonyloxy)-1-propyne. H & E × 38.

of some degree either at the margin or within the immediate vicinity of the myocardial tumor or at some distance from it. Figures 13 and 14 illustrate one such myocardial tumor. The endocardium showed marked subendothelial proliferation. We have, however, no example of a heart with a tumor of any dimension in which the endocardium was completely free of the proliferative lesion. This, of course, is apart from the non-endocardial type tumors listed near the bottom of Table 3.

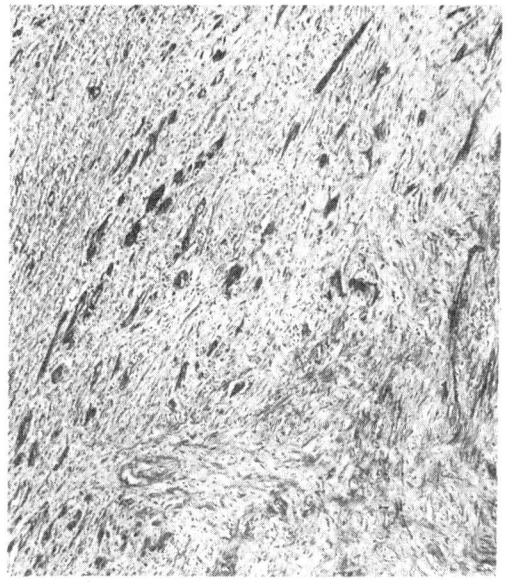

Figure 14. Details at the upper margin of the tumor shown in Figure 13. The spindle-shaped tumor cells are separated by numerous collagen bundles. H & E × 120.

The rarity of tumors of the heart in untreated rats has been explained in part by the relative weight of the heart to total body weight; in man, the heart constitutes 0.4 to 0.5% of the body weight (6). However, the adrenal gland weighs much less than the heart, yet primary tumors and metastases, e.g., of pulmonary cancer to adrenal gland are common. Genetic factors, such as strain and sex, physical factors such as the continuous movement of the heart, and biochemical factors, such as the specific tissue metabolism of the myocardial tissue, may influence the development of cardiac tumors.

In studies of the manner by which nitrosourea, nitrosamines and related compounds may exert, at the molecular level, their carcinogenic activity, Druckrey and associates (24, 25, 30) and Preussmann and associates (90) demonstrated that enzymatic dealkylation, probably initiated by α-C-hydroxylation and subsequent degradation of the resulting alkyl compound, produce the respective alkyldiazonium as the proximate carcinogen. The production of alkyldiazonium is a common feature of this group of indirect carcinogens. MNU is, however, unstable and does not require enzymatic activation to react with cellular components. Magee and Farber (79) had shown that DMN is enzymatically degraded to the diazonium compound, with consecutive methylation of guanine in the nucleic acid, a process assumed to represent the formation of the ultimate carcinogen. The proximate carcinogen for AAF and related compounds is the 7-OH derivative of these chemicals (85).

The increasing number of spontaneous endocardial tumors reported since 1973 suggests the possibility of the introduction into the laboratory environment of rats of an agent or agents not previously present. In this connection the ubiquitous asbestos and other durable fibrous materials which had been shown to induce tumors in the lung and the pleura (17, 113, 133) were found by us to be associated with the induction of cardiac tumors (51). The dimensions of the fibers associated with the induction of cardiac tumors were in the same range as those found to be carcinogenic for the lung and pleura of rats (113).

Hemangioendothelioma

Among the accessions of the Registry of the AFIP is a hemangioendothelioma within the cardiac septum. In 1968, Schardein and associates described under the term endothelioma a cardiac tumor in a 455-day-old female Sprague-Dawley rat which according to their statement "consisted of a small focus of vascular spaces lined by hyperplastic and hypertrophied endothelial cells and was classified as endothelioma." From their description we would designate the tumor as hemangioendothelioma.

Tumors of the pericardium

Primary tumors of the pericardium are exceedingly rare, while tumors primary in the mediastinum, pleura or lung of rats may secondarily invade cardiac tissues. Stula (117) reported an unusual combination of a pulmonary adenocarcinoma with extension into the pleural cavity and in addition the rat "had a benign pleural and epicardial meso-

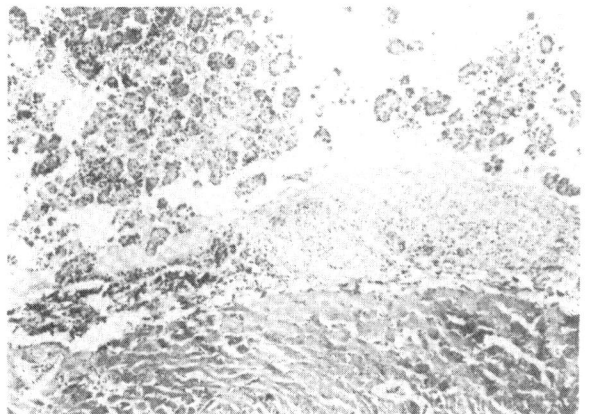

Figure 15. Visceral pericardium of the left ventricle covered by biphasic mesothelioma. Female Osborne-Mendel rat, 16 months of age, received an intrathoracic implant of a pellet of aluminum-zirconium. H & E × 80.

thelioma." The photomicrograph illustrates a biphasic, papillary and fibrous tumor covering the visceral pericardial surfaces. This rat was one of 6 with primary pulmonary tumors, out of a group of 365 untreated Charles River rats about 2 years of age. Accessed at the NCI Registry are 2 rats with fibro-papillary tumors, which cover the visceral pericardium. They had been treated with MOCA (4,4′-methylene-bis-2-chloroaniline), both had pulmonary tumors, one of which was confined to the lung, while other infiltrated the mediastinum.

In an Osborne-Mendel female rat treated with intrathoracic implantation of aluminum-zirconium, accessed in the NCI Registry, a diffuse biphasic tumor lined the visceral pericardium (Figure 15). The papillary formations were generally capped by a single layer of flattened or cuboidal cells, which only rarely were in mitosis, while the sarcomatous areas consisted of multiple layers of elongated fibroblast-like cells, many of which were in mitosis. This rat also had an adenocarcinoma of the lung. Whether a tumor of the pericardium in the presence of a primary tumor in a neighborhood structure can be accepted as being a primary mesothelioma reopens an old problem. After studying tumors diagnosed as mesotheliomas in man and in domestic animals, Willis (139) and Leinati (69), respectively, concluded that many such tumors are misdiagnosed and are instead metastatic from primary tumors elsewhere. Saphir (100) insisted that tumors designated as mesothelioma of a serosal surface should be only when tumors of other primary sites had been excluded. Since 1961, owing to the detailed morphological and chemical studies of mesotheliomas of humans exposed to asbestos (17, 133) and of rodents exposed to asbestos (113, 132) or treated with polyoma virus (112), pathologists nowadays have become more confident in the differential diagnosis of mesothelioma than were those of earlier years. With humans, the differential diagnosis rarely involves more than the distinction between the serosal tumor and a primary tumor of one other site. By contrast, in dealing with rodents with mesotheliomas, the problem is more complicated, since treatment with carcinogenic agents usually results in the induction of tumors at multiple primary sites. Particularly complicating its differential diag-

nosis in rodents is the combination of a primary lung tumor with mesothelioma of the pericardium or pleura.

Atrio-caval epithelial mesothelioma (primary epithelial tumor, endodermal inclusion, atrioventricular node tumor)

This unusual cardiac tumor occurs in the right atrium or inferior vena cava of certain rats. From the examination of the smallest detectable lesions, Goodall and associates (38, 39) determined that the tumor arises in equal numbers at either of two sites, in the endocardial aspect of the right atrium involving the atrioventricular node or in the inferior vena cava. From these locations, the early growth, as it enlarges, spreads within the wall of the atrium to form a large tumor. The tumors are composed of cystic, alveolar or tubular structures embedded in fibrous stroma. These structures are lined by single or multiple layers of flattened cuboidal, columnar or squamoid epithelial type cells. The cell nuclei are large, centrally located, and have a single prominent nucleolus. Many epithelial cells contain mucus, several are ciliated. On electron-microscopic study, the epithelial cells have microvilli and a well developed basal membrane surrounding the alveoli. Fine reticulin fibers surround the cells. Groups of epithelial-like cells, similar to those which line the alveolar structures, may be found scattered through the fibrous stroma. The lumen of the alveolar and tubular structures may contain mucus, granular or amorphous acidophilic material and desquamated cells. In areas, the histologic pattern of the tumor resembles hemangioendothelioma, but the channels do not contain blood.

This histologic type of tumor was first described in the heart of a man by Armstrong and Mönckeberg (3), who classified it as a lymphangio-endothelioma. Although the morphology of every reported tumor of this type is the same, the proper designation and histogenesis are matters of disagreement. Rezek (93) opined that the tumor develops as a dysgenetic endodermal tumor, derived from fetal inclusion of neighboring endodermal tissues, such as the thyroid gland or the tracheo-bronchial tract. This theory of Rezek (93), that the tumor originates from embryonal displacement of endodermal tissues was supported by Willis (140), who considered the foregut as the possible origin of these elements foreign to the heart. The endodermal origin of the tumor *versus* a mesothelial origin, which was suggested by Mahaim (80) is now more generally accepted (9, 54, 71, 109). The mucin-producing and ciliated columnar epithelial cells are difficult to explain as of mesothelial or endothelial derivation, and their presence in this location strongly suggests an endodermal origin. The subject was recently reviewed by Travers (126). As with the atrio-caval tumor in man, the origin of this tumor in the rat is thought to lie in an embryonic anomaly which occurs at the earliest development of the cardiovascular system before the thoracic mesenchymal block divides.

In the inbred strain NZR/Gd rat, a genetically determined occurrence of these tumors was reported by Goodall and associates (38, 39). The tumor was present in several consecutive generations in about 12% of the male and 4% of the female rats over one year of age. The tumor could be diagnosed clinically when it caused cardiac failure, as it often did. The localizations of this tumor of the rat differ from

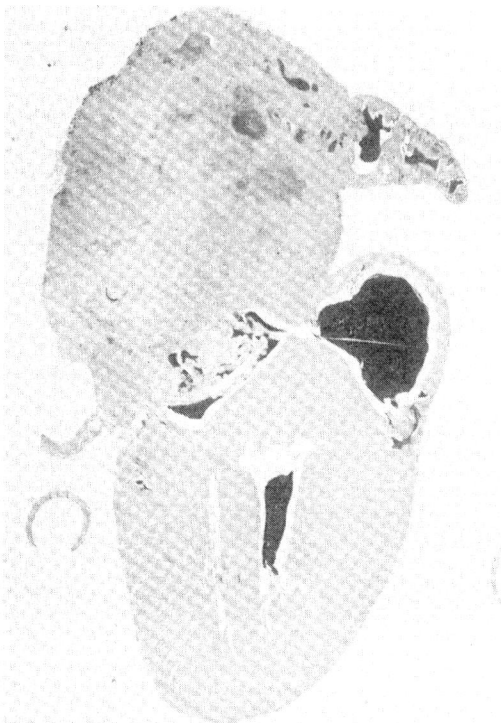

Figure 16. Right atrium with atrio-caval "mesothelioma." The right atrium is largely replaced by a large tumor mass. The wall of the right ventricle is hypertrophied. Male Charles River rat, 18 months of age had ingested a diet containing 25 ppm ETU (ethylthiourea). H & E × 9.5.

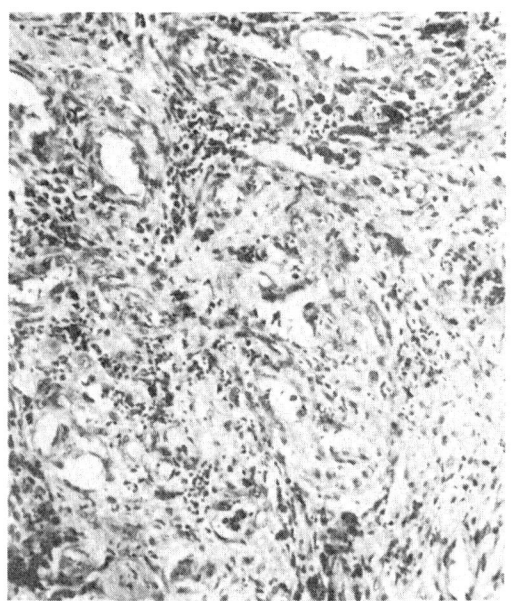

Figure 17. Details of tumor shown in Figure 16. There is a mixed vascular and glandular pattern with infiltration of small round cells. H & E × 220.

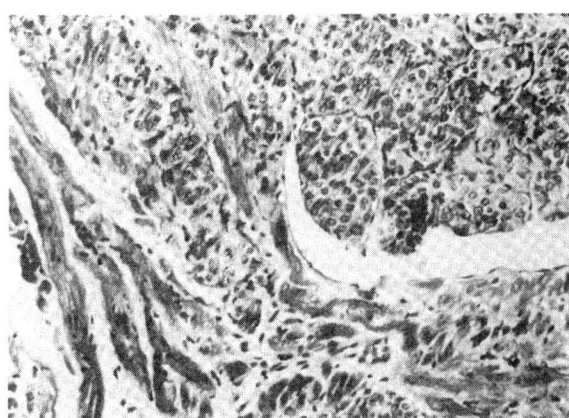

Figure 18. Aortic body tumor. The pattern consists of cell-balls delineated by thin connective tissue. The tumor has invaded the myocardium of the right auricle. WAG/Rij rat, 23 months of age, treated with 15 meV neutrons, 50 rad. H & E × 220.

those of the human counterpart. In the human they are located always in the atrioventricular septum. In the rat they are located in about equal numbers in the atrioventricular septum or in the inferior vena cava. Large tumors in rats often involve the pericardium and are the cause of voluminous blood-stained pericardial effusions. Occasionally, small tumor nodules are situated on the pericardium. The tumor spread in 11 (22%) of NZR/Gd rats to several different sites including lung, pleura, pericardium, mesentery, lymph nodes, liver and bone. In about one third of the number of rats with the cardiac tumor, there were associated primary tumors at other sites. Remarkably, a hepatic collagen storage disease was also found to be hereditary in the inbred strain NZR/Gd rat (39).

Only relatively few examples of the isolated occurrence of this atrioventricular tumor in other strains of rats have been reported. Sharma (105) reported, under the designation mesothelioma, a tumor in the right atrium of an untreated 543-day-old Charles River-COBS-CD rat.

Among the accessions at the NCI Registry is an unpublished example of the atrio-caval tumor of a rat, which demonstrates well the morphology of this tumor (Figures 17 and 18). The tumor developed in an 18-month-old male Charles River rat, which had ingested drinking water containing 25 ppm ETU (ethylthiourea). The occurrence of this single cardiac tumor among a group of rats similarly treated argues against the treatment as being the cause of the tumor. This type of tumor had never previously been induced.

We think that, of the numerous designations applied to this tumor, mesothelioma is the least fortunate and should be avoided, since a mesothelial origin of the tumor is not proven and the term mesothelioma is regularly applied to tumors of the serosal surfaces of the pleura, peritoneum and pericardium.

Tumors of the aortic body (paraganglioma, chemodectoma, glomus tumor)

Gilbert and Gillman (36) reported a paraganglioma of the heart in one of 1342 Wistar rats, between 20 and 22 months of age. Trevino and Nessmith (127) reported an aortic body tumor in a 3-year-old albino rat, strain not given. In both reports, a description of the tumors was not detailed.

The morphology of the normal aortic body of the rat and the hyperplastic and neoplastic changes that develop in it were described by van Zwieten and associates (130). Van Zwieten studied the aortic-pulmonary paraganglia in untreated rats, maintained for aging studies, and in rats that were subjected to different experimental procedures in connection with a study of the development of mammary tumors. Aortic bodies were investigated in 56 rats of 3 strains. Paraganglia in man are formed by two types of cells (37). The most numerous are the chief, or type 1, cells which are round, oval or polygonal, rather large, with well defined cytoplasmic borders and slightly basophilic, often foamy or granular cytoplasm. Argyrophilic cytoplasmic granules are demonstrable in the chief cells. The nuclei are oval and contain a single nucleolus with finely stippled chromatin. Fine reticulin and collagen fibers surround the cells. Type 2 or sustentacular cells have scanty basophilic cytoplasm with small hyperchromic lenticular or oval nucleus. The cells are arranged in small nests, "Zellballen," separated by thin fibrous tissue in which numerous small vessels are present. Formalin-induced fluorescence, although present in some paraganglia could not be demonstrated in the aortic body tumors. Electron-dense membrane-bound granules were shown in the chief cells, which indicates that these cells belong to the APUD cell system. The cells in a hyperplastic nodule of the aortic body are vacuolated, a feature lacking in the neoplastic nodule. The majority of the tumors is benign, and the cells are infrequently in mitosis. Tumors classified as malignant show increasing nuclear abnormalities and large numbers of mitotic figures and they invade the surrounding tissue. Van Zwieten and associates (130) did not identify metastases at remote sites, but they did quote a personal communication from Quast and Jersey, who found pulmonary metastases of an aortic chemodectoma in rat descendent of the Sprague-Dawley line. A strong strain and sex predilection for development of aortic body tumors was evidenced by the occurrence of hyperplastic and neoplastic lesions in the aortic body of 33 of 34 WAG/Rij strain rats; 32 were females. A genetic control of these lesions awaits study.

An aortic body tumor in a rat exposed to X-rays is accessed at the NCI Registry (Figure 18).

Secondary tumors of the heart

Wilens and Sproul (138), in a report of 17 rats with leukemia, identified 2 small collections of neoplastic cells in the subendocardial and interstitial tissues of the heart. These authors also reported a cardiac metastasis from an osteosarcoma.

The almost non-occurrence of secondary tumors of the heart in the rat is surprising, in view of the fact that both in man and in mice the number of secondary tumors greatly exceeds that of primary tumors of the heart.

CARDIAC TUMORS IN MICE

Primary cardiac tumors in mice, whether spontaneous or

induced, are exceedingly rare. This fact is the more noteworthy because spontaneous tumors of the heart of rats have been reported with increasing frequency since 1973, and beginning in 1967, cardiac tumors have been induced with nitrosourea, nitrosamine and other carcinogenic agents.

Cloudman, (19), was the first to report a primary cardiac tumor in a mouse. The tumor arose in an untreated mouse and was diagnosed rhabdomyosarcoma. In 1975, Szepsenwol and Boschetti (121) reported rhabdomyosarcomas of the heart of one male 405 days of age and one female 604 days of age 2TM strain of mouse. These had been maintained on a Purina chow diet, supplemented in one with refined corn oil, and in the other with corn oil and fatty acid. The tumors metastasized to the lung in both mice, and to the kidney of the female. The same authors reported two mice with subcutaneous tumors which had metastasized to a number of sites one of which was the heart. One of these subcutaneous tumors, which they diagnosed as rhabdomyosarcoma, arose at the site of an injection of 30ug Delestrogen (estradiol 17-n-valerate).

The largest number of primary cardiac tumors in mice, 7 in all, and all from the NCI Registry accessions, was reported by Hoch-Ligeti and Stewart in 1984 (52). Five were from the experiments of Lorenz and associates (72) and had received a cumulative dose of whole body irradiation which ranged up to 1500 R (Roentgens).

Mesenchymal cell sarcoma

There were 3 mesenchymal cell sarcomas, two of which arose in irradiated mice, and one in a mouse treated with 2,5,7-dibenz(a)-anthracene. The tumors infiltrated deeply

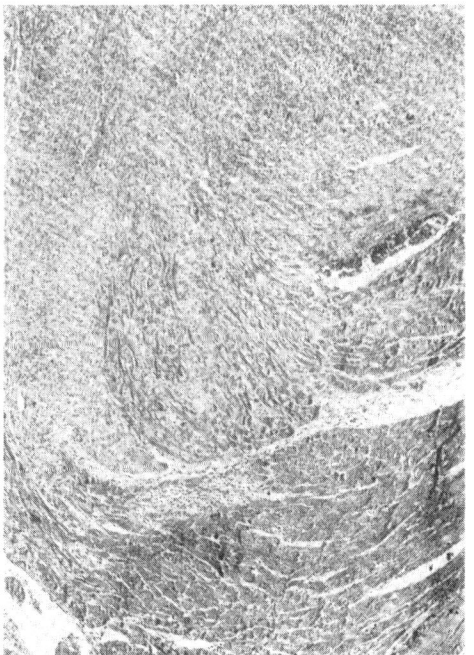

Figure 19. Apex, right ventricle with large mesenchymal cell sarcoma infiltrating myocardium. (C57XA) F_1 male mouse, 25 months of age, received a total of 179 R gamma radiation. H & E × 54.

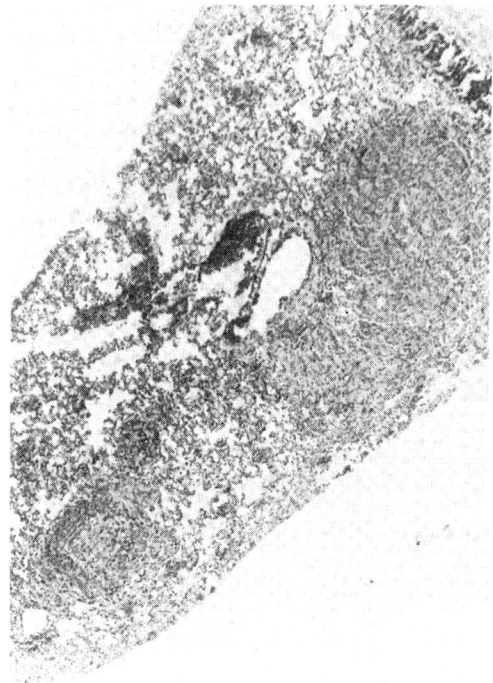

Figure 20. Lung. Multiple metastases from the cardiac tumor shown in Figure 19. H & E × 54.

the cardiac musculature and one of these formed multiple deposits in the left ventricular myocardium (Figures 19–23). All three metastasized to the lung, two to the kidney, and one to the spleen. These highly malignant tumors were composed of poorly differentiated loosely arranged cells, which varied from round to elongated, and from quite small to very large, bizarre giant cells (Figure 24). Hyperchromatic nuclei nearly filled the small cells to the exclusion of the cytoplasm, whereas the large cells had abundant acidophilic cytoplasm, which was often elongated into a strap-like formation. No PAS positive material and no longitudinal or cross striation could be demonstrated in the cytoplasm.

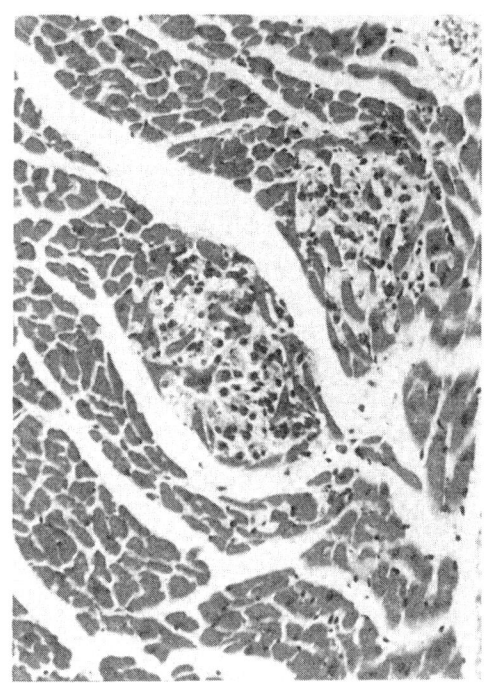

Figure 22. Left ventricular myocardium with multiple tumor deposits. Same mouse as in Figure 21. H & E × 220.

Many large cells were multinucleated, the single hyperchromic nuclei were often ballooning, and the nucleoli were dense and prominent. Mitotic figures were numerous and generally confined to the small cell type. Very scanty collagen and few reticulum fibers were present.

Mesenchymoma

A well circumscribed mesenchymoma in the heart of a $B_6C_3F_1$ male mouse treated with gamma radiation was located in the interatrial septum and protruded into the

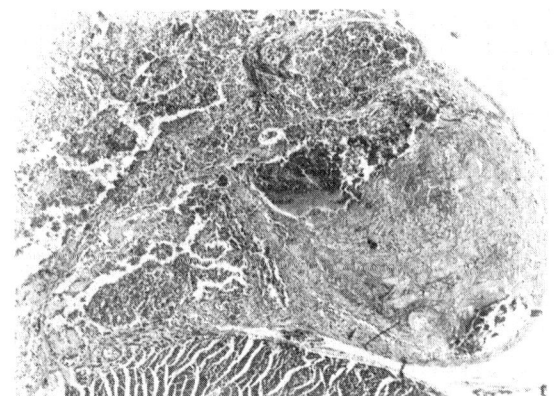

Figure 21. Right atrium with mesenchymal cell sarcoma. Tumor tissue has infiltrated the wall of the atrium and along with a thrombus fills the chamber. C_3HB female mouse, 25 months of age, received whole-body irradiation of 4.4 R X-rays daily. H & E × 38.

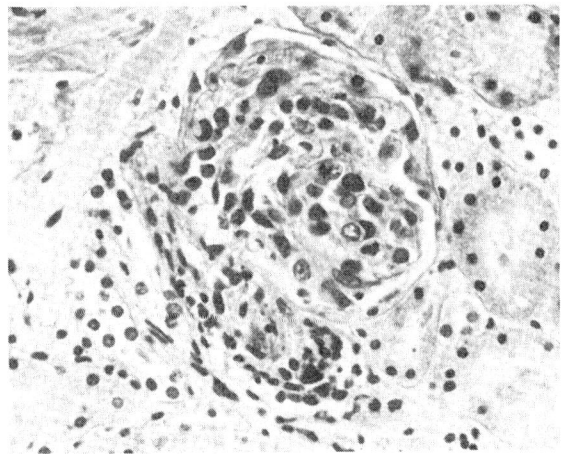

Figure 23. Mesangium of the renal glomerulus contains large, bizarre cells from the mesenchymal cell sarcoma of the heart. Same mouse as in Figures 21 and 22. H & E × 500.

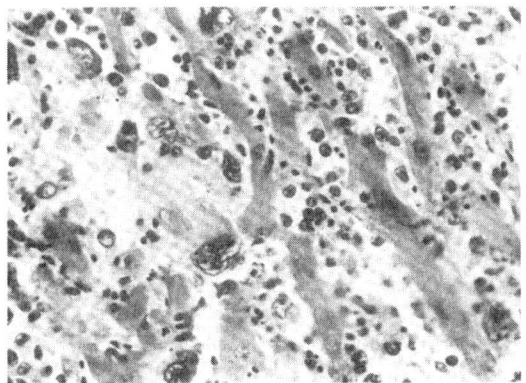

Figure 24. Wall, left ventricle with mesenchymal cell sarcoma. The tumor cells vary greatly in size and shape and have bizarre nuclei. Male DBA mouse, 13 months of age, had for 11 months ingested 0.2 mg DBA/ml of aqueous olive oil emulsion substituted for drinking water. H 7 E × 240

distended right atrium (Figure 25). The tumor was composed of an irregular arrangement of fibrous and vascular tissue with foci of cartilage and calcifying osteoid and with an intermingling of round, oval, spindle-shaped and stellate neoplastic cells that exhibited a moderate range of variation in size and staining characteristics. There was an associated infiltration of lymphocytes, plasma cells and iron-containing histiocytes.

Hemangioendothelioma

Three mice, one untreated and two irradiated had hemangioendothelioma of the myocardium (Figure 26). In one

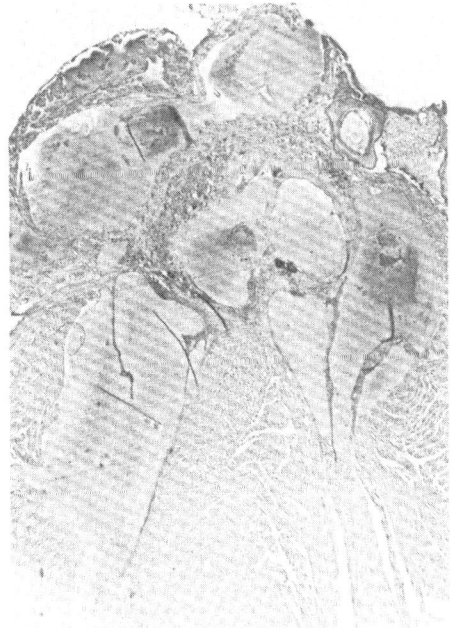

Figure 25. Base of heart. A mesenchymoma, located cranial to the atrio-ventricular septum, protrudes into the right atrium. Male $B_6C_3F_1$ mouse treated with gamma radiation. H & E × 16.

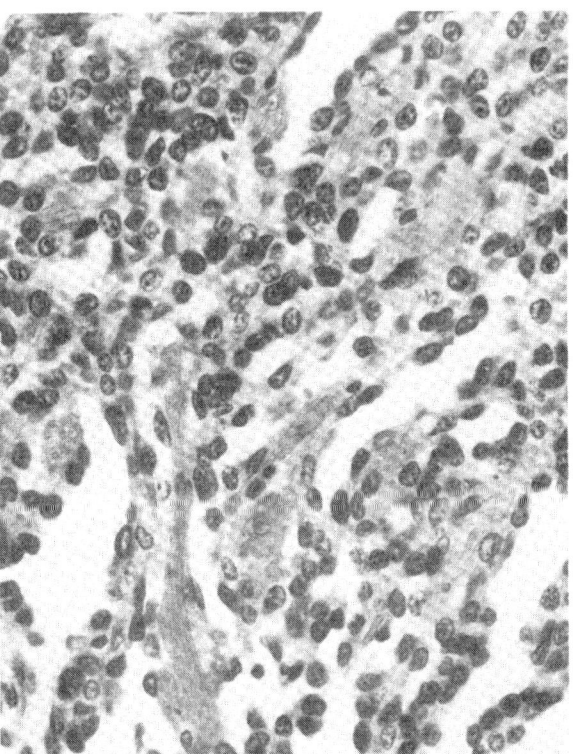

Figure 26. Wall of right ventricle with hemangioendothelioma. Female C_3Hb mouse, 13 months of age, treated with 100 R X-rays. H & E × 500.

mouse the heart and no other site was involved by hemangioendothelioma. The other two mice had in addition to the cardiac tumor, hemangioendotheliomas in the liver, intestine, kidney, spleen, adrenal gland and bone marrow. Since all the tumors were of similar size, the probability of multicentric tumors of these different sites was strongly suggested. The possibility could not, however, be ruled out that a single primary hemangioendothelioma had yielded multiple metastases, including those to the heart.

In mice, exposed to inhalation of air which contained 1,3-butadiene in concentration of 0.625 or 1250 parts per million, large numbers of cardiac hemangiosarcomas were induced (55a). Hemangiosarcomas were present also in the liver, lung and kidney, and these tumors were considered to be metastatic from the heart. Several other types of primary tumors were induced in many organs.

Reticulum cell neoplasms and lymphomas of the heart

Two tumors of the heart were classified as reticulum cell neoplasm type B, and one other as reticulum cell neoplasm, not otherwise specified (Figure 27). This latter tumor was similar histologically to a neoplasm given this diagnosis by Dunn (31). Of the former two neoplasms, one arose in a strain I male mouse 6 months of age that had ingested methylcholanthrene, and the other in a strain $B_6C_3F_1$ female mouse exposed to fast neutrons. The mouse with the reticulum cell neoplasm NOS, was a 23-month-old untreated BALB/c mouse. One reticulum cell type B neoplasm, a large

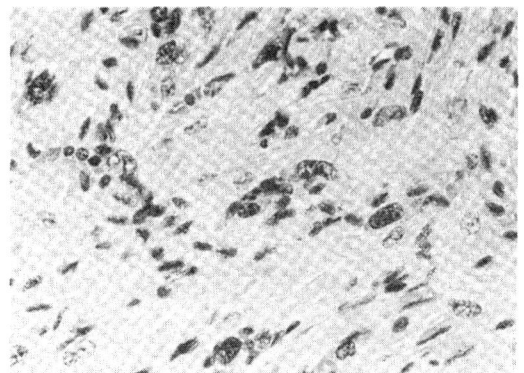

Figure 27. Wall, left ventricle, infiltrated with reticulum cell sarcoma (NOS) along the course of the vessel. BALB/c mouse, 23 months of age, untreated. H & E × 330.

circumscribed tumor, occurred in the right auricle of a female mouse. The other two tumors diffusely infiltrated the myocardium of all cardiac chambers. The blood in the sections of two mice contained neoplastic cells. The question arises, in dealing with disseminated tumors of these types, whether a single deposit at a given site like the heart represents a spread from tumor deposits at other sites in the same mouse or an original tumor of multifocal origin. One thing is striking, that despite the frequency with which mice of various strains are affected with disseminated neoplasms of the hematopoietic lympho-reticular types, the only mice with tumors of this classification involving the heart to be reported to date are the 3 reported herein.

Huff and associates (1985) found that the malignant lymphomas, induced by inhalation of 1,3-butadiene, which appeared to originate in the thymus, involved also the heart together with spleen, lymph nodes, liver, pancreas and stomach (55a).

Mesothelioma of the pericardium

Stanton and associates, (112), described wart-like papillary mesotheliomas involving the serosal surfaces of the peritoneum, pleura and pericardium in strain Swiss Albino mice which in late fetal life had been inoculated with tissue-culture preparations of polyoma virus. The authors did not give the relative frequencies of tumors of the three different sites, although apparently the pleura was the site most commonly involved. The tumors were never very large or numerous, and often showed evidence of regression.

Secondary cardiac tumors in mice

With mice, as with some other animal species secondary tumors of the heart, while infrequent, occur more often than do primary tumors. In mice the majority of the tumors, that have metastasized to the heart were primary in the lung. Campbell, (14), reported the first such example in a mouse among a group in which he had induced pulmonary tumors in 26/78 by exposure to inhalation of tar-free road dust. The tumors in two mice had metastasized, in both to the kidneys and one also to the heart.

Wells, Slye and Holmes (137) reported the spontaneous tumors in 147,132 mice that were allowed to live out their entire life span. Lung tumors were found in 2,865(2%), and of these 104(3.6%) metastasized, all to the mediastinal lymph nodes, chest wall and diaphragm, and 10 to distant sites, 3(0.1%) of which had metastasized to the heart.

Biancifiori (10) induced pulmonary tumors in 25/25 breeding female mice with daily intragastric administration of hydrazine sulfate in a 1.3% aqueous solution. Fifteen of the tumors spread locally, 3 metastasized to the adrenal gland and one metastasized to the heart.

Turusov and associates (128) reported an uncommonly high frequency of cardiac metastases from pulmonary tumors in CF_1 mice. In the largest group of 668 untreated CF_1 mice, 281(42%) developed lung tumors and of these, metastases to other sites were present in 5(1.8%), in one of which the heart was a site of metastasis (0.36% of the lung tumors). Pulmonary tumors developed in 1,206(43.7%) of 2,764 mice treated with DDT, and of these 43(3.6%) metastasized, 12(1.0%) to the heart. Urethan treatment of 555 mice induced pulmonary tumors in 442(80%), of which 17(3.9%) metastasized, 10(2.3%) to the heart.

In mice of two strains, squamous cell carcinoma and alveolar cell adenocarcinoma were induced by intratracheal administration of 3-methylcholanthrene (48). Of 234 $B_6C_3F_1$ mice examined, 172 had squamous cell carcinomas of the lung, of which 90 either invaded adjacent tissues or metastasized: "The most prominent route of metastases was by direct invasion of the pulmonary vein with extension to the left atrium of the heart." The number of mice with heart tumor or how many heart tumors was the result of direct invasion was, however, not stated.

Reznik (94) reported that out of an unstated number of $B_6C_3F_1$ mice, two developed pulmonary tumors that metastasized to the left cardiac chamber.

Among the accession of the NCI Registry, are 12 mice of

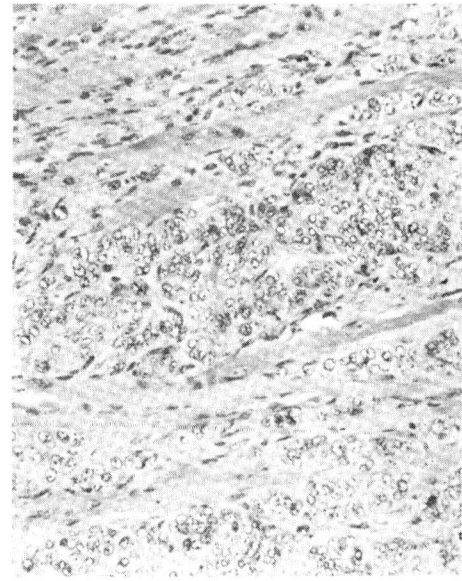

Figure 28. Interventricular septum, with metastases of pulmonary alveologenic carcinoma. Male $B_6C_3F_1$, 24 months of age, untreated. H & E × 220.

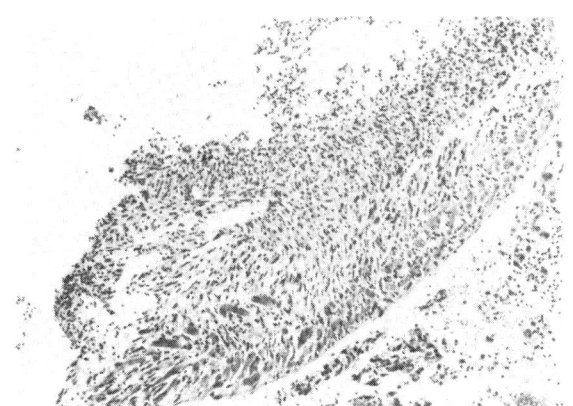

Figure 29. Right ventricle. Metastases from subcutaneous sarcoma. Female C₅₇bl mouse, treated twice weekly for 8 months with topical applications of 5,9,10-trimethyl-1,1-benzanthracene (0.06% in benzene). H & E × 130.

a number of different strains with metastatic tumors of the heart, from alveologenic carcinoma, squamous cell carcinoma, or carcinoasarcoma of the lung (Figure 28). The three mice with squamous cell carcinoma had received intratracheal instillations of 3-methylcholanthrene. Of the remaining 9 mice, five had been treated with ionizing radiation, two underwent some type of surgical procedure, and two were untreated. With two exceptions, the metastases to the heart were associated with extension of the pulmonary tumor onto the pleura and with metastases to lymph nodes and remote organs. Tumors at sites other than lung have also metastasized to the heart. One 6th-generation subcutaneous transplant of a uterine sarcoma metastasized to the heart. Subcutaneous sarcomas in four mice metastasized to the heart; two mice had been irradiated (400R), and two had been painted on the skin with 5,9,10-trimethyl-1,2-benzanthracene (Figure 29). Topical application of this chemical carcinogen induced, in a large number of mice, squamous cell carcinoma, sarcoma and mixed carcinosarcomas (46); it also stimulated an increase in the number of

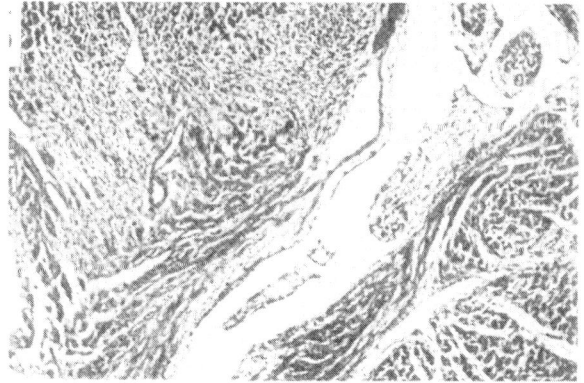

Figure 30. Left ventricle. Poorly defined nodule of rhabdomyoma with vacuolated cells. Male hybrid guinea pig, 14 months of age, ingested DEN in drinking water (calculated total 160 mg). H & E × 35.

melanoblasts in the dermis, resulting in the accumulation subcutaneous tissue of large collections of melanophores filled with melanin pigment (61/90 tumor-bearing animals). With one possible exception, none of the induced tumors were classified as melanomas.

It is noteworthy to consider that over the years many of the subcutaneous sarcomas which have been induced with benzanthracene derivatives have metastasized to various sites, but only these two have metastasized to the heart. The question whether subcutaneous sarcomas induced by 5,9,10-trimethyl-1,2-benzanthracene possess a unique ability to metastasize to the heart because of their association with stimulated melanoblasts and the presence of melanotic foci in the subcutaneous tissues, is intriguing if one recalls the high degree of metastatic potentialities of melanoma in man.

CARDIAC TUMORS IN GUINEA PIGS

Lymphosarcoma, sarcoma

The first cardiac tumor reported in a guinea pig was diagnosed as a lymphosarcoma (7). The tumor consisted of a large white mass that replaced much of the left ventricle and considerably enlarged the heart of a young male guinea pig of about 400 g body weight. Except for a small tumor deposit in the portal vein, no tumors were present elsewhere. On histologic examination, Bender (7) described the tumor as composed of "large round cells that infiltrated the cardiac muscle in every direction." Numerous small polypoid excrescences extended into the chamber of the left ventricle. There was a possible increase in the lymph cells of the lung, but the lymphoid tissues were unaffected.

The second cardiac tumor to be reported, Athias (4) diagnosed as polymorph and giant-cell sarcoma. The tumor was located in one of the auricles of a female guinea pig that died 110 days following the first of two intracerebral injections of 0.4 ml methylcholanthrene. The tumor infiltrated the cardiac tissues, and histologically consisted of "small polymorph cells, fusiform, triangular or star-shaped" with round or oval vesicular nuclei with numerous chromatin granules. Many intermediate cell forms were present. Cells with blood pigment were disseminated throughout the tumor tissue. The stroma was sparse and contained numerous giant cells. In the wall of the auricle were calcified material, areas of metaplastic bone and small well-circumscribed nodules of cartilage. Tumors were not found at any other site. Since none of the other 33 guinea pigs similarly treated developed any neoplasm, the author concluded that the cardiac tumor was spontaneous.

Mesenchymoma

Toth (125) reported that out of 40 guinea pigs, which he treated at birth and twice later with 3 mg of 7,12-dimethylbenz(a)anthracene, 1 male developed 42 weeks later a sarcoma of the heart. He did not further describe the morphology of this tumor.

This tumor reported by Athias bears certain resemblances to the cardiac tumors diagnosed as mesenchymoma and described by McConnell and Ediger (74). Out of 3698 Hartley-

Dunkin guniea pigs, maintained at Fort Detrick, Maryland, 4 females had tumors of the heart. The tumors were composed "of fibrous, angiomatous, adipose, cartilaginous, hematopoietic, myxomatous and, possible, smooth muscle tissue."

Ediger and Kovatch, (32), reported a number of spontaneous tumors identified among a total of 8700 Dunkin-Hartley strain guinea pigs younger than 27 months of age, and of these, 10 had mesenchymoma of the heart; amongst 34 guinea pigs older than 27 months, 2 had mesenchymoma of the right atrium.

Rhabdomyoma

Rhabdomyoma is the most commonly observed tumor of the heart of the guinea pig. Whether this tumor represents a congenital hamartoma or is an expression of glycogen storage disease, or a genuine neoplasm, is still under consideration (47, 56, 141). In the human, cardiac rhabdomyoma is frequently associated with tuberous sclerosis of the brain (62, 114). In the guinea pig heart, rhabdomyomas are usually poorly circumscribed with histologically indistinct borders, and consist of large vacuolated cells, containing one, and occasionally two large nuclei, encircled by weakly acidophilic cytoplasm. Fine strands of the cytoplasm extend from the nucleus to the cell membrane, resulting in the characteristic "spider cell" appearance. Silverman and associates (106) examined 3 human rhabdomyomas by electron microscopy and reported that their cells exhibited features characteristic of both Purkinje cells and myocardial muscle cells. Already in 1906, Knox and Schorer (64) had called attention to the resemblance of the cells of these tumors to Purkinje cells. The designation "purkinjoma" was later suggested for them.

Rhabdomyomas of the heart of guinea pigs are frequently multiple, as indeed was the case with the first example reported by Hueper (55). He observed grossly a single nodule in the wall of the left ventricle and on microscopic examination, multiple additional nodules in the right ventricle, right and left auricles, intraventricular septum and papillary muscles. Weber (134), in 1949, also described multiple rhabdomyomas in the heart of guinea pigs. The tumors are quite common in certain breeds of guinea pigs, in which they may be present in the wall of every chamber, located subendocardial, intramural or subpericardial. Rooney (96) observed among 193 Hartley guinea pigs, 24 (12%) with cardiac rhabdomyomas, which were single in 11, and multiple in the others. Cintorino and Luzi, in 1970, counted 11 heart tumors among 24 guinea pigs that belonged to a breed in Siena, Italy (18).

Argus and Hoch-Ligeti, (2), found rhabdomyomas of the heart, which they believed to be spontaneous and not induced, in 2 male hybrid guinea pigs, treated with diethylnitrosamine (Figure 30). One of these guinea pigs also had a liver nodule composed of large, glycogen-filled cells.

Vink, (131), counted 22 guinea pigs with rhabdomyosarcomas, all confined to the wall of the left ventricle, out of a total of 1400 dissected guinea pigs of the randombred closed colony at the Rijks Instituut voor de Volksgezondheid, Bilthoven-Utrecht, The Netherlands.

Cardiac rhabdomyomas have not been identified among

the accessions at the NCI Registry that include 249 Strain 2, 64 Strain 13, and 229 noninbred male or female guinea pigs, either exposed to whole-body irradiation with gamma or X-rays, or serving as controls (72). There are, however, one animal with subendocardial inflammatory fibrosis, one with a perithelioma of the myocardium and 24 others with proliferative, tumor-like, lesions of the cardiac valves.

The subendocardial lesion in the guinea pig (Figure 31) differs from that of the rat described in the foregoing by exhibiting necrosis, inflammatory cell infiltrates and fibrosis in the deep layers of the subendocardium associated with myocarditis. This lesion, therefore, resembles the endomyocardial fibrosis of the natives in Uganda, described by Davies and Ball (22).

The myocardial perithelioma presented as a white nodule within the wall of the left ventricular chamber of a 40-months-old noninbred guinea pig, that had been irradiated with 4.4 R daily. Histologically (Figures 32 and 33), the tumor was poorly circumscribed and consisted of multiple groups of fusiform cells with elongated nuclei and pale cytoplasm arranged concentrically, often about a small vessel. In the adventitia of two neighboring vessels, focal proliferation of the fibroblast-like cells was observed. Mitotic figures were not seen. Several small groups of cells extended into the adjacent myocardium.

Papillary tumors of the heart valves (valvular fibroma, fibromyxoma, elastofibroma)

Among the accessions of the NCI Registry are tissues from 24 guinea pigs with proliferative lesions of the heart valves,

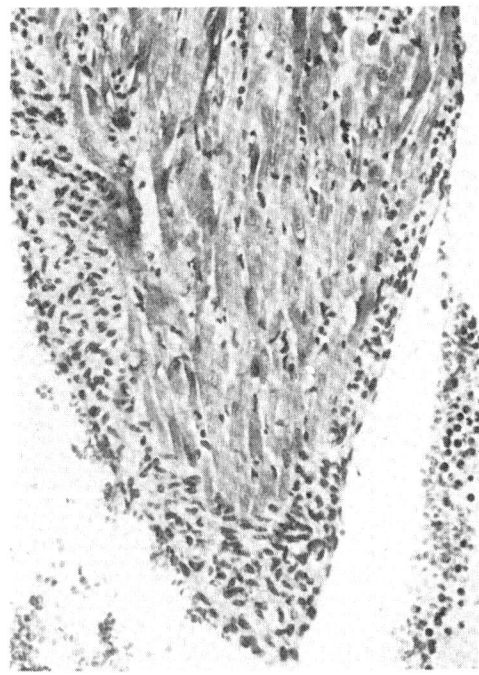

Figure 31. Papillary muscle showing myocarditis and endocardial fibrosis. Male Strain 13 guinea pig, 29 months of age, untreated. H & E × 220.

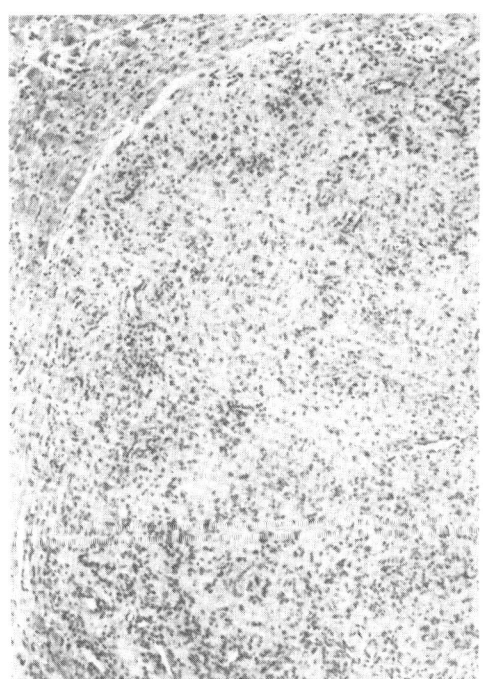

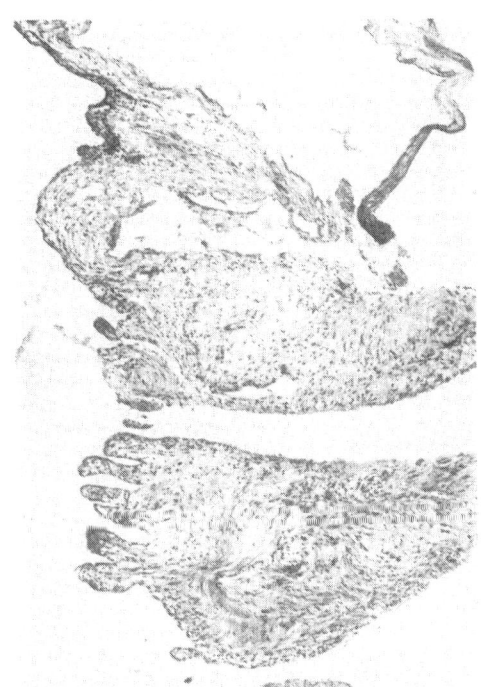

Figure 32. Wall, left ventricle with perithelioma in myocardium. The tumor cells are oriented around small vessels. Noninbred male guinea pig, 40 months of age, treated with 4.4 R X – rays daily. H & E × 80.

Figure 34. The two positions of one leaflet that occupy the lower 2/3rd of the field are joined together beyond the right margin of the illustration. Male Strain 2 guinea pig, 46 months of age, untreated. H & E × 54.

mostly the mitral valve, occasionally also the aortic cusps. Usually, only one valve or cusp was involved, although lesions might be present on both the mitral and aortic valves. The leaflets or cusps of the respective valve were not necessarily involved to the same degree. The affected guinea pigs, ranging in age from 25 to 65 months were from inbred Strains 2 and 13, or from noninbred stock, and about equal numbers had been subjected to total body irradiation with gamma or X-rays or had served as controls.

The valvular lesions were located on the free margin of the elongated valve and consisted of nodular accumulation of myxomatous and edematous fibroblastic tissue (Figures 34–37). The surface of the lesions was covered generally by a single layer of cells, but occasionally the layers were multiple. Numerous polypoid or finger-like excrescences, oriented usually in the direction of the bloodstream, gave the border of the valve a serrated appearance (Figures 35 and 36). A few inflammatory cells were usually present at the base of the affected valve and occasionally small thrombotic excrescences adhered to the surface (Figure 37). These lesions in guinea pigs closely resembled the lesion of a patient designated papillary fibroma of the cardiac valve reported by Hertzog (49), who noted its resemblance to Lambl's excrescences (68). Whether this lesion in humans is neoplastic has been the subject of debate ever since. Raeburn, (92), considered it to be a hamartoma. Others noted its similarity to the cardiac myxoma. In the guinea pig, valvular papillary lesions have not been found in animals younger than 25 months of age, thus a hamartomatous origin is unlikely. Pomerance (88) presents evidence that in the human "the lesion is entirely thrombotic in nature." In the guinea pig, thrombi were but rarely observed adjoining or around the

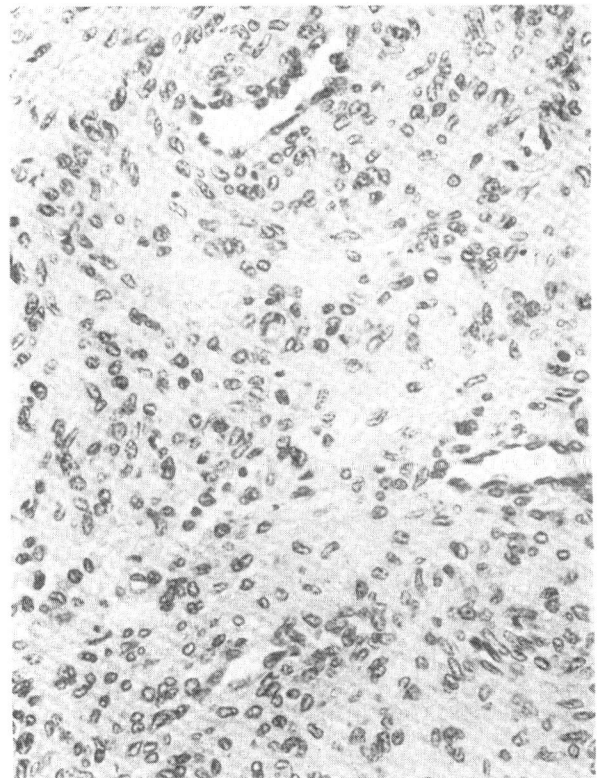

Figure 33. High-power view of perithelioma of Figure 32. The elongated tumor cells are oriented around vessels. H & E × 330.

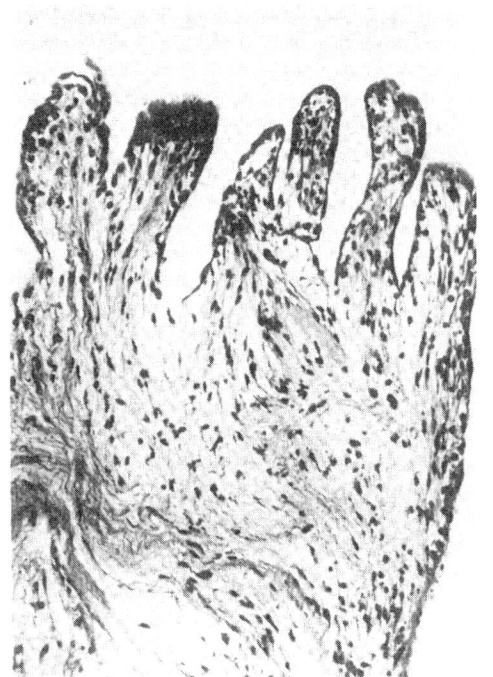

Figure 35. Same lesion as in Figure 34. The proliferating fibroblasts are separated by loose, edematous, mucoid stroma. The finger-like projections appended to the ventricular surface are covered in most areas by a single layer, in others by multiple layers of endothelial cells. H & E × 220.

valvular lesion, and did not appear to play any role in its genesis; the presence of inflammatory cells was, however, common. The guinea pigs in the same age group as those with cardiac lesions, had many different types of primary tumors, but there was no preferential association with any one type.

Spatz (110), during the course of series of experiments, aimed at the clarification of the pathogenesis of the carcinoid syndrome, identified another type of valvular lesion of the heart of guinea pigs. The lesion was most commonly localized to the pulmonary valve, and consisted of a cellular fibrous proliferation beneath the endothelial lining. Her experimental protocol included elevation of the blood serotonin levels, periodic tryptophan deficiency and alteration of liver function.

CARDIAC TUMORS IN HAMSTERS

In the survey of Squire and associates (111) of the tumors of laboratory animals, no cardiac tumors in hamsters were reported. Ketkar and associates (61), in a report on 120 European hamsters, captured in the wild and subsequently treated by injection of MNU into the sublingual vein, described a significantly higher frequency of cardiac tumors in males (22/45) than in females (8/45). By contrast, the females (22/45) had a higher incidence of gastric tumors than males (16/45). The exact location of the tumors within the heart was not given, except for one massive tumor which involved the right atrium. The gross and histologic features

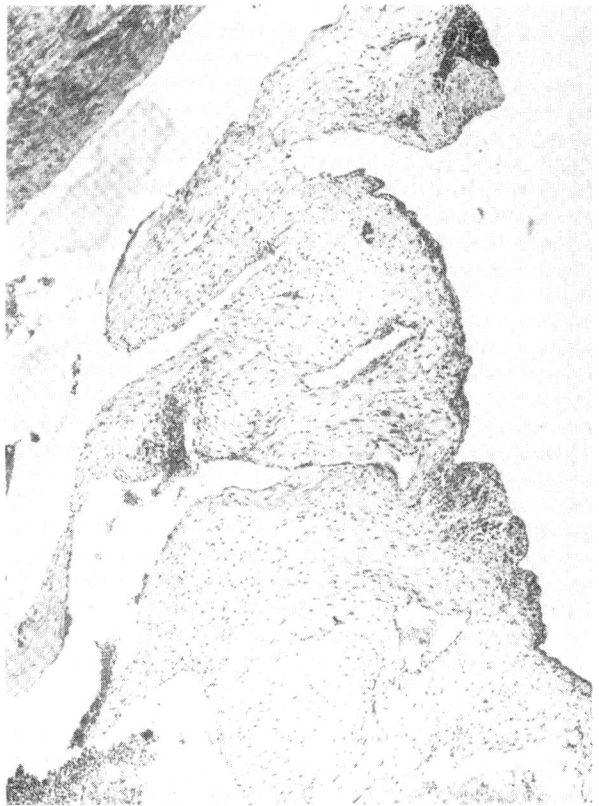

Figure 36. Thickened leaflet of mitral valve with proliferative lesion is covered by single or multiple layers of endothelial cells. Male Strain 2 guinea pig, 46 months of age, treated with 8.8 R daily to an approximate total of 1,500 R. H & E × 110.

of this tumor was illustrated, and the authors stated that it was located in the myocardium of a male hamster autopsied 26 weeks following treatment. Histologically, the tumors were classified as fibrosarcomas, but the possibility that they may have been schwannomas was discussed. Metastatic tumors were observed, but the authors did not state whether from cardiac tumors or from the gastric tumors.

On intrapleural injection of harsh chrysotile and of amosite, Smith and associates (107) induced mesotheliomas in hamsters. In one harsh chrysotile-treated hamster, a tumor that had infiltrated the wall of the thorax was located "between the heart and the vertebral column and displacing the lung downward." No tumors arose in the tissues bordering the pleural cavity of hamsters treated with soft chrysotile.

In the heart of 2 hamsters treated with diethyl stilbestrol, polypoid papillary lesions were present, involving the mitral valve and the endocardium immediately distal from it. The lesions distal from the valve bore close resemblance to cardiac myxomas (unpublished observation).

CARDIAC TUMORS IN *PRAOMYS (MASTOMYS) NATALENSIS*

Primary tumors of endocardium or myocardium in *Praomys (Mastomys) natalensis* are not accessed in the large collection of specimens from this species at the NCI Registry, nor are such tumors reported in the literature.

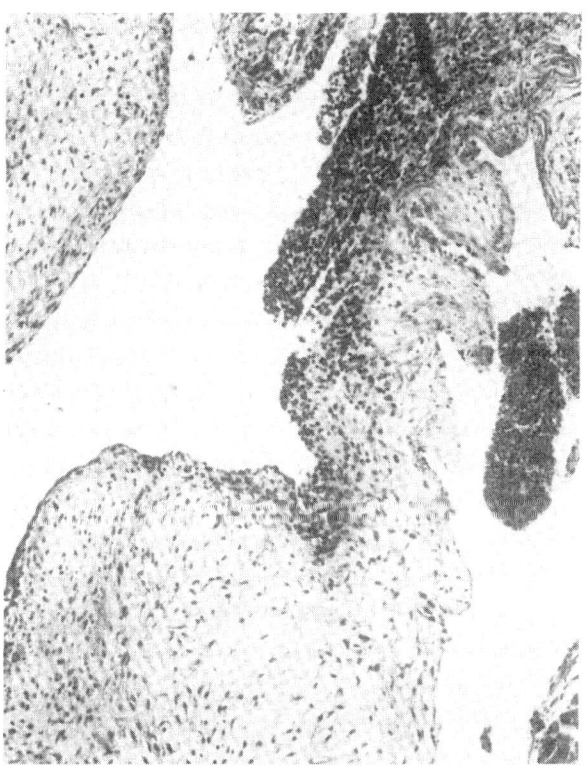

Figure 37. The proliferative lesion of the mitral valve is covered in areas by fresh thrombus. Female strain 13 guinea pig, 42 months of age, treated with 4.4 R daily. H & E × 220.

On the leaflets of the cardiac valves, fibromyxomatous lesions are found in all *Mastomys* older than 18 months (108). The lesions resemble in all respects those described herein for the cardiac valves of the guinea pig.

A frequent finding in the auricles of the heart is the occurrence of large bizarre nuclei with prominent nuclear inclusions in some muscle fibers. The nature and cause of these are unclear. These altered cardiac cells develop independent of the presence or absence of thymoma or the associated myosites of skeletal muscle and myocarditis, lesions that suggestively resemble those of myasthenia gravis in man.

Of the tumors primary at various sites that metastasized to the heart, one was an ovarian adenocarcinoma in a 28-month-old untreated female that metastasized to the right ventricular myocardium; metastases were also present in ribs, peritoneum, spleen and intestine. A sacral sarcoma NOS of an untreated female 35 1/2 months of age formed metastatic deposits over the larger portion of the visceral pericardium with extension into the myocardium of the right atrium. A mediastinal teratoma in an untreated male 27 months of age invaded the right ventricle.

A 5th-generation transplant of a gastric carcinoid, 3 months after transplantation formed minute deposits of tumor cells in the myocardium and the free-floating groups of tumor cells in the right ventricle. Metastases were also present in the lung. Quite similar findings were present in a *Mastomys* bearing a 6th-generation transplant of a gastric carcinoid.

COMPARISONS OF CARDIAC TUMORS OF LABORATORY RODENTS AND HUMANS

Comparisons of primary cardiac tumors of laboratory rodents with those of man reveal differences in frequency of occurrence, histologic classification and location within the heart. Since it is not known what genetic, environmental, dietary, or other factors influence the occurrence of cardiac tumors in man, a comparison of these features with those of laboratory rodents with so-called spontaneous and induced cardiac tumors seems appropriate. In humans assessment of the frequency of primary cardiac tumors relative to tumors primary at all other sites is difficult because of the small percentage of necropsies. A difficulty with rodents is that the total number of animals in a colony in which one or a few cardiac tumors occurred is often not available. In man the number of cardiac tumors found at necropsy is given as 0.017% (115) to 0.1% (47, 91). During the last 2 to 3 decades, due to improved techniques, more cardiac tumors are being diagnosed clinically; this, however, cannot be taken as an indication of an increase in the frequency of their occurrence.

Regarding the histologic classification of primary cardiac tumors, some types have been observed only in man, some only in a single rodent species, some in man and in one or two rodent species, and some in two species of rodents but not in man.

The most common tumor in man is the myxoma, which accounts for 50% of all his cardiac tumors (91). By contrast, cardiac myxoma has not been reported in any laboratory rodent species. In rats the subendothelial endocardial tumor is the most frequent, and, possibly, the only type of tumor which is inducible in this species. This subendothelial endocardial tumor has not been observed in any other rodent species or in man. In rats, the neoplastic proliferation of the tissue underlying the layer of endothelial cells might be thought to resemble the endocardial fibrosis type 1, the most common cardiac disease in parts of Africa (21, 22). In man, however, inflammatory granulation tissue characteristically involves the deeper layers of the lesion, which never evolves into cancer. Endomyocardial fibrosis has been described in rats treated with N-nitrosomorpholine (83). In the rat there is no inflammatory reaction in their cardiac lesion which is a neoplasm *ab initio*. In a sole instance in a guinea pig, we described endocardial fibrosis in association with necrosis in the deeper endocardial layers and myocarditis, and pointed to its comparability to the non-neoplastic cardiac disease in Africans. Endocardial tumors have not been found in the guinea pig.

Since the histogenesis of the subendothelial endocardial tumor of the rat is as yet unresolved, a comparison cannot usefully be made between the induced endocardial tumors variously designated as of connective or of neurogenic tissue origin, with the human cardiac tumors, classified as fibromas, fibrosarcomas, neurolemmomas or neurosarcomas.

The second most common cardiac tumor in man is rhabdomyoma. This type of tumor also occurs in the guinea pig, but not in other rodents. In man the nature of this lesion, whether neoplastic or hamartomatous, is still incompletely resolved. Hamartomatous origin of the lesion is supported by electron-microscopic studies (Fenoglio, et al., 1976). In the guinea pig, cardiac rhabdomyoma occurs in a high percentage of some strains (131), while in man, cardiac rhabdomyoma occurs in association with tuberous sclerosis (114), a familial disease. In the guinea pig, lesions in the brain in association with cardiac rhabdomyoma have not been observed. The cells of the cardiac rhabdomyoma in man and in the guinea pig, and the cells of the cerebral lesion in tuberous sclerosis in man contain large quantities of glycogen, and are thought to represent disturbance of glycogen metabolism (5).

The genetically determined atrio-caval mesothelioma of the rat was also shown to be associated with a disturbance of glycogen metabolism. This tumor in the NZR/Gd strain of rat (39), as well as hepatic glycogen deposition in the same animal is hereditarily transmitted with male preponderance. By contrast, in man tumors at the atrioventricular septum, which have been reported under a variety of designations (54, 67, 93, 109) have shown no hereditary tendency. Another difference is, that in man this type of tumor is always located at the atrioventricular septal junction, whereas in the rat the tumor occurs with about equal frequency in the atrioventricular septum and in the inferior vena cava.

Hemangioendotheliomas of the heart occur in dogs (63), in man (73, 91), rarely in the mouse (52) and rat (101), and have not been reported in the guinea pig.

Papillary valvular fibroma consisting of a tumor-like growth most often located on the mitral valve, was described in man by Hertzog (49), Pomerance (88) and Fishbein et al. (33). This lesion was reported for the *Praomys* (*Mastomys*) *natalensis* (108) and is described herein for the guinea pig for the first time.

The exact nature of the cardiac mesenchymoma is still unresolved. Tumors with this designation were reported in guinea pigs (74) and in a mouse (52). For the guinea pig, Ediger and Kovatch (32) reported a hereditary tendency for this tumor with female preponderance.

Malignant mesenchymal cardiac tumors were reported both in man (15, 45) and in the mouse (52). In the mouse this tumor metastasized to distant sites.

Aortic body tumors are not cardiac tumors in the strict sense of the word, but, because of their location at the base of the heart, their inclusion in a study of the groups of cardiac tumors is justified.

Carotid body chemodectomas in man and aortic body chemodectomas in the rat each infiltrate locally, but exhibit a low tendency to metastasize to distant sites. In the WAG/Rj strain of rat, chemodectomas of the aortic body were found predominantly in the female (130). In humans chemodectomas of the carotid body were found to be familial and sex-bound. Del Fante and Watkins (23) reported an aortic body chemodectoma in association with carotid body chemodectoma. This is the only report of the occurrence of a chemodectoma in the heart in man. The familial occurrence of chemodectomas was first reported by Chase (16), and Kroll and associates (66) established the autosomal dominant inheritance of the tumor. Familial bilateral occurrence of carotid body chemodectomas was reported by Rush (97), Wilson (142) and Pratt (89). Saldana and associates (99) found the female-to-male ratio of occurrence of carotid body tumor to be 6.3.

Pericardial mesotheliomas have been reported in rats and mice in association with exposure to asbestos or other durable fibrous materials (51, 113). In man, Churg and asso-ciates (17) described a pericardial mesothelioma which was associated with surgical dusting of the pericardium with asbestos and fiberglass. Another example of the rare pericardial mesotheliomas in man was attributed to exposure to asbestos while working in shipyards 30 years earlier (60).

In regard to the frequency with which primary tumors at other sites metastasize to the heart, there is also a considerable difference among species. In man, mice and mastomys, metastatic tumors from other sites to the heart are considerably more common than are primary tumors. In man, a metastatic tumor of the heart is approximately 20 to 40 times more frequent than is a primary cardiac tumor (91). By contrast, a metastasis of a tumor from elsewhere to the heart of a rat is exceedingly rare. Wilens and Sproul (138) reported the metastasis of an osteosarcoma and of two lymphomas to the heart. Tumors metastatic to heart have not been reported in the guinea pig or hamster, this despite the fact that primary tumors of many different sites are common in these two species.

REFERENCES

1. Altman NH, Goodman DG: Neoplastic diseases. *In*: The Laboratory Rat, Academic Press (Baker HJ, Lindsey JR, Weisbroth ST, eds.) 1:334, 1979
2. Argus MF, Hoch-Ligeti C: Induction of malignant tumors in the guinea pig by oral administration of diethylnitrosamine. *J Natl Cancer Inst* 30:533, 1963
3. Armstrong H, Mönckeberg JG: Herzblock bedingt durch primären Herztumor bei einem 5-jährigen Kind. *Dtsch Arch Klin Med* 102:144, 1911
4. Athias M: Sarcome du coeur chez un cobaye après injection, dans le cerveau, de methylcholanthrene. *Comptes Rendues Soc Biol* 126:585, 1937
5. Batchelor TM, Maun ME: Congenital glycogenic tumors of the heart. *Arch Pathol* 39:67, 1945
6. Beck CS: An intrapericardial teratoma and a tumor of the heart: removed operatively. *Ann Surg* 116:161, 1942
7. Bender L: Sarcoma of the heart in a guinea pig. *J Cancer Res* 9:384, 1925
8. Berman JJ, Rice JM, Reddick R: Endocardial schwannomas in rats. *Arch Pathol Lab Med* 104:187, 1980
9. Bharati S, Bicoff JP, Fridman JL, Lew M, Rosen KM: Sudden death caused by benign tumor of the atrioventricular node. *Arch Intern Med* 136:224, 1976
10. Biancifiori C: Ovarian influence on pulmonary carcinogenesis by hydrazine sulfate in BALB/c/Cb/Se mice. *J Natl Cancer Inst* 45:965, 1970
11. Bode G, Hartig F: Primary neoplasms of the heart. *Exp Pathol* 19:31, 1981
12. Boorman GA, Zurcher C, Hollander CF, Feron VJ: Naturally occurring endocardial disease in the rat. *Arch Pathol* 96:39, 1973
13. Burek JD, Hollander CF: Incidence patterns of spontaneous tumors in BN/Bi rats. *J Natl Cancer Inst* 58:99, 1977
14. Campbell JA: The effects of road dust "freed" from tar products upon the incidence of primary lung tumors of mice. *Brit J Exp Pathol* 18:215, 1937
15. Ceretto WJ, Miller ML, Shea PM, Gregory CW, Vieweg WVR: Malignant mesenchymoma obstructing the right ventricular outflow tract. *Amer Heart J* 101:114, 1981
16. Chase WH: Familial and bilateral tumours of the carotid body: *J Pathol Bact* 36:1, 1933
17. Churg A, Warnock ML, Bensch KG: Malignant mesothelioma arising after direct application of asbestos and fiber glass to the pericardium. *Amer Rev Resp Dis* 118:419, 1978

18. Cintorino M, Luzi P: Myocardial rhabdomyomas in the guinea pig. *Beitr Pathol* 142:407, 1970

19. Cloudman AM: Spontaneous neoplasms in mice. *In*: Biology of the Laboratory Mouse. Jackson Laboratory. (Snell GD, eds). Philadelphia: The Blakiston Company, p. 169, 1941

20. Conley FK, Rubinstein LJ, Spence AM: Studies on experimental malignant nerve sheath tumors maintained in tissue and organ culture systems. II Electron microscopy observations. *Acta neuropath (Berl)* 34:293, 1976

21. Davies JNP: Some considerations regarding obscure diseases affecting the mural endocardium. *Amer Heart J* 59:600, 1960

22. Davies JNP, Ball JD: The pathology of endomyocardial fibrosis in Uganda. *Br Heart J* 17:337, 1955

23. Del Fante FM, Watkins E Jr: Chemodectoma of the heart in a patient with multiple chemodectomas and familial history. *Lahey Clinic Foundation Bull* 16:224, 1967

24. Druckrey H: Specific carcinogenic and teratogenic effects of 'indirect' alkylating methyl and ethyl compounds, and their dependency on stages of ontogenic developments. *Xenobiotica* 3:271, 1973a

25. Druckrey H: Chemical structure and action in transplacental carcinogenesis and teratogenesis. *In*: L. Tomatis and U. Mohr (eds). Transplacental Carcinogenesis. IARC Scientific Publications No. 4, p. 45. Lyon, France: International Agency for Research on Cancer, 1973b

26. Druckrey H, Kruse H, Preussman R, Ivankovic S, Landschutz Ch, Gimmy J: Cancerogene alkylierende Substanzen IV. 1,3-Propansulton und 1,4-Butansulton. *Z Krebsforsch* 75:68, 1970a

27. Druckrey H, Ivankovic S, Preussman R: Neurotrope carcinogene Wirkung von Phenyl-dimethyl-triazen an Ratten. *Naturwissenschaften* 54:171, 1967

28. Druckrey H, Landschutz Ch: Transplacentale und neonatale Krebserzeugung durch Äthylnitrosobiuret (ÄNBU) an BD IX-Ratten. *Z Krebsforsch* 76:45, 1971

29. Druckrey H, Schagen B, Ivankovic S: Erzeugung neurogener Malignome durch einmalige Gabe von Athyl-nitrosoharnstoff (ANH) und neugeborene und junge BD IX-Ratten. *Z Krebsforsch* 74:141, 1970b

30. Druckrey H, Steinhoff D, Preussmann R, Ivankovic S: Erzeugung von Krebs durch eine einmalige Dosis von Methylnitroso-Harnstoff und verschiedenen Dialkylnitrosaminen an Ratten. *Z Krebsforsch* 66:1, 1964

31. Dunn TB: Normal and pathologic anatomy of the reticular tissue in laboratory mice. With a classification and discussion of neoplasms. *J Natl Cancer Inst* 14:1281, 1954

32. Ediger RD, Kovatch RM: Spontaneous tumors in the Dunkin-Hartley guinea pig. *J Natl Cancer Inst* 56:293, 1976

32a. Fenoglio, JJ, McAllister HA, Ferrans V: Cardiac rhabdomyoma: A clinicopathologic and electron microscopic study. *Ann J Cardiol* 38:241, 1976

33. Fishbein MC, Ferrans VJ, Roberts WC: Endocardial papillary elastofibromas. *Arch Pathol* 99:335, 1975

34. Frith CH, Farris HE, Highman B: Endocardial fibromatous proliferation in a rat. *Lab Animal Science* 27:114, 1977

35. Ghadially FN: Ultrastructural Pathology of the Cell. A Text and Atlas of Physiological and Pathological Alterations in Cell Fine Structure. Butterworth (London and Boston) p. 463, 1977

36. Gilbert C, Gillman J: Spontaneous neoplasms in the albino rat. *S Afr J med Sci* 23:257, 1958

37. Glenner GG, Grimley PM: Tumors of the extra-adrenal paraganglion system (including chemoreceptors). Atlas of Tumor Pathology, Second Series, Fascicle 9. Armed Forces of Pathology, Washington, D.C., 1974

38. Goodall CM, Christie GS, Hurley JV: Primary epithelial tumour in the right atrium of the heart and inferior vena cava in NZR/Gd inbred rats; pathology of 18 cases. *J Pathol* 116:235, 1975

39. Goodall CM, Doesburg RMN: Age-specific incidence of neoplasms in untreated NZR/Gd rats: an inbred strain with cardiovascular tumours and liver glycogen storage disease. *J Pathol* 135:147, 1981

40. Goodman DG, Ward JM, Squire RA, Chu KC, Linhart MS: Neoplastic and nonneoplastic lesions in aging F344 rats. *Toxicol and Appl Pharmacol* 48:237, 1979

41. Goodman DG, Ward JM, Squire RA, Paxton MB, Reichardt WD, Chu KC, Linhart MS: Neoplastic and nonneoplastic lesions in aging Osborne-Mendel rats. *Toxicol and Appl Pharmacol* 55:433, 1980

42. Haas H, Hilfrich J, Mohr U: Induction of heart tumours in Wistar rats after a single application of ethylmethanesulfonate and dimethylnitrosamine. *Z Krebsforsch* 81:225, 1974

43. Habs M, Schmähl D, Wiessler M: Carcinogenicity of acetoxymethyl-methyl-nitrosamine after subcutaneous, intravenous and intrarectal applications in rats. *Z Krebsforsch* 91:217, 1978

44. Habs M, Schmähl D, Kretzer H: Effect of disulfiram on acetoxymethyl-methyl-nitrosamine-induced tumors in rats. *Oncology* 38:18, 1981

45. Hagström L: Malignant mesenchymoma in pulmonary artery and right ventricle. *Acta Pathol Microbiol Scand* 51:87, 1961

46. Hartwell JL, Stewart HL: Action of 5,9,10-trimethyl-1,2-benzanthracene on the skin of the mouse. *J Natl Cancer Inst* 3:277, 1942

47. Heath D: Pathology of cardiac tumors. *Amer J Cardiol* 21:315, 1968

48. Henry CJ, Billups LH, Avery MD, Rude TH, Dansie DR, Lopez A, Sass B, Whitmire CE, Kouri RE: Lung cancer model system using 3-methylcholanthrene in inbred strains of mice. *Cancer Res* 41:5027, 1981

49. Hertzog AJ: Papillary fibroma of cardiac valve. *Arch Pathol* 22:222, 1936

50. Hoch-Ligeti C, Harris PN, Stewart HL: Endocardial tumors induced by carbamate or fluorenylacetamide derivatives in rats. *J Natl Cancer Inst* 71:211, 1983a

51. Hoch-Ligeti C, Sass B, Sobel JH, Stewart HL: Endocardial tumors in rats exposed to durable fibrous materials. *J Natl Cancer Inst* 71:1067, 1983b

52. Hoch-Ligeti C, Stewart HL: Cardiac tumors in mice. *J Natl Cancer Inst* 72:1449, 1984

53. Holzhausen HJ, Schreiber D: Elektronmikroskopische Untersuchungen an Frühstadien experimenteller Herztumoren bei Ratten: *Exp Pathol* 13:20, 1977

54. Honey M, Axelrad MA: Intracardiac endodermal heterotopia. *Br Heart J* 24:667, 1962

55. Hueper WC: Rhabdomyomatosis of the heart in a guinea pig. *Amer J Pathol* 17:121, 1941

55a. Huff JE, Melnick RL, Solleveld MA et al: Multiple organ carcinogenicity of 1,3-butadiene in B6C3F, mice after 60 weeks of inhalation exposure. *Science* 227:548, 1985

56. Humphreys EM, Kato KK: Glycogen-storage disease. Thesaurismosis glycogenica (von Gierke). *Amer J Pathol* 10:589, 1934

57. Ivankovic S: Tumours of the heart. *In*: Pathology of Tumors of Laboratory animals. IARC Scientific Publications No. 6, Part 2, p. 313, 1976

58. Ivankovic S, Wohlenberg H, Mennel HD, Preussmann R: Erzeugung von Herztumoren durch chronische orale Gabe des Carcinogens 1-Pyridyl-3,3-Diathyl-Triazen und BD-Ratten. *Z Krebsforsch* 77:217, 1972

59. Jänisch W, Lageman A, Dietz W, Schreiber D: Experimentelle Nerventumoren bei Ratten durch Induktion mit N-Methyl-N-nitrosoharnstoff. *Exp Pathol* 4:317, 1970

60. Kahn EI, Rohl A, Barrett EW, Suzuki Y: Primary pericardial mesothelioma following exposure to asbestos. *Environmental Res* 23:270, 1980

61. Ketkar M, Reznik G, Haas H, Hilfrich J, Mohr U: Tumors of the heart and stomach induced in European hamsters by intravenous administration of N-methyl-N-nitrosourea. *J Natl Cancer Inst* 58:1695, 1977

62. Kidder LA: Congenital glycogenic tumors of the heart. *Arch Pathol* 49:55, 1950

63. Kleine LJ, Zook BC, Munson TO: Primary cardiac hemangiosarcomas in dogs. *J Amer Vet Med Assoc* 157:326, 1970

64. Knox JHM, Schorer EH: A multiple rhabdomyoma of the heart muscle. *Arch Pediat* 23:561, 1906

65. Kommineni VRC, Greenblatt M, Mihailovich N, Vesselinovitch SD: The significance of perinatal age periods and the dose of urethan on the tumor profile in the MRC rat. *Cancer Res* 30:2552, 1970.

66. Kroll AJ, Alexander B, Chochios F, Pecket L: Hereditary deficience in clotting factors VII and X associated with carotid body tumors. *New Eng J Med* 270:6, 1964

67. Lafargue RT, Hand AM, Lev M: Mesothelioma (Coelothelioma) of the atrioventricular node. *Chest* 59:571, 1971

68. Lambl VA: Papillary Excrescenzen an der Semilunar-Klappe der Aorta. *Wien med Wochnschr* 6:244, 1856

69. Leinati L: Geschwülste des Bauchfells und des subperitonealen Gewebes. *In*: Handbuch der speziellen pathologischen Anatomie der Haustiere (Parey, ed). Berlin-Hamburg, 1970

70. Lewis DJ: Subendocardial fibrosis in the rat: A light and electron microscopical study. *J Comp Pathol* 90:577, 1980

71. Lie JT, Lufschanowski R, Erickson EE: Heterotopic epithelial replacement (so-called "mesothelioma") of the atrioventricular node, congenital heart block, and sudden death. *Amer J Forensic Med Pathol* 1:131, 1980

72. Lorenz E, Jacobson LO, Heston WE, Shimkin M, Eschenbrenner AB, Deringer MK, Doniger J, Schweisthal R: Effects of long-continued total-body irradiation on mice, guinea pigs and rabbits. III. Effects on lifespan, weight, blood picture, and carcinogenesis and the role of the intensity of radiation. *In*: Biological Effects of External X and Gamma Radiation, Part I (RE Zirkle, ed) New York: McGraw Hill, p. 24, 1954

73. McAllister HA, Fenoglio JJ: Tumors of the cardiovascular system. *In*: Atlas of Tumor Pathology. Second Series, Fascicle 15. Armed Forces Institute of Pathology, Washington D.C., 1978

74. McConnell RF, Ediger RD. Benign Mesenchymoma of the heart in the guinea pig. A report of four cases. *Pathol Vet* 5:97, 1968

75. MacKenzie W, Garner FM: Comparison of neoplasms in six sources of rats. *J Natl Cancer Inst* 50:1243, 1973

76. Maekawa A, Kurokawa Y, Takahashi M, Kokubo T, Ogiu T, Onodera H, Tanigawa H, Ohno Y, Furukawa F, Hayashi Y: Spontaneous tumors in F-344/DuCrj rats. *Gann* 74:365, 1983

77. Maekawa A, Odashima S: Spontaneous tumors in ACI/N rats. *J Natl Cancer Inst* 55:1437, 1975

78. Maekawa A, Ogiu T, Matsuoka C, Onodera H, Furuta K, Kurokawa Y, Takahashi M, Kokubo T, Tanigawa H, Hayashi Y, Nakadate M, Tanimura A: Carcinogenicity of low doses of N-ethyl-N-nitrosourea in F344 rats; a dose-response study. *Gann* 75:117, 1984

79. Magee PN, Farber E: Toxic liver injury and carcinogenesis. Methylation of rat-liver nucleic acid by dimethylnitrosamine. *J Pathol Bact* 84:19, 1962

80. Mahaim I: Le coeloepithelioma tawarien benin, une tumeur *sui generis* de noeud Taware avec block de coeur. *Cardiology* 6:57, 1942

81. Mahaim I: Les tumeurs et les polypes du coeur: Etude anatomique clinique. Paris, Masson & Cie, 1945

82. Manning PJ: Neoplastic diseases. *In*: The Biology of the Guinea Pig (J.E. Wagner, PJ Manning, eds). Academic Press, New York, p. 211, 1976

83. Mayer D, Bannasch P: Endomyocardial fibrosis in rats treated with N-nitrosomorpholine. *Virchows Arch (Pathol Anat)* 401:129, 1983

84. Mennel HD: Die Morphologie der mit neurotropen Karzinogenen erzeugten Herztumoren bei Ratten. *Beitr Pathol* 144:221, 1971

85. Miller EC, Miller JA, Makoto E: The comparative carcinogenesis of 2-acetylaminofluorene and its N-hydroxy metabolite in mice, hamsters, and guinea pigs. *Cancer Res* 24:2018, 1964

86. Moore BW: A soluble protein characteristic of the nervous system. *Biochem Biophys Res Communications* 19:739, 1965

87. Morris HP, Wagner BP, Ray FE, Snell KC, Stewart HL: Comparative study of cancer and other lesions of rats fed N,N′-2,7-fluorenylene-bisacetamide or N-2-fluorenylacetamide. *Natl Cancer Inst Monogr No. 5* p. 1, 1961

88. Pomerance A: Papillary "tumours" of the heart valves. *J Pathol Bact* 81:135, 1961

89. Pratt LW: Familial carotid body tumors. *Arch Otolaryngol* 9:334, 1973

90. Preussmann R, von Hodenberg A, Hengy H: Mechanism of carcinogenesis with 1-aryl-3,3-dialkyltriazenes. Enzymatic dialkylation by rat liver microsomal fraction *in vitro*. *Biochem Pharmacol* 18:1, 1969

91. Prichard RW: Tumors of the heart. *Arch Pathol* 51:98, 1951

92. Raeburn C: Papillary fibro-elastic hamartomas of the heart valves. *J Pathol Bact* 65:371, 1953

93. Rezek P: Über eine primare epitheliale Geschwulst in der Gegend des Reizleitungssystems beim Menschen. *Virchows Arch Pathol Anat Physiol* 301:305, 1938

94. Reznik G: Unusual sites of lung tumor metastases in $B_6C_3F_1$ mice and F344 rats. *Anticancer Res* 1:159, 1981

95. Robertson JL, Garman RH, Fowler EH: Spontaneous cardiac tumors in eight rats. *Vet Pathol* 18:30, 1981

96. Rooney JR: Rhabdomyomatosis in the heart of the guinea pig. *Cornell Veterinarian* 51:388, 1961

97. Rush BF: Familial bilateral carotid body tumors. *Ann Surg* 147:633, 1961

98. Russell DS, Rubinstein LJ: Tumours of the nerve roots and peripheral nerves. *In*: Pathology of Tumours of the Nervous System. Fourth Ed. The Williams and Wilkins Company, Baltimore, p. 372, 1977

99. Saldana MJ, Salem LE, Travezan R: High altitude hypoxia and chemodectomas. *Human Pathol* 4:254, 1973

100. Saphir O: Spezielle Pathologie für die klinische und pathologische Praxis (Thieme). Stuttgart 1961

101. Schardein JL, Fitzgerald JE, Kaump DH: Spontaneous tumors in Holtzman-Source rats of various ages. *Pathol Vet* 5:238, 1968

102. Schreiber D: Die Erzeugung von Tumoren des Nervensystems mit Nitrosamiden bei verschiedenen Tierarten. *Habil-Schrift*, Erfurt 1969

103. Schreiber D, Batka H, Warzok R, Quentin E: Induktion von Herztumoren bei Ratten durch Methylnitrosoharnstoff. *Zbl allg Pathol* 115:31, 1972

104. Schreiber D, Gerlach H, Wessel H, Musil A: Experimentelle Herztumoren bei Ratten. *Arch für Geschwulstforschung* 46:169, 1976

105. Sharma RN: Naturally occurring mesothelioma in the right atrium of the heart of an albino rat. *The Bulletin, Soc Pharmacol Environm Pathol* 5:2, 1977

106. Silverman JF, Kay S, McCue CM, Lower RR, Brough AJ, Chang CH: Rhabdomyoma of the heart. Ultrastructural study of three cases. *Lab Invest* 35:596, 1976

107. Smith WE, Miller L, Churg J, Selikoff IJ: Mesotheliomas in hamsters following intrapleural injection of asbestos. *J Mount Sinai Hosp* 32:1, 1965

108. Solleveld HA: *Praomys (Mastomys) natalensis* in Aging Research. Doctoral Thesis. Publication of the Institute for Ex-

perimental Gerontology TNO, Rijswijk, The Netherlands, 1981

109. Sopher IM, Spitz WU: Endodermal inclusions of the heart. *Arch Pathol* 92:180, 1971
110. Spatz M: Pathogenetic studies of experimentally induced heart lesions and their relation to the carcinoid syndrome. *Lab Invest* 13:288, 1964
111. Squire RA, Goodman DG, Valerio MG, Fredrickson TN, Strandberg JD, Levitt MH, Lingeman CH, Harshbarger JC, Dawe CJ: Tumors. *In*: Pathology of laboratory Animals, Vol. II (K. Benirschke, F.M. Garner, T.C. Jones, eds) Springer-Verlag, New York p. 184, 1978
112. Stanton MF, Stewart SE, Eddy BE, Blackwell RH: Oncogenic effect of tissue-culture preparations of polyoma virus on fetal mice. *J Natl Cancer Inst* 23:1441, 1959
113. Stanton MF and Wrench C: Mechanisms of mesothelioma induction with asbestos and fibrous glass. *J Natl Cancer Inst* 48:797, 1972
114. Steinbiss W: Zur Kenntnis der Rhabdomyome des Herzens und ihrer Beziehungen zur tuberosen Gehirnsklerose. *Virchows Arch Pathol Anat Physiol und für klin Med* 243:22, 1923
115. Straus R, Merliss R: Primary tumor of the heart. *Arch Pathol* 39:74, 1945
116. Strandberg JD, Goodman DG: Neoplasms of the cardiovascular system. *In*: The Mouse in Biomedical Research. Vol. IV. Experimental Biology and Oncology. (H.L. Foster, J.D. Small, J.G. Fox, eds) Academic Press, p. 539, 1982
117. Stula EF: Naturally occurring pulmonary tumors of epithelial origin in Charles River-CD rats. *Bull Soc Pharmacol Environm Pathol* 3:3, 1975
118. Swenberg JA, Clendenon N, Denlinger R, Gordon WA: Sequential development of ethylnitrosourea-induced neurinomas: morphology, biochemistry, and transplantability. *J Natl Cancer Inst* 55:147, 1975b
119. Swenberg JA, Koestner A, Wechsler W, Brunden MN, Abe H: Differential oncogenic effects of methylnitrosourea. *J Natl Cancer Inst* 54:89, 1975a
120. Sytman AL, MacAlpin RN: Primary pericardial mesothelioma: Report of two cases and review of the literature. *Amer Heart J* 81:760, 1971
121. Szepsenwol J, Boschetti NV: Primary and secondary heart tumors in mice maintained on various diets. *Oncol* 32:58, 1975
122. Tamaschke C: Die Spontantumoren der kleinen Laboratoriumssäuger in ihrer Bedeutung für die experimentelle Onkologie. *Strahlentherapie* 96:150, 1955
123. Thomas C, Bollmann R: Untersuchungen zur Organotropie der krebserzeugenden Wirkung des N-Nitroso-N-methyl-Harnstoffes (NMH) an Ratten. *Experientia* 25:50, 1969
124. Thompson JH: N, N'-2,7-fluorenylenebisacetamide (2,7-FAA)-induced rat bowel cancer. *Internatl J Med Sciences* 2:565, 1969

125. Toth B: Susceptibility of guinea pigs to chemical carcinogens: 7,12-dimethyl-benz(a)anthracene and urethan. *Cancer Res* 30:2583, 1970
126. Travers H: Congenital polycystic tumor of the atrioventricular node. *Human Pathol* 13:25, 1982
127. Trevino GS, Nessmith WB: Aortic body tumor in a white rat. *Vet Pathol* 9:243, 1972
128. Turusov VS, Day NE, Tomatis L, Gati E, Charles RT: Tumors in CF-1 mice exposed for six consecutive generations to DDT. *J Natl Cancer Inst* 51:983, 1973
129. Vesselinovitch SD, Mihailovich N: The development of neurogenic neoplasms, embryonal kidney tumors, harderian gland adenomas, Anitschkow cell sarcomas of the heart, and other neoplasms in urethan-treated newborn rats. *Cancer Res* 28:888, 1968
130. van Zwieten MJ, Burek JD, Zurcher C, Hollander CF: Aortic body tumours and hyperplasia in the rat. *J Pathol* 128:99, 1979
131. Vink HH: Rhabdomyomatosis (nodular glycogenic infiltration) of the heart in guinea pigs. *J Pathol* 97:331, 1969
132. Wagner JC, Berry G: Mesotheliomas in rats following inoculation with asbestos. *Br J Cancer* 23:567, 1969
133. Wagner JC, Berry G, Timbrell V: Mesothelioma in rats after inoculation with asbestos and other materials. *Br J Cancer* 28:173, 1973
134. Weber G: Rhabdomyom multiple de cuore in *cavia cobaya*. *Arch Vecchi Anat Path e Med Clin* (Florence) 13:1049, 1949
135. Wechsler W, Pfeiffer SE, Swenberg JA, Koestner A: S-100 protein in methyl- and ethylnitrosourea induced tumors of the rat nervous system. *Acta Neuropathol* (*Berl*) 24:287, 1973
136. Weiss SW, Langloss JM, Enzinger FM: Value of S-100 protein in the diagnosis of soft tissue tumors with particular reference to benign and malignant schwann cell tumors. *Lab Invest* 49:299, 1983
137. Wells HG, Slye M, Holmes HF: The occurrence and pathology of spontaneous carcinoma of the lung in mice. *Cancer Res* 1:259, 1941
138. Wilens SL, Sproul EE: Spontaneous cardiovascular disease in the rat. *Amer J Pathol* 14:177, 1938
139. Willis RA: A metastatic deposit of bronchial carcinoma in a hydrocele misdiagnosed "endothelioma," with a review of supposed "endotheliomas" of serous membranes. *J Pathol Bact* 47:35, 1938
140. Willis RA: The borderline of embryology and pathology. Butterworth, London p. 321, 1958
141. Willis RA: Pathology of Tumors. Appleton-Century-Croft, Inc. New York, 1967
142. Wilson H: Carotid body tumors: familial and bilateral. *Ann Surg* 171:843, 1970
143. Zaidi I, Sullivan DJ, Seiden D: Endocardial thickening in the Sprague-Dawley rat. *Toxicol Pathol* 10:27, 1982

PROGRESSION OF CANCER IN DOMESTIC ANIMALS
(EXCEPT POULTRY)

W. MISDORP

INTRODUCTION

As in man, relatively little is known of the natural history of tumors in domestic animals.

This paucity of knowledge holds especially true for the earliest phases of development (initiation, promotion) of the carcinomas, the most common cancer types.

On the other hand, studies of virus-induced tumor diseases such as feline lymphosarcoma, enzootic bovine lymphosarcoma, feline fibrosarcoma and papillomas (in many species) have provided useful information concerning virus-host cell interaction and tumor development.

The evolution from one or more transformed cells to a full-blown generalized cancer can proceed along various pathways, which will be discussed in this review.

The course of an established tumor disease is the result of the interaction of multiple variables such as tumor-associated antigens and immunological host factors, hormone responsive cells, hormonal environment and factors influencing growth, vascularization, invasion and metastasis. The interaction of these factors may lead to either continuous tumor growth, regression, or progression. Many tumor diseases are, at the moment of detection, already in an advanced stage of development. Superficially situated tumors, both benign and malignant, are as a rule surgically removed and as a consequence, the further course of the tumor disease is interrupted. Other, deeper-situated tumors are difficult to diagnose clinically and therefore little is known of their course. In most cases of untreatable recurrence or metastasis, euthanasia on humane or economic grounds is carried out in small and large domestic animals, respectively, before the disease has run its full course. In spite of the limiting factors, mentioned before, it seems worthwhile to discuss the present knowledge concerning the different pathways by which cancers in domestic animals can develop with special emphasis on progressive changes in one or more tumor characteristics. Where possible, mention will be made of comparable data in man. This comprehensive review might be of comparative interest since tumors in domestic animals, as in man, are mostly of spontaneous nature arising in outbred animals sharing many of man's environmental factors.

De novo development of cancer

In many cases no preceding phase or precursor lesion is known.

There is no doubt that infiltrative carcinomas of skin, mucosa and glandular structures are preceded by a *non-infiltrative* (*in situ*) phase. Non-infiltrating carcinoma can also be found around infiltrating carcinomas, for instance, in cases of bovine ocular carcinoma and feline and canine mammary carcinoma. In the latter cases, spread of carcinoma along pre-existent ductules and acini has to be differentiated from true *in situ* carcinoma. Little is known about the factors which determine whether a non-infiltrative carcinoma will progress to an invasive carcinoma, remain stationary, spread to adjacent ducti or eventually will regress.

Experimentally-induced (FeLV) feline lymphosarcoma was found to be particularly useful to study the earlier stages of tumor development (43). Early intestinal lymphoid neoplasia was detected in germinal centers of Peyer's plaques (B cell type). In contrast, nodal involvement in the thymic and multicentric forms began with infiltration and proliferation of neoplastic cells in paracortical zones of the lymph nodes (T cells).

Early lesions of adult multicentric lymphosarcoma in cattle were reported to occur in the loose subepicardial tissue by Järplid (34). It seems debatable, however, whether these lesions represent early tumorous or rather inflammatory lesions.

Cancer in association with a preneoplastic condition

A pretumorous condition is defined as a condition, indicating a relatively high risk of cancer development. Such a condition is often, but not always related to the site of the future tumor development.

The presence of unpigmented skin is associated with two main groups of lesions: cutaneous melanomas and a range of plaques-papillomas-squamous cell carcinoma.

Depigmentation of hair or vitiligo of aging grey or white horses is associated with equine melanotic disease, a progressive pigmentory disorder best considered as a special manifestation of the blue nevus phenomenon (42). Depigmentation in miniature swine is also associated with the formation of cutaneous melanoma (20). The lesions in horse and swine begin with excess production of melanin in the basal layer of the epidermis followed by the migration of pigment producing cells from the epidermis into the dermis. The pigment is partly phagocytized by macrophages which accumulate causing the dermis to be elevated.

Lightly pigmented skin, when exposed to sunlight, was

H. E. Kaiser (ed.), Comparative aspects of tumor development.
© 1989, Kluwer Academic Publishers, Dordrecht. ISBN-13:978-0-89838-994-4

found to predispose to proliferative and neoplastic lesions in several species:

a) In the perilimbal conjunctiva of Beagle dogs a variety of mostly vascular lesions (ectasia, hemangioma and hemangiosarcoma), solar keratosis and squamous cell carcinomas was found (29).

b) In cows which lack any pigment around the eye, increased susceptibility for epithelial plaques, papillomas and squamous cell carcinoma of the corneal limbus and conjunctivae has been demonstrated. The absence of pigment is a genetic trait in the Hereford cattle, known for their high susceptibility to eye cancer (40).

c) Non-pigmented skin was found to be associated with the development of acanthosis, papillomas and carcinomas in the vulval region of Ayrshire cows in Kenya, of the ear, muzzle and perineum of Merino sheep in New South Wales and in Angora goats in South Africa (9).

Approximately 50 bone sarcomas were reported to be associated with previous fractures in dogs (and a single cat) in the United States and Europe. These fracture-associated sarcomas, developing several years (mean interval 5 years) after fracture constitute only a small fraction (< 10 per cent) of the total number of reported bone sarcomas. Most of the fracture-associated sarcomas were osteosarcomas, the site of which (diaphysis) contrasted with that of spontaneously developing osteosarcomas (metaphysis). The majority of these bone sarcomas was associated with internal fixation devices but at least four sarcomas developed following external fixation or no fixation at all. The possible role of corrosion of the device in the genesis of the sarcomas was emphasized (64). However, by atomic absorption analysis of tissue specimens adjacent to implants only low amounts of chromium and nickel were found (68). These authors consider the possibility of the metal implant as a nidus for continuing inflammation and repair. In man, astonishingly, little information about the association of fracture and bone sarcomas is available.

Bone sarcomas in dogs are also associated with multiple bone infarctions characterized by medullary necrosis and osteonecrosis possibly caused by occlusions of intramedullary arteries. The 14 dogs reportedly developing bone sarcoma (13 osteosarcoma, 1 fibrosarcoma) associated with bone infarctions, differ in distribution of breed, weight, class and site of primary tumor when compared with other dogs with bone tumors (15, 59). Also in man, bone sarcomas associated with preexisting medullary bone infarctions have been reported (14, 23).

In cats, the development of osteosarcomas might be associated with osteodystrophy due to beef liver diet with excess of vitamin A and phosphorus and a low calcium content. In man, twenty of 600 patients had osteosarcoma that developed in Paget disease, and sixteen had osteosarcoma that arose in bones that had been irradiated previously (12).

Cryptorchidism was shown to be a pretumorous condition in dogs in two studies. Reif and Brodey (58) found 53 percent of Sertoli cell tumors and 34 percent of seminomas in cryptorchid testes as compared with a 10 and 12 percent prevalence in breed-matched control dogs. In another study (30) cryptorchid dogs were found to have a significantly higher risk of testicular tumors than normal dogs. Cryptorchid dogs have about equal risk for the seminoma and Sertoli cell tumor. Male dogs with an inguinal hernia exhibit an increased risk for testis tumors. In cryptorchid humans, the relative risk has been calculated to be 14 (48). Among cryptorchid men seminomas are the major cell type.

Cancer in association with a preneoplastic lesion

A preneoplastic lesion (syn. precancerous, premalignant, precursor lesion) is defined as a proliferative (dysplastic) lesion, which is known to progress to a malignant lesion in a percentage of cases. The border line between a preneoplastic lesion and condition is somewhat arbitrary.

Chronic dermatosis resembling preneoplastic actinic dermatosis in man, developed in lightly pigmented sparsely haired, ventral body skin exposed to ultraviolet (sun)light in a large proportion (423/1733) of Beagles. In 13 of these affected dogs squamous cell carcinoma developed, 3–5 years after the onset of dermatosis (29). The metastatic rate (1/13) was low as in solar induced neoplasms in the skin of man and cat. The lesions of solar damage in Beagle skin are morphologically and histochemically identical to those seen in human skin with two exceptions.

Solar elastosis and abnormal pigmentary accumulation commonly found in man, were not found in solar exposed dog skin nor have they been mentioned in cattle, cats or goats.

In the pseudoepitheliomatously altered regions of the skin five years after severe heat burn two squamous cell carcinomas were reported to occur in a dog (24). Burn scar malignancies in human beings are predominantly of the squamous cell variety. Basal cell carcinoma, sarcoma, carcino-sarcoma and carcinoma *in situ* have been identified arising from scar tissue in man (31).

Granulomas are known to occur in the esophagus of *Spirocerci lupi* infected dogs. The development of osteosarcomas and fibrosarcomas in these granulomas and transition between granulomas and sarcomas have been reported (1). Also in a lung, granuloma with foci of invasive fibrosarcoma containing fragments of *S. lupi*, was reported (67).

Ocular sarcomas were reported to occur many years after trauma in cats. Mixtures of granulation tissue, metaplastic bone and spindle cell sarcoma were demonstrated in the affected eyes (16).

In cats infected with feline leukemia virus non-regenerative anemia may progress to leukemia as was demonstrated in 12 cats (44). However, not all FeLV positive anemic animals progress to malignancy. In man, the hematologic abnormalities that precede the development of acute myeloblastic leukemia, have been categorized into a recognizable syndrome: preleukemia. Polycythemia vera, pancytopenia and myelofibrosis belong to this syndrome.

In humans, clones with chromosomal translocations, monosomies, deletions and trisomies known to occur in leukemia, have been described in these disorders (50). Half of 30 patients with chromosomally abnormal clones developed true leukemia, whereas of patients with preleukemia with normal chromosomal constitution only 18 per cent developed leukemia.

Persistent lymphocytosis (PL) of the peripheral blood has been shown, as is the case with enzootic lymphosarcoma (leucosis) in cattle, to be associated with bovine leukemia virus (19). Lymphocytosis often precedes clinical lymphosarcoma in many but not in all affected cows. It is still uncertain whether PL is a preleukemic lesion, a subclinical manifestation of bovine lymphosarcoma or rather a concomitant condition.

In the mammary glands of untreated Beagle bitches aged 8 years, without palpable tumors, hundreds of hyperplastic lesions were demonstrated by using whole mounts techniques (7). In another study, mammary hyperplastic lesions were studied in young Beagle bitches. The hyperplastic lesions appeared before palpable tumors arose. The gradient for early onset of lesions coincided with the gradient for tumor frequency (71). In cats, hyperplastic lesions including epitheliosis were found to accompany mammary carcinomas but the relationship between hyperplastic and neoplastic lesions is not yet clear (74).

In women, the presence of benign proliferative lesions of the breast is associated with an average 2–3-fold increase of risk for a subsequent mammary carcinoma. There are differing views over the possibility of a linear histogenetic pathway from normal to carcinoma (73).

It is impossible to distinguish by light microscopy between proliferative lesions which will progress to cancer, those remaining stationary, or those that will regress. In older dogs hyperplasias of the liver, spleen, adrenal cortex and prostate, are very frequent but association with cancer has never been demonstrated.

Preneoplastic lesions have been studied in several organs (bladder, colon, liver, lung, mammary gland, pancreas, and thyroid) of rats and mice in initiation-promotion studies (54). Alkaline phosphatase-deficient foci were reported to occur in bladders of dogs treated with the initiating agent 2-naphthylamine in combination with the promotor D.L.-tryptophan (57).

Cancer through malignant transformation of a benign tumor

Skin papillomas in many species (rabbit, goat, sheep, cattle and man) are believed to be the precursor lesions of squamous cell carcinomas. Skin papillomas are induced by papilloma-viruses (e.g. Shope's virus in the rabbit). Exposure to sunlight is likely to be the etiologic factor in the transformation of papillomas to carcinomas (21, 70). This hypothesis has been supported by morphologic observations. Bovine ocular squamous cell carcinomas of the orbit frequently arise from a sequence of non-malignant precursor lesions. The initial hyperplastic lesions have been reported as plaques when they occur on the skin of the eyelid. Papillomas may arise at the site of either plaques or acanthosis, and cells within the papillomas sometimes transform to yield squamous cell carcinoma (21, 61). Papilloma virus found in conjunctival plaque and papillomas of the bovine eye appear to be site-specific. This type of virus differs from the 4–5 types of bovine papilloma of the skin, teats and udder, genital organs and gastrointestinal tract, respectively (21).

A squamous cell carcinoma arising in naturally occurring papillomatosis of the oral and pharyngeal cavities of an 18 months old dog, is probably the only reported case of malignant transformation of virus induced oral papilloma in the dog (72). Epidemiologic studies have shown a high incidence of squamous cell carcinoma of the upper alimentary tract of cattle in several parts of the world, including Scotland (35) and Kenya (55). In Scotland the alimentary tract tumors were associated with the presence in the food of bracken fern and with the occurrence of hematuria and bladder tumors. Another interesting finding was the concomitant presence of squamous cell carcinomas and multiple papillomas in the upper part of the alimentary tract and of adenomas or polyposis and adenocarcinoma of the lower intestinal tract. Transformation of the virus-containing and transmittable papillomas to carcinomas was evident in many of the Scottish cattle (35).

Although benign and malignant pigmented lesions of skin and oral mucosa are rather frequent in dogs, reports on premelanomatous lesions in dogs (as well as in other animals) are extremely rare. One report deals with a malignant melanoma developing in association with precancerous melanosis (Hutchinson's type) in the membrana nicticans of a poodle. Metastasis was lacking (42).

In man, development of skin melanomas in benign lesions is a well-known phenomenon.

Severe epithelial atypia, likely carcinoma in situ, was focally apparent in 5 out of 10 tubular adenomas of the rectal mucosa but not in papillary adenomas, or hyperplastic polyps in 17 dogs (62). In one of two adenomatous polyps of the rectal ampulla of a dog, a carcinoma invading the stroma was found (63). It is now believed that, in man, few adenomatous polyps become malignant. However, most carcinomas of the colon and rectum probably evolve through the polyp-cancer sequence (17).

Fibrosarcomas in the canine mammary gland were reported to be situated in conjunction with fibroadenomas (46). Later observations indicate that fibrosarcomas can arise in canine mammary fibroadenomas. Also, benign mixed mammary tumors in the canine mammary gland can progress to cancer.

Multiple skeletal osteochondromas are relatively rare tumors in the dog. The number of reported cases does not exceed ten. In two of these cases a malignant bone tumor, of chondrosarcoma type (2) and a metastasizing osteosarcoma (51) were reported to arise. The incidence of malignant change of this condition in man is uncertain. Approximately 3 percent of solitary osteochondromas and 25 percent of multiple osteochondromas are suspected to give rise to chondrosarcoma but the selection factor makes firm conclusions unwise (12).

In 4 out of 32 dogs irradiated for acanthomatous epulis, malignant tumors (3 carcinomas, 1 osteosarcoma) developed in the irradiated area (69). The intervals between radiation and the appearance of the malignancies ranged from 30–78 months. The most likely explanations for this phenomenon are: a) radiation induced de novo neoplasms; b) radiation induced progression from rests of the epulis to cancer.

Cancer after progression of an already malignant tumor into a different histologic and biologic type

Indication of histological progression of canine skeletal chondrosarcoma to fibrosarcoma was noticed in 3 out of 25 dogs (6). In 33 out of 370 human patients with well-differentiated skeletal chondrosarcoma dedifferentiated zones of fibrosarcoma or osteosarcoma were reported. The rapid deterioration of most of these 33 patients after operation was determined by the dedifferentiated portion of the tumors (11).

A single case of terminal blastic crisis was documented in a dog suffering from chronic myelogenous leukemia for more than a year (56). The occurrence of a blast crisis was documented in 4 out of 7 dogs with chronic myelogenous leukemia. The specific origin of the blastic cells could not be established (41). In man, chronic myelogenous leukemia usually terminates in a blastic crisis with changes, clinically and hematologically indistinguishable from acute myelogenous leukemia (52).

Cancer after progression of one or more tumor characteristics of an already existing cancer

Little is known of progressive changes of characteristics of untreated spontaneous primary cancers in domestic animals. This is partly due to the fact that most animals bearing a tumor, are either treated or killed. The control (nontreated) animals in a clinical trial lend themselves for study of tumor progression.

In the control group of untreated cows with bovine eye carcinoma in a recent immunotherapy study evidence for tumor progression was lacking (47). In this group a remarkable heterogeneity of an important tumor characteristic, the growth rate, was noticed. The growth rate was found not only to differ considerably between tumors, but some tumors also failed to show a constant growth rate.

Tumor growth rate in a non-treated group of sheep with *squamous cell carcinoma* of the skin was reported to be slow and regular (90 percent increase in tumor volume in 24 weeks) (37), but no individual growth curves were given. The growth rate is determined among other things by the ratio of the fractions of dividing, nondividing resting cells and cell loss.

Moreover, in some tumors like bovine cancer eye, and canine transmissible venereal tumor, the "tumors" consist partly of reactive lymphocytes and plasma cells.

There is little evidence, in domestic animals, of morphological signs of progression (increased anaplasia, infiltrative growth) when comparing recurrent and metastatic tumors with the initial primary ones. But thus far, with a few exceptions, no systematic studies on this item were reported (47).

Transplantation of cultured canine osteosarcoma cells into canine fetuses caused multiple sarcomata which, in contrast to the original tumor, were of undifferentiated type (5).

A single injection of allogeneic tumor vaccine causes regression of many eye carcinomas in cattle, whereas multiple injections cause progression or enhancement (66).

An extensive study on specific immunotherapy of ovine squamous cell carcinoma of the skin showed that large amounts of protein in the allogeneic tumor extracts were associated with severe progression of growth rate and metastatic potential in the treated group (37).

Discussion

Neoplasia was discussed by Foulds (22) as developing through discontinuous stages as a result of progression, characterized by irreversible, heritable changes in neoplastic cells.

Some general principles of progression based primarily on mammary neoplasia in mice, proved applicable to many other kinds of neoplasia in animals and in man (22).

One rule stresses the independent progression of multiple tumors. Another points to the independent progression of various tumor characteristics.

According to Pitot (53) it is not always possible to distinguish between the phase of tumor promotion and tumor progression since these two blend with each other in the natural history of many neoplasms. Furthermore, a number of neoplasms upon induction may already represent a fully progressed population of neoplastic cells. On the other hand, Pitot stresses that in the vast majority of so-called spontaneous neoplasms in man and animals, the natural history of the neoplasms involves all of the stages of initiation, promotion and progression.

Tumor progression is characterized by a more aggressive behavior often with concomitant loss of specific differentiated properties. According to Nowell (49), tumor progression results from genetic instability in the neoplastic population which permits sequential selection, over time, of increasingly mutated subpopulations within the original clone of cells.

Papillomas are known to undergo malignant transformation in at least four species (man, cattle, sheep, and rabbit). The first factor is infection with a papilloma virus and secondly, the presence of a co-factor, initiating malignant transformation, is necessary.

The co-factors including hydrocarbons in the rabbit system, bracken-fern and sunlight in the cattle system, and sunlight in sheep (65). Plausible co-factors in humans are irradiation (laryngeal papilloma → carcinoma) and sunlight (epidermo-dysplasia verruciformis → carcinoma).

The genesis and development of the range solar keratosis-plaque-papilloma-squamous cell carcinoma in unpigmented regions (not protected by melanin) of the thick epidermis, is associated with the influence of sunlight (ultraviolet light). In animals with a thinner type of unpigmented epidermis (including the dog), ultraviolet rays might reach deeper layers where mesenchymal lesions, inducing vascular tumors, develop.

The mechanism by which sunlight induces lesions in the skin, has been debated. Ultraviolet absorption is related to molecular structure. By far the most susceptible are the pyrimidine bases of the DNA molecule. Other types of damage include DNA-protein cross links, damage to bases other than pyrimidine and single strand breaks (33). Because much ultraviolet-induced damage is repairable in normal individuals it has been proposed that lack of DNA-repair is not responsible for most neoplastic development but rather it is faulty DNA-repair or replication which leads to mutation, and possibly integration of oncogenic viruses (33). The genesis of skin cancers, associated with ultraviolet irradiation, can be prevented in part by selective breeding of animals with pigmented skin. Precursor lesions, plaques and papillomas, of orbital carcinoma in cattle either were caused to regress or prevented to progress by intralesional injection of active BCG (38).

The observations from the bracken fern districts in Scotland are very interesting. The high incidence of intestinal papillomas was found to be associated with a new type of papillomavirus (8). In high cancer areas there is a marked increase in the overall incidence of the virus infection and an increase in the number of specific sites of infection. There is strong circumstantial evidence that the factor associated with the increased multiplicity of papillomas and the subsequent malignant transformation is the ingestion of bracken fern (35). Bracken fern is known to possess radiomimetic, mutagenic and carcinogenic activity. The system seems to present a dissectable model for investigating the mechanistic relationship between the viral infection and the ingestion of an environmental carcinogen (8). In cattle, papillomatosis of the alimentary tract and the induction of bladder cancer have been reproduced experimentally after infection with bovine papilloma virus and after either feeding bracken-fern or treatment with the immunodepressant, azathioprine. There seems also to be a correlation between Bovine Papilloma Virus-2, and bladder cancer in cattle (65).

Skeletal osteosarcomas arise preferentially in those parts of the skeleton of the respective animal species (dog, cat, horse, cattle) where the mechanical stress is greatest (32). In man, a relationship between favorite tumor localization and osteoblastic activity in these favorite sites was demonstrated by Johnson (36), who designed a general theory of bone tumors. The propensity for excessive cellular proliferation to progress to neoplasia is illustrated by the occasional development of bone sarcomas in actively proliferating bone diseases and benign tumors in man and animals. The mechanism by which the proliferating cells are transformed to cancer cells is unknown.

The phenomenon of piezoelectricity might help in clarifying many aspects of oncogenesis in bone. Piezoelectricity has been generated under the influence of mechanical stress in crystals of collagen and bone as shown in experiments with rabbits (3). Mechanical stress induced a negative potential, associated with osteoblastic activity at the concave, compression part of the bone, whereas at the convex, tension part, osteolytic activity was demonstrated. Charge transfers of electrons have been associated with mutagenic effects (45).

Chromosome studies in bovine lymphosarcoma ("bovine leucosis") have shown that within individual cases a consistent pattern of change consists as evidenced by the presence of the same cell line, or lines, in different lymph nodes or other tumor sites, and in a number of cases in the peripheral blood as well. These observations seem to indicate a unicentric origin with metastases rather than a multicentric origin for the tumor (27). Could cytogenetic studies help us to detect subsets of diseases which might be preleukemic in cattle and cats? Or should we accept the statement of Hare and Feeley (26), that "when cells of lymphoid origin in an otherwise chromosomally normal animal can be shown to have persistent chromosome changes, it can be stated with confidence, in the light of the present knowledge, that the animal has leukemia"?

In human patients with hematopoietic "preleukemic" dis-orders the emergence of a chromosomally abnormal clone enhances the risk of leukemia (50).

In polycythemia vera, a preleukemic disease in all six human patients examined, deletion of the long arm of chromosome 20 was found. But in the true, chronic myelogenous leukemia translocation of the Philadelphia chromosome was recognized. In the terminal acute blast crisis, patients showed a variegated pattern of chromosomal abnormalities (60).

Also Nowell (49) found progression of chronic myeloid leukemia via the blast crisis to result from a second mutation in a cell of an original clone also recognizable by additional chromosome alterations.

These findings indicate that the progression from a preleukemic disease → chronic leukemia → acute blast crisis, is associated with involvement of different chromosomes. By using recombinant DNA-techniques and chromosome banding it was demonstrated that Philadelphia chromosome translocation in patients with chronic myeloid leukemia is associated with activation of the C-*abl.* oncogene (de Klein et al., 1982).

Relatively little is known about the role of oncogenes in domestic animals. Oncogenes have been demonstrated in acute transforming retroviruses isolated from feline sarcomas (4).

It seems worthwhile to determine if, and to which extent, oncogenes play a role in the various stages of progression of tumors, including those in domestic animals.

REFERENCES

1. Bailey WS: Parasites and cancer: Sarcomas in dogs associated with *Spirocerca lupi. Ann NY Acad Sci* 108:890, 1963
2. Banks WC, Bridges CH: Multiple cartilaginous exostoses in a dog. *J Am Vet Med Assoc* 129:131, 1956
3. Bassett CAL, Becker RO: Generation of electrical potentials by bone in response to mechanical stress. *Science* 137:1063, 1962
4. Besmer P: Acute transforming feline retroviruses. Current topics in: *Microbiology and Immunology* 107:1, 1983
5. Bostock DE, Owen LN: Transplantation and tissue-culture studies of canine osteosarcoma. *Eur J Cancer* 6:499, 1970
6. Brodey RS, Misdorp W, Riser WH, Van der Heul RO: Canine skeletal chondrosarcoma: A clinicopathologic study of 35 cases. *J Am Vet Med Assoc* 165, 1:68, 1974
7. Cameron AM, Faulkin LJ: Hyperplastic and inflammatory nodules in the canine mammary gland. *J Natl Cancer Inst* 47:1277, 1971
8. Campo MS, Moar MH, Jarrett WFH, Laird HM: A new papillomavirus associated with alimentary cancer in cattle. *Nature* 286:180, 1981
9. Cotchin E: Some aetiological aspects of tumours in domesticated animals. *Ann R Coll Surg Engl* 38:92, 1966
10. Dahlin DC: Bone tumors. Thomas ChC, Springfield, Illinois, 27, 1967
11. Dahlin DC, Beabout JW: Dedifferentiation of low-grade chondrosarcomas. *Cancer* 28:461, 1971
12. Dahlin DC, Coventry MB: Osteogenic sarcoma. A study of 600 cases. *J Bone Joint Surg (Am)* 49A, 1:101, 1967
13. De Klein A, Geurts van Kessel A, Grosveld G, Bartram CR, Hagemeijer A, Bootsma D, Spurr NK, Heisterkamp N, Groffen J, Stephenson JR: A cellular oncogene is translocated to the Philadelphia chromosome in chronic myelocytic leukemia. *Nature* 300:765, 1982

14. Dorfman MD, Norman A, Wolff H: Fibrosarcoma complicating bone necrosis in a caisson worker. *J Bone Joint Surg (Am)* 48:477, 1965

15. Dubielzig RR, Biery DN, Brodey RS: Bone sarcomas associated with multi-focal medullary bone infarctions in dogs. *J Am Vet Med Assoc* 79, 1:64, 1981

16. Dubielzig RR: Ocular sarcoma following trauma in three cats. *J Am Vet Med Assoc* 184, 5:578, 1984

17. Ekelund G, Lindström C: Histopathological analysis of benign polyps in patients with carcinoma of the colon and rectum. *Gut* 15:654, 1974

18. Epstein WL, Fukuyama K, Epstein JH: Ultraviolet light, DNA repair and skin carcinogenesis in man. *Fed Proc* 30:1766, 1971

19. Ferrer JF, Abt DA, Bhatt DM, Marshak RS: Studies on the relationship between infection with bovine C-type virus, leukemia, and persistent lymphocytosis in cattle. *Cancer Res* 34:893, 1974

20. Flatt RE, Middleton CC, Tumbleson ME, Perez-Mesa C: Pathogenesis of benign cutaneous melanomas in miniature swine. *J Am Vet Med Assoc* 153, 7:936, 1968

21. Ford JN, Jennings PA, Spradbrow PB, Francis J: Evidence for papillomaviruses in ocular lesions in cattle. *Res Vet Sci* 32:257, 1982

22. Foulds L: *Neoplastic development.* Vol. 2. Academic Press Inc. New York, 549, 1975

23. Galli SJ, Weintraub MP, Proppe KH: Malignant fibrous histiocytoma and pleomorphic sarcoma in association with medullary bone infarcts. *Cancer* 41:607, 1978

24. Gourley IM, Madewell BR, Barr B, Ettinger SJ: Burn scar malignancy in a dog. *J Am Vet Med Assoc* 180, 9:1095, 1982

25. Grady HG, Blum HF, Kirby-Smith JS: Types of tumor induced by ultraviolet radiation and factors influencing their relative incidence. *J Natl Cancer Inst* 3:371, 1973

26. Hare WCD, McFeely RA: The present status of chromosome studies in bovine leukosis (leukemia). Proc 3rd Symp Comp Leukemia Res, Paris 1967. *Bibl Haematol* 31:231, 1968

27. Hare WCD, Yang TJ, McFeely RA: A survey of chromosome findings in 47 cases of bovine lymphosarcoma (leukemia). *J Natl Cancer Inst* 38:383, 1967

28. Hargis AM, Lee AC, Thomassen RW: Tumor and tumor-like lesions of perilimbal conjunctiva in laboratory dogs. *J Am Vet Med Assoc* 173, 9:1185, 1978

29. Hargis AM, Thomassen RW, Phemister RD: Chronic dermatosis and cutaneous squamous cell carcinoma in the Beagle dog. *Vet Path* 14:218, 1977

30. Hayes HM, Pendergrass ThW: Canine testicular tumors: Epidemiologic features of 410 dogs. *Int J Cancer* 18:482, 1976

31. Horton CE, Crawford HH, Lover HG: The malignant potential of burn scar. *Plast Reconst Surg* 22:348, 1958

32. Jacobson SA: *The comparative pathology of the tumors of bone.* Thomas ChC, Springfield, Illinois, 179, 1971

33. Jagger J: *Ultraviolet effects in medical radiation biology.* 1st ed. Dalrymple, Gaulden, Kollmorgen, Vogel, Eds. Saunders WB, Philadelphia, 44, 1973

34. Järplid B: Studies on the site of leukotic and preleukotic changes in the bovine heart. *Path Vet* 1:366, 1964

35. Jarrett WFH, McNeil PE, Grimshaw WTR, Selman IE, McIntyre WIM: High incidence area of cattle cancer with a possible interaction between an environmental carcinogen and a papilloma virus. *Nature* 274:215, 1978

36. Johnson LC: A general theory of bone tumors. *Bull NY Acad Med* 29:164, 1953

37. Jun MH, Johnson RH, Maguire DJ, Hopkins PS: Enhancement and metastasis after immunotherapy of ovine squamous-cell carcinoma. *Br J Cancer* 38:382, 1978

38. Kleinschuster SJ, Rapp HJ, Bier J, Musculpat CC, Swart RA, Van Kampen K: Immunoprophylaxis of an ocular solid malignant tumor in cattle. *J Natl Cancer Inst* 70:771, 1983

39. Koller L: The physics of the atmosphere in: *The biological effects of ultraviolet radiation.* 1st ed. Urbach Ed. Pergamon Press, Oxford, 329, 1969

40. Kopecky KE, Pugh Jr GW, Hughes DE: Biological effect of ultraviolet radiation on cattle, bovine ocular squamous cell carcinoma. *Am J Vet Res* 40, 12:1783, 1979

41. Leifer CE, Matus RE, Patnaik AK, MacEwen EG: Chronic myelogenous leukemia in the dog. *J Am Vet Med Assoc* 183, 6:686, 1983

42. Levene A: Equine melanotic disease. *Tumori* 57:133, 1971

43. Mackey LJ, Jarrett WFH: Pathogenesis of lymphoid neoplasia in cats and its relationship to immunologic cell pathways. *J Natl Cancer Inst* 49:853, 1972

44. Maggio L, Hoffman B, Cotter SM: Feline preleukemia: An animal model of human disease. *Yale J Biol Med* 51:469, 1978

45. Mason R: Electron mobility in biological systems and its relation to carcinogenesis. *Nature* 181:820, 1958

46. Misdorp W, Cotchin E, Hampe JF, Jabara AG, Von Sandersleben J: Canine malignant mammary tumours. I. Sarcomas. *Vet Path* 8:99, 1971

47. Misdorp W, Klein WR, Ruitenberg EJ, Hart G, Teppema JS, De Jong WH, Steerenberg PA: Immunotherapy by intralesional injection of BCG cell walls or live BCG in bovine ocular squamous cell carcinoma. *Cancer Immunol Immunother* 20:223–230, 1985

48. Mostofi FK: Testicular tumors. Epidemiologic, etiologic and pathologic features. *Cancer* 32:1186, 1973

49. Nowell PC: Chromosomes and tumor progression. In: *Differentiation and neoplasia.* Springer-Verlag, Heidelberg, 102, 1980

50. Nowell PC, Jensen J, Gardner F, Murphy S, Chaganti RSK, German J: Chromosome studies in "preleukemia". III. Myelofibrosis. *Cancer* 38:1873, 1976

51. Owen LN, Bostock DE: Multiple cartilaginous exostoses with development of a metastasizing osteosarcoma in a Shetland sheepdog. *J Small Anim Pract* 12:507, 1971

52. Pedersen B: The blastic crisis of chronic myeloid leukemia: acute transformation of a preleukemic condition? *Br J Haematol* 25:141, 1973

53. Pitot HC: The natural history of neoplasia. *Am J Pathol* 89:401, 1977

54. Pitot HC, Sirica AE: The stages of initiation and promotion in hepatocarcinogenesis. *Biochem Biophys Acta* 605:191, 1980

55. Plowright W, Linsell CA, Peers FG: A focus of rumenal cancer in Kenyan cattle. *Br J Cancer* 25:72, 1971

56. Pollet L, Van Hove W, Mattheeuws D: Blastic crisis in chronic myelogenous leukemia in a dog. *J Small Anim Pract* 19:469, 1978

57. Radomski JL, Krischer C, Krischer KN: Histologic and histochemical preneoplastic changes in the bladder mucosae of dogs given 2-naphthylamine. *J Natl Cancer Inst* 60(2):327, 1978

58. Reif JS, Brodey RS: The relationship between cryptorchidism and canine testicular neoplasia. *J Am Vet Med Assoc* 155, 12:2005, 1969

59. Riser WH, Brodey RS, Biery DN: Bone infarctions associated with malignant bone tumors in dogs. *J Am Vet Med Assoc* 160, 4:411, 1972

60. Rowley JD: Do human tumours show a chromosome pattern specific for each etiologic agent? *J Natl Cancer Inst* 52:315, 1974

61. Russell WO, Wynne ES, Loguvam GS: Studies on bovine ocular squamous carcinoma (Cancer Eye) I. Pathological anatomy and historical review. *Cancer* 9:1, 1956

62. Seiler RJ: Colorectal polyp of the dog: A clinicopathologic study of 17 cases. *J Am Vet Med Assoc* 174:72, 1979

63. Silverberg SJ: Carcinoma arising in adenomatous polyp of the rectum in a dog. *Dis Colon Rectum* 14:191, 1971

64. Sinibaldi K, Rosen H, SiKwang Liu, De Angelis M: Tumors

associated with metallic implants in animals. *Clin Orthop* 118:257, 1976

65. Smith KT, Campo MS: The biology of papillomaviruses and their role in oncogenesis. *Anticancer Res* 5:31, 1985

66. Spradbrow PB, Wilson BE, Hoffman D, Kelly WR, Francis J: Immuno-therapy of bovine ocular squamous cell carcinoma. *Vet Rec* 100, 18:376, 1977

67. Stephens LC, Gleiser A, Jardine JH: Primary pulmonary fibro-sarcoma associated with *Spirocerca lupi* infection in a dog with hypertrophic pulmonary osteoarthropathy. *J Am Vet Med Assoc* 182, 5:496, 1983

68. Stevenson S, Hohn RB, Pohler OEM, Fetter AW, Olmstead ML, Wind AP: Fracture-associated sarcoma in the dog. *J Am Vet Med Assoc* 180, 10:1189, 1982

69. Thrall DE, Goldschmidt MH, Biery DN: Malignant tumor formation at the site of previously irradiated acanthomatous epulides in four dogs. *J Am Vet Med Assoc* 178, 2:127, 1981

70. Vanselow BA, Spradbrow PB: Papilloma viruses, papillomas and squamous cell carcinomas in sheep. *Vet Rec* 110:561, 1982

71. Warner MR: Age incidence and site distribution of mammary dysplasias in young Beagle bitches. *J Natl Cancer Inst* 57:57, 1976

72. Watrach AM, Small E, Case MT: Canine papilloma progression of oral papilloma to carcinoma. *J Natl Cancer Inst* 45:915, 1971

73. Wellings SR, Misdorp W: Benign proliferative lesions of the breast: Workshop Report. *Eur J Cancer Clin Oncol* 19, 12:1721, 1983

74. Weijer K: Feline mammary tumours and dysplasias. Ph.D. Thesis. University of Amsterdam, 1979

CHEMORECEPTOR NEOPLASIA: COMPARATIVE FEATURES IN LABORATORY ANIMALS DOMESTIC ANIMALS, AND MAN

BERNARD SASS and HOWARD M. HAYES, Jr.

INTRODUCTION

The occurrence, epidemiology, gross, microscopic, and ultrastructural pathology of chemoreceptor neoplasms in laboratory animals, domestic animals and man are reviewed in this chapter. To understand better these aspects of chemoreceptor neoplasia, the normal gross, microscopic, and ultrastructural anatomy, and normal and abnormal physiology of this organ system are also discussed.

In an accompanying chapter, Grimley reviews recent knowledge of tumors of neuroendocrine tissue, including extra-adrenal medullary tissue and other paragangliomas, and a pertinent survey of literature on multiple endocrine syndromes. We have attempted to provide information pertinent to chemoreceptor neoplasia not duplicating that found in Grimley's review.

General characteristics of chemoreceptor organs and terminology

Chemoreceptor organs are so named because they are sensitive to changes in arterial oxygen and pH. In man, organs termed branchiomeric and intravagal paraganglia are rather widely distributed in various sites of the body including jugulo-tympanic, subclavian, laryngeal, coronary, aortico-pulmonary, intercarotid and interpulmonary locations (47). The most prominent and well studied of these in all species are the carotid and aortico-pulmonary groups. Some of the paraganglia have been shown to be part of the adrenal medullary endocrine system and some others, the carotid and aortic bodies, have chemoreceptor functions. The term branchiomeric paraganglia has validity since both the extra-adrenal medullary tissues and the chemoreceptor organs arise in the walls of the branchial arteries; however, their development is not related to embryonic origin from the gill arches (47).

The terms "glomus cell" or "glomus cell tumor" are inappropriate for tumors of the chemoreceptor organs, since true glomus cells are epithelial-like cells which appear to arise from smooth muscle and line arteriovenous anastomoses (137). Such anastomoses in man are located in the glomus coccygeum in the coccyx and the nail beds (48); in animals these anastomoses are found in the glomeruli caudales, located in the distal portions of the tail (144).

Kondo (76) studied the ultrastructure of the rat glomeruli caudales. The epitheliod cells did not contain granules and nerve endings were found only in the adventitia of the organ.

These features were considered proof that the glomeruli caudales had no endocrine function and were arteriovenous anastomoses.

Throughout this chapter, the anatomic location of the chemoreceptor bodies will be used as the prefix, followed by the term body, e.g. aortic body. This terminology will be used when making reference to the overall system of chemoreceptors. Similarly, when designating the location of neoplasms of the chemoreceptor system, the location of the tumor will be used as the prefix followed by the word tumor. The general term "chemodectoma" will also be used, as it appears in the veterinary literature, however, we recognize that new techniques are necessary to provide further information on the identity of such tumors. According to Rosai (130), the only structures thus far identified for certain as having chemoreceptor function in man are the carotid and aortic bodies. According to Grimley (personal communication) tumor cells of aortic body tumors may not be definitely assigned to the category of chemodectomas, but some authors have done so. Since the carotid body is the largest and most accessible of the chemoreceptor organs, most of the work cited deals with studies of this organ.

Embryology

The earliest stages of development of the human carotid body is an accumulation of cells around the third branchial artery (65, 74, 125, 150). Rogers (128) found the same pattern of development in the rat. Several different views were advanced as to the origin of chemoreceptor cells. Early workers (17, 125) believed that the perivascular accumulation of cells were derived in situ from mesodermal cells. Several investigators (65, 150) believed that the perivascular cellular accumulation was the stroma of the chemoreceptor organ, and that the chemoreceptor cells migrate into the carotid body from nearby nerves of ganglia.

Histologic studies alone are inadequate to ascertain with certainty the origin of the cells of the carotid body; the embryonic development of this structure was studied by a number of researchers (77, 91, 131). Their studies confirmed the existence of two types of cells in the carotid body: the chief (type I) cells and the sustentacular (type II) cells.

Kondo (77), conducted sequential light and electron microscopic examinations of the carotid bodies of 50 rat embryos ranging from 13 to 18 days gestation in order to study the differentiation of the two types of cells. The first development of rat carotid bodies was detected at 13.5–14 days gestation as a thickening of the anterior wall of the

H. E. Kaiser (ed.), Comparative aspects of tumor development.
© 1989, Kluwer Academic Publishers, Dordrecht. ISBN-13:978-0-89838-994-4

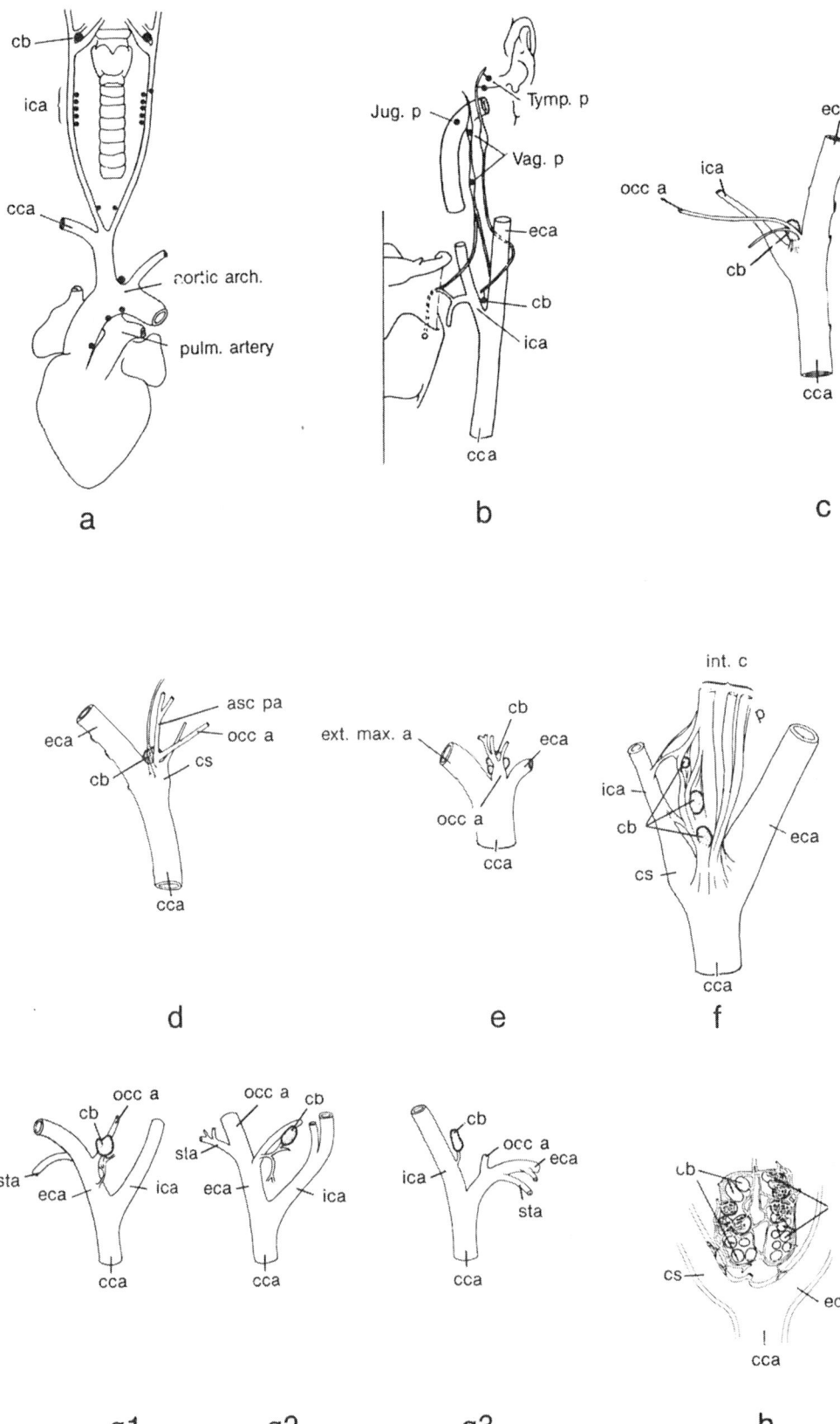

carotid artery which extended around the entire circumference of the vessel.

The cells comprising this early structure were elongated, and had large oblong nuclei with little chromatin. This morphology was similar to that of immature smooth muscle cells, but myofilamentous bundles were lacking, and in addition, the cytoplasm contained abundant granular and agranular endoplasmic reticulum, well-developed golgi and numerous vesicles. Unmyelinated nerve fibers containing both neurotubules and neurofilaments surrounded the undifferentiated cells (77).

With increased gestation time, the carotid body anlage grows in size and becomes separated by fibroblasts from the wall of the internal carotid artery. Fenestrated capillaries appear during this time also (77). Undifferentiated cells had a tendency to develop sheet-like processes which enveloped granule-containing cells. Synapse formation consisting of junctions between unmyelinated nerve fibers and granule-containing cells began at the 17th day of gestation and reached maximum development by the 20th day.

Gross anatomy

The positions of the various paraganglia including the chemoreceptor bodies of man were reviewed by Glenner and Grimley (47). The general location of chemoreceptor tissues and the comparative anatomy of the carotid bodies in man, (text Figure 1a and 1b) and selected domestic and laboratory animals is shown in text Figure 1.

In the monkey (*Macaca fascicularis*), the carotid bodies are located at the bifurcation of the common carotid artery into the external and internal carotid arteries (52).

The aortic bodies, which are the more prevalent chemoreceptor organs in the dog are located within the pericardial sac near the coronary arteries, dorsal, ventral and lateral to the aortic arch (text Figure 1c) between the aorta and the pulmonary artery (14, 114, 115). The carotid bodies of the dog are inconspicuous groups of cells located at the bifurcation of the carotid artery, intimately attached to or folded over and around the origin of the occipital and ascending pharyngeal arteries (2).

In the cat, the carotid body is oval or fusiform, reddish in color and is located in the carotid bifurcation rather than medial to it (text Figure 1d). It is intimately associated with the common occipito-ascending pharyngeal trunk and with the nerves coursing to the bifurcation (2).

In the cow, the carotid body consists of several lobes which are closely adherent to several branches of the ascending pharyngeal artery, (text Figure 1e) which is a branch of the external maxillary artery (2, 116).

In the horse, the carotid body is often multiple, ovoid or

General and comparative anatomy of chemoreceptor organs (paraganglia) including carotid bodies of man and selected domestic animals and laboratory animals.

a) General diagram to show the potential distribution of chemoreceptor tissue in mammals. The six black dots along the course of the common carotid artery represent "miniglomerula." The four lowermost black dots represent the locations of the aortic bodies (Adapted from Easton and Howe, 1983).

b) Location of the carotid bodies and vagal, jugular and tympanic paraganglia of man (Adapted from Glenner and Grimley, 1974).

c), d), e), f) Location of carotid body in dog, cat, cow and horse respectively and in that order (Adapted from Adams, 1958).

g-1, g-2, g-3 Variations in the location of carotid bodies in strain Wistar rats (Adapted from Habeck et al., 1981).

h) Location of guinea pig and rabbit carotid body. Multiple rabbit carotid bodies are shown.

asc pa = ascending pharyngeal artery
cb = carotid body
cca = common carotid artery
cs = carotid sinus
eca = external carotid artery
ext. max. a = external maxillary artery
ica = internal carotid artery
int. cp = intercarotid plexus
jug. p. = jugular paraganglia
occ a = occipital artery
pulm. artery = pulmonary artery
sta = superior thyroid artery
Tymp. p = tympanic paraganglia
Vag. p = vagal paraganglia

Figure 1a–h.

irregularly rounded and is located at the bifurcation of the common carotid artery, the lateral or medial wall of the carotid sinus, or within the perineurium of the intercarotid plexus (text Figure 1f) and of the vagus nerve (2).

In rats, the relative frequency of aortic bodies was studied, and considered inconstant and scarce by Easton and Howe (36). These authors found that in strain Wistar rats, only 2 of 7 had a full complement of aortic bodies and only 7 of 19 contained any aortic bodies (see text Figure 1a, g). van Zwieten et al. (148) identified histologically normal aortic bodies in 17 female and 2 male rats of strain WAG/Rij, in two female rats of strain Sprague-Dawley and in one male (WAG × BN)F₁ hybrid rat. The aortic bodies were present in the loose areolar connective tissue around the base of the aorta or pulmonary artery, or near the origin of a coronary artery (see text Figure 1a). They were frequently located adjacent to the cranial-most portion of the left ventricular wall. The carotid bodies of both the rat and the mouse (2, 24) are often recessed into the lateral aspects of the superior cervical ganglion, just caudal to the bifurcations of the external carotid arteries and at their medial aspects.

By the use of formalin-induced fluorescence coupled with electron microscopy small aggregates of chemoreceptor cells were found in the vagus nerve of rats (81). Similar aggregates were found in the recurrent laryngeal nerve of rats by Dahlqvist et al. (30) who used Evans blue dye coupled with electron microscopy. The use of Evans blue dye allows visualization of chemoreceptor cells because of its ability to readily fill the vessels of chemoreceptor bodies in man and other animals, and thus permits the study of species variations in the location, size, and number of such bodies.

Generally, the carotid bodies in the guinea pig and rabbit (see text Figure 1h) are located cranial to the bifurcation of the common carotid arteries, between the origins of the external and internal carotid arteries. They are intimately associated with the occipito-ascending-pharyngeal trunk. The carotid body of the domestic rabbit may vary somewhat in its location. It usually lies immediately distal to the bifurcation of the common carotid artery, but may be dorso-medial to the internal carotid (2). According to Clarke and Daly (24), the rabbit carotid body is not a compact structure and extends as strands or islands of tissue around the carotid bifurcation.

Histology

The histologic pattern of normal paraganglia including chemoreceptor organs is characterized by the presence of the predominant chief (type I) cells arranged as compact nests (see Figure 1) or "Zellballen" ("cell balls"). Chief cells are large, and rounded; they contain intracytoplasmic 0.1–0.2 micron diameter granules barely resolvable by light microscopy after fixation in glutaraldehyde. The granules fail to react with potassium dichromate, but stain by the Grimelius silver, McConail's lead-hematoxylin methods (47) or Bodian's stain ((86) see Figure 1). The nuclei are round and have abundant chromatin (47). Norepinephrine can be demonstrated in human chemoreceptor organs in both the free form and within the intracytoplasmic granules by fixation with hot formaldehyde vapors followed by exposure to ultraviolet radiation, yielding a blue green fluores-

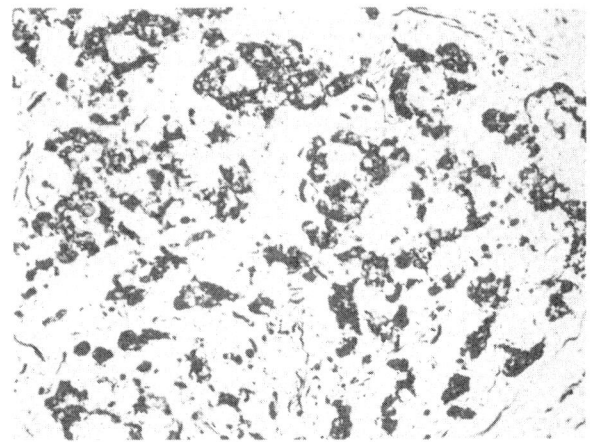

Figure 1. Normal carotid body from a 15 month old child. Several lobules contain cords and clusters of chief cells with distinct cytoplasmic argyrophilia. Bodian stain. 220 ×.

cence (39, 40). This staining reaction was first employed in the dog by Serafini-Francassini and Frasson (136). Efforts to obtain fluorescence of equine carotid body cells resulted in only faint fluorescence of the intracytoplasmic granules which was attributed, by the authors, to depletion of the contents of the granules by the anesthetic employed (61).

As mentioned in the foregoing, a second type of cell found in normal chemoreceptor organs is known as the sustentacular (type II) cell. The sustentacular cells surround the nests of chief cells. They are homologous to the satellite cells of autonomic ganglia, are distinguished by their peripheral location, and have oval or lenticular nuclei with condensed chromatin (61).

In cats, spherically shaped, 30–500 micron diameter micro-aggregates of chemoreceptor cells were described in the neck region by Matsuura (96). These tiny aggregates were located, by means of the response to electrical stimulation, at the level of the common carotid artery, between the carotid sinus and the thyroid artery. Clarke and Daly (24) demonstrated similar microscopic aggregates of chemoreceptor cells by serially sectioning the carotid bifurcations of 5 rabbits, 5 rats, 5 mice and the connective tissues around the wall of the ascending pharyngeal artery of the guinea pig. In rabbits only, such aggregates were also found in the connective tissues surrounding the internal carotid artery adjacent to the carotid bifurcation and common carotid artery.

Intravagal paraganglia in man are microscopic aggregates of cells within the vagus nerve (text Figure 1b) at or just below the level of the ganglion nodosum (47). Similar small aggregates of cells were located in the vagus nerve of rats by Kummer and Addicks (81) using formalin induced fluorescence and in recurrent nerve of rats (30), using Evans blue dye coupled with electron microscopy and formalin induced fluorescence.

Evans blue dye readily permeates vessels supplying chemoreceptor cells (100). Using this technique, the authors conducted a quantitative study in 10 rats to demonstrate the presence of (paraganglion) chemoreceptor cells in the vicinity of the glossopharyngeal, vagus, and sympathetic nerves.

An average of 92.5 of these aggregates (range 41–134) were found in the neck region and 41.5 (range 17–68) in the combined thorax and abdomen. On the basis of these studies, the authors postulated the existence of similar mini- and micro-chemoreceptor bodies in man and other animals, and the species variations in the location, size and number of such bodies.

Ultrastructure

Two forms of chief cells (type I) can be identified in human chemoreceptor organs and paraganglia. The first and predominant has a relatively pale cytoplasm with uniform, round dense granules. The second form appears as a dark cell with condensed cytoplasm and granules which are more angular and irregular than the granules of the first form. The dark cells often surround the light cells (47). The intracytoplasmic granules in man (47) and cat and rabbit (91) measure 0.1–0.15 mM and 0.15–0.20 mM in the horse and dog (61).

The satellite cells (type II) are analogous to Schwann cells; they have slender cytoplasmic processes which surround and interdigitate between the chief (type I) cells, separating small groups of chief cells from one another and from adjacent capillaries. There are occasional gaps between the satellite cell envelope; such gaps might permit contact of portions of the chief cells with the interstitium. Most of the satellite cells are separated from capillaries by two layers of basement membrane and, in addition, by both pericytes and satellite cells. Light and dark chief (type I) cells containing granules and sustentacular cells of the carotid body were demonstrated for the cat (10, 131), for the cat and rabbit by Lever et al. (91) and for the dog by Kobayashi (71).

Type I cells of the dog have a lower cytoplasmic density than do those of the horse. In the cat, dog and horse carotid body the endoplasmic reticulum is arranged in a Nissl-like fashion (10, 61) but such an arrangement of endoplasmic reticulum is absent in the guinea pig and rat (15, 75). In cats, Morita et al. (110) distinguished four types of chief cells based on the size, number and pleomorphism of the granules. Type I cells have large pleomorphic granules, while the granules of type II cells are small and dense and those of type III are small, homogeneous and less dense. Type IV cells are few in number, their cytoplasm is pale and the granules are sparse. In monkeys, Hansen (52) distinguished four types of chief cells based on size, density, number and pleomorphism of their dense core residues. The capillaries of the carotid body are similar in structure to the other endocrine organs, that is, they are of the fenestrated type. The innervation of the carotid bodies and the relationship of such nerves to the function of the carotid bodies continues to be the subject of further investigation. In this chapter only the ultrastructure of the innervation of the carotid bodies is considered; the physiologic and pharmacologic aspects will be considered in another chapter.

Glenner and Grimley (46), found, in human chief cell nests, unmyelinated axons which enter the chief cell nests accompanied by satellite cells. Ross (131) stated that, in the cat, nerve fibers are seen to be embedded in sustentacular cells. The sustentacular cells fold around nerve fibers where they have left Schwann cell sheaths en route to chief cells.

According to Hoglund (61), ultrastructural studies of the horse and dog carotid body showed synaptic vesicles, neurotubules and high concentrations of mitochondria located at the point of contact of a nerve fiber with glomus cells.

There is considerable controversy over the nature of the innervation of chief cells. Biscoe (9), as a result of experimental sectioning of the glossopharyngeal nerve, reported that all the synapses on type I cells were efferent in nature. The studies in rabbits (149), guinea pig (75), and mouse (73) affirmed the afferent innervation of the type I cell. A third group of investigators (1, 3, 61, 71) suggested that innervation of type I cells was by both afferent and efferent nerves. The chief cells of the rat carotid body (97) and dog (71) have dendrite like processes which extend 20–40 microns from the cell body. These processes contain smooth endoplasmic reticulum and scattered free ribosomes, very few polyribosomes, little ribosome-covered endoplasmic reticulum and few cytoplasmic granules. However, small clear vesicles, which are the hallmark of synapses within the chief cell are more numerous in the processes than in the remainder of the cytoplasm. Furthermore, the vesicles are more numerous as the distance from the cell body increases (97).

In the cat and rabbit, the synaptic vesicles are often fused with or bud from sacs of the golgi apparatus (10). Microfilaments of microtubules, mitochondria and lysosomes were demonstrated in the cytoplasm of chief cells (type I) of rabbits and cats (10) and in rats by Morgan et al. (109).

Cilia of the 9 + 0 fibril pattern were observed in both chief (type I) and satellite (type II) cells of the rabbit and cat by Biscoe and Stehbins (10), in the rat by Morgan et al. (109) and in the dog by Kobayashi (71). Biscoe and Stehbins (10), Kobayashi (71), and others observed variations in the density of the granular contents of synaptic vesicles. This change in density was considered to be related to secretion of neurotransmitters.

Some authors (102, 109) postulated on the basis of ultrastructural studies coupled with studies of denervation of several nerves, the existence of both efferent and afferent nerve endings. According to McDonald and Mitchell (102), in the rat carotid body two types of chief cells could be distinguished on the basis of the size of their dense cored vesicles. In cells classified as type A, the dense cored vesicles are 30% greater in diameter than those of type B. Furthermore, type A chief cells have at least two types of afferent nerve endings, which together make up 95% of the total. The remaining 5% of the nerve endings are preganglionic efferent axons from the cervical sympathetic trunk.

The ultrastructure of vessels supplying the rat carotid body presents three unique structures (101). The first of these structures is a large sphincter-like intimal cushion at the point of origin of the carotid body artery from the external carotid artery or occipital artery. The sphincters contain circular smooth muscle and constrict the diameter of the orifice to less than one-half. The second type of unique vascular structures resemble precapillary sphincters; these structures are located at the junction of the terminal arterioles and capillaries. The third type of unique vascular structures are the arteriovenous anastomoses, which bypasses capillaries and join directly to small venules. The authors postulate that these structures control carotid body blood flow and also serve to increase the hematocrit of the blood entering the carotid body.

Physiology

In this section the mechanisms for the activation of the chemoreceptor system are considered.

Deviation from the normal level of alveolar output is the level of alveolar ventilation; this in turn controls the levels of partial pressures of CO_2 (PCO_2) and O_2 (PO_2) in the blood. This alveolar output is monitored by the central chemoreceptors in the brain and the peripheral chemoreceptors in the aortic and carotid bodies (140).

The peripheral chemoreceptors maintain a tonic discharge, which increases as the level of dissolved oxygen in the blood falls. The respiratory rates increase only when the PO_2 is less than 5 mm of mercury. Therefore, the PO_2 is not a major factor in the control of respiration, but PO_2 does become important in life-threatening situations. In hypoxemia, ventilatory response is augmented by increased PCO_2 acting both on central (located in the ventral medulla) and on peripheral chemoreceptors. Changes in pH also activate the peripheral chemoreceptors, but a change of at least .1 unit is necessary before there is an increase in ventilation (140).

Since the cellular events by which chemoreceptor cells accomplish their regulatory task are not clear and since the literature is replete with numerous reports on the subject, several theories of the neurophysiology of the chemoreceptor organs will be presented here.

Heymans et al. (60) were the first investigators to demonstrate experimentally the chemoreceptive function of the carotid body. DeCastro (34) postulated, on the basis of axonal degeneration experiments, that carotid body cells are innervated by sensory axons of the glossopharyngeal nerve and that they are receptor cells that taste the chemical composition of the blood. Biscoe and Stehbins (10) demonstrated that nerve endings on chemoreceptor cells contain synaptic vesicles, suggesting that such nerves are motor and not sensory. Biscoe (9) proposed that chemoreceptor cells coupled with their motor innervation were parts of a feedback system regulating the sensitivity of chemoreceptor nerves.

Osborne and Butler (117) developed a theory of the mechanism of action of chemoreceptor cells based on their ultrastructural observations in ducks, those of Kobayashi (71) in dogs, and those of Hess and Zapata (59) in cats. This theory is as follows: sensory nerve fibers discharge spontaneously, possibly from a constant sodium current initiating action potentials. Dopamine acts as an inhibitory transmitter during conditions of normal CO_2 and O_2 concentrations in the blood. Thus, a high rate of dopamine would hyperpolarize the nerve endings and reduce the discharge frequency. In hypoxia, dopamine secretion is reduced and the nerve endings return to the depolarized state. Furthermore, depolarization causes release of a neurotransmitter (possibly acetylcholine) from the efferent synapses and this efferent neurotransmitter then acts to reduce dopamine secretion by the chemoreceptor cells. The decreased dopamine secretion results in a greater depolarization and, in turn, greater discharge.

McDonald and Mitchell (102) and McDonald (98, 99) postulated that there are reciprocal synapses between chemoreceptor cells and also between chemoreceptor cells and sensory nerves. The reciprocal synapses are thought to form an inhibitory loop, and sensory nerves release an excitatory transmitter when stimulated; the transmitter causes glomus cells to release dopamine and dopamine inhibits the sensory nerves.

The opioid enkephalin was localized, by immunologic means, in the chief cell granules of cat aortic and carotid bodies (53). The authors postulated that opioids, such as enkephalin may have a trophic influence on catecholamines which modulate chemoreceptor activity and are present in the same granules.

Arias-Stella (5) reported an increase in the size of carotid bodies in man and animals living at high altitude. Edwards et al. (37) demonstrated animals (guinea pigs) kept at high altitude had vacuolated and hyperplastic carotid body type I cells.

The carotid bodies of rats placed in hypobaric chambers develop hypoxia. The study of such rat carotid bodies was useful in elucidating the alterations brought on by hypoxia. A number of authors (6, 7, 88, 103) observed an increase in the size of the carotid bodies from hypoxic rats. Carotid body chief cells from hypoxic rats were increased in number and the nuclear diameter was increased (88, 89). Chief cell volume density was decreased (6) and the number of nuclear profiles decreased (103).

Increases in capillary lumen size were demonstrated ultrastructurally (6, 13). The mitochondria may be increased in number (88) or decreased (12) in hypoxia as is the amount of stromal collagen (13). Synaptic vesicle density is reduced (12).

The work of Korkala and Waris (78) with Sprague-Dawley rats subjected to hypovolemia caused by removal 1/4–1/3 of the total blood volume, induced an increased aggregation of granular vesicles which became closer to nerve endings. Biochemical changes in the carotid bodies of hypoxic rats include a decreased dopamine content, suggesting dopamine release during hypoxia. The norepinephrine levels in hypoxic rats remained constant (58). However, in the work of Pallot et al. (118) in which hypoxic rats received L-hydroxy dopamine or removal of the superior cervical ganglion, there was depletion of norepinephrine, but dopamine levels remained constant.

Hanbauer and Lovenberg (50) demonstrated, in the carotid bodies of hypoxic rats, a 2-fold increase in calcium dependent activator protein for cyclic ADP. The relationship of the activator protein to neurotransmission is based on the fact that membrane permeability for divalent calcium is the cause of neurotransmitter release and the amount of this release is directly proportional to influx of calcium ions.

Habeck et al. (49) and Honig et al. (62) studied the size, anatomic position and blood supply of the carotid bodies in rats of strains SHR (hypertensive) and NWR (normotensive, Wistar). The hypertensive rats had very few intimal cushions in the arteries supplying the carotid body and they developed respiratory alkalosis.

Hanbauer et al. (51) found an increase in the activity of tyrosine 3-monooxygenase in the carotid bodies of hypoxic rats. This enzyme was not induced in adrenal medulla, carotid artery or superior cervical ganglia of rats exposed to hypoxia.

Spontaneously occurring lesions of carotid or aortic bodies related to diseases characterized in hypoxia are reported in the literature for man, rats and dogs. Nissenblatt (113)

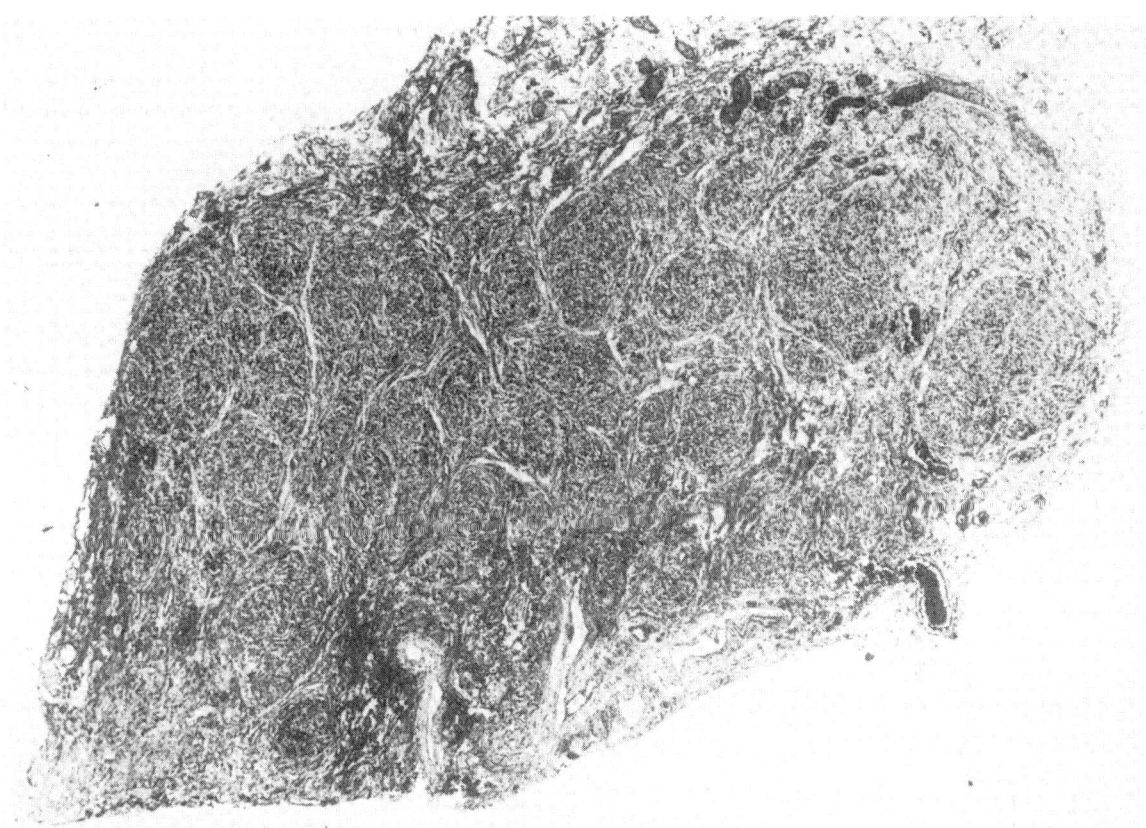

Figure 2. Carotid body from a 21-year-old girl with cystic fibrosis. Lobules ("Zellballen") are prominent, numerous and surrounded by a scant stroma. Hematoxylin and eosin. 28 ×.

reported on a case of hypoplastic right heart syndrome, polycythemia and carotid body tumor in a woman.

Lack (84) determined, at autopsy, the size and the histological characteristics of the carotid bodies of 69 patients with a variety of conditions which caused hypoxemia and examined these bodies histologically. The diseases included cystic fibrosis, cyanotic and congenital heart disease with or without chronic hypoxemia, sudden infant death syndrome and hyaline membrane disease. In 8 of 12 patients with hypoxemia, the carotid bodies were increased in width and length, but the diameter of the cell cords and the size of the individual cells was unaffected.

Lack et al. (86) examined morphologically, morphometrically, ultrastructurally and biochemically the carotid bodies of 85 humans. The cases included sudden infant death syndrome (38 cases), cystic fibrosis (30 cases, see Figures 2 and 3) and cyanotic heart disease (17 cases). Criteria used to judge alterations in the carotid bodies were presence or absence of intracytoplasmic argyrophilic granules and dopamine levels. The highest levels of dopamine occurred in the cases of cyanotic heart disease, in which argyrophilia was also increased. No measurable changes were made in sudden infant death syndrome, perhaps because of the short course of the disease.

Hopper et al. (63) reported on the occurrence of a carotid body tumor and an associated arteriovenous fistula in an 11-year-old female old English sheepdog which clinically showed congestive heart failure related to the shunting. The signs of congestive heart failure were diminished after excision of the fistula.

In rats of strains WAG/Rij, BN/Bi and (WAG × BN)F_1, aortic bodies were hyperplastic or neoplastic (Figures 4 and 5) in only strain WAG/Rij and in a preponderance of females (148). The authors suggested that since chronic respiratory disease was present in all three strains and, that in addition, myocardial fibrosis was present in strain BN/Bi, the occurrence of aortic body hyperplasia and neoplasia in only strain WAG/Rij may have a genetic basis. Unfortunately, the carotid bodies of the rats on this study were not systematically examined.

Gross pathology

Sites of occurrence and other features of paragangliomas and chemodectomas in man and chemodectomas of animals are shown in Tables 1 and 1a.

Carotid body tumors of man are usually adherent to the medial aspect of the adventitia of the common carotid artery. The tumor may be localized and displace the external and internal carotid arteries.

Carotid body tumors of the bovine (116, 138) were located in the neck, closely attached to the left carotid artery at the point of origin of the occipital artery. The two reported

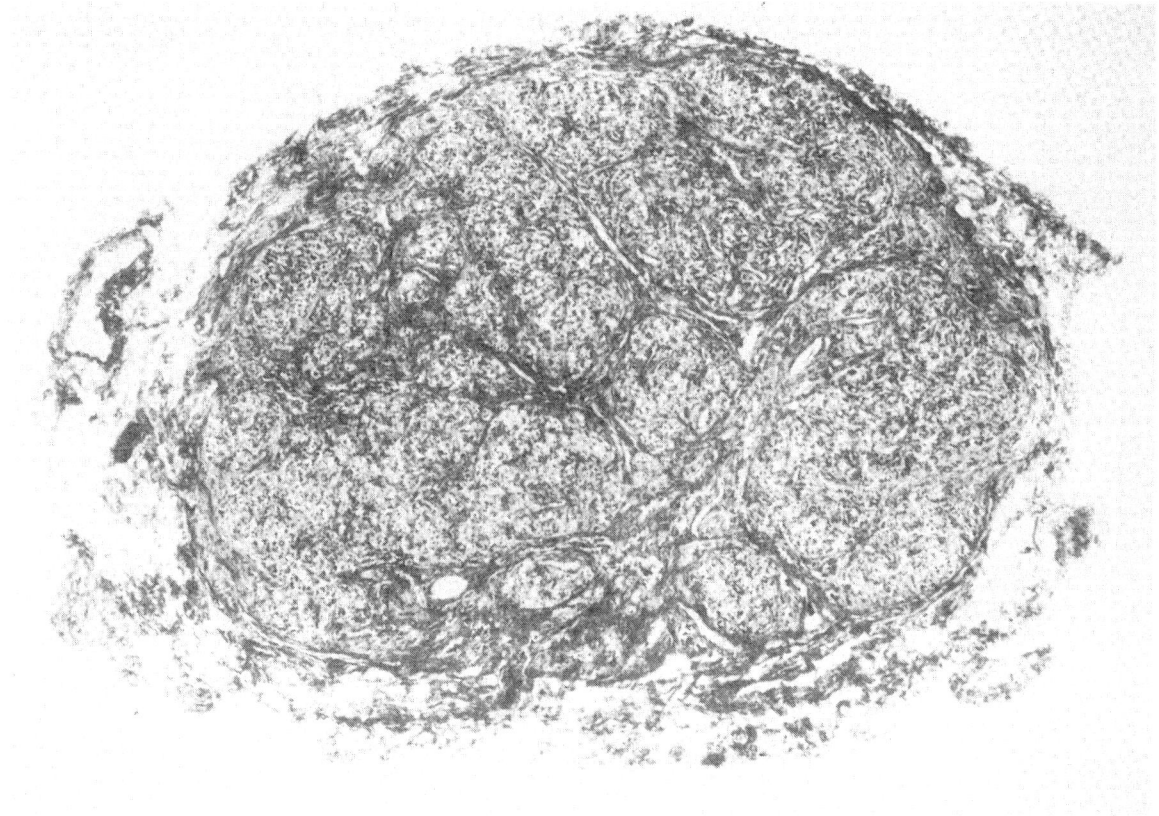

Figure 3. Carotid body from a 9-year-old girl with cystic fibrosis. The lobules are surrounded by a well vascularized stroma. Hematoxylin and eosin. 40 ×.

cases of bovine aortic body tumors (a.b.t.) were located as follows: 1) The tumor covered the right auricle and heart base extending between it and the pulmonary artery to which it adhered; the pulmonary artery contained tumor deposits when opened (93) 2) The tumor was situated "above the interventricular septum" and was also attached to the wall of the auricles (87). Unfortunately, a detailed necropsy was not performed and the gross illustration in the paper by Ladds and Daniels (87) does not illustrate the heart base and great vessels.

In man, paragangliomas of the jugulo-tympanic bodies occur in the middle ear and originate laterally in the temporal bone and erode through the floor of the tympanum, presenting clinically as a mass in the middle ear. Tumors of the laryngeal paraganglia usually arise on either side of the midline above the anterior end of the vocal cords or between the thyroid and cricoid or form within the recurrent branch of the vagus nerve. Aortic body tumors in man are often attached to or lie within the pericardium surrounding the left auricle or are associated with the ascending aorta. Occasionally, the tumor lies anterior to the aorta and extends to the left subclavian artery, but is not intimately attached to these vessels (47).

Canine carotid body tumors are located at the carotid bifurcation and may incorporate this structure, the external jugular vein and the left common carotid artery (64, 82, 135). Canine aortic body tumors are located within the

pericardial sac near the base of the heart, often intimately related to the ascending aorta and pulmonary arteries (14, 31, 67, 119, 127). Nilsson (112) cited 20 cases of a.b.t. located at the heart base between the left auricle and the pulmonary artery; in 7 cases the tumors were located between the left auricle and the pulmonary artery and in 4 other cases the tumors were located between the right auricle and the aorta. Patnaik et al. (119) studied the exact anatomic locations of 61 a.b.t. Thirty-four were located at the base of the aorta, 27 occurred in the space between the aorta and the pulmonary artery. Of the remainder, 4 were at the anterior surface of the aortic arch, 2 on the adventitia of the subclavian artery, 2 between the branches of the pulmonary artery, and 2 elsewhere on the adventitia of the pulmonary arteries.

Feline a.b.t. have been reported by Collins (26), Buergelt and Das (18) and by Yates et al. (153). The cat reported by Buergelt and Das (18) had three distinct a.b.t. The first was located between the left pulmonary artery and the ventral curvature of the aortic arch covering the free margin of the right auricle. The second tumor was located at the dorsal insertion of the pericardium, between the right pulmonary artery and the left atrium, and the third tumor was located ventral to the cranial portion of the thoracic aorta.

The single equine aortic body tumor (33) was located between the ascending aorta and the pulmonary artery; it was attached to the adventitia of the aorta.

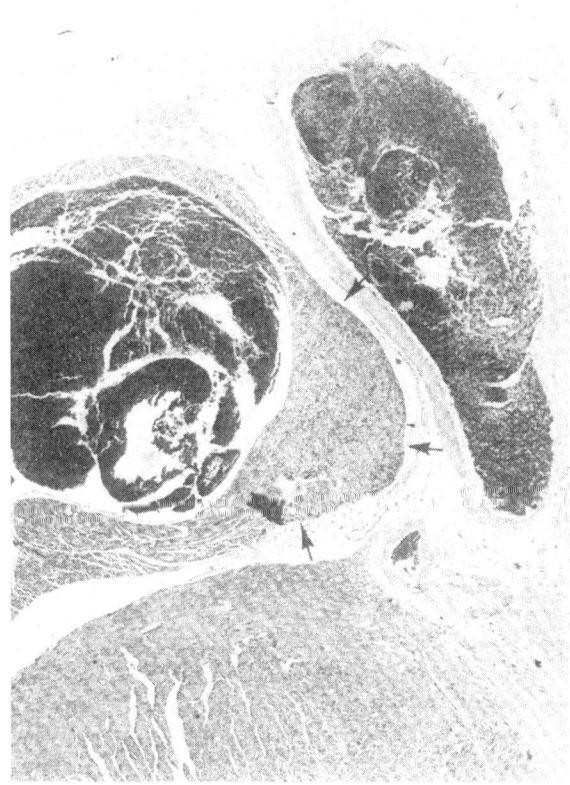

Figure 4. Chemoreceptor body tumor of left atrium in a strain WAG/Rij rat, female, 33 months of age. The animal had been ovariectomized and irradiated at between 6 and 8 weeks of age. The tumor (arrows) has invaded wall of the left atrium, center and left; the left ventricle is at bottom, aorta upper right. Hematoxylin and eosin. 15 ×.

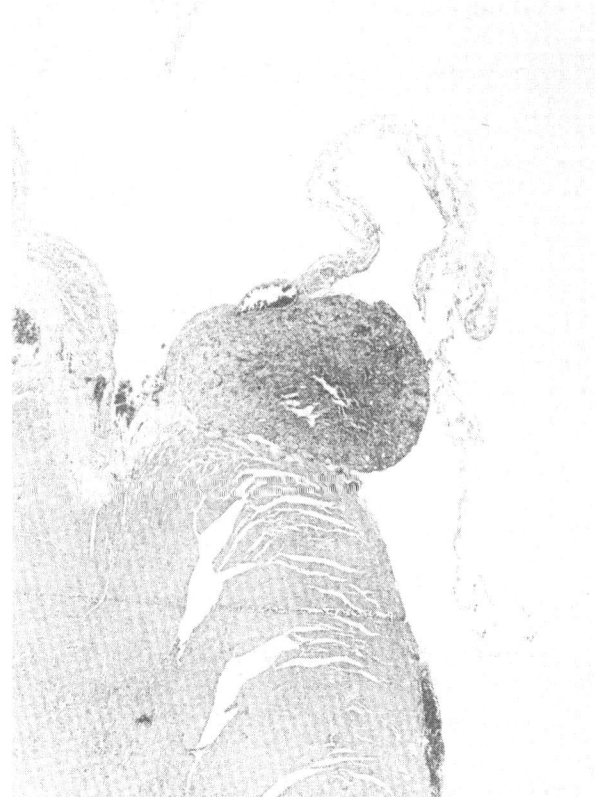

Figure 5. Chemoreceptor body tumor at base of left ventricle (lower left) in a strain WAG/Rij rat, female, 25 months of age. The animal had been ovariectomized and irradiated at between 6 and 8 weeks of age. The tumor is well-circumscribed and compresses the myocardium. A portion of the pericardium is at lower right (arrows). Hematoxylin and eosin. 16 ×.

Only two rat chemodectomas were described grossly (121, 145). The aortic body tumor of the first rat was 3 mm in diameter and was attached to the aortic adventitia. The chemodectoma of the second rat was located "near the primary bronchus."

Tumors of the pulmonary paraganglia in man are described as being in a subpleural location. Patnaik et al. (119) reported the occurrence of two canine pulmonary chemodectomas, but did not give their exact location.

Chemodectomas and paragangliomas of all species are firm, yellow-tan or white, and on cut surface contain red areas, are lobulated owing to their connective tissue content, and some (64) may contain central moist gelatinous areas.

Patnaik et al. (120) designated as chemodectoma a tumor of the urinary bladder in a dog. The tumor was located in dorsolateral part of the wall and extended into the ureter; it was soft, gray and lobulated.

Histology: Histopathology

Tumors of the paraganglia and chemoreceptor organs have the tendency to reproduce the architecture of the normal gland, thus imparting an organoid appearance (47). Many chemodectomas of man give the impression of proliferation or glandular hyperplasia. Poor preservation or fixation of the cellular component may increase difficulty of diagnosis (16, 47).

Chemodectomas of domestic animals are usually well encapsulated; the opposite is true in man (47). In paragangliomas of man and chemodectomas of both man and animals the neoplastic cells are usually arranged as nests or "Zellballen" (see Figure 6) (16, 47, 83, 85, 92), in canine chemodectomas in an alveolar pattern (14, 23, 64, 119) or as nests (32). In paragangliomas of man the neoplastic cells may be arranged as ribbons, festoons and rosettes (47), or as interlacing bundles of small spindle cells (85). The connective tissue stroma surrounds the groups of neoplastic cells and is highly vascular. Hemosiderin is frequently seen at the periphery of both human paragangliomas and animal chemodectomas; fibrosiderotic (Gamna-Gandy) nodules occurred in a single human carotid body tumor and a single human vagal body tumor (85). In human paragangliomas, sinusoids may be dilated, imparting a "lymphangiectoid" appearance (85). Mast cells are often present in perilobular tissues in hypertrophic human carotid bodies (84). In canine chemodectomas, palisading of the nuclei around sinusoids gives rise to a peritheliomatous appearance (14, 16, 64, 67,

Table 1. Paragangliomas in man: site, incidence and other features.

Race, Age, Sex	Site	Incidence	Comments	Reference
white, 27 yrs., 28 yrs., both F	c.b	2 cases	27 yr old F. had bilateral tumors. The patients were sisters; reviews early lit.	(22)
white, 50 yrs., M	c.b.	single case	Tumor extended from vicinity of thyroid to mediastinum. Vascular invasion. Metastases to multiple sites. Author reviewed 8 other cases with metastases	(129)
white, 43 yrs., M	c.b. (bilateral)	single case	Removed two well-differentiated carotid body tumors. Five relatives also had carotid body tumours	(132)
Irish, English, Dutch descent 5 M, 1 F	c.b. bilateral in 3 males	6 cases	Entire family had thick, short necks. The tumor in one family member arose at the carotid bifurcation and involved cranial nerves IX, X, XI, XII	(70)
Caucasian, aged 19–42, 11 females 3 males	c.b.	14/242 in a single family in 2 generations	The tumors were bilateral in 5 family members. Eight also had clotting defects	(79)
4th to 6th decade 16 F, 13 M	c.b. one patient had 4 tumors, 2 of carotid body; 2 of jugular body c.b. = carotid body	29 cases	This article emphasizes the clinical features of carotid body tumors	(27)
mean age 43 yrs. (range 30–53) 7 females, 3 males	c.b. tumors, all on left side	10 cases	Average size was 3–5 cm. in diameter. One tumor was considered inoperable because of its large size	(28)
43 years, F	c.b. right side	single case	Tumor metastasized to lung	(41)
33–66 yrs., 6 F, 5 M	c.b. tumors	11 cases	Two patients had locally invasive tumors requiring carotid artery prostheses; two patients had local recurrence of their tumors	(108)
65 yr. old male	c.b. tumors, bilateral	5/6 siblings and three of their children were affected	5.5 × 4.5 × 3 cm. tumor removed on right side. No metastases	(152)
av. age 47 yrs at 1st visit	c.b.	30 cases 28 followed for av. of 11 yrs.	7 cases with metastases. (1.n., lu., base of skull, ht.)	(95)
64 yr. old female	c.b.	single case (reviews 13 others	Metastasis to vertebral bodies of L2, L3, L4, L5, L10, L11, L12, femur and pubis	(134)
19–72 yrs. (c.b.) 20–71 yrs. (v.b.) 22–80 yrs. (j.-t.) females predominant in v.b. and j.-t.	21 c.b. (1t) 19 c.b. (rt) 7 v.b. (rt) 6 v.b. (1t) 5 j.-t. (1t) 4 j.-t. (rt) 3 nasal 1 ea.-aortico-pul. aortic arch laryngeal orbit	26 males 44 females of 13,400 autopsies (.012%)	3 carotid body tu. metastasized. (heart, lymph node, lung, vertebrae, ribs)	(84)
4 whites, 4 coloured, 1 black 31–70 yrs. 8 females, 1 male	petrous temporal bone, 2 tumors jugular bulb and middle ear 7 tumors	8 women, 1 man 1–2/20,000 otolaryngology cases	1 patient had extensive spread, the other had lung metastases	(43)
56 yr. old female, other cases ranged in age 13–66 yrs.	vertebrae L-3 to L-5	very rare	Reviewed 16 previously reported cases of cauda equina "paragangliomas." The author's case was positive for nonspecific enolase	(92)

Table 1. Continued.

Race, Age, Sex	Site	Incidence	Comments	Reference
white 38 yr. old female	retroperitoneum	single case	Reviewed 37 cases. Five metastasized to lung and pleura; 4 to bones, 2 to lymph node and 1 each to liver and kidney; 2 spread within the abdominal cavity	(80)
Japanese 37 yr. old female	right nasal cavity	single case only four cases in world literature	All recurred locally; none metastasized	(146)

v.b. = vagal body
j.-t = jugulo-tympanic
tu. = tumor

Table 1a. Chemodectomas in animals: site, incidence and other features.

Species	Strain, Breed Age and Sex	Site	Comments	Reference
Canine	Dachshund 13 yrs. male	heart base	Described osteochondrosarcoma of heart base and reviewed heart base tumors of man and animals	(8)
Canine	Alsation no age or sex given	a.b.	Tumor of heart base caudal to aorta; compressed atrium	(66)
	Sealyham terrier age and sex unk.	a.b.	As above; metastasized to lung	
	unknown	a.b.	No gross pathology given	
Canine	2 Boston terriers 14 and 9 yrs, males	a.b.	Tumors of heart base compressing atria	(14)
Canine	Boston terrier 10 yrs., male	c.b.	Mass in neck attached to carotid artery at level of hypoglossal nerve	(135)
Canine	2 Boston terriers 13 yr f. and 15 yr m.	c.b.	Both had ascites one had coronary artery disease	(64)
	1 Boxer, aged, f.	c.b. & a.b.	Had myocardial necrosis fibrosis of heart valves	
Canine	7 Boston Terriers 10 Boxers 1 Dachshund 1 Spitz 1 Mongrel mean age 10 yrs. 12/20 were males	a.b.	2/20 had lung metastases 5/6 male boxers also had interstitial cell tumors of the testis	(67)
		a.b. = aortic body c.b. = carotid body		
Canine	Boxer, castrated male, 12 yrs.	a.b.	Animal also had pancreatic adenocarcinoma with metastases	(82)
Canine	Boxer, female 9 yrs.	a.b., 3	Infiltrated wall of left ventricle and metastasized to lung, kidney adrenal	(127)
Canine	Boxers – males, 11 & 14 yrs; spayed female, 8 yrs., terrier male, 17 yrs. Saluki, female, 7 yrs.	a.b., 5 c.b.	527 dog carcasses examined and 6 had chemoreceptor neoplasms. There was no mention of metastasis	(154)
Canine	11/20 in boxers 28/45 were of thyroid origin 4 unclassified	69 heart base tumors	Identified in two cases, typical type I cells by electron microscopy	(16)
Canine	Fox terrier, female, 13 yrs.	wall of urinary bladder	Animal also had pheochromocytoma and mammary adenocarcinomas	(120)
Canine	Mongrel, terrier cross, male, 8 yrs.	a.b.	Tumor at heart base, compressing the left auricle	(31)

Table 1a. Continued

Species	Strain, Breed Age and Sex	Site	Comments	Reference
Canine	Boxers, Boston Terriers, 9 other breeds over 50% in Boxers 12% in Boston Ter. 15% in mixed breeds most frequent in 10–15 yr. age group	a.b. (71) c.b. (7) includes dogs with multiple tumors	Metastases to lung occurred in 6 Metastases to liver occurred in 4 Metastases to myocardium occurred in 4 Metastases to kidney occurred in 3 Metastases to lymph n., adr., brain occurred in 1 ea.	(119)
Canine	Basset, female, 6 yrs. Boxer, female, 12 yrs. Cocker, female, 8 yrs. Airdale, male, 7 yrs.	c.b.	All four were surgical cases, none were necropsied. Author reviews 22 previously reported cases, 9 of which also had aortic body tumors	(32)
Canine	Basset, female 3 yrs.	c.b.	Tumor metastasized to liver, pancreas, spleen and heart	(44)
Canine	Wire Haired Fox Terrier, male, 7 yrs	a.b.	Tumor invaded rt. atrium, metastasized to lymph node, spleen and arch of 8th thoracic vertebra	(21)
Canine	Doberman Pinscher	a.b. (2)	Clinical presentation for lesion of wing of left ileum. Tumor metastasized to the lung and wing of left ileum	(107)
Canine	Boston Terriers – 7 Boxers – 5 Collies – 5 Other Breeds and mongrels – 11 mean age 10 yrs. 16/28 were males	a.b. (24) c.b. (4)	9 cases with metastases 4 cases were locally invasive but were not tabulated as to primary site	(153)
Canine	Boxer, 7 yrs., f. Min. Schnauzer, 11 yrs., m.	a.b. a.b.	Both cases diagnosed as tumors at heart base by angiographic means. Histologic examination not performed on the boxer. The tumor of the Schnauzer invaded the atrial wall and lumen	(20)
Canine	Old English Sheepdog, 11 yrs., spayed female	c.b.	Animal had concomitant arteriovenous fistula, located in the cervical region	(63)
Canine	mixed breed, 7 yr. old castrated male	a.b.?	Tumors of anterior mediastinum, interatrial septum. Tumor adherent to 1st thoracic vertebra and invaded the intervertebral foramina of T1 and T2	(11)
Feline	Domestic shrtr. 12 yrs., female	c.b.	Tumor metastasized to lungs bronchi and mediastinal lymph nodes; there were tumor deposits in coronary vessels	(26)
Feline	Siamese, 7 yrs., female	a.b.	Three separate aortic body tumors. There was invasion of lymph vessels of the lung, pericardium, myocardium and epicardium	(18)
Feline	Breed not given, 12 yrs. sex unknown	c.b.	On cut surface cystic spaces were visible grossly	(153)
Bovine	Holstein, female, 1 yr.	c.b.		(138)
Bovine	Holstein female, 5 yrs., from abbatoir	c.b.	Tumor deposits in pulmonary artery were visible grossly. Tumor invaded the wall of the aorta	(87)
Bovine	Head of cow from abbatoir	c.b.	18 × 15 cm. mass attached to common carotid artery	(116)
Bovine	Specimen of bovine heart from abbatoir age and sex unknown	c.b.	Tumor located "above interventricular septum."	(87)
Equine	Breed not given, female, age not given	a.b.	Neoplasm localized at heart base	(33)
Rattine	Albino, 3 yrs. male	a.b.	Only case of 2552 tumors of rats. (N = 399925 rats). Animal also had a subcutaneous fibrosarcoma. Aortic body tumor was attached to the adventitia of the aorta, was round, smooth, tan and measured 3 mm. in diameter	(145)

Table 1a. Continued

Species	Strain, Breed Age and Sex	Site	Comments	Reference
Rattine	WAG/Rij, 22–47 mo.	a.b.		
	5 females (5.5%) - - - - - - - - - - - - -		untreated	(148)
	8 females- - - - - - - - - - - - - - - - -		treated by various means	
	Sprague Dawley, 23 months of age, 1 female Separated hyperplastic lesions from neoplastic lesions on the basis of local invasion		treatment status not given	

107, 112, 135). According to Patnaik et al. (119), all 6 of the carotid body tumors, but only half of the aortic body tumors (30 of 59) of the dogs studied by him had a distinct pattern. Nordstoga (116) observed a peritheliomatous pattern in his bovine case.

According to Glenner and Grimley (47) and Lack et al. (85), lymphocytic infiltrates occur in some human paragangliomas. Lymphocytic infiltrates of the tumor capsule were frequently found in the 69 canine chemodectomas studied by Bomhard et al. (16).

Stromal hyalinization occurred in about one-half of the 72 carotid body tumors and in the vagal body tumors described by Lack et al. (85) and in some cases of human paragangliomas described by Glenner and Grimley (47). In

man capillaries encircling individual groups of cells are demonstrable with silver stains.

The tumor cells are round, oval or polygonal, closely packed and have poorly defined borders in chemodectomas of all species studied by sections colored by hematoxylin and eosin. The cytoplasm is acidophilic and may be finely granular. The nuclei are centrally situated, generally vesicular, but sometimes hyperchromatic and pleomorphic (see Figure 6). In human paragangliomas multinucleated giant cells may be present (47, 85). Cells with giant nuclei are frequently seen in canine chemodectomas (14, 16, 64, 82, 112) and in the bovine a.b.t. reported on by Lombard and Sarrazy (93) and Ladds and Daniels (87). The nucleoli are often multiple and there may be intranuclear cytoplasmic inclusions (85). In human paragangliomas, there are cells which may vary greatly in density of cytoplasmic staining, so-called "light and dark" cells (47).

A second type of tumor cells occurs in both human paragangliomas and canine chemodectomas (16, 47). Such cells are elongated, resemble fibrocytes, and have scant cytoplasm and chromatin-rich nuclei.

Differential diagnosis

In man, the occurrence of neoplasms of the jugulotympanic, cauda equina and retroperitoneal necessitates a review of possible differential diagnoses for such tumors. Middle ear adenomas arising from lining epithelium, may on histologic examination, be confused with neuroendocrine tumors and previously were labeled as adenomatous neoplasms, adenomas, carcinomas, ceruminous carcinomas, adenocarcinomas and carcinoid tumors (105). The authors reviewed 7 cases of middle ear adenomas and demonstrated intracytoplasmic lysozyme immunocytochemically in all. Four of seven middle ear adenomas also contained intracytoplasmic granules demonstrable with the Grimelius stain. The authors considered immunocytochemical demonstration of lysozyme a useful tool for the separation of middle ear adenomas from neuroendocrine tumors of this region.

Lipper and Decker (92) described a case of paraganglioma of the cauda equina and reviewed 16 cases in the literature. They state that neuroendocrine tumors (paragangliomas) of the cerebrospinal axis occur in the pineal gland, pituitary gland and the filum terminale. Their patients, a 56-year-old female, had a tumor located within the dura mater of the cauda equina at the level of L-3. Histologically, the tumor cells were arranged as sharply circumscribed nests and surrounded by a richly vascular stroma. Argyrophilic intracytoplasmic granules were demonstrated with the Grimelius stain. Immunohistochemical staining

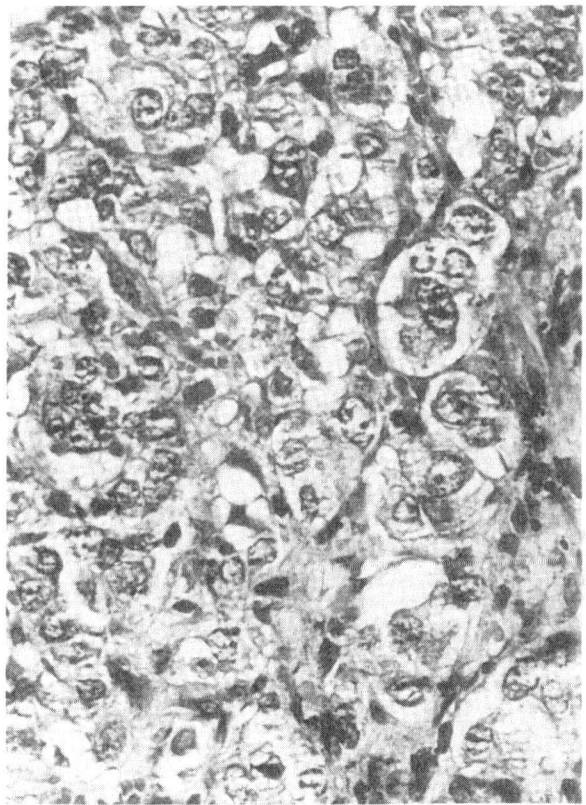

Figure 6. High power view of tumor shown in figure 5, above. The tumor cells are arranged as nests, upper and right, or single and in clumps, left center. The tumor cells vary markedly in size and shape; their cytoplasm is finely granular or vacuolated and the nuclei are round to oval. Hematoxylin and eosin. 330 ×.

utilizing an antiserum directed against neuron-specific enolase, S-100 protein and glial fibrillary protein was positive for only neuron specific enolase. Neuron-specific enolase is demonstrable in neuroblastomas, small cell lung carcinomas, thyroid medullary carcinomas, trabecular carcinomas of the skin, melanomas, carcinoids and paragangliomas (92).

Kryger-Baggesson et al. (80) described a single case and reviewed 37 cases of neuroendocrine tumors of the retroperitoneum of man. Their patient had a large tumor (15 × 7 × 7 cm) located anterior to the left kidney and it was in close relationship to the pancreas and spleen. By electron microscopy, dense core granules were noted but the tumor was negative for the chromaffin reaction. The authors stated that possible differential diagnoses to be considered are: large tumor of the abdominal cavity, malignant tumors of the stomach, colon and kidney, ovarian cysts, fibromyomas of the uterus, leukemias of the spleen or retroperitoneal lymph nodes and metastases to the lymph nodes or retroperitoneal fibrosis.

Heart base tumors of the dog include tumors of ectopic thyroid, parathyroid glands, aortic bodies or metastases of other tumors. In this section the differentiation of such tumors and of heart base tumors in other domestic species is discussed.

Barth (8) reviewed the literature on heart base tumors of man and domestic animals with an emphasis on the dog. Included was a single case of an extra-skeletal osteochondrosarcoma of the base of the heart in a dachshund. The author reviewed equine heart base tumors and quoted 1) Signol and Lavland (1869) who described a large sarcoma, 2) Doenecke (1900) who described an osteosarcoma, 3) Dexter (1892) a melanoma (probably metastatic), 4) Haubold (1907) and 5) Magnussen (1916) who both described single cases of lymphosarcoma.

In cattle, single cases of neurofibrosarcoma of the heart base were ascribed to kitt (1891), Magnussen (1916), Fehsenmeier (no date given) and 5 cases to Peters (1910). A single bovine myxosarcoma of the heart was attributed to Waldemann (1906) and a single case of lymphosarcoma to Huynen (1907). Numerous reports of lymphosarcoma, metastatic to the heart of bovines, are reviewed elsewhere (see chapter on bovine lymphosarcoma). Barth also reviewed a single case of "spindle cell sarcoma" in the heart of a sheep, described by Joest (1909) and in a tumor of the heart base in a dog designated as "adenoma" by the same author in 1912 and thought by Barth (8) to represent a thymoma. However, the tumor did not contain Hassal's corpuscles and this prompted Jackson (66) in his review to consider it as a true heart base tumor.

Jackson (66) reviewed the literature on canine heart base tumors and described 3 cases of his own, including them in a chapter on canine venereal tumors, and stated that canine venereal tumors and canine heart base tumors could not be distinguished microscopically (but this is not considered to be true now). Bloom (14) reviewed the work of Jackson and Barth and added two additional cases of his own. The gross and microscopic anatomy of the neoplasms and of normal aortic bodies was compared. The author concluded that the histologic appearance and cytology of both normal and neoplastic aortic bodies were similar. It was also concluded that aortic and carotid bodies were part of the chemoreceptor system and not paraganglia or arteriovenous anastomoses. Bloom also commented on the difficulties expressed by Jackson in distinguishing canine venereal sarcomas from aortic body tumors. The main criteria given for differentiating the two types of tumors are the absence of giant cells and the lack of a peritheliomatous pattern in canine venereal sarcomas. Small cell size, distinct cell outline and a greater number of mitoses were the other criteria used by Bloom for distinguishing aortic body tumors from canine venereal sarcoma.

Cohrs (25) found that ectopic thyroid tissue located at the heart base was enlarged in dogs with goiter and described what was felt to be medullary thyroid carcinoma at the heart base. Ectopic thyroid tissue embedded in the fat at the base of the aorta was found in 190/400 or 47.5% of normal dogs.

Nilsson (112) studied 40 cases of canine heart base tumors and classified them histologically into 2 groups: group 1 (33 cases) had considerable variation in the morphology of the tumor cells, and the presence of giant cells and necrosis; group 2 (7 cases) had a few giant cells, little necrosis, lacked a pattern and lacked differentiation. The tumors in these 7 cases were regarded as being of possible ectopic thyroid origin.

Cheville (23) compared the histologic and ultrastructural features of aortic and carotid body tumors with the features of tumors of ectopic thyroid or parathyroid origin. Chemoreceptor tumors could be differentiated from ectopic thyroid tumor tissues by the following criteria:

1) Neoplastic chemoreceptor cells contain dense osmiophilic membrane bound granules.

2) Chemoreceptor cells contain biogenic amines which can be demonstrated by the use of the Falck test (formalin induced fluorescence).

3) The absence in neoplastic chemoreceptor cells of the criteria for ectopic thyroid tissue, namely follicles with PAS positive content or intracellular PAS positive droplets.

Aortic body tumors of rats (148) and normal aortic body cells of the horse did not react to the Falk test. Therefore the use of this criterion may be useful only in identifying human and canine tumors.

Thake et al. (142) examined both histologically and ultrastructurally, three ectopic thyroid adenomas of the canine heart base. All three tumors were located between the ascending aorta and the pulmonary artery. Histologically, they were composed of areas of well-differentiated follicles containing PAS positive material and less well-differentiated solid groups of cells, some of which contained PAS positive granules. Ultrastructurally, the most striking characteristic was the presence of long tubular structures within the cisternae of the endoplastic reticulum. The tubular structures were randomly distributed and on cross section were round with central dense cores; they were symmetrically arranged in units of 6 surrounding a single central tubule. The tubules were found in the cytoplasm of cells in both differentiated (follicular) and undifferentiated portions of the tumors. A single tumor designated by Cheville (23) as ectopic thyroid adenoma contained, histologically, cystic and solid areas composed of tumor cells arranged in cords. The rod-like structures earlier described by Thake et al. (142) in three other ectopic thyroid tumors of the canine heart base were not mentioned for the tumor described by Cheville. However, both Cheville (23) and Deutschlander (35) found similar tubular structures in the cytoplasm of neoplastic epithelial cells of canine thyroid adenocarcinomas located at the usual site surrounding the first two tracheal rings.

Bomhard et al. (16) reported on 69 cases of canine heart base tumor. Sixty-seven of the cases were examined by light microscopy using conventional and semi-thin toluidine blue stained sections; two cases were examined by both light and electron microscopy. Forty-five of the 69 cases (65%) were regarded as ectopic thyroid tumors of the heart base and 20 as chemodectomas; 4 could not be classified because of poor preservation. The authors applied the histologic criteria of Cheville (23) to their classification and stated that the finding in semi-thin sections of large granules (1.5 microns or larger) in the cytoplasm could be used as an additional criterion for the identification of undifferentiated neoplastic cells of ectopic thyroid origin. Such granules are regarded as lysosomes and were different from the PAS positive droplets described by Cheville (23). The authors mention that granules of smaller size (0.3 microns) occur in both c cells and in chemoreceptor cells. None of the tumors designated thyroid adenomas of the heart base were subjected to electron microscopy, nor was there any mention of the gross or microscopic appearance of the thyroids. The authors suggested that endemic iodine deficiency could have caused the high rate of occurrence of ectopic thyroid adenomas.

Metastasis

Metastasis of carotid body tumors in man (the most frequent chemoreceptor tumor of man) generally occurs in less than 10% of cases (27, 85, 95) but the tumor often invades the periadventitial tissue in the area of the carotid bifurcation. The most frequent sites of metastasis are the regional nodes and the lung; liver, heart and bone are less frequent sites.

Aortic body tumors, the most frequent chemoreceptor tumor in animals, frequently invade the heart (16, 119), pericardium (119) veins and lymphatics (23, 29, 66, 68, 111). Metastases of canine aortic body tumors occur less frequently than metastases of carotid body tumors, but metastases are found in lung, liver, mediastinal and tracheobronchial lymph nodes, and rarely in kidney, other nodes, adrenal cortex and brain (119).

Nilsson (112), Jubb and Kennedy (68) and Cheville (23) reported on cases of canine aortic body tumors with widespread pleural carcinomatosis, which Cheville (23) regarded as characteristic of aortic body tumors. Other authors (32, 112, 119) did not mention this feature as characteristic of aortic body tumors.

Patnaik et al. (119) reported that 15 of 67 canine chemodectomas they studied by them metastasized, consisting of 4 of the 6 carotid body tumors and 11 of 59 aortic body tumors. Two pulmonary chemodectomas did not metastasize. Nilsson (112) claimed that 3 of 7 canine heart base tumors, designated as being of ectopic thyroid origin, showed infiltrative growth and other indications of a malignant tumor, but metastasis was not mentioned.

Bomhard et al. examined and described 69 canine heart base tumors but did not mention metastasis, probably because only two of the cases were necropsied at their laboratory; only slides and blocks of the remaining cases were submitted by other laboratories. There are three reported cases of canine aortic body tumors which metastasized to bone (21, 107, 141). The dog of Carlisle et al. (21) showed signs of spastic paraplegia, and at necropsy a tumor was located in the dorsal arch of the 8th thoracic vertebra and compressed the spinal cord. The patient of Montgomery et al. (107) presented with lameness and soft tissue swelling of the left hemipelvis. The tumor destroyed most of the ala of the left ilium.

Collins (26) reported on the occurrence of the only known case of metastasizing chemoreceptor tumor in a cat. The primary tumor was located at the bifurcation of the trachea. The metastases were described grossly as involving "the large coronary vessels, parietal pleura, which was granular, with granular whitish proliferations particularly prominent over each rib. About two-thirds of the lung tissue was involved."

Aortic body tumors of bovines and equines have not been reported to metastasize, although the bovine case reported by Ladds and Daniels (87) invaded the left ventricular wall. None of the aortic body tumors of rats reported on by Van Zwieten et al. (148) metastasized, however all the lesions classified as neoplasms invaded the left or right atrium (Figure 4).

Epidemiologic aspects of chemodectomas

In man, most chemodectomas commonly arise in the carotid body; others have been reported in the glomus jugulare, and rarely in the aortic, vagal, femoral, retroperitoneal, and ciliary bodies (19). Spontaneously occurring chemodectomas have been reported frequently in dogs and rarely in any other domestic animal species (153). In dogs, the typical sites of origin have been the aortic body and the carotid body, in a ratio of about 5:1 (55).

Several retrospective veterinary hospital studies have related their diagnoses to a referent population drawn from patients seen at medical teaching facilities. The largest (54) published to date involved 73 dogs seen at 12 North American veterinary university facilities collaborating in the Veterinary Medical Data Program (VMDP) (54). That study provided statistical evidence of a familial predisposition among dogs with English bulldog ancestry (e.g., Boston terrier, Boxer) and a male risk, also confined to bulldog breeds, particularly to the Boston terrier (54). A review of 2 million computerized abstracts representing canine hospital episodes reported to the VMDP through June, 1983, by 17 participating North American veterinary university facilities yielded 278 [including the 73 previously reported by Hayes (54)] patients with microscopically confirmed chemodectomas (Hayes and Sass, 57)). Of these, 224 dogs had an aortic body tumor, 48 a carotid body tumor, and 6 dogs had both. Because of sufficient numbers, separate statistical analyses were performed to characterize the epidemiologic features of patients with each neoplasm.

A familial aggregation in English bulldog relatives continued to predominate, representing 43% of those dogs with an aortic body tumor and 26% of those with a carotid body tumor. Relative risk (*RR*) values (45) were significantly (P (0.01) higher than expected by chance for aortic body and carotid body tumors individually in the Boston terrier and Boxer, and related English bulldog breeds collectively. No other canine breed was detected with a statistically significant elevated risk. Other purebreds, a category composed of all other purebreds not individually tested, showed for chemodectomas about the same relative risk as mongrel dogs. This suggests that, outside the English bulldog family, genetic inducement plays little, if any role in etiology. In man, familial aggregations are uncommon but have been reported in people with chemodectomas of the carotid body (70, 79, 139) glomus jugulare (147) and vagal body (69); those of the carotid body have been attributed to an autosomal dominant form of inheritance (4).

A male risk in dogs was evident with chemodectomas of both aortic and carotid body origin. This was confined only to English bulldog related breeds. In man, chemodectomas have been reported with about equal frequency among those with carotid body tumors, except in Peruvians who live at high altitudes in the Andes where a 6-fold excess was recorded in women (133). In smaller case series of vagal body (83) and glomus jugulare tumors (126) women have predominated in a ratio of 4:1 or greater, but these studies were not analyzed relative to a referent population.

The average age of dogs with chemodectomas is 10 years. The rate of diagnosis of both carotid and aortic body tumors increases in dogs as they get older. This age relationship is similar to that seen for canine neoplasia generally (123). Comparable age-specific data in humans are unavailable; however, most patients have been middle aged at time of first diagnosis (122).

As in man (151) dogs exhibit examples of multiple endocrine neoplasia in association with chemodectomas. However, these primary endocrine tumors were particularly evident in dogs with aortic body tumors; about half occurred in bulldog breeds suggesting the association was independent of a familial risk for chemodectoma. Most frequent were thyroid carcinomas and adrenocortical neoplasms; there were 2 cases with pheochromocytoma. The latter combination was reported rarely in man and always associated with carotid body tumors (124). Four autosomal dominant familial syndromes have been associated with human pheochromocytomas; one involves multiple endocrine neoplasia (94).

Epidemiologically, canine chemodectomas should not be considered as one nosological entity since the pattern of disease differs between English bulldog related animals and other dogs. The English bulldog, and its relatives, display the prominent phenotypic characteristic of an "undershot" jaw in conjunction with a shortened muzzle relative to the size of its skull (brachycephaly) (104). Most commonly associated with this physical trait are soft tissue anomalies of the nasal and oral cavities, and pharynx. These include oversize tongue, elongation of the soft palate, and stenotic nares (42, 90). The airway restriction of the latter two anomalies can be so severe that, during stress, they collapse the larynx because of the greatly increased negative intrapulmonary pressure created on inspiration (90). Thus, the presence of these anomalies may compel brachycephalic dogs to compensate throughout life for respiratory distress by increased respiratory effort and other physiological changes.

Emphysema, a condition associated with long standing respiratory disease and a cause of chronic hypoxia, has been positively correlated with carotid body hyperplasia (38). Studies have reported that the carotid bodies of several mammalian species, including dogs (37) and humans (5), undergo hyperplasia when subjected to chronic hypoxia by living in a natural high altitude environment. Further investigation has shown that humans living at high altitudes (2000 meters) have 10 times the incidence of chemodectomas as those living at sea level (133). Thus, hyperplasia and neoplasms of chemoreceptor tissue have been associated with the same etiological exposure-chronic hypoxia.

It has been proposed that the elevated risk for chemodectomas in English bulldog breeds is the result of a genetic predisposition aggravated by chronic hypoxia (54). Other common brachycephalic breeds (the Pekingese and Pug) have not been reported as having chemodectomas or a high frequency of other neoplasms (123).

The epidemiologic features of canine chemodectomas bear a similarity to that in man. Whatever the environmental exposure or genetic mechanism involved, the dog appears to be a suitable model to further our understanding of human chemodectomas in familial aggregation, in association with chronic hypoxia, or in association with other primary endocrine neoplasms.

ACKNOWLEDGEMENTS

The author wishes to thank Dr. Ernest E. Lack, NCI who contributed figures 1, 2 and 3. Drs. C. Hollander, H. Solleveld of the Institute for Experimental Gerontology, TNO, Rijswijk, the Netherlands and M. van Zwieten of Merck and Co. West Point, PA. are herewith acknowledged for contributing sections of rat chemodectomas.

REFERENCES

1. Abraham A: Electron microscopic investigations on the human carotid body. (preliminary communication) *Z Mikrosk-Anat Forsch* 79:309, 1968
2. Adams WE: *The Comparative Morphology of the Carotid Body and Carotid Sinus.* C.C. Thomas, Springfield, IL. 1958
3. Al-Lami F, Murray RG: Fine structure of the carotid body of normal and anoxic rats. *Anat Rec* 160:697, 1968
4. Anderson DE: Genetic varieties of neoplasia. In: *Genetics, Concepts and Neoplasia.* pp. 85–104. Williams and Wilkins, Baltimore. 1970
5. Arias-Stella J: Human carotid body at high altitude. *Am J Pathol* 55:82a, 1969
6. Barer GR, Walsh M: Chronically hypoxic rat carotid bodies. *J Physiol (Lond.),* 290:38, 1979
7. Barer GR, Edwards CW, Jolly AI: Changes in the carotid body and the ventilatory response to hypoxia in chronically hypoxic rats. *Clin Sci and Mol Med* 50:311, 1976
8. Barth A: Ein Beitrag zur Kenntnis der Herzbasisgeschwülste beim Hund. Inaug. Diss. Univ. Leipzig. pp. 1–52, 1920
9. Biscoe TJ: Carotid body: Structure and function. *Physiol Rev* 51:437, 1971
10. Biscoe TJ, Stehbens WE: Ultrastructure of the carotid body. *J Cell Biol* 30:563, 1966
11. Blackmore J, Gorman NT, Kagan K, Hines S, Spencer C: Neurologic complications of a chemodectoma in a dog. *J Am Vet Med Assoc* 184:475, 1984
12. Blakeman N, Pallot DJ: Ultrastructural changes in the rat

carotid body in response to hypoxia and hyperoxia. *J Anat* 135:839, 1982

13. Blessing MH, Kaldeweide J: Light and electron microscopic observations on the carotid bodies of rats following adaptation to high altitude. *Virchows Arch (Cell Pathol)* 18:315, 1975

14. Bloom F: Structure and histogenesis of tumors of the aortic bodies in dogs. *Arch Pathol* 36:1, 1943

15. Blumcke S, Rode I, Niedorf HR: The carotid body after oxygen deficiency. *Z Zellforsch Mikrosk Anat* 80:52, 1967

16. Bomhard Dv, Luderer M, Hanichen T, Sandersleben Jv: Zur Histogenese der Herzbasistumoren beim Hund. *Zbl Vet Med-A* 21:208, 1974

17. Boyd JD: The development of the human carotid body. *Contrb Carnegie Inst* 26:1, 1937

18. Buergelt C-D, Das KM: Aortic body tumor in a cat. *Path Vet* 5:84, 1968

19. Byrne JJ: Carotid body and allied tumors. *Am J Surg* 95:371, 1958

20. Cantwell HD, Blevins WE, Weirich WE: Angiographic diagnosis of heartbase tumor in the dog. *J Am An Hosp Assn* 18:83, 1982

21. Carlisle CH, Kelly WR, Samuel J, Robins GM: Spinal cord compression caused by a metastatic lesion from an aortic body tumor. *Aust Vet J* 54:311, 1978

22. Chase WH: Familial and bilateral tumors of the carotid body. *J Pathol Bacteriol* 36:1, 1933

23. Cheville NF: Ultrastructure of canine carotid body and aortic body tumors. *Vet Pathol* 9:166, 1972

24. Clarke JA, Daly M de Burgh: A comparative study of the distribution of carotid body type-I cells and periadventitial type-I cells in the carotid bifurcation regions of the rabbit, rat, guinea-pig and mouse. *Cell Tissue Res* 220:753, 1981

25. Cohrs P: Beitrag zur Kenntnis der intrapericardialen akzessorisch Schilddrüsen und Epithelialkörperchen beim Hund. *Berl tierärztliche Wochenschrift* 46:683, 1930

26. Collins DR: Thoracic tumor in a cat. *Vet Med Small An Clin* 59:459, 1964

27. Conley JJ: The carotid body tumor. A review of 29 cases. *Arch Otolaryngol* 81:187, 1965

28. Cordell AR, Myers RT, Hightower F: Carotid body tumors. *Ann Surg* 165:880, 1967

29. Cotchin E: Neoplasms of the domesticated animals. A review. *Commonwealth Bur An Hlth Rev Ser No. 4*, pp. 21–22, 1956

30. Dahlqvist A, Carlsoo B, Domeij S, Hellstrom S: Morphometric analysis of glomus cells within the recurrent laryngeal nerve of the rat. *J Neurocytol* 13:407, 1984

31. Damodaran S, Thanikachalam M: Aortic body tumor in a dog. *Indian Vet J* 52:747, 1975

32. Dean MJ, Strafuss AC: Carotid body tumors in the dog: A review and report of four cases. *J Am Vet Med Assoc* 166:1003, 1075

33. de Barros CSL, dos Santos MN: Aortic body adenoma in a horse. *Aust Vet J* 60:61, 1983

34. de Castro F: Sur la structure et l'innervation du sinus carotidien de l'homme et des mammiferes. Nouveaux faits sur l'innervation et la fonction du glomus caroticum. Etudes anatomiques et physiologique. *Trav Lab Invest Biol Univ Madrid* 25:331, 1928

35. Deutschlander N: Ungewöhnliche Tubuli im Endoplasmatischen Retikulum von Schilddrüsentumorzellen. *Virchows Arch (Cell Pathology)* 11:11, 1972

36. Easton J, Howe A: The distribution of thoracic glomus tissue (aortic bodies) in the rat. *Cell Tissue Res* 232:349, 1983

37. Edwards C, Heath D, Harris P, Castillo Y, Kruger H, Arias-Stella J: The carotid body in animals at high altitude. *J Pathol* 104:231, 1971a

38. Edwards C, Heath D, Harris P: The carotid body in emphysema and left ventricular hypertrophy. *J Pathol* 104:1, 1071b

39. Falck B: Observations on the possibility of the cellular localization of monoamines by a fluorescent method. *Acta Physiol Scand* 56: suppl. 197, 1962

40. Falck B, Owman CA: A detailed methodological description of the fluorescence method for the cellular demonstration of biogenic amines. *Acta Univ Lund Sec II* 7:1, 1965

41. Fanning JP: Metastatic carotid body tumor. Report of a case with review of the literature. *J Am Med Assoc* 185:49, 1965

42. Fox MW: Developmental abnormalities of the canine skull. *Can J Comp Med Vet Sci* 27:219, 1963

43. Gertler R, Sellars SL: Paragangliomas of the petrous temporal bone. *SA Med J* 66:614, 1984

44. Garand M: Histoire de cas. Chemodectome malin du corps carotidien chez une chienne Basset Hound. *Can Vet J* 18:228, 1977

45. Gart JJ: Point and interval estimation of the common odds ratio in the combination of the 2 × 2 tables with fixed marginals. *Biometrika* 57:471, 1970

46. Glenner GG, Grimley PM: Histology and ultrastructure of carotid body paragangliomas. Comparison with the normal gland. *Cancer* 20:1473, 1967

47. Glenner GG, Grimley PM: Tumors of the extra-adrenal Paraganglion system (including chemoreceptors) in: *Atlas of Tumor Pathology*. 2nd series, Fascicle 9. Armed Forces Institute of Pathology, Bethesda, MD. 1974

48. Gray H: Neurology. Anatomy of the Human Body. pp. 1014, 1339. Edited by Goss CM, Lea and Febiger, Philadelphia, PA. 1948

49. Habeck J-O, Honig A, Pfeiffer C, Schmidt M: The carotid bodies in spontaneously hypertensive and normotensive rats. A study concerning size, location, and blood supply. *Anat Anz (Jena)* 150:374, 1981

50. Hanbauer I, Lovenberg W: Presence of a calcium^{2+}-dependent activator of cyclic-nucleotide phosphodiesterase in rat carotid body: effects of hypoxia. *Neuroscience* 2:603, 1977

51. Hanbauer I, Lovenberg W, Costa E: Induction of tyrosine 3-monooxygenase in carotid body of rats exposed to hypoxic conditions. *Neuropharmacology* 16:277, 1977

52. Hansen JT: Ultrastructure of primate carotid body; a morphometric study of the glomus cells and nerve endings in the monkey (*Macaca fascicularis*). *J Neurocytol* 14:13, 1985

53. Hansen JT, Brokaw J, Christie O, Karasek M: Localization of enkephalin-like immunoreactivity in the cat carotid and aortic body chemoreceptors. *Anat Rec* 203:405, 1982

54. Hayes HM Jr: An hypothesis for the etiology of canine chemoreceptor system neoplasms, based upon an epidemiological study of 73 cases among hospital patients. *J Small Animal Pract* 16:337, 1975

55. Hayes HM Jr, Fraumeni JF Jr: Chemodectomas in dogs: Epidemiologic comparisons with man. *JNCI* 52:1455, 1974

56. Hayes HM Jr, Wilson GP, Moraff H: The veterinary medical data program (VMDP): past, present, and future. In: Proceedings of the International Symposium on Animal Health and Disease Data Banks. pp. 127–132. Technical Information Service, Science and Education Administration, U.S. Department of Agriculture, Beltsville, MD. 1979

57. Hayes HM Jr, Sass B: Epidemiologic features of canine chemodectomas by site of origin. Manuscript in preparation.

58. Hellstrom S, Hanbauer I, Costa E: Selective decrease of dopamine content in rat carotid body during exposure to hypoxic conditions. *Brain Res* 118:352, 1976

59. Hess A, Zapata P: Innervation of the cat carotid body. Normal and experimental studies. *Fed Proc* 31:1365, 1972

60. Heymans C, Boouckeart JJ, Dautreband L: Sinus carotidien et reflexes respiratoires. II Influences respiratoires reflexe de

l'acidose de l'alkalose, de l'anhydride carbonique, de l'ion hydrogen et l'anoxemie: Sinus carotidien et exchanges respiratoires dans les poumons et au dela des poumones. *Arch Int Pharmacodyn* 39:400, 1930

61. Hoglund R: An ultrastructural study of the carotid body of horse and dog. *Z f Zellforsch* 76:568, 1967

62. Honig A, Habeck J-O, Pfeiffer C, Schmidt M, Huckstorf Chr, Rotter H, Eckermann P: The carotid bodies of spontaneously hypertensive rats (SHR): A functional and morphological study. *Acta Biol Med Germ* 40:1021, 1981

63. Hopper PE, Jongward SJ, Lammerding JJ: Carotid body tumor associated with an arteriovenous fistula in a dog. *Comp Cont Ed* 5:68, 1983

64. Hubben K, Patterson DF, Detweiler DK: Carotid body tumor in the dog. *J Am Vet Med Assoc* 137:411, 1960

65. Ito T: On the origin of the carotid body in the rabbit. *Folia Anat Jap* 23:117, 1950

66. Jackson C: The contagious (transmissible venereal) neoplasm of the dog and heart-base tumours of the dog. 2- Tumours of the base of the heart in the dog. *Onderstepoort J Vet Sci and An Ind* 6:399, 1936

67. Johnson KH: Aortic body tumors in the dog. *J Am Vet Med Assoc* 152:154, 1968

68. Jubb KVF, Kennedy PC: Endocrine System. In: Pathology of Domestic Animals. Vol. I, p. 340. 1st Ed. Academic Press, New York, NY. 1963

69. Kahn LB: Vagal body tumor (non-chromaffinic paraganglioma, chemodectoma and carotid body-like tumor) with cervical lymph node metastasis and familial association. *Cancer* 38:2367, 1976

70. Katz AD: Carotid body tumors in a large family group. *Am J Surg* 108:570, 1964

71. Kobayashi S: Fine structure of the carotid body of the dog. *Arch Histol Jap* 30:95, 1968

72. Kobayashi S: Comparative cytology studies of carotid body. Ultrastructure of synapses on the chief cell. 2. Ultrastructure of synapses. *Arch Histol Jpn* 33:397, 1971

73. Kobayashi S, Uehara M: Occurrence of afferent synapses in the carotid body of the mouse. *Arch Histol Jap* 32:193, 1970

74. Kohn A: Uber den Bau und die Entwicklung der sog. Carotisdruse *Arch Mikr-Anat Anat Entwickl* 56:81, 1900

75. Kondo H: An electron microscopic study on innervation of the carotid body of the guinea pig. *J Ultrastruct Res* 37:544, 1971

76. Kondo H: An electron microscopic study on the caudal glomerulus of the rat. *J Anat* 113:341, 1972

77. Kondo H: A light and electron microscopic study on the embryonic development of the rat carotid body. *Am J Anat* 144:275, 1975

78. Korkala O, Waris T: Ultrastructural changes in the rat carotid body in severe hemorrhagia. *Cell Tissue Res* 158:355, 1975

79. Kroll AJ, Alexander B, Cochios F, Pechet L: Hereditary deficiencies of clotting factors VII and X associated with carotid-body tumors. *N Engl J Med* 220:6, 1964

80. Kryger-Baggesen, Kjaergaard T, Sehested M: Nonchromaffin paraganglioma of the retroperitoneum. *J Urol* 134:536, 1985

81. Kummer W, Addicks K: The paraganglion vagi: An intravagal paraganglion in the rat. *Cell Tissue Res* 224:455, 1982

82. Kurtz HJ, Finco DR: Carotid and aortic body tumors in a dog – A case report. *Am J Vet Res* 30:1247, 1969

83. Lack EE: Carotid body hypertrophy in patients with cystic fibrosis and cyanotic congenital heart disease. *Human Pathol* 8:39, 1976

84. Lack EE, Cubilla AL, Woodruff JM, Farr HW: Paragangliomas of the head and neck region. A clinical study of 69 patients. *Cancer* 39:397, 1977

85. Lack EE, Cubilla AL, Woodruff JM: Paragangliomas of the head and neck region. A pathologic study of tumors from 71 patients. *Human Pathol* 10:191, 1979

86. Lack EE, Perez-Atayde AR, Young JB: Carotid body hyperplasia in cystic fibrosis and cyanotic heart disease. A combined morphometric, ultrastructural and biochemical study. *Am J Pathol* 119:301, 1985

87. Ladds PW, Daniels PW: Aortic body tumor in an ox. *Aust Vet J* 51:43, 1975

88. Laidler P, Kay JM: The effect of chronic hypoxia on the number and nuclear diameter of type I cells in the carotid bodies of rats. *Am J Pathol* 79:311, 1975

89. Laidler P, Kay JM: A quantitative study of some ultrastructural features of the type I cells in the carotid bodies of rats living at a simulated altitude of 4300 metres. *J Neurocytol* 7:183, 1978

90. Leonard HC: Collapse of the larynx and adjacent structures in the dog. *J Am Vet Med Assoc* 137:360, 1960

91. Lever JD, Lewis PR, Boyd JD: Observations on the fine structure and histochemistry of the carotid body in the cat and rabbit. *J Anat* 93:478, 1959

92. Lipper S, Decker RE: Paraganglia of the Cauda equina. A histologic immunohistochemical, and ultrastructural study and review of the literature. *Surg Neurol* 22:415, 1984

93. Lombard CH, Sarrazy J: Deuxieme cas de tumeur du corps aortique chez la vache. *Bull Acad Vet* 38:209, 1965

94. Manager WM, Gifford RW Jr: Pheochromocytoma. Springer Verlag, New York, NY. 1977

95. Martin CE, Rosenfeld L, McSwain B: Carotid body tumors: A 16 year follow-up of seven malignant cases. *Southern Med J* 66:1236, 1973

96. Matsuura S: Chemoreceptor properties of glomus tissue found in the carotid region of the cat. *J Physiol* 235:57, 1973

97. McDonald DM: Structure and function of reciprocal synapses interconnecting glomus cells and sensory nerve terminals in the rat carotid body. In: Chromaffin, Enterochromaffin and related cells, Chapter 24, pp. 375–394. edited by Coupland RE, Fujita T. Elsevier Scientific Publishing Co. New York, NY. 1976

98. McDonald DM: Structure-function relationships of chemoreceptive nerves in the carotid body. *Adv Biochem Psychopharmacol* 16:193, 1977a

99. McDonald DM: Role of glomus cells as dopaminergic interneurons in the chemoreceptive function of the carotid body. *Adv Biochem Psychopharmacol* 16:265, 1977b

100. McDonald DM, Blewett RW: Location and size of carotid body-like organs revealed in rats by the permeability of blood vessels to Evans blue dye. *J Neurocytol* 10:607, 1981

101. McDonald DM, Larue DT: The ultrastructure and connections of blood vessels supplying the rat carotid body and carotid sinus. *J Neurocytol* 12:117, 1983

102. McDonald DM, Mitchell RA: The innervation of glomus cells and blood vessels in the rat carotid body: a quantitative ultrastructural analysis. *J Neurocytol* 4:177, 1975

103. McGregor KH, Gil J, Smatresk NJ, Barnard P, Lahiri S: A morphometric study of the carotid body in chronically hypoxic rats. *Fed Proc* 42:978, 1983

104. Miller ME, Christensen GC, Evans HE: Anatomy of the Dog. p. 8. W.B. Saunders, Philadelphia, PA. 1964

105. Mills SE, Fechner RE: Middle ear adenoma. *Am J Surg Pathol* 8:677, 1984

106. Mirov AG: Benign and malignant carotid body tumors. *JAMA* 181:13, 1962

107. Montgomery DL, Bendele R, Storts RW: Malignant aortic tumor body tumor with metastasis to bone in a dog. *Vet Pathol* 17:241, 1980

108. Morfin E: Carotid-body tumors. *Arch Surg* 91:947, 1965

109. Morgan M, Pack RJ, Howe A: Nerve endings in rat carotid body. *Cell Tissue Res* 157:255, 1975

110. Morita E, Chiocchio SR, Teramessani JH: Four types of main cells in the carotid body of the cat. *J Ultrastruct Res* 28:399, 1969

111. Nieberle P, Cohrs P: Special Pathological Anatomy of Domestic Animals. Pergamon Press, Oxford, Great Britain. 1967

112. Nilsson T: Heart-base tumours in the dog. *Acta Path Microbiol Scand* 37:385, 1955

113. Nissenblatt MJ: Cyanotic heart disease: "Low altitude" risk for carotid body tumor? *J Hopkins Med J* 142:18, 1978

114. Nonidez JF: The aortic (depressor) nerve and its associated epithelioid body, the glomus aorticum. *Am J Anat* 57:259, 1935

115. Nonidez JF: Distribution of the aortic nerve fibers and the epithelioid bodies (Supracardial "paraganglia") in the dog. *Anatomy* 69:299, 1937

116. Nordstoga K: Carotid body tumor in a cow. *Path Vet* 3:412, 1966

117. Osborne MP, Butler PJ: New theory for receptor mechanism for carotid body receptors. *Nature* 254:701, 1975

118. Pallot DJ, Al Neamy KW, Mir AK, Nahorski SR: Rat carotid body catecholamines: strain variations and the effects of sympathectomy and hypoxia. *J Anat* 133:703, 1981

119. Patnaik AK, Liu S-K, Hurvitz AJ, McClelland AJ: Canine chemodectoma (extra-adrenal paragangliomas) – a comparative study. *J Small Animal Pract* 16:785, 1975

120. Patnaik AK, Lord PF, Liu S-K: Chemodectoma of the urinary bladder of the dog. *J Am Vet Med Assoc* 164:797, 1974

121. Peck HM: Design of experiments to detect carcinogenic effects of drugs. In: Carcinogenesis Testing of Chemicals. p 1. Edited by: Goldberg L, CRC Press Inc., Cleveland, OH. 1974

122. Pratt LW: Familial carotid body tumors. *Arch Otolaryngol* 97:334, 1973

123. Priester WA, Mantel N: Occurrence of tumors in domestic animals. Data from 12 United States and Canadian colleges of veterinary medicine. *JNCI* 47:1333, 1971

124. Pritchett JW: Familial occurrence of carotid body tumor and pheochromocytoma. *Cancer* 49:2578, 1982

125. Rabl H: Die Entwicklung der Carotisdrüse beim Meerschweinchen. *Arch Mikr Anat* 96:315, 1922

126. Reddy EK, Mansfield CM, Hartman GV: Chemodectomas of glomus jugulare. *Cancer* 52:337, 1983

127. Richards MA, Mawdesley-Thomas LE: Aortic body tumours in a boxer dog with a review of the literature. *J Pathol* 98:283, 1969

128. Rogers DC: The development of the rat carotid body. *J Anat* 99:89, 1965

129. Romanski R: Chemodectoma (Non-chromaffinic paraganglioma) of the carotid body with distant metastases. *Am J Pathol* 30:1, 1954

130. Rosai J: Adrenal gland and paraganglia. In: Ackerman's Surgical Pathology. pp. 717–727. C.V. Mosby Co., St. Louis, MO. 1981

131. Ross L: Electron microscopic observations of the carotid body of the cat. *J Biophys Biochem Cytol* 6:253, 1959

132. Rush BF: Familial bilateral carotid body tumors. *Ann Surg* 157:633, 1963

133. Saldana MJ, Salem LE, Travezen R: High altitude hypoxia and chemodectomas. *Hum Pathol* 4:251, 1973

134. Say CC, Hori J, Spratt J: Chemodectoma with distant metastasis: Case report and review of the literature. *Am Surg* 39:333, 1973

135. Scotti TM: The carotid body tumor in dogs. *J Am Vet Med Assoc* 132:413, 1958

136. Serafini-Francassini A, Frasson P: Histochemical observations on the carotid body of the dog. *Acta Anat* 63:240, 1966

137. Simeonescu N, Simeonescu M: Circulatory System. Histology – Cell and Tissue Biology. p 420. Edited by Weiss L. Elsevier Biomedical, New York, NY. 1983

138. Smith HA, Jones TC: Veterinary Pathology. Lea and Febiger, Philadelphia, PA. 1961

139. Sprong DH, Kirby FG: Familial carotid body tumors. *Ann West Med Surg* 3:241, 1949

140. Steffey EP, Robinson NE: Respiratory System-Physiology and Pathophysiology. In: Textbook of Veterinary Internal Medicine. Edited by: Ettinger SJ. W.B. Saunders, Philadelphia, PA. 1983

141. Szczech GM, Blevine W, Carlton W, Cutlen G: Chemodectoma with metastasis to bone in a dog. *J Am Vet Med Assoc* 162:376, 1973

142. Thake DC, Cheville NF, Sharp RK: Ectopic thyroid adenomas at the base of the heart of the dog. *Vet Path* 8:421, 1971

143. Tisseur H: Les tumeurs du système chemorecepteur chez le chien. *Econ et Med Anim* 5:257, 1964

144. Trautman A, Fiebiger J: The circulatory system. Fundamentals of the Histology of Domestic Animals. pp 114–115. Translated by Habel RE and Biberstein EL, Comstock Publishing Associates, Ithaca, NY. 1952

145. Trevino GS, Nessmith WB: Aortic body tumor in a white rat. *Vet Path* 9:243, 1972

146. Ueda N, Yoshida A, Fukunushi R, Fujita H, Yanagihara N: Non-chromaffin paraganglioma in the nose and paranasal sinuses. *Acta Pathol Jpn* 35:489, 1985

147. Van Baars F, Broek PV, Cremers C, Veldman J: Familial non-chromaffinic paragangliomas (glomus tumors): clinical aspect. *Laryngoscope* 91:988, 1981

148. van Zwieten MJ, Burek JD, Zurcher C, Hollander CF: Aortic body tumours and hyperplasia in the rat. *J Pathol* 128:99, 1979

149. Verna A: Terminations nerveuses afferentes et efferentes dans le glomus carotidien du lapin. *J Microscopie* 10:59, 1971

150. Watzka M: Über die Entwicklung des Paraganglion Caroticum der Säugetiere. *Z ges Anat L Z Anat Entwickl Gesch* 108:61, 1938

151. Weichert RF III: The neural ectodermal origin of the peptide-secreting endocrine glands. *Am J Med* 49:232, 1970

152. Wilson H: Carotid body tumors: Familial and bilateral. *Ann Surg* 171:843, 1970

153. Yates WDG, Lester SJ, Mills JHL: Chemoreceptor tumors diagnosed at the Western College of Veterinary Medicine 1967–1979. *Can Vet J* 21:124, 1980

154. Zakarian B, Naghshineh R, Sanjar M: Aortic body and carotid body tumours in dogs in Iran. *J Small Animal Pract* 13:249, 1972

BOVINE LYMPHOMA – EPIDEMIOLOGY, DIAGNOSIS, TRANSMISSION, PATHOLOGY

BERNARD SASS

Bovine leukemia is a malignant neoplastic disease which was first reported in the 1870's (74, 101). Bovine lymphosarcoma is also known as bovine leukemia, even though leukemia in the classical sense rarely occurs. According to the classification of Dunn (20), however, a systemic neoplastic process of blood-forming tissues denotes leukemia, irrespective of whether there is an increase in the number of peripheral blood leukocytes.

Ellerman and Bang (23) used the term leukosis to designate leukemic and pseudoleukemic disorders of the leukocyte-forming tissues of chickens. Dobberstein (17) proposed this term for the corresponding disorders in cattle, including lymphosarcoma (lymphocytic neoplasm) and persistent lymphocytosis (PL), which is a condition that may precede or accompany lymphosarcoma.

Lymphosarcoma is the most frequently disgnosed neoplastic disease of cattle (4, 10, 11, 58, 74, 110). Studies have shown that per 100,000 cattle slaughtered, there are 14 condemnations for lymphosarcoma in North America (118), 40 in the Sjaelland and Lolland-Fallster Islands of Denmark, and 1,000 in S. E. Sweden (10). Since affected animals could serve as a reservoir of the virus believed to cause the disease, and since milk and meat consumed by humans may contain the agent (26), bovine leukemia is believed important from the public health standpoint.

Guralnick (49) reported a high incidence of lymphoid tumors among rural residents; Fasal (24) found that farmers and farm workers as a combined group had a leukemia mortality risk greater than the general population; Kohklova and Rakhmanin (65) found high mortality rates of bovine and human leukemia in the Baltic Republic of the U.S.S.R. Cases of leukemia in people who lived in close contact with leukotic cattle and drank raw milk from a herd of leukotic cattle were reported (68, 81, 95, 120). A cluster of cases of nonlymphocytic leukemia in adult humans was reported in an area surrounding a small Wisconsin dairy farm with a high incidence of bovine leukemia (26). Evidence also exists for a lack of correlation between infection by Bovine Leukemia virus (BLV) the causative agent of bovine leukemia and human leukemia. Antibody to BLV could not be detected in farmers, some of whom drank raw milk from BLV-infected cattle, workers who handled BLV infected materials, veterinarians, cancer patients or members of high incidence families. Molecular hybridization studies failed to detect BLV-related sequences in human tumors (62). Pasteurization destroys the infectivity of BLV, thus posing no risk of drinking milk which often contains infectious BLV (8).

Studies in chimpanzees fed raw milk from bovine leukemia virus (BLV)-infected cattle indicated that a myeloproliferative disorder was induced, but not all pathologists agreed on the diagnosis, and the illnesses in the chimpanzees, which also included pneumocystis pneumonia and anemia, made an unequivocal diagnosis of BLV-induced disease difficult (75).

Clinical forms of bovine lymphosarcoma

The clinicopathologic and epidemiologic characteristics of the enzootic and sporadic forms of bovine lymphosarcoma are detailed below:

1) Enzootic form. This is the most common form of bovine lymphosarcoma in the United States, Europe (26) and Venezuela (72). It is caused by a type C virus (22, 26, 29), and occurs in geographic and herd aggregations in cattle three years old and older, with a peak incidence at 5–8 years of age.

The disease is manifested clinically by weight loss, anemia, decreased milk yield, and enlargement of one or more lymph nodes usually in the pelvic area. Leukemic infiltrates of periorbital tissues may cause exophthalmos. Signs of respiratory, digestive, reproductive, urinary, and neurological disorders may occur when these specific organ systems are involved. Sudden death may occur in animals with cardiac involvement (26, 74). The sites most commonly found to be affected at necropsy are lymph nodes, heart, abomasum, and uterus (67, 74).

Only one-third of affected cattle manifest leukemia – an increase in the number of circulating lymphocytes. In such animals, there is a high proportion of atypical lymphoblasts. Since a high proportion of atypical lymphoblasts in blood and at tumor sites also have abnormal karyotypes consisting of hyperploidy, this suggests a unicentric origin of the disease (52, 74).

So-called persistent lymphocytosis (PL) occurs in many cattle from high incidence lymphosarcoma herds (4, 10, 74, 110). PL is defined as an increase in the absolute lymphocyte count by three or more standard deviations above the normal mean for that respective breed and age (73). Supposedly, PL can be distinguished from transient lymphocytosis associated with conditions not related to lymphosarcoma by demonstrating an elevation in the circulating lymphocytes for at least 3 months (73). PL in a given animal can continue for several years, and may remain the same or develop into

H. E. Kaiser (ed.), Comparative aspects of tumor development.

lymphosarcoma (34, 35). Several European authors (61, 96) consider persistent lymphocytosis the first phase of a biphasic disease, and claim that 90% of animals with lymphocytosis go on to the lymphosarcoma phase. Bendixen (10, 11) developed an eradication program for enzootic leukosis for use in Denmark, based on a hematologic key.

Lymphocytes from animals with PL differ from lymphocytes of animals with leukemia in that they do not show aneuploidy (52, 74). These PL lymphocytes are termed "atypical" or "unusual" and the majority have B cell markers (26, 82, 108), but such cells are not unique for PL, since they occur in both normal cattle and those with nonneoplastic diseases (26).

Bendixen (11) postulated that adult lymphosarcoma and PL are caused by the same agent, a hypotheses that was confirmed after the discovery of BLV. Since Bendixen also considered PL a pretumor phase of bovine lymphosarcoma followed by a second phase during which leukotic tumors occurred, the term bovine leukosis is used for both conditions. This is unfortunate, since PL is considered a benign proliferative response to BLV (27, 34, 35).

The relationship between the occurrence of lymphocytosis, lymphosarcoma, and bovine leukosis virus is far from clear. Abt et al. (1, 2) observed that in 25 leukosis herds, PL occurred in 7% of the cows tested, and in 24 leukosis-free herds the PL rate was 4.2%, suggesting that PL is not a good screening tool for predicting the development of lymphosarcoma, contrary to the findings in Denmark of Bendixen (10, 11). Although few cattle without PL developed lymphosarcoma, a large number (42/64 or 65%) that developed lymphosarcoma also developed PL previously.

Ferrer et al. (34, 35) reviewed the relationship between BLV infection, PL and lymphosarcoma. BLV is believed to be the cause of both PL and lymphosarcoma and, based on studies of different cow families, both conditions tend to aggregate in different cow families even within the same herd, pointing to a separate genetic predisposition for each condition.

Since BLV infected lymphocytes become transformed much less commonly than in leukemias of other species, the mere presence of the virus is insufficient for such cells to be considered neoplastic (28). However, if, as Ihle has postulated (56), the theory of chronic immunostimulation is operative, the virus may cause, in certain cow families, an overgrowth of antigen-specific lymphocytes capable of producing lymphokines in response to antigen stimulation. Lymphosarcoma could then result from continual production of more lymphocytes, some of which will undergo proviral integration.

Although the mechanism of BLV induced leukemogenesis is unknown, it was recently demonstrated that expression of the C-myc gene is elevated in all BLV induced tumors, but not in BLV infected nonleukemic or BLV free neoplastic bovine cells. The results indicate that BLV probably enhances the expression of the C-*myc* gene through a transacting regulatory element (45).

2) Sporadic form. This rare form of lymphosarcoma usually affects cattle under the age of 3 years, and encompasses 3 clinicopathological configurations:
a) The calf, or juvenile form, occurs in calves less than 6

months of age (27, 54). There is generalized lymph node involvement and the bone marrow is frequently infiltrated. The frequency of this form is 6.9/100,000 in the U.S. and 5.4/100,000 in Sweden (10, 11, 26).
b) The thymic form occurs in cattle less than 2 years old and is characterized by thymic enlargement; generalized lymph node enlargement may be present. This form is rare in the United States, but is the most common form of lymphosarcoma in Great Britain (4, 5, 6). Smith (102) reported on the occurrence of 7/1,113 cases of bovine lymphosarcoma. In 5 of those cases in which there was involvement of the thymus, he considered only 2 to be true thymomas. Dungworth et al. (18) reported on the occurrence of thymic lymphosarcoma in 14 California cattle.
c) The cutaneous form occurs in cattle 1 to 3 years of age. The dermis of affected animals contains focal leukemic infiltrates. Involvement of lymph nodes and organs usually is seen in the late stages of the disease. Smith (102) reported that 7 of his 1,113 bovine lymphosarcoma cases had skin lesions; but the skin involvement was secondary to underlying neoplasms and was not considered analogous to the "skin leukosis" described in Europe.

The virus and its characteristics

Epidemiologic studies in Europe, demonstrating the enzootic occurrence of the adult form of bovine lymphosarcoma and PL led several workers to hypothesize a viral etiology (10, 11, 40, 97). This hypothesis was also used to document the spread of both disease states from enzootic to leukosis free areas (10, 11, 85, 94, 96, 97). Several workers (12, 56, 85) observed that bovine origin whole blood piroplasmosis vaccine from multiple cases herds was associated with lymphosarcoma and PL.

Dutcher et al. (21) found a few structures resembling C-type particles in milk from a multiple case herd. BLV-infected lymphocytes usually do not produce virus particles or express viral antigens *in vivo* (29), and detection of the virus depends on the use of *in vitro* systems (22, 31, 33, 80, 99). Distinct and numerous C-type particles were first seen in bovine leukemic lymphocytes cocultivated with human WI-38 or embryonic tracheal cells (14), and later, short term cultures of lymphosarcoma lymhocytes of PL lymphocytes from cattle (22, 27, 29, 60, 99). Long-term culture methods were developed by Stock and Ferrer (105). The latter systems provided evidence for replication and the viral nature of these particles (33, 105).

Monolayer cultures of bat lung Tb, Lu cells (16, 42) are now the preferred means of propagating BLV, since this system is free of bovine virus diarrhea virus (BVDV) and other adventitious agents often present in bovine origin cells. BLV infected-fetal lamb kidney (FLK) cells produce BLV abundantly and is extensively used as a source of BLV. However, it is contaminated with BVDV. Other cell lines such as human, simian, canine, caprine and equine cells (16, 42) can also readily be infected.

In vivo transmission studies demonstrated that BLV infects (53, 92, 116) and induces leukemia in sheep. This constitutes an important method of diagnosis. Calves are infected only with difficulty because of maternal antibodies derived from colostrum (26).

The use of numerous diagnostic methods, including immunofluorescence (25, 93) immunofluorescence absroption (25), immunodiffusion (25, 76), radioimmunoprecipitation (39, 76) showed that the major internal protein (p24 or p25) does not share any antigenic determinants present in any of the other known mammalian or avian oncornaviruses (77) with the exception of a C-type leukemia virus from sheep (87). It is not clear if this agent is a virus indigenous to sheep or if it was transmitted from sheep to cattle. Recently, however, Thiry et al. (113) showed cross reactivity between BLV antigens p24 and p51 with p13 of the lymphadenopathy syndrome associated virus (LAV) derived from Zairian acquired immunodeficiency syndrome (AIDS) patients and grown in human lymocyte culture.

Reverse transcriptase (121), gp (15) and the p15 (63) antigens are also distinct characteristics of BLV. A nonglycosylated p65 BLV protein thought to be the precursor of p25, p15, p12, and p10 (70) subsequently was shown to be a 27,000 molecular weight polypeptide containing the 3 antigenic components, p24, p15, and p12. (48). Molecular hybridization with BLV and other oncornaviruses (13, 64) failed to show homology. Hybridization was not observed with DNA from uninfected cattle, goats, deer, elk, bison, horses, sheep, dogs, cats, and mice (26), man or birds. The authors concluded that BLV is not endogenous in the bovine or the other species tested. Several authors (14, 16) demonstrated syncytia formation to be a property unique to BLV when it was inoculated directly into monolayer cultures of a number of different cell lines derived from a number of species. Poste (90) treated UV irradiated cell lines infected with viruses other than BLV and showed that when infectivity was destroyed, but biochemical composition was intact, syncytia inducing capability remained intact indicating syncytia formation is medicated by a structural component of the virion.

The work of Ferrer and Cabrodilla (27) showed by the use of a cell line infected with BLV, but resistant to syncytia formation by BLV, produced syncytia when cocultivated with CC81 cells. The authors concluded that syncytia induced with BLV in cell cultures was due to a virus-induced product in the infected cells.

Transmission

Gross (43, 44) classified the natural transmission of oncornaviruses as 1) horizontal, meaning the spread of the virus among animals of the same generation, or 2) vertical, meaning that the spread of the virus is from one generation to the next. Thus, vertical transmission includes genetic, congenital, milk-borne and contact transmission from parents to offspring. Vertical transmission can thus be divided into prenatal and postnatal for the purposes of control and eradication (26).

The mechanisms of prenatal transmission incorporating of the viral genome in the gametes (genetic transmission) and transmission of complete virus to the embryo or fetus (epigenetic or extrachromosomal transmission). Postnatal transmission may occur via milk, by contact with excretions or secretions, or from the transfer of the virus by vectors or fomites.

Before identification of BLV as the infectious agent, Theilen et al. (111) reported the occurrence of PL in calves inoculated with preparations from cattle with lymphosarcoma, and several authors (10, 11, 85, 94, 96, 97) reported horizontal spread of PL and lymphosarcoma from high incidence areas to leukosis-free areas. Such spread is now interpreted as interaction between horizontal spread and genetic predisposition (26).

Prenatal vs. postnatal transmission of BLV

As mentioned previously, free BLV particles are seldom produced *in vivo* and most cattle are infected by exposure to infected lymphocytes rather than by exposure to virus particles. To test the frequency of infection with BLV before and after birth, the presence of virus and of antiviral antibodies was determined in cattle of various ages in a multiple case herd. Less than 20% of adult BLV-positive animals in a multiple case herd became infected before birth (37, 89). Antiviral antibodies were found in sera of all calves infected before birth, indicating that the virus was acquired some time after the fetus attained immunological competence (26). Since fetuses can produce antibody after the first 3 months of gestation (100), it is concluded that natural transplacental infection occurs during the last 6 months of gestation rather than through germ cell or transmission to the embryo. According to Piper et al. (89) some, but not all, calves born to BLC-infected dams are infected, showing that ability of the dam to transmit the virus to the fetus is not a constant feature.

After the age of 3 years, all cattle were infected with BLV (1, 37, 89). Because only 18% of the calves at birth and after first nursing were positive for virus even though they were born to infected dams, it was concluded that most animals in a multiple-case herd were infected after birth. Between the age of 1 and 3 years, virtually all animals studied became positive (37, 88). This was attributed to mixing the calves with the adults after 1 year of age.

Straub and Lorenz (106) studied rates of BLV infection in colostrum-derived calves derived by cesarean section from leukotic dams and raised in isolation. Twelve of 18 animals developed lymphocytosis due to BLV infection. Ferrer (26) belived this high infectivity rate was most likely explained by transmission during the course of the cesarean operation.

Preliminary evidence, based on competitive radioimmunoassay (RIA), showed intermittence shedding of viral particles in the urine of infected cattle (47, 79). Thus, aerosols created by unrination may constitute a potential route of BLV spread (26).

Preliminary experiments for the detection of BLV in the semen of infected bulls were negative (79); however it was suggested that BLV-infected lymphocytes might be present in the semen from bulls with inflammation of the genital tract. Incidence of BLV infection in off-spring of BLV-positive bulls was no greater than in offspring of BLV-negative bulls. (7).

Ingestion of milk cannot be incriminated as a natural mode of transmission because the design of the studies used to determine if milk-borne transmission occurs did not allow the distinction between milk-borne, prenatal, or contact transmission. The work of Miller and Van Der Maaten (79) demonstrated that milk or colostrum from 5 infected cows induced BLV when inoculated into sheep. Ferrer et al. (32) demonstrated that inoculation of milk-derived lymphocytes from cows with lymphosarcoma could be used to infect lambs. Although BLV is present in milk and colostrum of infected dams, shedding of virus is intermittent (109). Ferrer and Piper (30) showed that if calves free of BLV at birth nursed infected dams by 3 months of age they were free of virus but had serum antibody. Of 17 such calves kept in isolation for 27–29 months, only 3 were infected with BLV; of 17 other calves kept in continual contact with infected cattle for $2\frac{1}{2}$ years, all 17 were infected. Thus, colostrum has a protective effect and BLV or BLV-infected lymphocytes do not cross the protective barrier of intestinal mucosa, which is impermeable after the first 24–36 hours of life. Large numbers of BLV-infected lymphocytes administered experimentally to calves at various times after birth showed this to be true (117). Under natural conditions, in which small numbers of infected lymphocytes enter the milk, it would be unlikely that calves receiving colostrum during the first day of life would be infected. Kettman et al. (61) found proviral sequences of BLV in tumor tissues from cows with enzootic form of bovine lymphosarcoma, but not in tissues without lymphocytic infiltrates. Ohnuma et al. (84) demonstrated, *in vitro*, a serum derived release inhibiting factor produced by BLV-infected cells. Recently, Gupta and Ferrer (46) characterized as a nonimmunoglobulin, noninterferon protein molecule, a BLV release-inhibiting factor from the plasma of leukotic cattle. This factor is believed to act at the cell surface, thus possibly explaining the failure to detect viral-specific, RNA-infected lymphocytes, and also the failure to isolate the virus from plasma. Since antibody is found in serum of most BLV-infected animals, this may also explain the difficulty of isolation of the virus from the serum of BLV-infected cattle. It is not known if the factor described by Onuma et al. is the same factor described by Gupta and Ferrer.

Since the basic mechanism of the leukemogenic process is unknown, the search for such a mechanism should answer the question of why such a small fraction of BLV-infected cattle develop lymphosarcomas.

Role of vectors

In BLV-free calves exposed to BLV-infected cattle under controlled conditions, contact transmission in 90% at the end of a $4\frac{1}{2}$ to 6 year observation (1, 9, 37, 88, 89). It is possible that calves found to be serologically positive by the immunodiffusion test during the winter months following exposure to BLV-infected animals became infected in the summer, but did not become seropositive until winter since it takes several months between the time of infection and the development of serological response (119).

Calves from a BLV-free herd, when introduced into a small holding area containing 25–30 BLV-infected, nonlactating cows, became infected within 4 months if contact occurred in midsummer, but did not become infected if exposed in winter (9). Insect vectors are believed to play a role in contact transmission of BLV, since the midguts of horseflies (*Tabanus nigrovitatus*, Marcquart) feeding on

BLV-infected cattle contained BLV-infected lymphocytes (9). Cattle in a high-incidence (70% BLV-infected) herd (1, 34, 37, 89) were also infected with Trypanosoma theileri (51). This parasite is nonpathogenic and is transmitted by Tabanus and Stomoxys (103). Thus, BLV may share a vector with one or both agents.

Bloodsucking insects are known to play a role in transmission of other C-type viruses, including Friend murine leukemia virus (38), and possibly feline leukemia virus (50). Transmission by mosquitos of both leukemic lymphocytes and sarcoma cells was reported (6).

In tropical areas of South America like Venezuela, bloodsucking insects are prevalent and BLV, PL lymphosarcoma are frequently found (72). Since bat cells can be infected with BLV *in vitro* (42), and since South American vampire bats feed on cattle, it is possible that bats could transmit BLV, either as biological or as mechanical vectors. As mentioned previously, piroplasmosis vaccine made with blood of BLV-infected cattle was implicated in the spread to previously leukosis-free areas (12, 55, 85), and in the occurrence of leukemia in some sheep flocks (24). Attempts to transmit BLV from infected cattle to sheep by use of saliva, nasal secretion, and urine failed (79), but the sensitivity of the method of transmission to sheep was not determined.

Diagnosis

Most cattle infected with BLV do not develop PL or lymphosarcoma; therefore, a diagnosis of BLV infection cannot be used to ascertain whether an animal will develop leukosis. To establish a diagnosis of lymphosarcoma in an animal, lymphoid tumors or neoplastic lymphocytes must be demonstrated. Several procedures for the diagnosis of BLV infection i.e., detection of BLV or antigens associated with BLV are discussed briefly. Demonstration of BLV and BLV antigens require *in vitro* cultivation of lymphocytes, which are the only BLV-infected cells in the bovine (5, 105).

The detection of BLV antibody is the most reliable, specific and inexpensive procedure for the identification of BLV-infected cattle. The most sensitive of the tests available for detection of BLV antibody in serum is the radioimmunoassay (RIA) test and enzyme-linked immunosorbent assay (ELISA) test (26).

Electron microscopy was used in early studies for visualization of cultured peripheral blood lymphocytes (36, 80, 105). However, such studies are expensive, slow, cumbersome, and require specialized equipment.

Immunofluorescent markers, especially p25, for demonstrating BLV in cultured lymphocytes (5, 25) are useful but are now supplanted by competitive RIA. The RIA utilizes extracts of peripheral blood leukocytes cultured for 48 hours. The extracts are then examined for the presence of the antigen by assaying the ability to prevent binding of radiolabeled p25 with specific antibody.

Immunodiffusion (ID), regular (98) or radical (84), is used to detect BLV antigens in peripheral lymphocytes. According to Ferrer (26) both ID methods are the least sensitive procedures for the dectection of antigen.

Syncytia assay. As previously metioned, the discovery of syncytia formation in vitro using CC81 cells cocultivated with lymphocytes (27, 28) and more recently a feline cell line (31) led to the development of a sensitive viral assay. The method is more sensitive than immunofluorescence or electron microscopy.

An assay based on induction of BLV p25 in susceptible cells was reported (59). The method utilizes peripheral blood lymhocytes in monolayer cultures of indicator cells. After an incubation period of 5–7 days, the cells are examined for the presence of BLV p25 antigen using a specific antiserum with the immunoperoxidase technique. Aida et al. (3) recently developed a monoclonal antibody technique as a sensitive *in vitro* test for bovine leukemia tumor cell associated antigen. The test was specific in that it allowed detection of tumor cells from 19 cattle with enzootic leukosis but normal tissues from the same animals and blood lymphocytes or fetal liver and kidney cells were negative.

The authors divided the reactivity of cells from the 19 tumors with the 13 monoclonal antibodies into 3 groups. Antibodies of the first group reacted with cells from all 19 tumors. Antibodies of the second group reacted with cells from several, but not all tumors; the third group of antibodies reacted only with homologous tumor cells. This system shows promise in the early detection of bovine lymphosarcoma.

Histomorphology and cytomorphology

Smith (102) studied 1,113 cattle with lymphomas: 5 were the giant follicular type, and the remainder were the diffuse type. The predominant cell types in bovine lymphosarcoma are regarded as lymphocytic, prolymphocytic, and lymphoblastic (54, 107, 112). There are individual cases, however, in which variable types of lymphoid cells are found which makes classification difficult.

Marshak et al. (74) gave the sites of localization and identified two types of cells in 59 cases of bovine lymphosarcoma: lymphocyte and lymphoblast. Although the cell population may be mixed, one type is usually predominant. Squire (104) studied bovine malignant lymphomas and concluded that the variable cell types represented "a broad spectrum of development." Valli et al. (115) studied the histocytology of bovine lymphomas, and classified them histologically according to the Rappaport system and cytologically according to the method of Lukes and Collins (69). Histologically, 82 of the tumors were diffuse and 8 were nodular. Smith (102), in his series of 1,113 cases of bovine lymphosarcomas (1,000 from the U.S. Department of Agriculture and 113 cases from the files of the Armed Forces Institute of Pathology) classified the tumors into lymphocytic (32 cases), histiocytic (375 cases), stem cell (566 cases) or mixed (indeterminate) (27 cases). The histiocytic type was described as composed of cells "having been caught up in the process of amoeboid movement, stretched into long and bizarre shapes". Other features described for the histiocytic group are the starry sky effect, and variability in size and shape. The histiocytic group also included what the author felt were 42 cases diagnosed as having cytologic features of Hodgkin's disease of man, including eosinophils, giant cells, and cells resembling Reed-Sternberg cells. Areas of necrosis were often present in these tumors.

In the study by Valli et al., 57 animals with lymphomas that were cytologically classified as noncleaved lymphomas died at a mean age of 3.4 years; 33 animals with cleaved cell lymphomas died at a mean age of 6 years. Thus, there was a statistically significant different age at death for the two types of tumors as reported with lymphomas in man (69). Raich et al. (91) classified bovine and ovine lymphomas using enzyme cytochemical and immunologic markers on both peripheral blood lymphocytes and lymph node impression smears. The smears and imprints were stained with Wright's stain and with the following special cyto-chemical stains: Sudan black B (SBB),-periodic-acid-Schiff (PAS), combined naphhthol AS-D chloracetate (ANA) esterase, naphthol AS-D acetate (NASDA) esterase with and without sodium fluoride, and acid phosphatase (ACP) with and without tartrate inhibition. According to Mann (71) and Gralnick et al. (41), SBB, PAS, and NASDA are used to separate granulocytes from cells of the lymphocyte series. NASDA esterase with fluoride inhidits esterase of monocytes and without fluoride is a marker for granulocytes or lymphoid cells and ACP a T cell marker with and without tartrate inhibition is a marker for hairy cell leukemia of man (71).

Tests for the immunologic separation of T and B lymphocytes included surface immunoglobulin labeling, erythrocyte antibody complement and the test for E rosettes.

The findings of Raich et al. were as follows: SBB, PAS, and NASDA esterase reaction were negative in normal and both calf and adult lymphosarcoma cells, while ANA esterase was moderately positive for all 3 groups. The NASDA esterase reaction was weekly positive with partial inhibition by fluoride in both normal and lymphosarcoma cattle. A larger percentage of lymphosarcoma cells (83%) than normal cells (30%) reacted positively with ACP, but most of this activity was lost following tartrate inhibition.

Both peripheral blood lymphocytes and thymic cells from animals with the rare thymic type lymphosarcoma reacted positively with ANA enterase, but SBB, PAS and NASDA esterase reactions were negative.

Peripheral blood lymphocytes from 5 sheep with lymphosarcoma induced by BLV were strongly positive for ANA esterase and ACP as in bovine thymic lymphosarcoma, which is compatible with T lymphocyte origin, since several authors (71, 41) have recommended this marker for T lymphocytes for man. However, in sheep with lymphoma, 87–97.5% of peripheral blood mononuclear cells were surface immunoglobulin positive, but in bovine thymic lymphosarcoma only 10% of the neoplastic cells had this marker. Raich et al. (91), stated that specimens prepared from the calf and thymic forms had a low percentage of B cells and of T cells by the surface immunoglobulin and erythrocyte antibody complement tests for B cells and by the E rosette tests for T cells in both lymph nodes and blood. This was considered compatible with a non-B, non-T cell (null cell) lymphoma. Unfortunately, the authors made no mention of the use of anti-theta serum for the identification of T-lymphocytes.

Previous studies (108), using Ficoll membrane filtration, E rosetting, erythrocyte complement receptors, and IgS surface markers, showed the adult type of bovine lymphosarcoma to be of the B cell type, since there were increased numbers of cells with surface immunoglobulin and erythrocyte antibody complement receptors, compared with normal controls.

Muscoplat et al. (82) examined 4 cows with persistent lymphocytosis and 12 normal cows for the presence of lymphocyte cell surface immunoglobulin (IgS) by fluorescence micrography and found 63% of peripheral lymphocytes had IgS, whereas the normal cattle had 28% of peripheral lymphocytes with this marker. The fluorescent antibody technique was claimed by the authors to be fairly specific for B lymphocytes, but the authors state that the fluorescence method was not sufficiently sensitive to detect T cells with surface immunoglobulin.

Thorell (112) stained suspensions of leukotic bovine cells derived from tumorous lymph nodes with acridine orange and quantified, by flow cytofluorimetry, the green and red fluorescence of double-(mostly DNA) and single-stranded (mostly RNA) nucleic acids, respectively. The green fluorescence was used to distinguish normal diploid lymphocytes from a second peak which is of aneuploid lymphocytes in the S and G_2 phase. The red-RNA (protein) fluorescence was more variable and distinct between cells. The green fluorescence peak attributed to diploid cells was postulated to be a surveillance reaction against aneuploid neoplastic cells. Such a phenomenon was described in lymphomas of man by several authors (71, 41).

Initial lesions of enzootic leukosis

There is little agreement as to the site and morphology of initial lesions in bovine lymphoma. Uebershar (114) reported "lymph node lesions located in the extra follicular regions and which extended along the sinuses." Some workers (17, 18) recognized the accumulation of neoplastic cells in the cortex and medullary cords of affected lymph nodes, and other workers (19, 66, 74, 102) reported initial lesions in the medullary and intermediate sinuses. Jarplid (57) and Theilen (110) reported small, solitary lesions in the atrial and abomasal wall. None of these authors studied cattle of defined status with regard to BLV or anti-BLV antibody.

Ohshima et al. (83) studied 13 cattle (aged 1.5–9 years of Holstein-Friesian, Japanese Shorthorn, or Japanese Black breed), all of which were affected by bovine lymphosarcoma and were seropositive for BLV antibody or considered hematologically positive by use of the European Community key. Ten of the animals had lymphocytosis. Blood smears, histologic sections and thin sections were prepared from representative lymph nodes and hemolymph nodes.

Grossly, lymph nodes in the least affected animals were slightly enlarged and irregular in shape, and in the more severely affected group were swollen up to the "size of a hen's egg." Lymph nodes ranged in weight form 40–170 g. On the cut surface, the cortex was wider than normal and focal white areas were present. One animal had very large lymph nodes and was considered to have advanced lymphoma.

The earliest histological changes in affected lymph nodes observed by Ohshima et al. were considered to be an increased number of follicles and the medullary sinuses contained lymphoblasts. Pallaske (86) recognized accumulations of neoplastic cells in the cortex and medullary cords as

the initial lymph node change, while Smith (102) regarded neoplastic cells in the sinusoids as the earliest change. Eosinophils were often numerous, as in the cases reported by Smith (102) and in the author's experience. The hemolymph nodes had marked follicular hyperplasia.

In the lymph nodes from the more severely affected animals, moderate to marked follicular hyperplasia was noted with increased number and size. Cellular infiltrates composed of plasma cells and eosinophils were seen in the medulla, trabeculae and capsule. There was splenomegaly.

Electron microscopy was used to confirm the presence of lymphocytes, lymphoblasts and immature plasma cells. In addition, specimens from several animals contained reticulum cells.

The authors speculated about the possible origin in situ or peripheral blood of the proliferating cells in the perifollicular areas and medullary sinuses. The plasma cells were believed to play a role in antibody formation, and the eosinophils previously reported (102) were believed to be involved in an allergic response, possibly to the tumor cells or a product of the tumor cells.

Regression

Miller and Olson (78) reported on three cases of bovine lymphosarcoma that regressed: 2 of the cases were Holstein heifers, 8 and 19 months of age; the third animal was a Holstein cow, 2.5 years of age. The 8-month-old heifer had enlargement of a number of superficial lymph nodes and the 19-month-old heifer and the cow had lesions to limited areas of the skin.

The lesions in all 3 cases were histologically confirmed from biopsy material: the first case from lymph nodes and the other 2 cases from skin. The tumors were classified histologically as reticulum cell sarcoma. The first heifer was not followed beyond 18 months; the second heifer was free of lesions for 5 years and her single calf was also normal at the time of slaughter (31 months of age). The cow produced 6 normal calves, four of which were females. When necropsied at the age of 14 years, no tumors were found in the cow. The offspring had no clinical signs of lymphosarcoma when followed for 5 to 8 years. The authors reviewed previous reports which described temporary regression. The authors cite a single unpublished case of regression of an apparent thymic lymphosarcoma in a heifer. None of the cases cited as being examples of regression was studied with regard to BLV or BLV antibody or other correlates of BLV infection.

REFERENCES

1. Abt. DA, Marshak RR, Ferrer JF, Piper CE, Bhatt DM: Studies of the development of persistent lymphocytosis and infection with the bovine C-type leukemia virus. *Vet Microbiol* 1:287, 1976
2. Abt DA, Marshak RR, Kulp HW, Pollock RJ: Studies on the relationship between lymphocytosis and bovine leukosis. *Bibl Haematol* 36:527, 1969
3. Aida Y, Onuma M, Ogawa Y, Mihami T, Izawa H: Tumor-associated antigens on bovine leukemia virus-induced bovine lymphosarcoma identified by monoclonal antibodies. *Cancer Res* 45:398, 1985

4. Anderson LJ, Jarrett WFH: Lymphosarcoma in cattle, sheep and pigs. *Cancer* 22:398, 1968

5. Baliga V, Ferrer JF: Expression of the bovine leukemia virus and its internal antigen in blood lymphocytes. *Proc Soc Exptl Biol Med* 156:388, 1977

6. Banfield WG, Woke PA, Mackay CM, Cooper HL: Mosquito transmission of a reticulum cell sarcoma of hamsters. *Science* 148:1239, 1965

7. Baumgartener LE, Crawley J, Entine S, Olson C, Hugoson G, Hansen HJ, Dreher WH: Influence of sire on BLV infection in progeny. *Zentralbl Veterinarmed B* 25:202, 1978

8. Baumgartener LE, Olson C, Onuma M: Effect of pasteurization and heat treatment on bovine leukemia virus. *J Am Vet Med Assn* 169:1189, 1976

9. Bech-Neilsen S, Piper CE, Ferrer JF: Natural mode of transmission of the bovine leukemia virus: role of blood sucking insects. *Am J Vet Res* 39:1089, 1978

10. Bendixen HJ: Thesis: "Studies of leukosis enzootica bovis-with special regard to diagnosis, epidemiology and eradication." U.S. Dept. Health, Education and Welfare Public Health Serv. *Natl. Cancer Inst*, 1965

11. Bendixen HJ: Bovine enzootic leukosis. *Adv Vet Sci* 10:129, 1965

12. Bodin S, Enhorning G, Olson H, Wingvist C: Die Anzahl der Lymphozyten im Blut von Rindern bei lymphatischer Leukose und Piroplasmose. *Acta Vet Scand 2* (suppl. 2):47, 1961

13. Callahan R, Lieber MM, Todaro GJ, Graves DC, Ferrer JF: Bovine leukemia virus genes in the DNA of cattle. *Science* 192:1005, 1976

14. Cornefort-Jensen FR, Hare WCD, Stock ND: Studies on bovine lymphosarcoma: formation of syncytia and detection of virus particles in mixed cell cultures. *Int J Cancer* 4:507, 1969

15. DeVare SG, Stephenson JR: In: The serological diagnosis of enzootic bone leukosis. p. 44, edited by: A.A. Ressang, Commission of the European Communities, Luxemburg, 1977.

16. Diglio CA, Ferrer JF: Development of an *in vitro* infectivity assay for the C-type bovine leukemia virus. *Cancer Res* 36:1068, 1976

17. Dobberstein J, Paarman E: Die sogenante Lymphadenose des Rindes (Rinderleukose). *Z Infektionskr Parasit kr Hyg Haustiere* 46:65, 1934

18. Dungworth DL, Theilen GH, Lengyel J: Bovine lymphosarcoma in California. II. The thymic form. *Path Vet* 1:323, 1964

19. Dungworth DL, Theilen GH, Ward JM: Early detection of the lesions of bovine lymphosarcoma. *Proc. 3rd Int Symp Comp Leukemia Res Bibl Haematol* 31:206, 1967

20. Dunn TB: Normal and pathologic anatomy of the reticular tissue in laboratory mice. *J Natl Cancer Inst* 14:1281, 1954

21. Dutcher RM, Larkin EP, Marshak RR: Virus-like particles in cow's milk from a herd with a high incidence of lymphosarcoma. *J Natl Cancer Inst* 33:1055, 1964

22. Dutta SK, Larson VL, Sorenson DK, Berman V, Weber AL, Hamer RF, Shope RO: Isolation of C-type virus particles from leukemic and lymphocytotic cattle. *Bibl Haematol* 36:548, 1970

23. Ellerman N, Bang O: Experimentelle Leukemie bei Hühnern. *Zbl Bacteriol* Sec. I 46:595, 1908

24. Fasal E, Jackson EW, Klauber MR: Leukemia and lymphoma mortality and farm residence. *Am J Epidemiol* 87:1871, 1968

25. Ferrer JF: Antigenic comparison of bovine type-C virus with murine and feline leukemia viruses. *Cancer Res* 32:1871, 1972

26. Ferrer JF: Bovine lymphosarcoma. *Adv Vet Sci* 24:1, 1980

27. Ferrer JF, Cabrodilla C: The phenomenon of polykaryocytosis induced by BLV in mixed cultures: specificity, mechanisms and application to the diagnosis of BLV infection in cattle. *Ann Rech Vet* 9:721, 1978

28. Ferrer JF, Diglio CA: Development of an *in vitro* infectivity assay for the C-type bovine leukemia virus. *Cancer Res* 36:1068, 1976

29. Ferrer JF, Lin PS: C-type virus in cell lines originating from lymphocytes of leukemic cattle. *Proc Am Assoc Cancer Res* 12:53, 1971

30. Ferrer JF, Piper CE: An evaluation of the role of milk in the natural transmission of BLV. *Ann Rech Vet* 9:803, 1978

31. Ferrer JF, Cabrodilla C, and Gupta P: Use of a feline cell line in the syncytia infectivity assay for the detection of bovine leukemia virus infection in cattle. *Am J Vet Res* 42: 9–14, 1981

32. Ferrer JF, Kenyon SJ, Gupta P: Milk of dairy cows frequently contains a leukemogenic virus. *Science* 213:1014, 1981

33. Ferrer JF, Stock ND, Lin PS: Detection of replicating C-type viruses in continuous cell cultures established from cows with leukemia: effect of culture medium. *J Natl Cancer Inst* 48:985, 1971.

34. Ferrer JF, Abt DA, Bhatt DM, Marshak RR: Studies on the relationship between infection with bovine C-type virus, leukemia and persistent lymphocytosis in cattle. *Cancer Res* 34:893, 1974

35. Ferrer JF, Marshak RR, Abt DA, Kenyon SJ: Relationship between lymphosarcoma and persistent lymphocytosis in cattle: A review. *J Am Vet Med Assn* 175:705, 1979

36. Ferrer JF, Bhatt DM, Abt DA, Marshak RR, Baliga VL: Serological diagnosis of infection with putative bovine leukemia virus. *Cornell Vet* 65:527, 1975

37. Ferrer JF, Piper CE, Abt DA, Marshak RR, Bhatt DM: Natural mode of transmission of the bovine C-type leukemia virus. *Bibl Haematol* 36:504, 1976

38. Fisher RG, Luecke DH, Rehacek J: Friend leukemia virus activity in certain arthropods. III Transmission studies. *Neoplasma* 20:255, 1973

39. Gilden RV, Long CW, Hanson M, Toni R, Charman HP, Oroszlan S: Characteristics of the major internal protein and RNA dependent DNA polymerase of bovine leukemia virus. *J Gen Virol* 29:305, 1975

40. Gotze R, Rosenberger G, Ziegenhagen G: Die Leukose des Rindes. Ihre haematologische und klinische Diagnose. *Münch. Vet Med* 9: 517, 1954

41. Gralnick HR: Classification of acute leukemia. *Ann Intern Med* 87:740, 1977

42. Graves DC, Ferrer JF: *In vitro* transmission and propagation of the bovine leukemia virus in monolayer cell cultures. *Cancer Res* 36:4152, 1976

43. Gross L: "Oncogenic Viruses." 2nd Ed. Pergamon, Oxford, 1970.

44. Gross L: Viral etiology of cancer and leukemia: A look into the past. present, and future. G. H. A. Clowes Memorial Lecture. *Cancer Res* 38:485, 1978

45. Gupta P: Unpublished observations, 1985

46. Gupta P, Ferrer JF: Expression of bovine leukemia virus genome is blocked by a nonimmunoglobulin protein in plasma from infected cattle. *Science* 215:405, 1982

47. Gupta P, Ferrer JF: Detection of bovine leukemia virus antigen in urine of naturally infected cattle. *Int J Cancer* 25:663, 1980

48. Gupta P, Ferrer JF: Detection of a precursor like-protein of bovine leukemia virus structural polypeptides in purified virions. *J Gen Virol* 47:311, 1980

49. Guralnick L: In: "Vital Statistics Special Reports," p. 480, U.S. Dept. Health, Education and Welfare, 1963

50. Hardy WD, Old LJ, Hess PW, Essex M, Cotter S: Feline leukemia virus field study on horizontal transmission. *Nature* 244:266, 1973

51. Hare WCD, Soulsby EJL, Abt DA: Bovine trypanosomiasis and lymphocytosis parallel studies. *Bibl Haematol* 36:504, 1970

52. Hare WCD, Yang TJ, McFeely RA: A survey of chromosome findings in 47 cases of bovine lymphosarcoma (leukemia). *J Natl Cancer Inst* 38:383, 1967

53. Hoss HE, Olson C: Infectivity of bovine C-type virus for sheep and goats. *Am J Vet Res* 35:633, 1974

54. Hugoson G: Juvenile bovine leukosis. An epizootiological, pathoanatomical and experimental study. *Acta Vet Scand Suppl* 22:1, 1967

55. Hugoson G: The occurrence of bovine leukosis following the introduction of Babesiosis vaccination. *Bibl Haematol* 30:157, 1968

56. Ihle JN, Rein A, Mural R: "Immunologic and virologic mechanisms in retroviurs-induced murine leukemogenesis." In: Advances in Viral Oncology, p. 95. Edited by G Klein. Raven Press, NY., 1984

57. Jarplid B: Studies on the site of leukotic and preleukotic changes in the bovine heart. *Path Vet* 1:366, 1964

58. Jarrett WFH, Crighton GW, Dalton RG: Leukemia and lymphosarcoma in animals and man. *Vet Rec* 79:693, 1966

59. Jerabek L, Gupta P, Ferrer JF: An infectivity assay for bovine leukemia virus using the immunoperoxidase technique. *Cancer Res* 39:3952, 1979

60. Kawakami TG, Moore AL, Theilen GH, Munn RJ, Comparisons of virus-like particles from leukotic cattle to feline leukosis virus. *Bibl Haematol* 36:471, 1970

61. Kettman R, Burny A, Cleuter Y, Ghysdael J, Mammerickx M: Distribution of bovine leukemia virus proviral sequences in tissues of animals with enzootic bovine leukosis. *Leuk Res* 2:23, 1978

62. Kettman R, Burney A, Cleuter Y, Ghysdael J, Mammerickx M: Distribution of bovine virus leukemia proviral sequence in tissues of bovine, ovine and human origin. *Ann Rech Vet* 9:837, 1978

63. Kettman R, Marbaix G, Cleuter Y, Portetelle D, Mammerickx M, Burney A: Genomic integration of bovine leukemia provirus and lack of viral RNA expression in the target cells of cattle with different responses to BLV infection. *Leuk Res* 4:509, 1982

64. Kettman R, Portetelle D, Mammerickx M, Cleuter Y, De-Kegel D, Galoux M, Ghysdael J, Burny A, Cantrenne H: Bovine leukemia virus: An exogenous RNA oncogenic virus. *Proc Natl Acad Sci U. S. A.* 73:1014, 1976

65. Kohklova MP, Rakhmanin PP: Comparative study on the geographical distribution of human and cattle leukosis. *Bibl Haematol* 36:654, 1970

66. Kramer A: Zum Problem der Frühdiagnose der tumorösen Leukose des Rindes durch histologische Lymphknotenuntersuchung. *Arch Exp Veterinarmed* 21:77, 1967

67. Lappnow H, Niepage H, Loliger H-Ch: In: Pathologische Anatomie der Leukosen der Haustiere. p. 339, Verlag Paul Parey, Berlin und Hamburg, 1971

68. Lemon HH, Twiehous MJ, Wilson RB, Rigby PG, Mebus CA, Nimocks W: Symbiotic human and bovine lymphoma. *Proc Am Assoc Cancer Res* 7:41, 1966

69. Lukes RJ, Collins RD: New approaches to the classification of the lymphomata. *Br J Cancer* 31: Suppl. II:1, 1975

70. Mamoun RZ, Astier T, Guillemain T, Duplan JF: Bovine lymphosarcoma: Expression of BLV-related proteins in cultured cells. *J Gen Virol* 64:1895, 1983

71. Mann RB, Jaffe ES, Berard CW: Malignant lymphomas: A conceptual understanding of morphologic diversity. *Am J Pathol* 94: 103, 1979

72. Marin C, Lopez N, Lozano O, Palencia L, Espana W, Costanos H, Leon A: Epidemiology of bovine leukemia in Venezucla. *Ann Rech Vet* 9:743, 1978

73. Marshak RR, Chairman: Criteria for the determination of the normal and leukotic state in cattle. Prepared by an International Committee on Bovine Leukosis. *J Natl Cancer Inst* 41:243, 1968

74. Marshak RR, Coriell LL, Lawrence WC, Crowshaw JE, Jr, Schryver HF, Altera KP, Nichols WW: Studies on bovine lymphosarcoma. I Clinical aspects, pathological alterations and herd studies. *Cancer Res* 22:202, 1962

75. McClure HM, Kelling ME, Custer RP, Marshak RR, Abt DA, Ferrer JF: Erythroleukemia in two infant chimpanzees

76. McDonald HC, Ferrer JF: Detection, quantitation, and characterization of the major internal virion antigen of the bovine leukemia virus by radiommunoassay. *J Natl Cancer Inst* 57:875, 1976

77. McDonald HC, Graves DC, Ferrer JF: Isolation and characterization of an antigen of the bovine C-type virus. *Cancer Res* 36:1251, 1976

78. Miller LD, Olson C: Regression of bovine lymphosarcoma. *J Am Vet Med Assoc* 158:1536, 1971

79. Miller JM, Van Der Maaten MJ: Infectivity tests of secretions and excretions from cattle infected with bovine leukemia virus. *J Natl Cancer Inst* 62:425, 1979

80. Miller JM, Miller LD, Olson C, Gillette KG: Virus-like particles in phytohemagglutinin stimulated lymphocyte cultures with reference to bovine lymphosarcoma. *J Natl Cancer Inst* 43:1297, 1969

81. Mitscherlich E, Plunnecke A, Schmidt FW, Schimmelpfennig IR: Untersuchungen zur Übertragbarkeit von Leukosen des Menschen auf das Rind. *Berl Münch Tierärztl Wochenschr* 86:404, 1973

82. Muscoplat CC, Johnson DW, Pomeroy KA, Olson JM, Larson VL, Stevens JB, Sorenson DK: Lymphocyte surface immunoglobulin: frequency in normal and lymphocytotic cattle. *Am J Vet Res* 35:593, 1974

83. Ohshima K, Sato S, Okada K: A pathologic study on initial lesions of enzootic bovine leukosis. *Jpn J Vet Sci* 44:249, 1982

84. Onuma M, Olson C, Baumgartener LE, Pearson LE: Inhibition of bovine leukemia virus release. *J Natl Cancer Inst* 54:1199, 1975

85. Olson H: Studien über das Auftreten und die Verbreitung der Rinderleukose in Schweden. *Acta Vet Scand* 2 Suppl. 2:13, 1961.

86. Pallaske G: Pathologische Anatomie der Säugetier-Leukosen. *Monatsschr Veterinaermed* 13:65, 1958

87. Paulsen J, Thies L: Bovine leukosis: various methods in molecular virology. Edited by A. Burney, p. 95. Commission of the European Communities, Luxembourg, 1977.

88. Piper CE, Abt DA, Ferrer JF, Marshak RR: Seroepidemiological evidence for horizontal transmission of bovine C-type virus. *Cancer Res* 35:2714, 1975

89. Piper CE, Ferrer JF, Abt DA, Marshak RR: Postnatal and prenatal transmission of the bovine leukemia virus natural conditions. *J Natl Cancer Inst* 62:165, 1979

90. Poste G: In: "Advanced Virus Research 161," p. 303. Edited by Smith KM, Lauffer MA, Bang FB: Academic Press, New York, 1970

91. Raich PC, Takashima I, Olson C: Cytochemical reactions in bovine and ovine lymphosarcoma. *Vet Path* 18:494, 1983

92. Ressang AA, Boars IC, Calafet J, Maastenbroek N, Quak J: Studies on bovine leukemia. III. The hematological response of sheep and goats to infection with whole blood from leukemic cattle. *Zentralbl Veterinaermed B* 23:662, 1976

93. Ressang AA, Mastenbroek N, Quak J, Van Griensven LJLD, Calafat J, Hilgers J, Hageman PhC, Soussi T, Swen S: Studies on bovine leukemia. I. Establishment of C-type virus-producing lines. *Zentralbl Veterinaermed. B* 21:602, 1974

94. Ritter H: Über die Verbreitung der Rinderleukose. *Deutsch Tierärztl Wochenschr* 69:329, 1962

95. Ritter H: Studien über die Übertragungswege bei der enzootischen Rinderleukose. *Deutsch Tierärztl Wochenschr* 72:56, 1965

96. Rosenberger G: Ergebnisse zwölfjähriger Leukose-Untersuchungen an der Rinderklinik Hannover. *Deutsch Tierärztl Wochenschr* 70:410, 1963

97. Schottler F, Schottler H: Über Aetiologie und Therapie der leaukämischen Lymphadenose des Rindes. *Berl Tierärztl Wochenschr* 50:497, 1934

98. Schmidt FW, Mitscherlich E, Garcia de Lima E, Milczewski

KEV, Lembke A: Cultivation of bovine C-type leukemia virus, its transmission to calves and the development of leukemia as determined by hematological, electron microscopical and immunodiffusion tests. *Vet Microbiol* 1:231, 1976

99. Schmidt FW: Uebershar S, Tiefenau M: Virus-Partikel in Leukozyten-Kulturen von experimentell infizierten Leukose-Rindern. *Deutsch Tierarztl Wochenschr* 77:451, 1970.

100. Schultz RD: Developmental aspects of the fetal bovine immune response. *Cornell Vet* 63:507, 1973

101. Siedamgrotsky O: Leukemie bei Tieren. Bericht des Veterinärwesens, Königreich Sachsen. 23:16, 1878

102. Smith AH: The pathology of malignant lymphoma in cattle-a study of 1,113 cases. *Path Vet* 2:68, 1965

103. Soulsby EJL: "Helminths, Arthropods and Protozoa of Domesticated Animals" (Monnig). 6th Ed. Williams and Wilkins, Baltimore, 1975

104. Squire RA: A cytologic study of malignant lymphoma in cattle, dogs and cats. *Am J Vet Res* 26: 97, 1965

105. Stock ND, Ferrer JF: Replicating C-type virus in phytohemasglutinin treated buffy-coat cultures of bovine origin. *J Natl Cancer Inst* 48:985, 1972

106. Straub OC, Lorenz RJ: The influence of colostrum and milk on the development of lymphocytosis in the bovine. *Vet Microbiol* 1:327, 1976

107. Straub OC, Weiland P: Studies on different types of leukosis In: "Bovine Leukosis: Various Methods of Molecular Virology," p. 291. Commission of the European Community, Luxembourg, 1977

108. Takashima I, Olson C, Driscoll DM, Baumgartener LF: B lymphocytes and T lymphocytes in three types of bovine lymphosarcoma. *J Natl Cancer Inst* 59:1205, 1977.

109. Takatori I, Itohara S, Yonaiyama K: Difficulty in detecting in vivo extracellular infective virus in cattle naturally infected with bovine leukemia virus. *Leuk Res* 6:511, 1982

110. Theilen GH, Appelman RD, Wixom HG: Epizootiology of lymphosarcoma in California cattle. *Ann NY Acad Sci* 108:1203, 1963

111. Theilen GH, Dungworth DL, Harrold JE, Straub OC: Bovine lymphosarcoma transmission studies. *Am J Vet Res* 28:373, 1967

112. Thorell B: Characterization of lymphoid cell populations in bovine lymphosarcomas by flow cytofluorimetry. *Leuk Res* 5:235, 1981

113. Thiry L, Sprecher-Goldberger S, Jaquemin P, Cogniaux J, Burny A, Bruck C, Portetelle D, Cran S, Clumeck N: Bovine leukemia virus related antigens in lymphocyte cultures infected with AIDS-associated viruses. *Science* 227:1482, 1984

114. Ueberschar S: Histologische Untersuchungen an Lymphknoten und Organen von Rindern mit tumoröser lymphatischer Leukose unter vergleichender Berücksichtigung von Tieren mit reaktiven und präleukotischen Lymphoytosen. *Arch Exp Veterinaermed* 25:285, 1971

115. Valli VE, McSherry BJ, Dunham BM, Jacobs RM, Lumsden JH: Histocytology of lymphoid tumors of the dog, cat and cow. *Vet Path* 18:494, 1981

116. Van Der Maaten M J, Miller JM: Induction of lymphoid tumors in sheep with cell-free preparations of bovine leukemia virus. *Bibl Haematol* 43:377, 1975

117. Van der Maaten MJ, Miller JM: In: "Bovine Leukosis: Various Methods of Molecular Virology," p. 209. Edited by A. Burney. Commission of the European Communities, Luxembourg, 1977

118. Van Der Maaten MJ, Boothe AD, Malmquist WA: Bovine lymphosarcoma. *J Dairy Sci* 53:614, 1970

119. Wilesmith JW, Straub OC, Lorenz RJ: Some observations on the epidemiology of bovine leukosis virus infection in a large dairy herd. *Res Vet Sci* 28:10, 1980

120. Wisniewski D, Weinreich J: Lymphatische Leukämie bei Vater und Sohn. *Blut* 12:241, 1966

121. Wuu KD, Graves DC, Ferrer JF: Inhibition of the reverse transcriptase of bovine leukemia virus by antibody in sera from leukemic cattle and immunological characterization of the enzyme. *Cancer Res* 37:1438, 1977

GEOLOGIC AND TECHNOLOGIC-CULTURAL CHANGES AND THEIR IMPLICATIONS FOR SPECIES-SPECIFIC CANCER PROGRESSION

H.E. KAISER

THE APPEARANCE OF ANIMALS AND PLANTS DURING THE HISTORY OF THE EARTH: FOSSILS AND INDEX FOSSILS

The life forms and their relationships to the environment are constantly changing. The time difference of geologic changes to man made changes is so large that in a person's life only the man-made changes are visible. We distinguish therefore between the geologic development in a period of more than 500 million years since the Cambrian and the changes of the centuries even decades produced by man. The pre-Cambrian era is worthless because no morphologic fossils are known from this era due to the fact that they were destroyed by metamorphosis of the sediments.

With exception of echinoderms and insects, the majority of important invertebrate groups had developed in pre-Cambrian era and marine algae as well. The phylogenetic development proven by fossils indicates the sequence of the organismic groups and their duration. This way it is possible to distinguish between fossils of types which exhibit a long duration such as the type Lingula of the brachiopods. The class of pelecypods of the molluscs is a larger group which remained stable during the history of the earth. In contrast the index fossils exhibit a geologically rapid change and are therefore used for stratigraphic purpose. Table 1 gives a brief review of the historic appearance of the organismic groups.

The index fossils enable us to distinguish among the various layers of the sediments. The most interesting mammals appeared in the Triassic. Small three-rooted teeth as sign of mammalian development were found since this time. The real uprise of the mammals started with the Oligocene epoch. The last important animal class to appear was this one of the birds in the Upper Jurassic. The flowering plants appeared with the Jurassic period and grasses and cereals followed later; the primitive vascular plants were on earth since the Devonian period. In a later section the immense duration of time and the slow progression during phylogeny and the swift devastating destruction of large portions of the environment on earth by man are mentioned.

Phylogenetic and present tissue dependence of neoplasms

Well preserved soft tissues of invertebrates appeared in British Columbia in the Burgess shale belonging to the Cambrian strata. From then on the different types of organisms have left their marks on the crust of the earth. The phylogenetic age and the diversification of life in each phylo-genetic period have embossed the phylogenetic development of the tissues and their abnormalities up to the present tissue and disease spectrum.

The neoplasms were dependent on their parent tissue throughout the phylogenetic period, proven by the few fossils with signs of neoplastic affection. If a large phylo-genetic gap exists as between entoprocta and ectoprocta and mammals, myoepithelial musculature must have developed at different tissue intervals. Accordingly, with a few exceptions, stratified epithelia may not have been developed monophyletically, but closer together in one main group where they succeeded, the vertebrates.

The ways of fossilization as an explanation of the scarcity of preservation of oncologic specimens

At least 95% of the life of the past has not been fossilized by remnants, impressions or traces. Plants generally are chopped up and the pieces separately fossilized. Even different parts of the same plant were often named as different genera. Animal or human specimen with various diseases will have earlier fallen prey to the predator or escaped in various ways from fossilization. If it is considered that 5% of carcasses and other material from fossil life may fossilize and of these, perhaps, 1% may be afflicted with diseases the expectation of finding neoplastic fossils becomes even smaller. If only a variable percentage of all fossils afflicted with diseases will have had neoplasms then the percentage of neoplasms in fossils becomes even smaller. From vertebrate fossils, in general, only the hard tissues such as bones, teeth, horns, hooves, and claws fossilize. Besides this, not all trends of fossilization permit preservation of the signs of neoplastic diseases.

Summarizing it can be stated that for the scarcity of fossilized neoplasms or their traces are responsible: (1) rarity of fossilization, (2) falling prey of diseased organisms, (3) small percentage of affliction with neoplasms among other diseases, (4) not all types of fossilization preserve diseases, (5) fossilization generally of hard portions only. The last two points are especially responsible for the increase of the scarcity of signs of neoplasms of vertebrates dating from earlier periods.

A part from neoplasms in human remains a hemangioma occurred in a Jurassic Apatosaurus, an osteoma in a Creta-ceous mosasaur, an osteosarcoma in a Pleistocene *Hyaena, spelaea*, an odontoma in *Ursus splaeus* and a bone invading carcinoma in *Microtus* sp., both from the same period.

H. E. Kaiser (ed.), Comparative aspects of tumor development.
© 1989, Kluwer Academic Publishers, Dordrecht. ISBN-13:978-0-89838-994-4

Table 1. Brief review of the historic appearance of organisms, animal and plant tissues.

Eras	Periods and systems	Absolute time	Appearance of animals	Appearance of plants	Comments
Cenozoic	Quaternary		Man		* Trilobites were the index-fossils of the early Paleozoic periods, especially the Cambrian on the one hand and the highly developed arthropods (Arthropoda amandibulata), related to recent Amandibulata the Chelicerata such as Merostomata (e.g. *Limulus polyphemus* L., the horseshoe crab), Arachnida (scorpions, spiders, mites) and Pantopoda, on the other hand, indicating a long phylogeny in the Proterozoic and even Archeozoic eras
	Tertiary	60/70,000,000	Placental Mammals		
	Cretaceous				
Mesozoic	Jurassic	160,000,000	Birds	Angiosperms	
	Triassic		Earliest Mammals		
	Permian	230,000,000			
	Pennsylvanian		Insects		
	Mississippian		Reptiles	Gymnosperms	
Paleozoic	Devonian	390,000,000	Amphibians		** The earliest vascular plants, such as *Cooksonia* from the Pridolian of the Silurian period in Wales indicate clearly the phylogenetically later appearance and development of plant tissues as compared to those of the Trilobites, even of the Cambrian period
	Silurian			Earliest vascular plants**	
	Ordovician	500,000,000	Fishes		
				Brophyta	
	Cambrian	620,000,000	Trilobites*		
Proterozoic	Precambrian (Lacking morphologically recognizable fossils)	1,420,000,000	Invertebrates	Fungi? Algae	
			Protista	Monera	
Archeozoic		2,300,000,000		Virus?	

Neoplasms are an old disease group: Theoretical and practical aspects

Theoretically neoplasms can not be phylogenetically older than the tissues they derive from. But they can be traced also from the fossils with afflicted parts. Neoplasms from invertebrates have the oldest history followed from those of vertebrates with fishes from the Ordovicium and finally the vascular plants. Animal tissues are older than plant tissues, with exception of the breast tissue and the hair of mammals. The development of metastatic growth is restricted up to birds and becomes then the dominating spreading of tumors in the mammal with its abundant lymphatic metastasis. The development of mammalian lymphatic metastasis may have been uprising in the Oligocene epoch and slowly beginning from the upper Triassic. The development during phylogeny was slow if compared to our own life span and our man-made environmental changes.

The immense increase in man-made changes of the environment

The influence of man on the environment in the Pleistocene was nearly nil. It began at this time with the cutting of the forests and building with the first agricultural endeavors. The next step can be seen in the rising of the different empires in the Euphrat-Tigris region in Egypt, in the Greek and Roman empires the state of Carthage and the civilization of the Aztecs. More destructive to nature were the times of the medivial age, suddenly changing into the time of revolution, the foundation of the United States in the 18th century. The killing of the buffaloes and the near extermination of the American Indians are important examples. In Europe, the industrial revolution in 1848 was followed by the Soviet revolution in 1917. In the last decades, Japan became an industrial world power; other countries followed. These historic events are of signicance to our problem because they were followed by a rapid industrialization which has led in a number of years to the most drastic change in the environment accompanied by a massive increase in world population. The results are dramatic changes in the world we live in; some of which have to be dseen as positive others as negative. The old diseases which are known as the neoplastic ones have increased not in the types of neoplasms, in general, but in the number of discased persons. The dog is the typical animal in this regard; the boxer is the most cancer prone dog.

Man undermines the natural balance in the environment (1) destruction of normal fauna and flora - destruction of forest and interspecies barrier; (2) promoting of continued extinction; (3) air pollution; (4) water pollution; (5) soil pollution; (6) change of nutrition in different ways in different populations; (7) endangering his chemical environment by paints, tar products, smoking of chimneys; (8) accumulation of toxic trash; (9) influence of chemical industry releasing many products into the environment; (10) atomic mishaps as possibility; (11) acid rain; (12) change of the ozone layer and increasing ultraviolet radiation.

The results of human intervention are sometimes disastrous: hunger, disease, overpopulation, even the extinction of whole species. Worldwide lack of adequate education exacerbates these difficulties.

The species-specific reaction of these processes

Some factors of man-made changes on earth have been outlined. It is known from epidemiology that different human populations exhibit a different frequency of neoplasms. Species differences exist also. The results of these factors is a number of chain reactions in different compartments of the environment.

REFERENCES

1. Kaiser HE: Das Abnorme in der Evolution (Abnormal Facts in the Evolution). Leyden/The Netherlands: Brill Publisher, 1970
2. Kaiser HE: Species-specific Potential of Invertebrates for Toxicological Research. Baltimore: University Park Press, 1980
3. Kaiser HE: Neoplasms – Comparative Pathology of Growth in Animals, Plants, and Man. Baltimore: Williams & Wilkins, 1981

POSTSCRIPT

A combined effect of tobacco, alcohol, diet, and occupation exists in the initiation and promotion of esophageal cancer. This chain reaction of the risk factors includes also higher consumption of fried bacon or ham, less fresh fruits and raw vegetables, and less whole grain bread by the patients if compared to controls. The different unequal risk factors of the man-made environment as exhibited in the epidemiology of this type of cancer are not equal, but additive.

POSTSCRIPT REFERENCE

Yu, MC et al: Tobacco, alcohol, diet, occupation and carcinoma of the esophagus. *Cancer Res* 48(13): 3843–3848, 1988.

26

SPONTANEOUS TUMORS OF FREE-RANGING TERRESTRIAL MAMMALS OF NORTH AMERICA

ELIZABETH S. WILLIAMS and E. TOM THORNE,
with a contribution of THEODORA STEINECK

Published information on tumors of free-ranging wild animals is limited. Case reports are scattered throughout the literature in journals as well as project reports from wildlife management agencies, preceedings of meetings and theses and dissertations. Much information on occurrence of tumors in wildlife remains buried in files of wildlife biologists, veterinary pathologists and diagnostic laboratories.

Among free-ranging wild animals, age structure of most populations is such that young animals are far more numerous than aged individuals. As a consequence of predation, competition, hunting, and diseases, relatively few free-ranging animals live long enough to develop tumors associated with advanced age. The situation is somewhat different for animals in zoological collections where they are protected from many of the hazards that lead to short life spans. As a result, captive animals may live their biological life expectancy and conseqently have a longer period of time to develop neoplasms.

When tumors develop in free-ranging animals to the point of recognition by biologists, hunters, or the public, the animals are seldom examined by diagnosticians capable of classifying the tumors. This results in poor and essentially useless records of the disease. An unfortunate problem with the study of wildlife disease in general, and neoplasia in particular, is that when wild animals are found dead, autolysis is often advanced, making accurate diagnoses impossible. Often diagnostic facilities are located at some distance from personnel in the field and carcasses or tissues are frozen, again resulting in less than desirable specimens for diagnostic evaluation.

Frequently, the behavior of sick or debilitated wild animals results in decreased likelihood of finding the individual or carcass. Sick animals usually segregate themselves from others, seek dense shelter, or, if fossorial, stay underground. Also, debilitated animals are easier for predators to kill and consume than healthy animals.

A number of biases are assumed when reviewing case reports of neoplasms of free-ranging animals. Tumors of the skin are more readily recognized than internal neoplasms, consequently the literature contains numerous reports of cutaneous tumors. Generally there is more interest in diseases and neoplasms of game animals than in non-game species. In these cases, wildlife biologists and hunters may observe tumors and report them, but tumors of non-game animals are seldom carefully examined.

Tumors induced by viruses are commonly reported in the wildlife literature (14, 16, 27, 34, 36, 37, 43–45, 47, 50, 53, 57, 66, 70, 71, 74, 75, 81–83, 85, 86, 88) for several reasons.

Generally these tumors are on the skin which increases recognition; younger animals are most commonly affected and are usually numerous in the population; and many animals are affected at one time which leads to increased opportunity for diagnosis.

This discussion will include only neoplasms diagnosed in wild free-ranging terrestrial mammals and will be arranged by body systems. When the information is available, gross and microscopic descriptions will be included. A number of excellent reviews of neoplasms of animals in various zoological parks are published (1, 23, 32, 52).

Neoplasms of the skin

As mentioned above, skin tumors are probably the most frequently recognized and reported neoplasms of free-ranging species. Papilloma-viruses commonly induce skin tumors in cervids (50, 71, 81, 83) and these viruses appear to be relatively species specific (53, 83, 86). Fibromas are the most common cutaneous neoplasm in deer (81). They have been reported in white-tailed deer (*Odocoileus virginianus*) from all parts of their range (3, 16, 26, 29, 41, 71, 81); mule deer (*Odocoileus hemionus*) (35, 39, 40, 81, 83, 90); black-tailed deer (*Odocoileus hemionus columbianus*), (27, 81); moose (*Alces alces*) (18, 27, 80, 81, 90) caribou (*Rangifer tarandus*) (6, 18, 72) and elk (*Cervus elaphus canadensis*) (90).

Fibromas rarely cause significant disease in affected animals but occasionally tumors may be very large, numerous or located in a site that interferes with sight or ability to feed. Fibromas of deer are self-limiting and usually regress without residual after a course of several months (29). Tumors are most frequently observed on the head, neck and medial aspect of the forelimbs (81). Males are affected more often than females (16, 29, 82) and the individuals are usually young (29, 82). Information gathered at hunter check stations revealed a 1.4% (29) to 8.5% (82) prevalence of the tumors.

The morphology of fibromas is similar in all cervid species. Grossly the tumors are firm, generally rounded and have a smooth, wrinkled or papillomatous surface. They may be single or multiple, sessile or pedunculated, and range in size from several mm to 25 cm in diameter. The surface epithelium is usually pigmented, though unpigmented fibromas are occasionally reported. The superficial epithelium is often ulcerated and inflamed. Cut surfaces are white to tan and fibrous and areas of mineralization or ossification may be present ((16); Williams and Thorne, unpublished data).

H. E. Kaiser (ed.), Comparative aspects of tumor development.

Microscopically fibromas from most cervids are similar, and these features are well described (14, 16, 81). The connective tissue element is composed of stellate to spindle shaped fibroblasts in a dense interlacing matrix of collagen. The cells tend to be perpendicular to the epithelium at the surface but become irregularly arranged deeper in the mass. There is low to moderate vascularity and widely separated adnexal structures may be present. Occasionally, areas of necrosis and hemorrhage occur. Mitotic figures are rarely observed in the fibrous component.

Epidermal changes vary somewhat depending on the gross characteristics of the tumors. In papillomatous types, the epithelium is acanthotic, hyperkeratotic and often parakeratotic, with a folded irregular surface and irregularly arranged basal cells. Basal cells frequently contain melanin. In the smoother surfaced forms, epithelial rete pegs may extend into the fibrous component. The overlying epithelium may vary considerably in thickness. Mitotic figures are observed in basal cells. Eosinophilic intranuclear inclusion bodies have been described in the outermost layer of the stratum granulosum and throughout the parakeratotic areas of stratum corneum in white-tailed deer (86); however, they are seldom mentioned in other histologic descriptions of these tumors.

Fibrosarcomas of the skin are rarely reported from free-ranging cervids. Wadsworth (89) described multiple skin masses which were especially numerous on the head and neck of a white-tailed deer. Two marble-sized fibrotic masses were found on the margins of the right lung. Microscopically, the tumors were characterized by numerous fibroblasts arranged in an irregular pattern and there was active mitosis. Sundberg and Nielsen (81) suggest this may have been fibromatosis with pulmonary involvement as was described in another white-tailed deer (47). The pulmonary tumors may have represented "multiple hits" by the deer papillomavirus (81) or may have been initiated during a viremic state (47).

Virally induced skin tumors are also commonly reported in squirrels and rabbits. These include squirrel fibroma, rabbit fibroma, and rabbit papilloma.

Fibromas in rabbits are caused by a pox virus (70) of the Leporivirus genus which is closely related to myxoma virus. The tumors are reported in free-ranging wild cottontail rabbits (*Sylvilagus floridanus*) in the eastern and midwestern United States (36, 51, 85, 93). The virus causes localized, single or multiple tumors which regress after several months. Grossly, the cutaneous growths are firm, spherical and range from 1 to 4 cm in diameter. The surface may be smooth to irregular and frequently is ulcerated (85). Following initial inflammatory reaction to the virus in the corium, fibroblast-like cells appear which have abundant cytoplasm, vesicular nuclei and contain granular cytoplasmic inclusion bodies. There is epidermal hyperplasia and epidermal rete pegs extended into the fibrous component. At the time of regression, necrotic foci appear with an infiltrate of lymphocytes and neutrophils (92).

Fibromas in squirrels are similar to those in rabbits (92). Gray squirrels (*Sciurus carolinensis*) (37, 44, 45) and western gray squirrels (*Sciurus griseus griseus*) (62) are most commonly affected, but the disease has been diagnosed in eastern fox squirrel (*Sciurus niger*), black squirrel (species not given) and red fox squirrel (species not given) (9). Tumors

are most common on juveniles, may be scattered over the body, range from minute to 2.5 cm in diameter and are elevated, flattened and firm. Involvement of internal organs has been described (44, 45, 57). The epidermis is hyperkeratotic and rete pegs extend into the dermal mass of fibroblastic cells. Viral inclusions bodies are present in the epithelial cells. Chronic dermal inflammation is common, especially during regression. In systemic infections, fibromas or fibromatous proliferations are often seen in lung (45), but they may be present also in intestines, heart, mesentery and testes (57).

Rabbit papillomas are hard, horn-like, often multiple and frequently pigmented protrusions from the skin. These tumors also are virally induced (43). They are reported most often in cotton-tail rabbits but also occur in jack rabbits (*Lepus* sp.). The tumors are typical papillomas with a pink fleshy cut surface (34) and microscopically composed of proliferating epithelium thrown into folds. Hyperkeratosis is prominent and mitotic figures may be common. Occasionally, papillomas may progress to squamous cell carcinomas (54).

Oral papillomatosis is a viral disease of wild and domestic canids caused by a papovavirus. Coyotes (*Canis latrans*) and wolves (*Canis lupus*) have been reported with this disease (66, 87, 90). These oral tumors are discrete, usually unpigmented and flat, smooth, pedunculated, or cauliflower-like. Lesions may involve gums, palate, lips, tongue, epiglottis, and esophagus. Microscopically, the lesions are typical papillomas with hyperplastic, hyperkeratotic epithelium thrown into folds and supported on vascular connective tissue. Mitotic figures may be numerous in the basal cells of the epithelium and ballooning degeneration may occur in acanthocytes. The tumors usually regress in 1.5 to 3 months.

Cutaneous fibropapillomas have been reported in pronghorn antelope (*Antilocapra americana*) from Wyoming (40, 84). Grossly and microscopically the fibromas in pronghorn were similar to those described in deer. The covering epithelium was acanthotic, hyperkeratotic and heavily pigmented. Small dark eosinophilic intranuclear inclusion bodies were observed in epithelial cells. Papillomavirus genus-specific structural antigens were demonstrated in cells of the stratum granulosum and corneum of the fibropapilloma (84).

A proliferative mass from the foot of a nine-banded armadillo (*Dasypus novemcinctus*) was diagnosed as a fibroma (59). The mass was cauliflower-like with a fissured, verrucose surface. The epidermis was hyperkeratotic with slight acanthosis. The dermal fibrous component was arranged in dense whorls and mitotic figures were not observed. Evidence of viral etiology was not found.

Additional reports of fibromas and papillomas are in the literature, but they were poorly described and etiology was not examined. Skin fibromas were mentioned as naturally occurring neoplasms of raccoons (*Procyon lotor*) in Connecticut (19). Squamous papillomas were seen in beaver (*Castor canadensis*) (10) and in river otter (*Lutra canadensis*) (13) in Michigan. Dodge (20) reports heavily pigmented papillomas being common on upper lips of adult porcupines (*Erethizon dorsatum*). These tumors apparently cause little problem to the animal but may be extensive. Dieterich (18) reported a papilloma on an insular vole (*Microtus abbreviatus fisheri*) in Alaska.

Large subcutaneous lipomas were described on the rear

leg of a cottontail rabbit in Michigan (51). The tumors were composed of variably sized and shaped fat cells with areas of fat necrosis primarily at the periphery of the neoplasms. Lipomas in the skin have been reported twice in white-tailed deer (9, 26).

Two additional benign tumors of skin have been reported but not described. A melanoma was diagnosed in the skin of an elk in Colorado (90) and a sebaceous gland adenoma was seen in a yellow cheeked vole (*Microtus xanthognathus*) in Alaska (18).

Only a few malignant skin neoplasms are reported in free-ranging species and these are not described. Dieterich (18) reported squamous cell carcinomas in a tundra vole (*Microtus oeconomus macfarlani*) and an arctic ground squirrel (*Spermophilus parryii plesius*) and an adnexal carcinoma in a northern red backed vole (*Clethrionemys rutilus dawsoni*). A squamous cell carcinoma was seen in a skunk (*Mephitis mephitis*) from Ontario (73).

Soft tissue neoplasms

A rapidly growing invasive subcutaneous fibrosarcoma was described in an aged white-tailed deer (25). The mass was 8 cm in diameter and extensively infiltrated the supraorbital process of the left frontal bone. The tissue was well vascularized and composed of proliferating fusiform to stellate cells forming bundles and whorls, many plump larger cells with pale ovoid nuclei and occasionally multinucleated cells. Fibrosarcomas were reported from the jaw of a white-tailed deer (16) and from a muskox (*Ovibos moschatus niphoecus*) (18). These neoplasms were not described.

Mesotheliomas were reported twice in free-ranging white-tailed deer; both cases involved the abdomen (16, 26). Fay (26) described a 9-year-old doe as having generalized malignant mesotheliomas throughout the abdominal viscera.

Lipomas involving the mesenteries and kidneys of a white-tailed deer in Pennsylvania have been reported (26). A porcupine and a black bear (*Ursus americana*) were reported to have liposarcomas (20, 58). The liposarcoma in the porcupine was present in a uterine horn where it was initially thought to be a developing fetus (20).

A description of a myxosarcoma in an adult male elk from Colorado is given by Snyder (76). A large mass (25 × 5 cm) was present on the medial aspect of the right thigh near the pubis. The mass was invasive, nonencapsulated, and was gray to pink, with regions of mucinous material on cut surface. Strands of fibrous tissue subdivided the mass into lobules. Microscopically the neoplasm was composed of fusiform to stellate cells in a mucinous stroma. Moderate numbers of mitotic figures were observed.

Musculoskeletal system

Only a few neoplasms of muscle are reported in free-ranging species. Dieterich (18) lists a rhabdomyoma in a beaver and a rhabdomyosarcoma in a northern red backed vole from Alaska. A highly undifferentiated sarcoma was described from the rear leg of an aged white-tailed deer doe (46). The neoplasm was firm, white with gray areas of necrosis and replaced much of the normal musculature. Similar tissue was present in inguinal lymph nodes, adrenal glands, kidney, liver and lung. The neoplasm was composed of undifferentiated, variably sized cuboidal to polygonal cells with acidophilic granular cytoplasm. Neoplastic cells had single to multiple nucleoli and mitotic figures were common. Minimal connective tissue stroma and vascularity were present. As is unfortunately often the situation with the study of tissues of free-ranging animals, freezing artifact precluded definitive statements about the tissue origin of the neoplasm.

Osteomas are uncommon. Dieterich (18) lists an osteoma in a tundra vole. An osteoma was mentioned in a white-tailed deer but location and description were not given (91). We have diagnosed an osteoma protruding from the head of a 3-year-old white-tailed deer doe from Wyoming. The mass was 22 × 21 × 16 cm, weighed 4.8 kg, and involved the frontal bone and squamous temporal bone with indentation of the cerebral cortex. Microscopically, the mass was composed of mature bone spicules lined by well differentiated osteoblasts and osteoclasts. Islands of cartilage and fibrous connective tissue were observed. There was no evidence of metastasis.

An osteosarcoma in an elk was mistakenly diagnosed as actinomycosis until microscopic examination revealed the lesion's true nature (22). Grossly the mass contained areas of necrosis and secondary infection, with spicules and small masses of bone interspersed with solid areas of fibrous and myxomatous tissue. The microscopic description was not given, but the neoplasm was reported to be of a low order of malignancy. An osteosarcoma was reported, but not described in a white-tailed deer in Michigan (11).

Lymphohemopoietic system

Lymphosarcomas, malignant lymphomas and leukemias have been reported from a variety of wildlife species. The etiology of most of the neoplasms was not determined; however, as is true in humans and domestic animals, viruses may play a role in some types of lymphoid tumors.

Malignant lymphomas were reported in six cotton-tail rabbits from Michigan (51). The neoplasms involved spleen, abdominal wall, liver, kidney, adrenal gland and gastrointestinal tract. Lymphomas classified as lymphocytic type consisted of mature lymphocytes infiltrating normal tissue structures or completely destroying the architecture. Histiocytic lymphomas were composed of large pleomorphic cells with large vesicular nuclei and prominent nucleoli.

Several authors describe lymphosarcomas in white-tailed deer (14, 16, 17, 90). The lymphosarcoma reported by Debbie and Friend (17) was characterized by a 20 cm diameter mass at the pelvic inlet and smaller solid masses in other areas of the abdominal and thoracic viscera. The neoplasm was composed of pleomorphic lymphoid cells. Many had pale eosinophilic cytoplasm resembling that of histiocytes. Occasional giant cells were observed. Additional cases of lymphosarcomas in deer and moose are listed but not described (31). Lymphosarcoma in a bison (*Bison bison*) (63) and a thymic lymphosarcoma in a wolverine (*Gulo gulo*) (18) are mentioned in the literature. A lymphoblastic lymphosarcoma involving kidneys, brain, and meninges was described in an adult female raccoon (64). The kidneys were enlarged and cut surface of the cortices appeared mottled. Microscopically, sheets of invading large lymphoblasts were present. The cells had scant basophilic cytoplasm and large nuclei with single large nucleoli. Some cells had deeply indented nuclei. Mitotic figures were numerous.

Hodgkin's disease was reported in four striped skunks from Ontario (73). It was not clear from the report if the disease occurred in free-ranging or captive skunks. The descriptions of the disease were thorough and the diagnosis of Hodgkin's disease was based on the presence of Sternberg-Reed cells, the cellular pattern and the malignant behavior of the neoplasms.

Reticuloendothelial neoplasms, without description, were mentioned as occurring in the Virginia opossum (*Didelphis virginiana*) (30).

Respiratory system

There are very few reports of tumors in the respiratory tract of wild animals. Pulmonary adenomatosis was described in opossums in North Carolina (68) and Gardner (30) mentions the occurrence of respiratory neoplasia in opossum. Adenomas were found in the lungs of 17 of 68 animals; most were not recognized on gross examination. The lesions were well circumscribed, papillary, and mitotic activity was not observed. Origin of the neoplasms was felt to be bronchial epithelium.

Bronchoalveolar adenomas were described in a gray squirrel with systemic poxviral infection (57). The epithelial cells of the neoplasms contained large eosinophilic inclusion bodies.

Digestive system

Only a few neoplasms have been reported from the tubular portion of the digestive tract. A large oral fibroma apparently interfered with mastication and swallowing leading to starvation and death in a wild mountain goat (*Oreamnos americanus*) (28). Microscopically the tissue changes were consistent with a well differentiated highly collagenous fibroma.

A 3.5-year-old white-tailed deer from Wisconsin was found to have an oral-nasal squamous cell carcinoma (79). A large necrotic ulcer was present on the hard palate, there was erosion of underlying bone and a pathologic fracture of the frontal bone was present. Nasal turbinates were thickened and surrounding structures were invaded by a cream to white, firm, rubbery growth which extended through the cribriform palate and into the retrobulbar space causing exophthalmia. The mass was composed of invasive cords of epithelial cells on a variably dense stroma with areas of necrosis. Cells varied in size, had one to three nucleoli and contained keratinaceous material. Bizarre mitotic figures were present and metastatic lesions were in a retropharyngeal lymph node.

Only two reports of neoplasms involving stomach could be found. Papillary tumors, composed of hyperplastic squamous epithelium, were associated with the nematode (*Synhimantus longigutturatus*) in the stomachs of muskrats (*Onda-*

tra zibethicus ripens) (15). A gastric adenoma was identified in a Michigan beaver (10).

A number of neoplasms are reported and described in the liver of free-ranging wild animals. Hepatic neoplasms are associated with a hepatitis virus in woodchucks (*Marmota monax*). A high prevalence of antibodies to woodchuck hepatitis virus was found in a survey of wild woodchuck populations, (88) Woodchuck hepatitis virus belongs to the same class of viruses as hepatitis B virus of humans. Hepatocellular carcinomas are common in some captive populations of woodchucks (74, 75) but are less common in free-ranging animals (33, 74).

A lymphangioma was reported in the liver of a white-tailed deer (8). The mass contained large raised cysts lined by low flattened endothelium. Several adenocarcinomas are reported in white-tailed deer (16, 60). A 1 year old buck had nodules and fibrosis involving two-thirds of the light brown to yellow-brown liver. Necrotic regions and hemorrhages were observed on cut surface. Neoplastic hepatocytes were arranged in acinar and trabecular patterns with abundant stroma. Nuclei were pleomorphic, multinucleated cells were numerous and few mitotic figure were seen. Groups of neoplastic cells were within vessels but metastases were not detected.

An adenocarcinoma of bile duct origin was reported in a 2-year-old doe mule deer from Wyoming (40). Multiple discrete white foci involved most of the liver.

Urinary system

A variety of species are reported having neoplasms of the urinary system. An embryonal nephroma was diagnosed in a young free-ranging elk from Colorado (Snyder (76). A soft mass (30 × 20 × 15 cm) weighing 6.6 kg was present in the position of the left kidney and infiltrating adjacent tissue. On cut surface, large areas of necrosis and hemorrhage and small cysts were seen. Epithelial and mesenchymal tissue elements were present in the neoplasm. Neoplastic cells formed tubules and glomerulus-like structures and the stroma occasionally formed myxomatous, cartilaginous and adipose tissue. Metastatic foci occurred in the lung.

An aged female moose was found to have a large (30 × 15 cm) multinodular mass replacing the right kidney and adrenal and extending into the caudal vena cava. The mass was composed of grey-white tissue with areas of necrosis and hemorrhage. Several small nodules were in liver and lung. Neoplastic epithelial cells formed alveolar and tubuloalveolar patterns on a fibrous stroma. The cells varied from columnar to cuboidal and had acidophilic to clear cytoplasm. Mitotic figures were rare. A diagnosis of renal adenocarcinoma was made (5).

Roher (65) reported a neoplasm in the urinary bladder of a white-tailed deer in New York. The 9 × 6 cm yellow-white lobulated mass involved the wall of the urinary bladder and areas of necrosis were observed within the tumor. The neoplasm was composed of large epithelial cells, with prominent nuclei and nucleoli and granular eosinophilic cytoplasm; which invaded connective tissue of the submucosa and muscularis of the bladder.

Renal tubular adenomas were associated with poxvirus

infection in a gray squirrel. The tumors involved the renal cortex and had a papillary growth pattern. Ballooning degeneration and cytoplasmic inclusions were observed in some epithelial cells (57). A discrete, white, 1 cm diameter cystic nodule was discovered in the renal cortex of an adult male fox squirrel from Wyoming (Williams, unpublished data). Microscopically, the mass was encapsulated and well-differentiated cuboidal epithelial cells formed papillary and tubular structures on a light stroma. Mitotic figures were not observed. Adjacent renal tissue was compressed. There was no evidence of viral infection in this individual.

Several renal tumors have been reported in cotton-tail rabbits. Lopushinsky and Fay (51) report a nephroblastoma in a rabbit from Michigan. The mass, located in the region of the right kidney, weighed 55 grams and was dark red, pulpy and faintly lobulated. Fibroblastic tissue made up the bulk of the tumor with a lining of epithelial cells. Carlton and Dietz (7) describe a hamartoma of urogenital origin and a renal adenocarcinoma in two wild cotton-tails. In addition, a transitional cell carcinoma was reported in a wolverine (*Gulo gulo*) and a renal adenocarcinoma listed in an arctic ground squirrel (18).

Genital system

Only one description is available of genital neoplasia in wild mammals. A seminoma was described in an elk from Oregon (67). The enlarged testicle was from a 10-year-old animal. The tumor was composed of sheets and packets of cells with round or polyhedral vesicular nuclei. Cytoplasm was eosinophilic and mitotic figures were numerous. Scattered foci of lymphocytes were present. Gardner (30) reports occurrence of urogenital tumors in Virginia opossum.

Tumor of the mammary gland

Neoplasia of the mammary gland is common in some domestic species (55) but appears to be very rare in wild animals. A single report was found of a malignant mixed mammary tumor diagnosed in a gray squirrel (69). The female had a 7 × 6 × 4.5 cm subcutaneous mass on the ventral thorax. Cut surface was white and lobulated with areas of necrosis and hemorrhage. The left axillary lymph node was firm and enlarged. Neoplastic epithelial cells were characterized as polygonal and cuboidal with pleomorphic nuclei and multiple prominent nucleoli. Cells were arranged in clumps or lining alveolar structures. Mitotic index was moderate. Small islands or lobules of cartilage, lobules of chondromucinous material and large areas of necrosis occurred in the tumor. A metastatic lesion was found in the left axillary lymph node. Myoepithelial cells were not observed.

Endocrine system

Neoplasms of the endocrine system are also rarely reported. An adenoma of possible adrenal origin was found on a ureter of an antlered female white-tailed deer (21). The authors suggest the neoplasm had a masculinizing effect

causing antler growth in the doe. The mass was ovoid, encapsulated, orange and 12 × 18 mm. Microscopically, the neoplastic cells were large, polyhedral with accentrically placed nuclei. Mitotic activity was not described. Two additional neoplasms of endocrine origin in wild ruminants are reported but not described. A thyroid adenoma was seen in an elk calf from western Colorado (4) and a pheochromocytoma was diagnosed in the adrenal of a white-tailed deer (16).

An insulin-producing islet cell tumor in an ectopic pancreas was reported in a red fox (*Vulpes vulpes*) (24). The 3 × 3 × 3 cm mass was attached to the colon of a young female fox. The tissue was composed of polygonal cells with small nuclei, arranged in trabecular and alveolar structures on a sparse stroma. The cellular morphology did not suggest malignancy. Immunohistochemical preparations demonstrated the presence of insulin in the tumor cell.

Nervous system

In comparison to neoplasms reported in other systems (excluding skin), tumors of the brain of cervids are numerous. This suggests deer may have a relatively high incidence of brain tumors, or it may only reflect the fact that animals with these tumors, because of behavioral changes, are more readily observed and more closely examined. All the reports of brain tumors in cervids are in free-ranging animals. Kradel and Dunne (49) describe ependymomas in two white-tailed deer. In both animals the ventricles of the brain were enlarged and contained soft, friable, papillary masses. Only the fourth ventricle was involved in one animal. While both tumors were reported as ependymomas, Nettles and Vandeveld (56) suggest these may have been choroid plexus papillomas. These authors report a thalamic ependymoma in a white-tailed deer. A 3 cm diameter pink mass was present in the left thalamus. Microscopically, the tumor was highly cellular, infiltrative and contained necrotic hemorrhagic areas. Cells were uniform, with nonstaining cytoplasm and ovoid nuclei with multiple nucleoli; they often were arranged around vessels in palisades and occasionally formed rosettes. Clusters of cyst-like structures were numerous in some areas. Metastases occurred throughout the ventricular system and meninges. An additional ependymoma has been listed for white-tailed deer (16). A white-tailed deer in Tennessee was found to have a mixed glioma and rhabdomyosarcoma (38). The frontal lobes of the brain contained a 3.8 cm diameter gelatinous mass. Cells in the mass varied from a regular population with small round nuclei to voluminous pleomorphic spindle-shaped cells showing cross striations. Astrocytomas have been reported twice in white-tailed deer (42, 48). In one case, there was a 5 cm diameter mass ventral to the thalamus and anterior to the optic chiasm. Lateral ventricles were compressed. There is one listing of a medulloblastoma occurring in a white-tailed deer (16).

Snyder (78) describes two brain tumors in elk in Colorado. An old female had a poorly delineated 4 × 2 cm mass in the area around the optic chiasm and adjacent tissue. The tumor was pink to red–brown and infiltrated the hypothalamus. The cells were fusiform with indistinct margins and arranged in sheets and whorls. Necrosis and calcification present. Mitotic activity was moderate. This neoplasm was diagnosed as a meningeal sarcoma. A differentiated protoplasmic astrocytoma was diagnosed in a second elk. The brain of this animal contained a soft, gray to brown $7 \times 5 \times 5$ cm mass in the left pyriform lobe. Areas of necrosis occurred in the tumor. Microscopically, neoplastic cells were fusiform to stellate and loosely-arranged. Few mitotic figures were present. Adjacent neuropil was compressed but not invaded.

A fibrous astrocytoma in a raccoon was described as a small, solid mass in the cerebral hemisphere posterior to the olfactory bulb (19). The cells of the tumor were pleomorphic and arranged in a whorled pattern. Cytoplasm was lightly staining and cell margins indistinct. Mitotic figures were numerous.

Miscellaneous neoplasms

Unfortunately, many neoplasms from wildlife are reported in lists or discussions without description of the history of the animal, gross appearance or histopathology. For completeness this section will list neoplasms from free-ranging mammals that are poorly described but which may be of interest to oncologists or comparative pathologists.
Adenoma
    White-tailed deer (26)
    Arctic ground squirrel (18)
    Collared lemming (*Dicrostonyx stevensoni*) (18)
Mixed cell tumor
    Collared lemming (*Dicrostonyx stevensoni*) (18)
Carcinoma
    White-tailed deer (8, 61)
Adenocarcinoma
    White-tailed deer (9,16)
    River otter (9)
    Mink (*Mustela vison*) (18)
    Cotton-tail rabbit (12)
    Collared lemming (8 tumors) (18)
    Tundra vole (18)
Sarcoma
    White-tailed deer (9)

    Cottontail rabbit (9)
    Northern red backed vole (18)
Malignant tumors
    White-tailed deer (26)
    Coyotes (2)
Unidentified tumors
    Dall sheep (*Ovis dalli*) (18)
    Black bear (58)

Summary

As the previous discussion illustrates, many neoplasms have been reported in free-ranging wild mammals. These frequently involve isolated case reports and seldom address the question of prevalence of neoplasia in these populations. Unfortunately, due to the inherent difficulties in wildlife disease studies as described in the introduction, surveys to determine prevalence of neoplasia are seldom conducted. Information is available for the virally induced skin fibromas of deer (29, 82) where surveys have indicated a 1.4% to 8.5% prevalence of the tumors. Estimates of prevalence for other types of neoplasia have not been made and cannot be reliably estimated with the data presently available.

Neoplasia have been reported from most organ systems of wild mammals. Neoplasms of the brain of cervids are well represented especially considering the difficulties associated with obtaining these tumors for examination. Of comparative interest are the reports of lymphoid neoplasms in a variety of species and the reports of Hodgkin's disease in a group of skunks (73). Hepatic tumors in woodchucks are asociated with a hepatitis virus related to hepatitis B virus of humans (74).

There is increasing interest among wildlife biologists, managers, and veterinary pathologists in diagnosing diseases of free-ranging species. As information continues to accumulate and is published we should begin to have a better understanding of the type and prevalence of neoplasias in the various species of wild animals and how these neoplasms compare with those found in domestic species and humans.

NEOPLASMS IN FREE-RANGING SPECIES OF TERRESTRIAL MAMMALS IN AUSTRIA AND BORDERING COUNTRIES

T. STEINECK

Neoplasm in free-ranging terrestrial mammals of North America have been described in this chapter and comparison of the occurrence of neoplasms in the mammals of North America with free-ranging mammals of Europe could conceivably augment our understanding of which effects man himself. This has been done in the following table of the cases diagnosed in Austria from 1972 until 1986 in our Institute in Vienna (Steineck). Neoplasms in free-ranging animals of the species mentioned amount only approximately 1% of the cases investigated. According to the author's

experience, the number of undetected neoplasms is minute. Especially in Europe, wardens maintain such a careful watch over their territory that tumors of a larger size will not escape attention. In the submitted case material, the localization, indicated by the hunters may not be properly given but these cases, also, have been included in an effort to achieve completeness of the record.

A selection of additional cases also of the red fox (*Vulpes vulpes*), or old world badger (*Meles meles*) and the European pine marten (*Martes martes*) have been included. The neo-

Table 1. Neoplasms in free-ranging mammals of Austria and conterminous European countries.

Species	Epithelial	Mesenchymal	Benign	Malignant	Tumor	No of cases	Steineck	Literature
Roe deer (*Capreolus capreolus*)	+		+		Adenoma of pituitary gland	1	+	Von Braunschweig, A., 1963: Z. f. Jagdwiss. 9, 36
	+		+		Liver cell adenoma			
	+		+		Adenoma of hypophysis			Burgisser, H., 1983: Schweiz. Arch. Tierheilk. 125, 510–527
	+			+	Squamous cell cancer	1	+	
	+			+	Carcinoma of the wall of the rumen	1	+	
	+			+	Liver carcinoma	3	+	
	+			+	Adenocarcinoma of the mamma	1	+	
	+			+	Seminoma	1	+	
Roe deer	+			+	Cavernous hemangioma in solid liver adenoma			Hoffmann, W., P. Möller, 1984: Z. f. Jagdwiss. 30, 259–264
	+			+	Liver cancer			Becker, 1941: Deutsche Jagd, Nr. 41/42, 391
	+			+	Biliary duct carcinoma			Brunk, R., 1960: Z. f. Jagdwiss. 6, 121–185
	+			+	Liver cell and bile duct cancer	1		Brunk, R., 1965: Z. f. Jagdwiss. 11, 145–150
	+			+	Liver cancer			Goeke, H., 1958: Wild u. Hund 61, 432
	+			+	Liver adenoma, liver carcinoma			Krause, C., 1938: Arch. Tierheilkde. 73, 1–24
	+		+		Liveradenoma			Mentschel, H., 1937: Vet. Diss. Giessen
	+			+	Liver cancer	1		Jaenecke, R., 1941: Tierärztl. Rdsch. 47, 590
	+			+	Adenocarcinoma of kidney			Burgisser, h., 1983: Schweiz. Arch. Tierheilk. 125, 510–527
Doe	+			+	Leydig cell tumor of right ovary	1		Wurster, K., et al, 1983: Z. f. Jagdwiss. 29, 74–81
Roe buck	+		+		Skin papilloma	1		Von Braunschweig, A., 1985: Wild u. Hund 88, 6
Doe	+			+	Cornified squamous cell carcinoma of the udder (mamma)			Arch. Tierheilk. 77, 319–327
	+			+	Squamous cell carcinoma of mammary gland			Brunk, R., 1960: Z. f. Jagdwiss. 6, 121–185
	+			+	Malignant melanoma, forelimb			Burgisser H., 1983: Schweiz. Arch. Tierheilk. 125, 510–527
	+			+	Epidermoid carcinoma of orbital region			Burgisser H., 1983: ....
Roe deer (*Capreolus capreolus*)		+	+		Lipoma	1	+	
		+	+		Fibroma molle	1	+	
		+	+		Fibroma durum	2	+	
		+	+		Osteofibroma	1	+	
		+	+		Chondroma	1	+	
		+		+	Fibrosarcoma	3	+	
		+		+	Osteochondrosarcoma	1	+	
		+		+	Giant-cell-sarcoma	1	+	
		+		+	Sarcoma with mixed cellularity	1	+	
		+		+	Lymphoid-cellular sarcoma	1		

Species	Tumor	N	Reference
Roebuck	Round-cell-sarcoma of liver	1	Jahnke, H-D., 1980: Wild u. Hund, *83*, 4
	Unspecified sarcoma	2	Ganzinger, K. et al., 1986: Z. f. Jagdwiss. *32*, 125–128
	Malignant neoplasm	1	
	Liver tumor	1	
	Leydig's interstitial cell sarcoma		Brömmel, J., Zettel, K., 1979: Der praktische Tierarzt *60*, 386–388
	Osteoblastic sarcoma, orbital region	1	
	Lymphosarcomatosis		Burgisser, H., 1983: Schweiz. Arch. Tierheilk. *125*, 510–527
	Lymphosarcomatosis of liver		Burgisser, H., 1983: Schweiz. Arch. Tierheilk. *125*, 510–527
	Reticulosarcoma of nasopharynx		Burgisser, H., 1983: Schweiz. Arch. Tierheilk. *125*, 510–527
	Osteosarcoma, hindleg		Petersilie, E., 1959: Z. f. Jagdwiss. *5*, 150–152
	Osteosarcoma, head		
	Osteofibrosarcoma, head		Meyer, P., 1979: Z. f. Jagdwiss, *25*, 239–241
	Lymphogranulomatosis	3	Schellinger, H.P., 1982: Berl. Münch Tieraerztl. Wschr. *95*, 462–464
	Leukosis		Schulze, H., 1960: Z. f. Jagdwiss *6*, 68
	Oligodendroglioma	2	Burgisser, H., 1983: Schweiz. Arch. Tierheilk. *125*, 510–527
	Selected neoplasms		Zettel, K., Brömmel, J., 1978: Tieraerztl. Praxis *6*, 521–534
Chamois (*Rupicapra rupicapra*)	Adenoma of bile duct	1	
	Adenofibroma	2	
	Squamous cell carcinoma	2	
	Testicular cancer	2	
	Adenocarcinoma, liver		
	Scirrhous carcinoma of liver	1	Burgisser, H., 1983: Schweiz. Arch. Tierheilk. *125*, 510–527
	Carcinoma of lung	1	Burgisser, H., 1983: Schweiz. Arch. Tierheilk. *125*, 510–527
	Fibroma	3	
	Fibroma durum	1	Burgisser, H., 1983: Schweiz. Arch. Tierheilk. *125*, 510–527
	Fibrous lymphoma at angle of mandible	1	
	Fibroma, forehead	1	Burgisser, H., 1983 ....
	Fibroma, pylorus	1	Burgisser, H., 1983 ....
	Osteoid chondrosarcoma	1	
	Liver sarcoma with mixed cellularity	1	
	Lymphomatosis of liver	1	
	Osteosarcoma, forelimb	1	
	Medullary sarcoma	1	
	Spindle cell sarcoma	1	
	Lymphosarcoma, liver	1	Burgisser, H., 1983 ....
Red deer (*Cervus elaphus*)	Fibropapilloma	1	
	Papilloma	1	
	Papillomatosis	1	
	Seminoma	1	Von Braunschweig, A., 1966: Z. f. Jagdwiss. *12*, 30

Table 1. (Continued)

Species	Tumor			Steineck	Literature
	Hemangioma	+ +	+	+	Burgisser, H., 1983: Schweiz. Arch. Tierheilk. *125*, 510–527
	Lipoma	+ +	+	+	
	Fibrosarcoma	+ +	+	+	
	Reticulosarcoma, head	+			Schaal, E., H. Ernst, 1964: Z. f. Jagdw. *10*, 116–121
	Round cell sarcoma of lung	+			Zettl, K., J. Brömel, 1978: Tieraerztl. Praxis *6*, 521–534
	Selected neoplasms	+			
Fallow deer (*Dama dama*)	Fibroma molle	+ +	+	+	Kierdorf, H. et al., 1985: Z. f. Jagdwiss. *31*, 52–55
	Round-cell-sarcoma	+ +	+	+	
	Osteochondroma	+	+		Steen, M. et al., 1985: Acta vet. scand. 26:461–465
Ibex (*Capra ibex*)	Nasal tumor: malignant schwannoma, carcinoma	+	+		
	Fibroma molle	+	+	+	Burgisser, H., 1958: Rev. Pathol. Physiol. Clin. *697*, 481–496
	Various tumours	+			
European hare (*Lepus europaeus*)	Carcinoma	+	+	+	Burgisser, H., 1956:………………
	Lung adenoma	+ +		3	
	Hepatoma	+ +			
	Carcinoma of ovary	+ +			
	Osteosarcoma	+ +			Zoller, H., 1940: Dtsch. Tieraerztl. Wschr. 48, 142–145
	Osteosarcoma	+ +			
	Tumorlike leucosis	+ +			Herzog, A., 1963: Z. f. Jagdwiss. 9, 148–150
	Lymphatic leucosis	+ +			Weidlich, N., 1959: Berl. Muench. Tieraerztl. Wschr. 72, 21–24
	Lymphatic leucosis	+			Von Braunschweig, A., 1960: Z. f. Jagdwiss. 6, 67
	Generalized lymphoreticulosis	+			Von Braunschweig, A., 1961: Z. f. Jagdwiss. 7, 87
Red fox (*Vulpes vulpes*)	Lymphosarcomatosis	+ +	+		Brunk, R., 1960: Z. f. Jagdwiss. 6, 121–185
	Adenocarcinoma of lung	+	+		Burgisser, H., 1958:
	Undifferentiated carcinoma of pelvic cavity	+		2	
	Fibrosarcoma	+ +			
	Lymphatic leucosis	+ +			
Old World badger (*Meles meles*)	Hemangioma	+			Burgisser, H., 1958:………………
	Liver cell carcinoma	+ +			
	Adenocarcinoma, liver and spleen	+ +			
Martes martes (European pine marten)	Adenocarcinoma, mammary gland	+			
	Lymphatic leucosis	+			See also: Fiedler, W., 1963: Zum Vorkommen der Geschwuelste bei Wildsaeugern und Edelpelztieren. Vet. Diis. Leipzig. Joest, E., 1967: Handbuch der speziellen pathologischen Anatomie der Haustiere. Bd. 6, Verlag Paul Parey

plasms of European species are interesting in comparison with the North American ones because some species as the red deer/wapiti (*Cervus elephus*) occur in Europe, Southern Canada and most of the conterminous United States; the red fox (*Vulpes vulpes*) or the brown hare (*Lepus capensis*) have a distribution in both continents. The distribution of others such as the roe deer (*Capreolus capreolus*) the old world badger and the American badger (*Taxidea taxus*) are found either in one or the other continent. Comparative studies on the question of endemic occurrence of neoplasms are also known from other vertebrates such as fish.

The table presents the review of cases diagnosed in our institute from 1972 to 1986 of *Capreolus capreolus, Rupicapra rupicpra, Cervus elaphus, Dama dama, Capra ibex, Lepus europaeus.* * Selected neoplasms of free-ranging European species including *Vulpes vulpes, Meles meles* and *Martes martes*, described in the literature have been added.

REFERENCES

1. Appleby EC: Tumors in captive wild animals: Some observations and comparisons. *Acta Zool and Pathol*, Antverpiensia. 48:77, 1969
2. Bekoff M: Coyote. p. 454. In: Wild Mammals of North America. Chapman JA, Feldhamer GA (eds). Johns Hopkins University Press, Baltimore, 1982
3. Berry EC: Fibroma in a Virginia deer. *J Mammal* 6:130, 1925
4. Boyd RJ: Elk of the White River Plateau, Colorado. Colorado Division of Game, Fish, and Parks. Tech. Publ. No. 25. 126 pp. 1970
5. Bratberg B: Metastasizing renal adenocarcinoma in a moose. *J Wild Dis* 18:91, 1982
6. Broughton E, Miller FL, Choquette LPE: Cutaneous fibropapillomas in migratory barren-ground caribou. *J Wildl Dis* 8:138, 1972
7. Carlton WW, Dietz JM: Two renal tumors in cotton-tail rabbits (*Sylvilagus floridanus*). *Vet Pathol* 14:29, 1977
8. Chute HL, Chamberlain DM: Lymphangioma in the white-tailed deer, (*Odocoileus virginianus*). *J Mammal* 37:552, 1956
9. Cooley TM: Summary of diseases affecting Michigan wildlife 1933–1975. In: Michigan-Wildlife Disease Manual. Department of Natural Resources, East Lansing, 1975
10. Cooley TM: Summary of diseases affecting Michigan wildlife 1978. In: Michigan Wildlife Disease Manual. Department of Natural Resources, East Lansing, 1978
11. Cooley TM, Schmitt SM: Summary of diseases affecting Michigan wildlife 1981. In: Michigan Wildlife Disease Manual. Department of Natural Resources, East Lansing, 1981
12. Cooley TM, Schmitt SM: Summary of diseases affecting Michigan wildlife 1982. In: Michigan Wildlife Disease Manual. Department of Natural Resources, East Lansing, 1982
13. Cooley TM, Schmitt SM: Summary of diseases affecting Michigan wildlife 1983. In: Michigan Wildlife Disease Manual. Department of Natural Resources, East Lansing, 1983
14. Cosgrove GE, Fay LD: Viral tumors. pp. 424–428. In: Infectious Diseases of Wild Mammals. 2nd Ed. Davis JW, Karstad LH, and Trainer DO (eds). Iowa State University Press, Ames, 1981
15. Cosgrove GE, Lushbaugh WB, Humason G, Anderson MG: Synhimantus (Nematoda) associated with gastric squamous tumors in muskrats. *Bull Wildl Dis Assoc* 4:54, 1967
16. Cosgrove GE, Satterfield LC, Nettles VF: Neoplasia. pp. 62–71. In: Diseases and Parasites of White-tailed Deer. Davidson WR, Hayes FA, Nettles VF, Kellogg FE (eds). Tall Timbers Research Station, Miscellaneous Publication No. 7, Tallahassee, Florida, 1981
17. Debbie JG, Friend M: Lymphosarcoma in a white-tailed deer. *Bull Wild Dis Assoc* 3:38, 1967
18. Dieterich RA: Tumors. pp. 236–239. In: Alaskan Wildlife Diseases. Dieterich RA (ed). University of Alaska, Fairbanks, 1981
19. Diters RW, Kircher CH, Nielsen SW: Astrocytoma in a raccoon. *J Am Vet Med Assoc* 173:1152, 1978
20. Dodge WE: Porcupine. p. 363. In: Wild Mammals of North America. Chapman JA, Feldhamer GA (eds). Johns Hopkins University Press, Baltimore, 1982
21. Doutt JK, Donaldson IC: An antlered doe with possible masculinizing tumor. *J Mammal* 40:230, 1959
22. Drake CH: Mistaken diagnosis of actinomycosis for osteogenic sarcoma in an American elk (*Cervus canadensis*). *J Wildl Manage* 15:284, 1951
23. Effron M, Griner L, Benirschke K: Nature and rate of neoplasia found in captive wild mammals, birds and reptiles at necropsy. *J Natl Cancer Inst* 59:185, 1977
24. Elvestad K, Henriques UV, Kroustrup JP: Insulin-producing islet cell tumor in an ectopic pancreas of a red fox (*Vulpes vulpes*). *J Wildl Dis* 20:70, 1984
25. Elwell MR, Burger GT, Moe JB, White JD, Stookey JL: Fibrosarcoma in a white-tailed deer. *J Wildl Dis* 13:297, 1977
26. Fay LD: Neoplastic diseases of white-tailed deer. pp. 132–137. In: Proc. of the First Natl. White-tailed Deer Dis. Symp. University of Georgia, Athens, 1962
27. Fay LD: Skin tumors of Cervidae. pp. 385–392. In: Infectious Diseases of Wild Mammals. Davis JW, Karstad LH, Trainer DO (eds). Iowa State University Press, Ames, 1970
28. Foreyt WJ, Leathers CW: Starvation secondary to an oral fibroma in a wild mountain goat (*Oreamnos americanus*). *J Wildl Dis* 21:184, 1985
29. Friend M: Skin tumors in New York deer. *Bull Wildl Dis Assoc* 3:102, 1967
30. Gardner AL: Virginia Opossum. p. 29. In: Wild Mammals of North America. Chapman JA, Feldhamer GA (eds). Johns Hopkins University Press, Baltimore, 1982
31. Garner FM, Schwartz LW: Spontaneous hematopoietic neoplasms of free-living and captive wild mammals. *Natl Cancer Inst Monogr* 32:153, 1969
32. Griner LA: Pathology of Zoo Animals. Zoological Society of San Diego. 608 pp, 1983
33. Habermann RT, Williams FP, Eyestone WH: Spontaneous hepatomas in two woodchucks and a carcinoma of the testis in a badger. *J Am Vet Med Assoc* 125:295, 1954
34. Hagen KW: Papillomatosis in rabbits. *Bull Wildl Dis Assoc* 2:108, 1966
35. Herman CM, Bischoff AI: Papilloma, skin tumors in deer. *California Fish and Game* 36:19, 1950
36. Herman CM, Kilham L, Warbach O: Incidence of Shope's rabbit fibroma in cotton-tails at the Patuxent Research Refuge. *J Wildl Manage* 20:85, 1956
37. Hirth RS, Wyand DS, Osborne AD, Burke CN: Epidermal changes caused by squirrel pox virus. *J Am Vet Med Assoc* 155:1120, 1969
38. Holscher MA, Page DL, Netsky MG, Powell HS: Mixed glioma and rhabdomyosarcoma in brain of a wild deer. *Vet Pathol* 14:643, 1977
39. Honess RF: A freak deer head. *J Wildl Manage* 3:360, 1939

---

* *Lepus europaeus* is now more or less constant included into the species *Lepus capensis*, the brown hare inhabiting the entire Palearctic region south of the corniferous forest zone (with exception of China and Japan), all nonforested parts of Africa. (Nowak RM, Paradiso JL: (eds) *Walker's Mammals of the World*. 4th edition Baltimore and London: The Johns Hopkins University Press, 1983, p. 488, Vol. 1.

224   *Elizabeth S. Williams* et al.

40. Honess RF, Winter KB: Diseases of Wildlife in Wyoming. *Wyoming Game and Fish Comm Bull* 9:1, 1956
41. Hoover EE: Neurofibromatosis in white-tailed deer. *J Mammal* 18:104, 1937
42. Howard DR, Krehbiel JD, Fay LD, Stuht JN, Whitenack DL: Visual defects in white-tailed deer from Michigan. Six case reports. *J Wildl Dis* 12:143, 1976
43. Kidd JG, Rouse P: Cancers deriving from the virus papillomas of wild rabbits under natural conditions. *J Exp Med* 71:469, 1940
44. Kilham L, Herman CM, Fisher ER: Naturally occurring fibroma of gray squirrels related to Shope's fibroma. *Proc Soc Exp Biol Med* 82:298, 1953
45. King JM, Woolf A, Shively JN: Naturally occurring squirrel fibroma with involvement of internal organs. *J Wildl Dis* 8:321, 1972
46. Kistner TP, Hayes FA: Sarcoma in an aged white-tailed deer. *J Wildl Manage* 35:850, 1971
47. Koller LD, Olson C: Pulmonary fibroblastomas in a deer with cutaneous fibromatosis. *Cancer Research* 31:1373, 1971
48. Kradel DC, Dunne HW: Diseases of the brain and spinal cord observed in Pennsylvania deer and other wildlife. Proc. Northeast Wildl. Conf., Hartford, Conn. Mimeo. 7 pp. Cited by Cosgrove et al. 1981
49. Kradel DC, Dunne HW: Brain tumors (ependymomas) in deer. *J Am Vet Med Assoc* 147:1096, 1965
50. Lancaster WD, Sundberg JP: Characterization of papillomaviruses isolated from cutaneous fibromas of white-tailed deer and mule deer. *Virol* 123:212, 1982
51. Lopushinsky T, Fay LD: Some benign and malignant neoplasms of Michigan cotton-tail rabbits. *Bull Wildl Dis Assoc* 3:148, 1967
52. Montali RJ: An overview of tumors in zoo animals. pp. 531–547. In: The Comparative Pathology of Zoo Animals. Montali RJ, Migaki G (eds). Smithsonian Institution Press, Washington, D.C, 1979
53. Moreno-Lopez J, Pettersson V, Dinter Z, Philipson L: Characterization of a papilloma virus from the European elk (EEPV). *Virol* 112:589, 1981
54. Moulton JE: Tumors in Domestic Animals. University of California Press, Los Angeles. 279 pp, 1961
55. Moulton JE: Tumors in Domestic Animals. 2nd Ed. University of California Press, Berkeley. 465 pp, 1978
56. Nettles VF, Vandeveld M: Thalamic ependymoma in a white-tailed deer. *Vet Pathol* 15:133, 1978
57. O'Connor DJ, Kiters RW, Nielsen WS: Poxvirus and multiple tumors in an eastern gray squirrel. *J Am Vet Med Assoc* 177:792, 1980
58. Pelton MR: Black bear. p. 511. In: Wild Mammals of North America. Chapman JA, Feldhamer GA (eds). Johns Hopkins University Press, Baltimore, 1982
59. Pence DB, Tran RM, Biship ML, Foster SA: Fibroma in a nine-banded armadillo (*Dasypus novemcintus*). *J Comp Pathol* 93:179, 1983
60. Placke ME, Roscoe DE, Wyand DS, Nielsen SW: Hepatocellular adenocarcinoma in a white-tailed deer (*Odocoileus virginianus*). *Can J Comp Med* 46:198, 1982
61. Pocock RI: p. 301. Antlers of a Virginia deer affected by cancer. *Proc Zool Soc London*, 1915
62. Regnery RL: Preliminary studies on an unusual poxvirus of the western gray squirrel (*Sciurus griseus griseus*) of North America. *Intervirology* 5:354, 1975
63. Reynolds HW, Glaholt RD, Hawley AW: Bison. p. 994. In: Wild Mammals of North America. Chapman JA, Feldhamer GA (eds). Johns Hopkins University Press, Baltimore, 1982
64. Roher DP, Nielsen SW: Lymphosarcoma in a raccoon, *Procyon lotor* (L.). *J Wildl Dis* 20:156, 1984
65. Roher DP, Nielsen SW, Stone WB: Carcinoma in the urinary bladder of a white-tailed deer (*Odocoileus virginianus*). *J Wildl Dis* 18:361, 1982

66. Samuel WM, Chalmers GA, Gunson JR: Oral papillomatosis in coyotes (*Canis latrans*) and wolves (*Canis lupus*) of Alberta. *J Wildl Dis* 14L165m 1978
67. Seefeldt S, Helfer D: Seminoma in an elk (*Cervus canadensis*). *Vet Pathol* 17:248, 1980
68. Sherwood BF, Rowlands DT Jr, Hackel DB: Pulmonary adenomatosis in opossums (*Didelphis virginiana*). *J Am Vet Med Assoc* 155:1102–1107, 1969
69. Shivaprasad HL, Sundberg JP, Ely R: Malignant mixed (carcinosarcoma) mammary tumor in a gray squirrel. *Vet Pathol* 21:115, 1984
70. Shope RE: A transmissible tumor-like condition in rabbits. *J Exp Med* 56:793, 1932
71. Shope RE, Mangold R, MacNamara LG, Dumbell KR: An infectious cutaneous fibroma of the Virginia white-tailed deer (*Odocoileus virginianus*). *J Exp Med* 108:797, 1958
72. Skoog RO: Ecology of the caribou (*Rangifer tarandus granti*) in Alaska. Ph.D. Thesis. University of California, Berkely. 699 pp. (Cited by Miller FL 1982. Caribou (*Rangifer tarandus*). In: Wild Mammals of North America. Chapman JA, Feldhamer GA (eds). Johns Hopkins University Press, Baltimore.), 1968
73. Smith DA, Barker IK: Four cases of Hodgkin's Disease in striped skunks (*Mephitis mephitis*). *Vet Pathol* 20:223, 1983
74. Snyder RL: Longevity and disease patterns in captive and wild woodchucks. *Am Assoc Zool Parks and Aquariums*, Regional Workshop Proceedings 1977–78, Wheeling, West Virginia, 1977
75. Snyder RL, Ratcliffe HL: *Marmota monax*: A model for studies of cardiovascular, cerebrovascular and neoplastic disease. *Acta Zool and Pathol Antverpiensia* 48:265, 1969
76. Snyder SP, Davies RB, Keiss RE: Myxosarcoma in a wapiti. *J Wildl Dis* 15:307, 1979
77. Snyder SP, Davies RB, Spraker TR, Browning H: Embryonal nephroma in a wapiti. *J Wildl Dis* 15:303, 1979
78. Snyder SP, Davies RB, Stevens D: Brain tumors in two free-ranging elk in Colorado. *J Wildl Dis* 17:101, 1981
79. Stroud RK, Amundson TE: Squamous cell carcinoma in a free-ranging white-tailed deer (*Odocoileus virginianus*). *J Wildl Dis* 19:162 1983
80. Sundberg JP, Morris K, Lancaster WD: Cutaneous fibromas of moose (*Alces alces*). *J Wildl Dis* 21:181, 1985
81. Sundberg JP, Nielsen SW: Deer fibroma: A review. *Can Vet J* 22:385, 1981
82. Sundberg JP, Nielsen SW: Prevalence of cutaneous fibromas in white-tailed deer (*Odocoileus virginianus*) in New York and Vermont. *J Wildl Dis* 18:359, 1982
83. Sundberg JP, Williams ES, Hill D, Lancaster WD, Nielsen SW: Detection of papillomaviruses in cutaneous fibromas of white-tailed deer and mule deer. *Am J Vet Res* 46:1145, 1985
84. Sundberg JP, Williams E, Thorne ET, Lancaster WD: Cutaneous fibropapilloma in a pronghorn antelope. *J Am Vet Med Assoc* 183:1333, 1983
85. Szczech GM, Carlton WW, Hinsman EJ, Jacobsen JJ: Fibroma in Indiana cotton-tail rabbits. *J Am Vet Med Assoc* 165:846, 1974
86. Tajima M, Gordon DE, Olson C: Electron microscopy of bovine papilloma and deer fibroma viruses. *Am J Vet Res* 29:1185, 1968
87. Trainer DO, Knowlton FF: Karstad L: Oral papillomatosis in the coyote. *Bull Wildl Dis Assoc* 4:52, 1968
88. Tyler GV, Summers JW, Snyder RL: Woodchuck hepatitis virus in natural woodchuck population. *J Wildl Dis* 17:297, 1981
89. Wadsworth JR: Fibrosarcomas in a deer. *J Am Vet Med Assoc* 124:194, 1954
90. Williams ES: Neoplasias (tumors). pp. 261–274. In: Diseases of Wildlife in Wyoming. 2nd Ed. Thorne ET, Kingston N, Jolley WR, Bergstrom R (eds). Wyoming Game and Fish Dept., Cheyenne, 1982

91. Witter JF: Annual reports of animal disease diagnostic laboratory, University of Maine, Orono, Maine. (Cited by Chute and Chamberlain, 1956.), 1935–1954

92. Yuill TM: Myxomatosis and fibromatosis. pp. 154–177. In: Infectious Diseases of Wild Mammals. 2nd Ed. Davis JW, Karstad LH, Trainer DO (eds). Iowa State University Press, Ames, 1981

93. Yuill TM, Hanson RP: Infection of suckling cotton-tail rabbits with Shope's fibroma virus. *Proc Soc Exp Biol Med* 117:376, 1964

POLYNUCLEAR AROMATIC HYDROCARBON RESIDUES IN SHELLFISH: SPECIES VARIATIONS AND APPARENT INTRASPECIFIC DIFFERENCES

MICHAEL E. BENDER and ROBERT J. HUGGETT

INTRODUCTION

Concern over the occurrence of polynuclear aromatic hydrocarbons residues (PAHs) in marine animals originates from two areas. The first relate to the potential effects of these substances on the biota, and the second arises from the transfer of the residues to higher animals, e.g., man. Several authors including: Malins and Hodgins (12), Mix (13), Hargis and Roberts (5), and Huggett et al. (7), have implicated PAHs as being the causative factors in various diseases and/or abnormalities of marine animals. Howard and Fazio (6) reviewed the occurrence of PAHs in a variety of foods and Neff (14) summarized the information on PAHs in aquatic environments. However, Neff observed in 1979, that "comparatively little information is available concerning the presence of PAHs other than BaP [benzo(a)pyrene] or concerning the PAH homolog distribution in tissues of aquatic organisms". This paper provides updated information on these subjects from the recent literature and through original observations.

The methods section attempts to describe some of the difficulties in comparing results derived using different methodologies. The values presented are those reported (modified only by conversion from wet to dry weight): they must be evaluated in light of their consistency with the literature reports. We have excluded from this paper studies which include only values for total PAHs and/or BaP.

Methods

Detailed accounts of the chemical methodologies utilized to determine PAH residues in the studies discussed in this chapter can be found in the original references cited. None of the studies cited utilized identical methods and frequently differed in means of extraction, clean-up, quantification and compound identification. Results were also quantified differently, i.e., either on a wet or dry weight basis. In this paper we have converted wet-weights to dry-weights by assuming an 80% moisture content. Variations in percent moisture content of shellfish occur both between species and within species and seasonally. However, an 80% water content is a reasonable average approximation based on our experience.

Compound separations were usually made by gas chromatography or high pressure liquid chromatography preceded by one or more clean-up steps to remove biogenic and aliphatic compounds. Quantification was normally accomplished with the use of internal standards, however, some studies reported results uncorrected for recovery.

Compound identifications were made by retention time comparisons with authentic standards, relative retention indices, mass spectral identifications and combinations of these methods.

A detailed account of the methods utilized for the original data reported here can be found in Beri et al. (1) and Huggett et al. (7). Briefly, they include: Soxhlet extraction with methylene chloride; gel permeation chromatographic clean-up (GPC); high pressure liquid chromatographic fractionation; compound separation by glass capillary chromatography; quantification relative to an internal standard by GC/FID; tentative compound identification by relative retention indices with mass spectral confirmation on selected samples.

The river systems sampled in Virginia for PAH residues in oysters (*Crassostrea virginica*) and brackish water clams (*Rangia cuneata*) are shown in Figure 1. Sample collections were made in the fall of 1984 in the James, York and Rappahannock rivers. Two composite samples of between 4–8 animals each were collected at various stations along these estuaries.

The Elizabeth River study was conducted during the fall of 1983. In this field experiment oysters were collected from two locations, one in the Rappahannock River (~35 km) from the mouth and at Hospital Point in the Elizabeth River (Figure 1). Oysters from both locations were transplanted to a station in the Elizabeth which had been shown to be heavily contaminated with PAHs (7). The oysters were suspended in cages about 0.3 meters from the bottom and composite samples were collected for PAH analysis at intervals of 2, 4 and 9 weeks. Prior to analysis the oysters were depurated for 24 hours in the York River. PAH residues were also determined at the beginning of the experiment on both groups of oysters. Lipid levels in these oysters were estimated gravimetrically on a portion of the methylene chloride extract before GPC clean-up.

Results and discussion

Tables 1, 2 and 3 present residue data, summarized from the recent literature and through original observations, on selected PAH compounds in oysters, mussels and clams, respectively. In most cases the values represent means of several

H. E. Kaiser (ed.), Comparative aspects of tumor development.

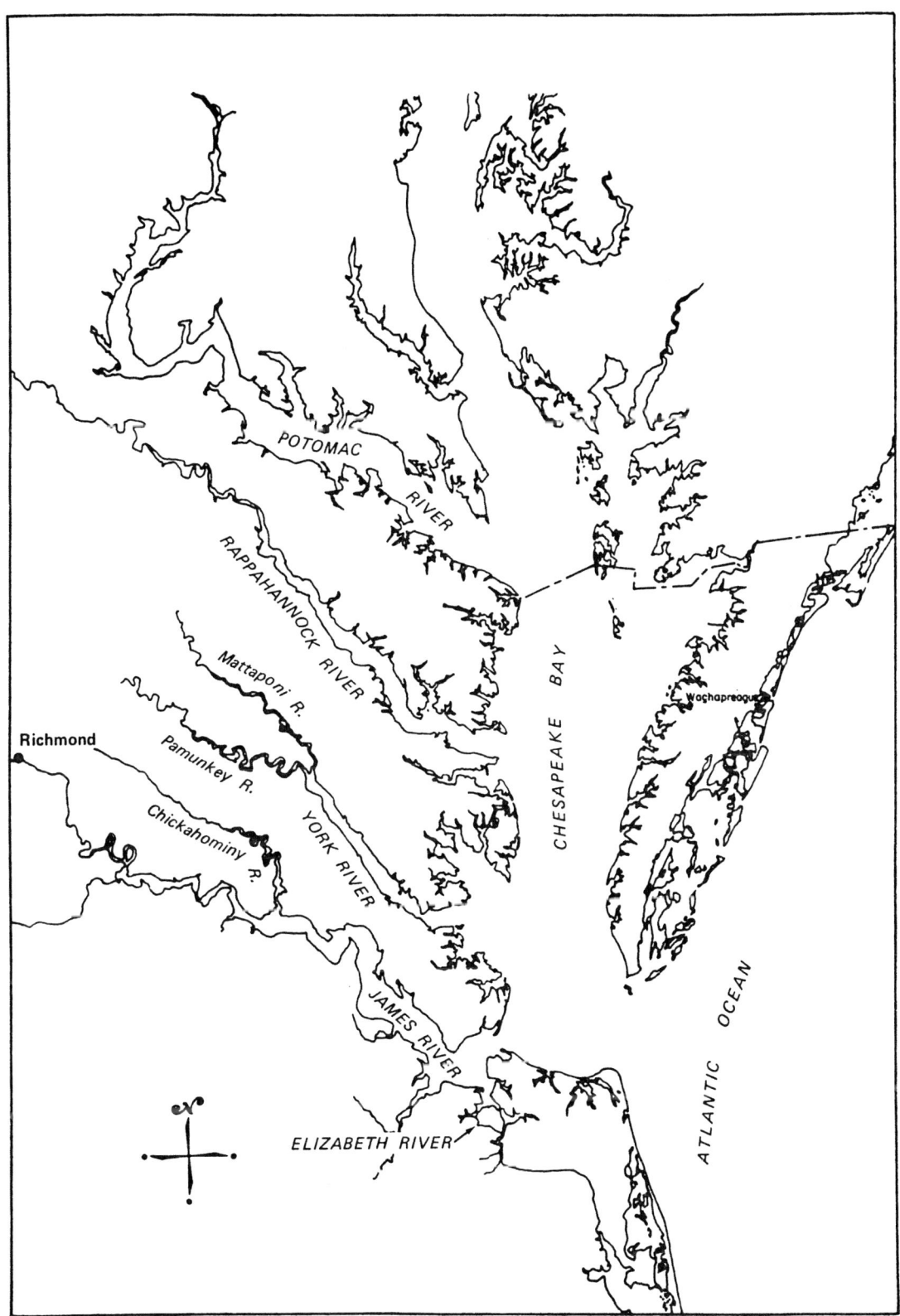

Figure 1. Lower Chesapeake Bay.

Table 1. PAH residues in oysters ng/g (dry wt.).

	Elizabeth River, VA	James River, VA	York River, VA	Rappahannock River, VA	Yaquina Bay, OR (1)	Biloxi, MS (2)	Mobile Bay, AL (3)	Cedar Key, FL (3)	Aransas Bay, TX (4)	Galveston Bay, TX-approved (4)	Galveston Bay, TX-closed (4)
Naphthalene	5	30	48	8	NR	9	170	176	NR	NR	NR
Subst. Naphthalenes	40	445	255	180	NR	103	85	105	NR	NR	NR
Phenanthrene	45	1	<1	<1	31	60	285	290	NR	NR	11
Subst. Phenanthrenes	690	20	60	<1	NR	464	NR	NR	NR	NR	NR
Anthracene	40	20	<1	<1	NR	NR	3	16	NR	NR	NR
Fluoranthene	450	15	20	<1	29	60	71	23	9	15	39
Pyrene	645	16	10	<1	19	90	41	31	5	9	33
Subst. Pyrene/Fluoranthene	295	10	6	<1	NR	NR	NR	NR	NR	NR	NR
Benzo(c)phenanthrene	70	<1	<1	<1	22	NR	NR	NR	NR	NR	NR
Benz(a)anthracene	135	<1	<1	<1	25	NR	2	ND	NR	NR	NR
Chrysene/Triphenylene	438	10	<1	<1	32	NR	3	13	3	1	3
Benzo(j,b,k)fluoranthene	850	<1	<1	<1	12[a]	NR	7[a]	ND	2	7	13
Benzo(e)pyrene	453	<1	<1	<1	NR	NR	NR	NR	1	6	10
Benzo(a)pyrene	285	108	75	50	7	NR	ND	ND	ND	ND	ND
Perylene	130	<1	<1	<1	NR	NR	NR	NR	ND	4	1
Dibenzo(a,h)anthracene	<4	20	<1	<1	2	NR	NR	NR	NR	NR	NR
Benzo(g,h,i)perylene	73	<1	<1	<1	2	NR	7	8	NR	NR	NR

[a] b+k (only), NR-not reported

References: (1) Mix, 1984; (2) Farrington, 1980, (3) Settine, et al., 1983; and (4) Fazio, 1971.

Notes: Elizabeth River x̄ of 2 samples from 1 station; James River x̄ of 2 samples from 5 stations; York River x̄ of 2 samples from 3 stations; Rappahannock River x̄ of 2 samples from 4 stations; Yaquina Bay x̄ of 14 samples taken over time from 1 station; Biloxi, 1 sample; Mobile Bay x̄ of 18 samples taken over time from 6 stations; Cedar Key x̄ of 6 samples over time from 2 stations; Aranas Bay x̄ of 2 samples; Galveston Bay approved areas x̄ of 13 samples; closed areas x̄ of 5 samples.

samples and include all specific compound data reported in the original source. Detailed information on the number of samples, etc., is shown in foot-notes to each table.

Generally the highest residues observed in oysters were for the lower molecular weight compounds, e.g. the substituted naphthalenes and phenanthrenes. Levels of the carcinogen BaP ranged between 285 ng/g in residues from the Elizabeth River to non-detectable at several other locations. The data tabulated in Table 1 also indicate that the more heavily urbanized and/or industrialized areas were more contaminated. A similar situation is shown in mussel residues (Table 2), i.e. generally higher concentrations of the lower molecular weight compounds and higher levels where anthropogenic sources are indicated. BaP residues ranged from non-detectable at several locations to ~ 500 ng/g at industrialized sites along the coast of Scotland. Concentrations of fluoranthene and pyrene also appeared to be quite high at some sites along the coasts of Scotland and Norway. Although only limited data are available on clams (Table 3) similar trends are indicated, i.e. higher residues at urbanized

stations and of compounds in the lower molecular weight range.

Table 4 compares residues found in various species of shellfish collected from either the same station or from adjacent stations, usually within 2–8 kilometers. Along the Norwegian coast mussels, *M. edulis*, had considerably higher residues than the snail, *L. littorea* or the limpet, *P. vulgate* and limpets showed higher concentrations than snails. In Tillamook Bay, Oregon mussels (*M. edulis*), clams (*M. arenaria*) and oysters (*C. gigas*) all contained similar residues generally differing by no more than a factor of 2. Comparisons between the brackish water clam (*R. cuneata*) and the Eastern oyster (*C. virginica*) from two Virginia estuaries indicate some differences between these species for specific compounds. Oysters contained somewhat higher levels of naphthalene and substituted naphthalenes than the clams, while the reverse was indicated for phenanthrene and substituted phenanthrenes. Residues for the other compounds usually differed by no more than a factor of 2 or 3.

Mussels collected from Wachapreague, on the Eastern

Table 2. PAH residues in mussels ng/g (dry wt.).

	Narragansett Bay, RI (2)	Boston Harbor, MA (2)	Tillamook Bay, OR (1)	Yaquina Bay, OR (1)	Thermaikos Gulf, Greece (3)	Norway-clean (4)	Norway-polluted (4)	Scottish Coast-clean (5)	Scottish coast-urban (5)	Scottish Coast-Industrial (5)	Gdansk Bay (6)	Slupsk-Bank (6)
Naphthalene	10	4	NR	NR	NR	ND	ND	19	91	18	56	75
Subst. Naphthalenes	21	209	NR	NR	NR	63[a]	234[a]	172	129	453	452	190
Phenanthrene	23	87	70	535	45	175	545	75	88	968	86	67
Subst. Phenanthrenes	88	2022	NR	NR	NR	363[b]	1290[b]	95[c]	82[c]	566[c]	790	110
Anthracene	NR	NR	NR	NR	NR	NR	NR	NR	NR	NR	6	5
Fluoranthene	81	239	47	235	35	180	1927	67	230	1082	370	88
Pyrene	59	327	37	125	20	77	1150	34	219	998	240	38
Subst. Pyrene/fluoranthene	NR	NR	NR	NR	NR	NR	NR	NR	NR	NR	140	27
Benzo(c)phenanthrene	NR	NR	24	130	NR	NR	NR	NR	NR	NR	NR	NR
Benz(a)anthracene	NR	NR	12	150	15	57	165	78[d]	352[d]	1357[d]	NR	NR
Chrysene/triphenylene	NR	NR	35	135	65	222	615	NR	NR	NR	NR	NR
Benzo(j,b,k)fluoranthene	NR	NR	10	20	NR	67	190	NR	NR	NR	NR	NR
Benzo(e)pyrene	NR	NR	NR	NR	NR	71	188	NR	NR	NR	NR	NR
Benzo(a)pyrene	NR	NR	2	6	5	11	47	32	192	506	NR	NR
Perylene	NR	NR	NR	NR	40	NR	NR	NR	NR	NR	NR	NR
Dibenz(a,h)anthracene	NR	NR	1	10	10	NR	NR	NR	NR	NR	NR	NR
Benzo(g,h,i)perylene	NR	NR	1	2	20	11	29	NR	NR	NR	NR	NR

[a] Naphthalene and substituted naphthalenes combined
[b] Includes subst. anthracenes
[c] Includes methyl anthracenes
[d] Includes benzo phenanthrenes
NR-not reported

References: (1) Mix, 1984; (2) Farrington, 1980; (3) Iosifidou, et al., 1982; (4) Knutzen & Shortland, 1982; (5) Mackie, et al., 1980; and (6) Law & Andrulewicz, 1983.

Notes: Narragansett and Boston one sample each; Tillamook Bay x̄ of 2 samples; Yaquina Bay x̄ of 16 samples taken over time from 1 station; Thermakos Gulf x̄ of 57 samples from 2 areas; Norway-clean sites x̄ of 6 samples from 6 sites; Norway-polluted sites x̄ of 3 samples from 3 stations; Scottish coast-clean sites, x̄ of 7 samples from 7 sites; Scottish coast-urban x̄ of 12 samples from 12 sites; Scottish coast-industrialized x̄ of 6 samples from 6 sites; Baltic Sea- Gdansk Bay-1 sample, Slupsk Bank-2 samples.

Shore of Virginia, contained residues about 3 times higher than those in oysters from the same area (Figure 1).

In general, it appears that while residue levels in mussels, oysters and clams collected from the same area differ slightly, they are usually within a factor of 2 or 3. More data contrasting residues in various shellfish species collected from the same station and/or from laboratory exposures would be very helpful in clarifying species variations. A better knowledge of these between species variations would be particularly valuable in estuarine monitoring where different species must be used as one progresses along the salinity gradient.

However, the utility of shellfish for monitoring PAHs in estuaries is demonstrated in Figures 2 and 3. These figures compare residues in oysters and brackish water clams from the James River in Virginia, beginning near its mouth and progressing upstream to near Hopewell. Figure 2 shows the concentrations of total resolved aromatics and the unresolved complex mixture in oysters and clams along the estuary and at one station on an undeveloped tributary river, the Chickahominy. Residues of total aromatics in oysters declined with increasing distance from the river mouth, while residues in clams, although generally higher than oysters, showed no distinct trends with distances. Residues in clams collected from the Chickahominy were considerably lower than those from the James River stations. Concentrations of hydrocarbons in the unresolved envelopes (mixtures of degraded aromatic hydrocarbons) are also shown in Figure 2, clams evidenced much higher UCMs than did oysters in the James. Substantial increases in the UCM were observed in clams collected near the turbidity maximum zone in the estuary. Clams collected from the Rappahannock River, a fairly pristine environment, showed no evidence of a UCM. This observation and the relatively

Table 3. PAH residues in clams ng/g (dry wt.).

	York River, VA, *M. mercenaria*	York River System, VA, *R. cuneata*	James River, VA, *R. cuneata*	Rappahannock River, VA, *R. cuneata*	Coos Bay, Oregon (1), *M. arenaria* (1) Site 3	Coos Bay, Oregon (1), *M. arenaria* (1) Site BF
Naphthalene	2	<1	5	10	NR	NR
C1-Naphthalene	2	17	11	10	NR	NR
C2-Naphthalene	3	60	108	21	NR	NR
C3-Naphthalene	<1	125	196	45	NR	NR
Phenanthrene	18	<1	15	<1	60	775
C1-phenanthrene	13	80	60	<1	NR	NR
C2-phenanthrene	5	130	50	<1	NR	NR
Fluoranthene	17	Int.	52	<1	53	550
Pyrene	23	165	45	17	32	308
Benzo(c)phenanthrene	<1	<1	9	<1	15	275
Benz(a)anthracene	<1	5	6	<1	25	208
Chrysene/triphenylene	9	60	228	16	75	275
Benzofluoranthene	18	<1	34	<1	12	90
Benzo(a)pyrene	<1	140	168	30	7	44
Perylene	36	10	6	<1	NR	NR
Benzo(g,h,i)perylene	3	10	<1	<1	2	21

NR - Not reported
Int. - Interference

References: (1) Mix, 1984.

Notes: York River (M. mercenaria) $\bar{x}$ of 4 replicates each from 4 stations;
York River (R. cuneata) $\bar{x}$ of 5 samples from 5 sites; James River $\bar{x}$ of
2 replicates from each of 5 sites; Rappahannock River $\bar{x}$ of 2
replicates from 1 station; Coos Bay (Site 3) $\bar{x}$ of 6 samples taken over
time from 1 location; Coos Bay (Site BF) $\bar{x}$ of 6 samples taken over
time from 1 location.

served in the Chickahominy samples, suggest anthropogenic origins for the envelopes.

Residues of hydrochrysenes (Figure 3), natural products believed to be derived mainly from terrestrial plant tissues, were relatively constant in clams from the most upstream stations but decreased dramatically in the turbidity maximum zone, declining to still lower levels in oysters. Concentrations in clams from the Chickahominy were considerably below those found in the upper James but approximated the residues in clams from the lower river. These data suggest an upstream source with decreasing residues as dilution with sea water occurs in the estuarine segment of the estuary.

The residues of dibenzofurans found in these animals, also shown in Figure 3, are almost a mirror image of the data on hydrochrysenes. Levels were substantially higher and relatively constant in oysters and then decreased dra-

matically in clams as the sampling progressed upstream, indicating a downstream source for the dibenzofurans.

Intraspecific differences

Figure 4, shows the change in residues as a function of time, for total resolved aromatics and the UCM in two groups of oysters transplanted to a polluted station in the Elizabeth River, Virginia. While, Figure 5 shows the residue data in these oysters for benz(a)anthracene and benzo(a)pyrene. As can be seen in the Figure 4 the Rappahannock transplants attained residues of total aromatics about 2 times higher than the oysters from the Elizabeth River which were transplanted upstream to a more polluted station. Figure 5 demonstrates that the behavior of individual compounds va-

Table 4. PAH ratios vs species.

	M. edulis/L. littorea (1)	M. edulis/P. vulgata (1)	P. vulgata/L. littorea (1)	M. edulis/M. arenaria (2)	M. edulis/C. gigas (2)	R. cuneata/C. virginica	R. cuneata/C. virginica York River, VA	M. edulis/C. virginica Wachapreague, VA (3)
Naphthalene	ND	ND	ND	NR	NR	0.3	0.2	2.7
Subst. Naphthalenes	0.8[a]	ND[a]	ND[a]	NR	NR	0.6	0.5	2.0
Phenanthrene	1.3	14.4	4.1	1.2	1.8	7.5	>10	3.1
Subst. Phenanthrenes	1.6	31.2	7.2	NR	NR	6.0	4.0	3.0
Fluoranthene	2.5	8.8	5.7	1.2	1.5	1.0	IF	4.6
Pyrene	2.8	14.6	7.7	1.3	2.0	2.0	IF	3.0
Benz(a)anthracene	5.6	6.0	3.1	1.3	1.0	2.0	2.3	NR
Chrysene/Triphenylene	6.3	17.7	3.7	1.2	0.9	4.0	IF	NR
Benzo(j,b,k)fluoranthene	5.7	>200	1.1	1.8	0.8	ND	ND	NR
Benzo(e)pyrene	6.0	>100	>300	NR	NR	ND	ND	NR
Benzo(a)pyrene	6.2	>20	0.6	0.6	0.3	3.0	1.2	NR

[a]Naphthalene + methyl naphthalenes

NR - not reported
ND - not detected
IF - interfering peak

References: (1) Knutzen & Shortland, 1982; (2) Mix, 1984; and (3) Farrington, 1980.

Notes: M. Edulis/L. littorea - x̄ of 3 stations-Norway
M. edulis/P. vulgata - Station 11-Norway
P. vulgata/L. littorea - Station 9-Norway
M. edulis/M. arenaria & C. Gigas - Tillamook Bay, OR
M. edulis/C. virginica - Wachapreague, VA

ried. Benz(a)anthracene residues increased in both groups of oysters after transplantation and then remained relatively constant after 2 weeks of exposure. Concentrations of benzo(a)pyrene peaked 2 weeks after transplantation and then declined in both groups of oysters.

Approximately 50 different PAH compounds were identified in this field exposure study. During the data analysis we observed that the differences in residue levels, between the Rappahannock and Elizabeth River oysters were not constant, i.e. for all of the various compounds measured. Figure 6 shows the ratios of the residues found in Rappahannock River oysters to those detected in Elizabeth River oysters, as a function of the molecular weight of the compounds. Plots for the individual sampling dates, i.e. the 2, 4 and 9 week exposure periods, were similar. As can be observed in the figure, the Rappahannock River oysters had higher residues of the lower molecular weight compounds than did the Elizabeth River oysters. One possible explanation for this observation is that the Elizabeth River residents have enzymatic systems capable of metabolizing and eliminating the lower molecular weight compounds more rapidly

than the oyster populations transplanted from the "pristine" Rappahannock River. Another possibility is that variations in lipid levels might influence the body burdens for these compounds. Other investigators, e.g., Stegeman and Teal (16) and Burns and Smith (2) have advanced the hypothesis that lipid levels are important in determining the absolute residue levels for slightly water soluble organic compounds. However, to our knowledge no one has suggested that lipid variations, i.e. in animals, are responsible for compound specific variations in residues. Figure 7 displays the change in "lipid" levels for the two transplanted populations over a nine week period.

ACKNOWLEDGEMENTS

The authors wish to thank Slone HD, Greene JR, Hunt DB, Vadas G and deFur PO for technical assistance and Howard P for manuscript preparation. Financial support for this study was provided in part by the State Water Control Board of the Commonwealth of Virginia. VIMS contribution No 1286.

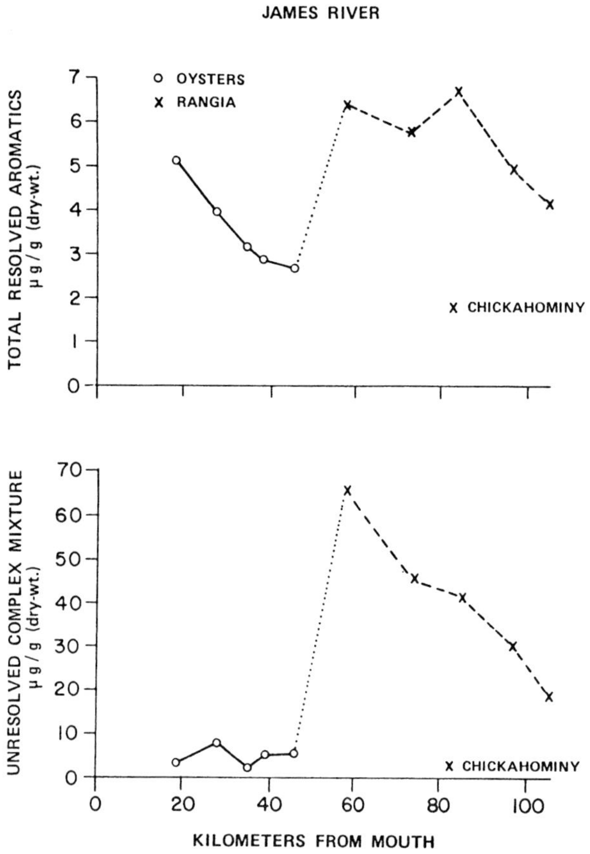

JAMES RIVER

TOTAL RESOLVED AROMATICS μg/g (dry-wt.)

○ OYSTERS
✕ RANGIA

✕ CHICKAHOMINY

UNRESOLVED COMPLEX MIXTURE μg/g (dry-wt.)

✕ CHICKAHOMINY

KILOMETERS FROM MOUTH

Figure 2. James River-Oysters and Rangia-total resolved aromatics and UCM.

JAMES RIVER

HYDROCHRYSENES (μg/g)

○ OYSTERS
✕ RANGIA

✕ CHICKAHOMINY

DIBENZOFURANS (ng/g)

KILOMETERS FROM MOUTH

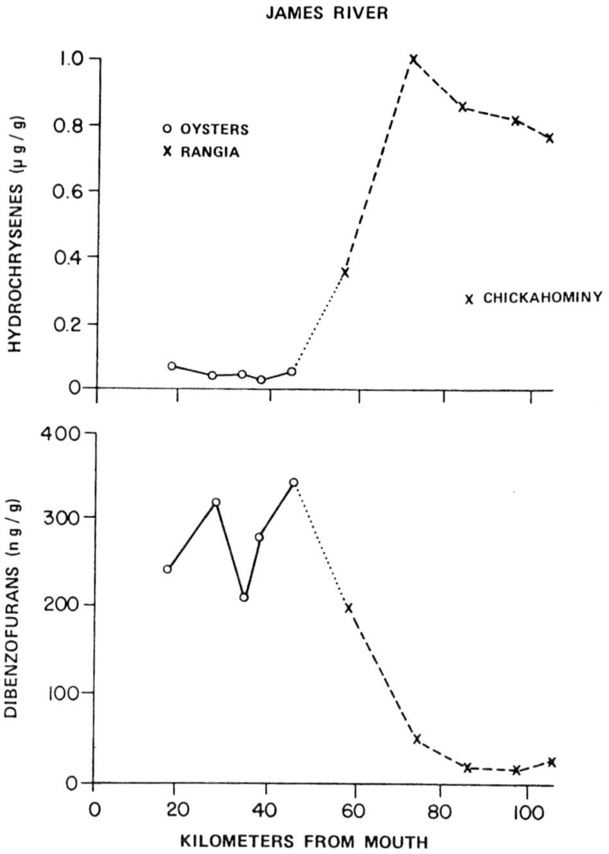

Figure 3. James River-Oysters and Rangia-hydrochrysenes and dibenzofurans.

○ RAPPAHANNOCK TRANSPLANTS
● ELIZABETH TRANSPLANTS

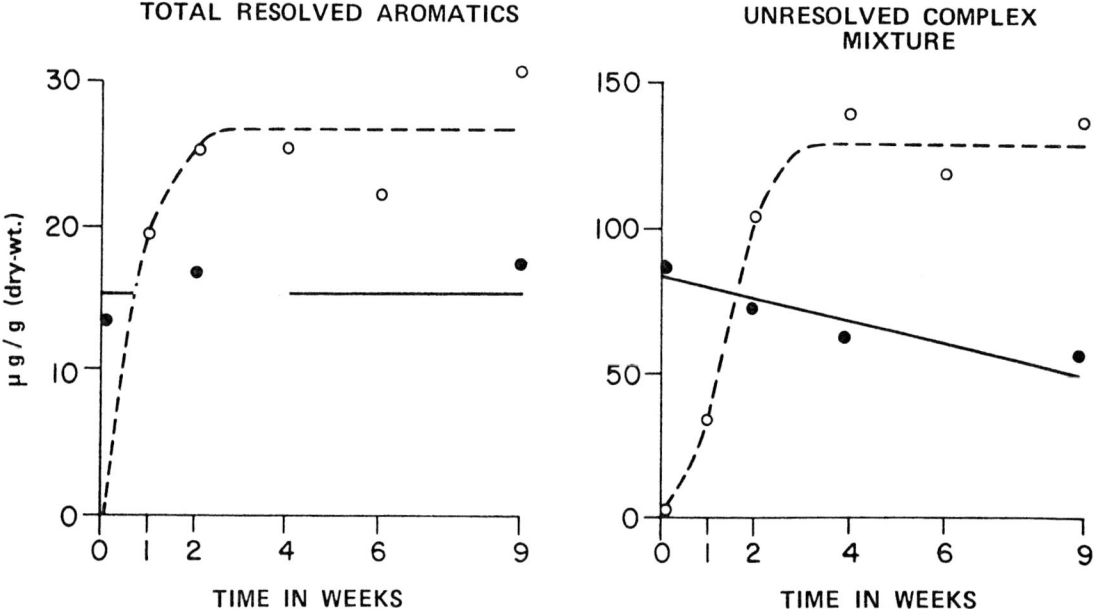

TOTAL RESOLVED AROMATICS

μg/g (dry-wt.)

TIME IN WEEKS

UNRESOLVED COMPLEX MIXTURE

TIME IN WEEKS

Figure 4. Transplant study-Elizabeth River-total resolved aromatics and UCM.

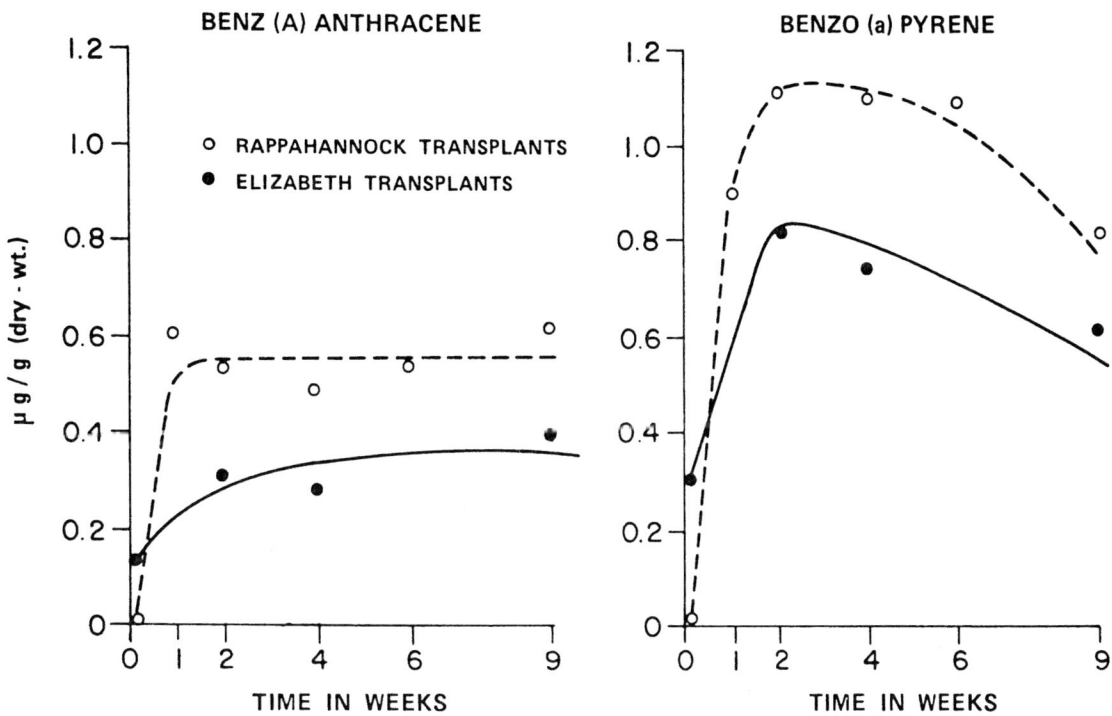

Figure 5. Transplant study-Elizabeth River-benz(a)anthracene and benzo(a)pyrene.

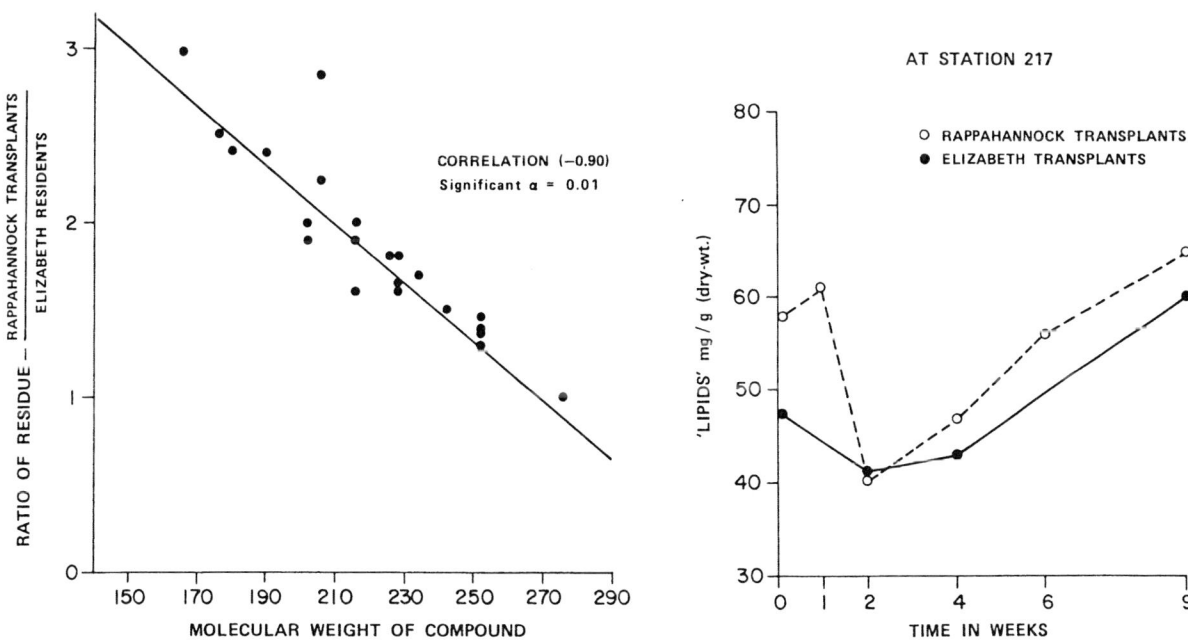

Figure 6. Ratio of residues vs compound molecular weight.

Figure 7. "Lipid" levels vs time.

REFERENCES

1. Bieri RH, Hein C, Huggett RJ, Shou P, Slone H, Smith C, Su-C-W: Polycyclic aromatic hydrocarbons in surface sediments from the Elizabeth River subestuary. *Intern J Environ Anal Chem* 26:97, 1986

2. Burns KA, Smith JL: Distribution of petroleum hydrocarbons in Westport Bay (Australia) results of chronic low level inputs. In: *Fate and Effects of Petroleum Hydrocarbons in Marine Environments and Ecosystems*. D. A. Wolfe (Ed). Pergamon Press. 442, 1977

3. Farrington JW: An overview of the biogeochemistry of fossil fuel hydrocarbons in the marine environment. In: *Petroleum in the Marine Environment*. L. Petraksis and F. Weiss (Eds). *Amer Chem Soc* Washington, D. C. p. 1, 1980

4. Fazio T: Analysis of oyster samples for polycyclic hydrocarbons. Proc. of the 7th Nat. Shellfish Sanit. Workshop. Washington, D.C.: FDA Div. of Shellfish Sanitation. p. 238, 1971

5. Hargis WJ Jr, Roberts MH Jr, Zwerner DE: Effects of contaminated sediments and sediment-exposed effluent water on an estuarine fish: acute toxicity. *Marine Environ Res* 14:337, 1984

6. Howard JW, Fazio T: Review of polycyclic aromatic hydrocarbons in foods. Analytical methodology and reported findings of polycyclic aromatic hydrocarbons in foods. *J Assoc Off Anal Chem* 63:1077, 1980

7. Huggett RJ, Bender ME, Unger MA: Polynuclear aromatic hydrocarbons in the Elizabeth River, Virginia. Proc. of the 6th Pellston Conf., Florissant, Colo., August, 1984 In: *Fate and effects of sediment bound chemicals in aquatic systems*. KL Dickson, AW Mackin, WA Brungs (eds). Setac Special Publications Series. 327, Oxford, Pergamon Press, 1987

8. Iosifidou HG, Kilikidis SD, Kamarianos AP: Analysis of polycyclic aromatic hydrocarbons in mussels (*Mytilus galloprovincialis*) from the Thermaibos Gulf, Greece. *Bull Environ Cotnam Toxicol* 28:535, 1982

9. Knutzen J, Shortland B: Polycyclic aromatic hydrocarbons (PAH) in some algae and invertebrates from moderately polluted parts of the coast of Norway. *Water Res* 16:421, 1982

10. Law R, Andrulewicz E: Hydrocarbons in water, sediment, and mussels from the southern Baltic Sea. *Mar Poll Bull* 14:289, 1983

11. Mackie PR, Hardy R, Whittle KJ, Bruce C, McGill AS: The tissue hydrocarbon burden of mussels from various sites around the Scottish coast. In: Bjorseth A, Dennis AJ, (Eds). PAHs: *Chemical and Biological Effects*, Battelle Press, Columbus, Ohio, 1980

12. Malins DC, Hodgins HO: Petroleum and marine fishes: a review of uptake, diposition and effects. *Environm Sci and Technol* 15:1273, 1981

13. Mix MC: Polycyclic aromatic hydrocarbons in the aquatic environment: Occurrence and biological monitoring. In: *Reviews in Environmental Toxicology* 1. E. Hodgson (Ed). Elsevier Press. p. 51, 1984

14. Neff JM: *Polycyclic aromatic hydrocarbons in the aquatic environment. Sources, Fates and Biological Effects*. Applied Science Pubs. Ltd London. 262 pp, 1979

15. Settine RL, Barker SA, Marion KA: Bivalves as indicators of environmental pollution: A pilot study of oysters (*Crassostrea virginica*) in Mobile Bay. Proc. Northern Gulf of Mexico Estuaries and Barrier Islands Res. Conf. Biloxi, Miss. June 13–14, p. 15, 1983

16. Stegeman JJ, Teal J: Accumulation, release and retention of petroleum hydrocarbons by the oyster, *Crassostrea virginica*. *Mar Biol* 22:37, 1973

28

THE HUMAN POPULATION – A FINAL RECEPTOR FOR CHEMICAL CONTAMINANTS

HAROLD E.B. HUMPHREY

Geographic circumstances and a series of events in Michigan have provided an opportunity to evaluate human exposure to environmental contaminants, especially the halogenated biphenyl compounds. Polychlorinated biphenyls (PCB) have been found in fish from the Great Lakes and in certain farm silos constructed in the 1940's and polybrominated biphenyls (PBB) contaminated domestic farm animals on over 500 Michigan farms in 1973. These situations have resulted in the exposure of thousands of residents who consume sport caught fish or food products from affected farms. They have also presented public health officials with the need and opportunity to quantitate those exposures and evaluate the short and long term human health outcomes from them. In Michigan, we have begun this process with the institution of several cohort studies which examine fisheaters (8, 9, 11), families from farms with the PCB coated silos (10) and families from farms contaiminated with PBB (Landrigan et al 1979). In this chapter, the focus will be on human populations exposed to PCB's primarily through consumption of contaminated fish.

There is experimental evidence of a carcinogenic effect of some polychlorinated biphenyls in rodents. Specifically, Aroclor 1254, and 1260 have induced benign and malignant liver-cell tumors in mice and rats respectively. For practical purposes "polychlorinated biphenyls should be regarded as if they were carcinogenic to humans" (12).

The Great Lakes which surround Michigan are located in a region inhabited by approximately 40 million people. These lakes represent a major sink for materials used in terrestrial activities. Nearly 1,000 chemical substances have been identified in the Great Lakes aquatic environment (IJC report 1983). Some of these substances have reported mammalian toxicity (IJC report 1981), are persistent and are known to bio-accumulate in the environment. A few of the contaminants have been detected in Great Lakes fish at greater than trace quantities. Of these, PCB dominates the spectrum of major contaminants likely to reach a person's dinner plate as shown by the concentrations recorded in Table 1. Although localized contamination may alter this spectrum at specific sites and in certain species, the compounds shown represent those generally encountered at higher concentrations in Great Lakes fish.

Fish therefore represent the principal link between contaminants in the acquatic environmental and humans. Although populations may receive exposure to a contaminant such as PCB from terrestrial, atmospheric or water column sources, these are minimal when compared to the potential dose present in fish (10, 11). Concentrations of lipid soluble

Table 1. Dinner plate exposure assessment.

| Contaminant | Median concentration* | | | |
	L. trout	Chinook	Coho	Other**
PCB	3,012	1,478	807	168
DDT	1,505	761	447	137
HCB	5	3	2	1
Oxychlordane	25	–	–	–
Trans nonachlor	195	107	55	–
Dieldrin	75	53	–	–

* Parts per billion
** Pike, perch, walleye, whitefish

contaminants are magnified to significant proportions in edible fish through food chain bioconcentration. Fish become accumulators of toxic organic chemicals representing a significant risk factor to humans who eat them on a regular basis. Carinogenic risk from eating fish contaminated with PCB and other organics such as DDT, dieldrin, toxaphene and chlordane have been reported to be 10–100 times greater than the risk associated with drinking groundwater contaminated with lower halogenated compounds such as chloroform, 1,1-dichloraethylene and other commonly encountered organics (6). Greater than average consumption rates and consumption of highly contaminated species contribute to the increased risk reported in these calculations. It was noted that fish tended to accumulate those lipophilic organics which have higher carcinogenic potency factors. The accumulation of these chemicals offsets the fact that far more water is consumed by humans than fish.

Connor stated that most of the known carcinogenic risk in his calculations was due to PCB (because of its higher concentration) and that other contaminants, even though some are more potent, provided only minor contributions to this risk because of their low concentrations in the fish. Our analysis of cooked fish caught from Lake Michigan substantiates this focus on PCB. Table 1 shows the concentration of the principal contaminants detected in fish dinners eaten by our study subjects and confirms that PCB is the dominant contaminant present. Although hundreds of chemicals have been detected in the Great Lakes and many may be present in raw fish at trace levels only a few represent significant dose factors for humans who eat prepared meals.

We initiated a study in 1973 (8) to quantitate exposure from fish in order to obtain a better understanding of fish contaminant dose factors. A cohort of 158 persons 90 of

235

H. E. Kaiser (ed.), Comparative aspects of tumor development.
© 1989, Kluwer Academic Publishers, Dordrecht. ISBN-13:978-0-89838-994-4

Table 2. Serum PCB levels found in the 1973 study participants.

Participants	No. people	Consumption pounds/yr	Serum PCB (ppb) Range	Serum PCB (ppb) Median
Non-eaters	29	0	< 5–41	15
Occasional eaters	39	0–26	< 5–41	20
Regular eaters	90	> 24	25–366	56

Table 3. Serum PCB levels found in the 1981 study participants.

Class	Comparison 0–6 lbs/yr	Exposed 24–270 lbs/yr*
Participants	419	572
Serum PCB Median (ppb)	6.6	21.4
Range (ppb)	< 3–59.5	< 3–202.7

* Median fish consumption, 38.5 lbs/yr

whom regularly ate Lake Michigan sport caught fish were enrolled. It was found that this group consumed an average of 32 pounds of sport-caught fish per year and some ate as much as 262 pounds per year. This average was nearly five times the national per capita fish consumption average commonly used in risk estimates. As shown in Table 1 regular consumption of these meals represents a significant source of exposure to fat soluble contaminants such as PCB and DDT. This was verified by comparison of PCB serum concentrations with fish consumption patterns for members of the study group (Table 2). Those who regularly ate sport-caught fish, 24 pounds per year or more, had serum concentrations significantly higher than persons who seldom or never ate such fish. Serum PCB was found to correlate directly with the quantity of salmon and lake trout consumed. As a result, persons in the upper range of consumption had serum concentrations up to twenty-four times the median value for the unexposed group.

Evaluation of human exposure to environmental contaminants is generally hindered by limited observations on a small number of subjects long after the event has occurred. The popularity of catching fish from the Great Lakes provides an opportunity to evaluate this relationship while

it is occurring. Funds provided by the U.S. Environmental Protection Agency in 1979–82 permitted expansion of the earlier study group and the establishment of a study cohort of 991 participants. Persons who regularly ate one or more meals of sport-caught fish per week (> 26 pounds/yr) were recruited from eleven communities along the Michigan shoreline of Lake Michigan. A group of 572 persons who met this criteria were identified and agreed to participate. A matched comparison group of 419 persons who ate little or no sport-caught fish (< 6 pounds/yr) were randomly selected from the same communities. Annual fish consumption rates were closely monitored over two seasons by field interviews and dietary logs. For the exposed group these rates were found to be similar to those stated previously. Serum PCB levels for the exposed and comparison groups are shown in Table 3. The analytical laboratory protocol developed for this study specifically quantitated PCB and ten other organochlorine compounds (9). The frequency of occurrence and concentration of these contaminants in the serum of the 572 exposed fisheaters are shown in Table 4.

PCB, DDT and DDE, lipid soluble compounds, were detectable in nearly every fisheater. These compounds were less frequently detected in the comparison group whose median concentrations of 6.6 ppb, 10.5 ppb and 9 ppb respectively, were significantly lower than those of the fisheaters. Except for polybrominated biphenyl (PBB), a contaminant unique to Michigan, the other seven compounds were detectable less than 50% of the time in fisheaters and seldom in the comparisons. The median concentration of PCB found in the comparison group is consistent with values reported in other studies of unexposed populations (9, 10, 15). The significant elevation of PCB concentration in Lake Michigan fisheaters confirm our earlier findings (8), correlates with fish consumption and has a higher upper concentration range than that reported for fisheaters at other geographic sites (16).

Ubiquitous sources of PCB contribute to a gradual increase in body burden over a life-time. Evaluation of serum PCB levels in a rural population with no specific source of exposure showed that 65–70 year olds had mean levels three times those of 1–19 year olds (15). Regular exposure to a known source of PCB (fish) adds to this baseline level as shown by the elevated serum concentrations reported for the fisheaters above. These additional body burdens are re-

Table 4. Chemical contaminants detected in the serum of 572 fisheaters, 1981 study.

Compound	Detection limit (ppb)	CV%	% of Cohort above detection	Concentration (ppb) Range	Concentration (ppb) Median
Total PCB	3	9.71	99.1	< 3–202.7	21.4
DDE	1	7.13	99.5	< 1–425.3	21.7
Total DDT	1	7.33	99.7	< 1–512.6	26.4
PBB	1	5.21	67.1	< 1–33.1	1.8
HCB	1	20.83	3.3	< 1–3.2	< 1
Beta BHC	1	–	18.4	< 1–4.8	< 1
Oxychlordane	2	–	4.2	< 2–5.5	< 2
Hept. epoxide	2	–	0.5	< 2–2.6	< 2
Trans-nonachlor	1	–	45.3	< 1–12.1	< 1
Dieldrin	1	–	19.6	< 1–6.0	< 1
Mirex	2	6.99	0.2	< 2–3.1	< 2

CV% = Coefficient of variation

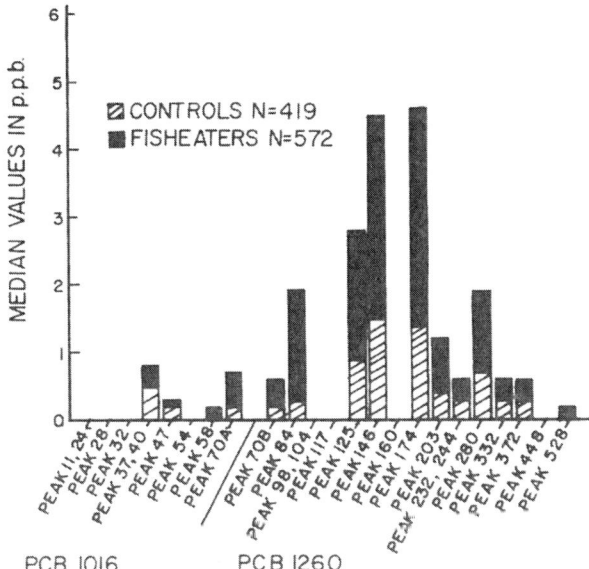

Figure 1. Median PCB levels for elution peaks found in human serum (11).

tained for decades (15). The reported correlation between serum concentrations and both quantity of fish eaten and duration (years) of regular sport-caught fish consumption (9, 10) show that these are significant factors contributing to increased serum levels and, accordingly, life-time body burdens.

Improvements in analytical chemistry have allowed a more precise evaluation of the PCB mixture in serum. For the 1981 study, the laboratory quantitated PCB using a temperature programmed gas chromatograph technique (Needham 1983) and the Webb and McCall isomer identificatiion method (24). This approach improved the separation of PCB and DDT avoiding inflated PCB values which were a problem with the laboratory methodology used in the 1973 study and allowed identification and quantitation of the major elution peaks associated with these standards. Figure 1 shows the median concentration calculated for each of the various PCB elution peaks found in the serum of the 1981 study fisheater and comparison participants. Peaks associated with the more highly chlorinated Aroclor 1260 standard dominate the PCB pattern seen in human serum. Persons exposed to contaminated fish had higher concentrations for each of the peaks and had two peaks which were not detected in the comparison group. Except for peak 47, the median concentrations for all peaks detected in fisheater

Table 5. Toxicity of several PCB congeners associated with prominent aroclor 1260 peaks found in human sera.

Peak no.	Congener assignment	Reported toxicity (safe 1984, safe 1985, aust 1981)
174	2342′4′5′	Cytotoxic+
146	2452′4′5′	Tumor promoter and PB inducer
125	2453′4′	Cytotoxic++ and mixed inducer
203	2342′3′4′	Mixed inducer
232, 244	2345 3′4′	Cytotoxic+++ and mixed inducer

serum were significantly higher (p < 0.001) than those for the comparison group.

Each of the PCB elution peaks contain one or more PCB homologs. Some of the specific congeners which are present and are major components in these elution peaks have been identified (23, 25). The toxicological properties for a number of the PCB congeners or structurally similar brominated congeners have been evaluated and reported (3, 20, 21). Table 5 identifies the seven elution peaks which constitute the major proportion of the total PCB quantified in human serum. Each of these peaks has at least one identified congener component for which the toxicological properties have been evaluated. As shown, the major proportion of the PCB mixture found in human serum contains more highly chlorinated PCB congeners which possess cytotoxic, enzyme induction or tumor promotion toxicological characteristics. The transfer of these toxic forms of PCB from the environment to humans is enhanced through consumption of contaminated fish. This data substantiates Connor's opinion that the organic contaminants found in fish are forms with higher carcinogenic potency and that their bio-accumulation in fish make them significant risk factors to humans (6).

Regular consumption of contaminated fish not only increases an individual's baseline body burden of PCB and its toxic congeners but each meal also causes a temporary rise in the blood serum concentration of these. Blood specimens were collected from 20 volunteers prior to and at 4, 6, 24, 48 and 168 hours after eating a 1/2 pound pan fried meal of fish. Ten persons ate lake trout (10.3 ppm PCB) and ten ate chinook salmon (3.7 ppm PCB). Following the meal, serum PCB levels immediately rose, peaked within ten hours and gradually declined returning to the pre-meal baseline level over the next seven days (Figure 2).

As shown, a contaminated fish dinner results in a large temporary elevation of circulating levels of the toxin. These increases averaged 230 to 500 percent of the mean baseline serum concentrations. The magnitude of this change was directly related to the concentration of the contaminant in the cooked meal. It was also noted that serum PCB concentrations following the meal reached higher levels in persons who regularly eat such fish than in comparison

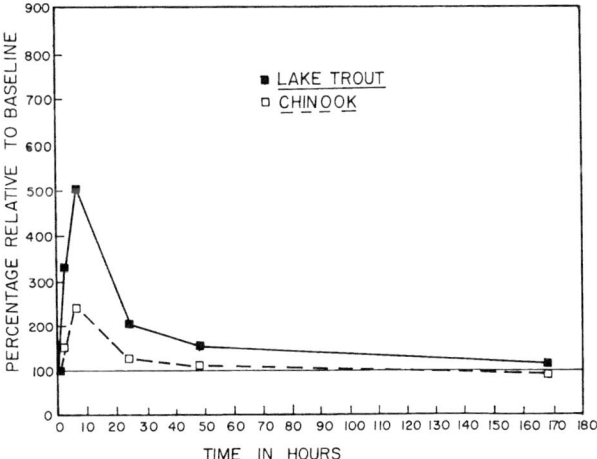

Figure 2. Percent change in baseline serum PCB levels following a meal (11).

persons who never ate these fish. The data indicate that regular consumers of contaminated fish receive repeated dose spikes significantly above their baseline. The long term toxicological significance of this for humans is unknown.

Consumption of fish represents an intermittent exposure to toxic contaminants, especially PCB. Consumption of milk and beef produced on a farm represents a more continuous exposure to any contaminants which may be present. Several thousand farm silos in the midwest were coated on the interior with PCB impregnated paint when they were built forty years ago. Over the years this coating flaked off and became mixed with silage and fed to farm animals, often dairy cows. Until ten years ago, regular maintenance included recoating the interior of the silo with the same material. As a result, members of the farm family who directly consumed milk and meat produced on these affected farms potentially received PCB contaminated food on a regular basis over a period of several decades. As described elsewhere (10) we have begun enrollment of families from the estimated 400 farms in Michigan which have such silos. Although enrollment and follow-up is not complete at this time preliminary observations indicate that this group has serum PCB concentrations similar to those found in the fisheater group illustrated above (10, 11). The silo farm participants represent persons who potentially received daily exposure to PCB for decades and therefore represent an opportunity to evaluate the long term health implications of such exposures.

Evaluation of this population group also provides a basis for estimating the possible health outcomes from regular consumption of contaminated Great Lakes fish, the availability of which is a relatively recent phenomenon compared to the farm silo exposure source. As reported (10), the development of cancer among persons living on the PCB coated silo farms should be followed up to determine whether or not a correlation exists between the cancer cases being observed and association with this long term source of exposure to PCB. This is especially important because neoplasms are reported to account for the largest number of deaths in Japanese Yusho patients ten years following that episode (22).

The Michigan cohort investigations have clearly demonstrated an association between significant contamination sources and human exposure. Although exposure assessment has primarily been on the basis of serum concentration, related work (7, 10, 15) has shown that this serves as an estimator for body burden. In addition, other body tissues especially breast milk and cord blood have been found to contain the halogenated lipophilic contaminants detected in serum indicating that female body burdens can become multi-generational as the contaminants are passed to the unborn and newborn offspring. More importantly, these studies demonstrate that halogenated biphenyl contaminants such as PCB have a long half life in exposed humans (15). Persistence in the human body, opportunity for repeated exposure and the accumulative effects of multiple doses create a situation where the contaminant has a long period of time within the body to express its toxic effect alone or in combination with other contaminants which may be encountered.

Persistence and latency are important factors because some of the PCB congeners believed to be associated with the dominant PCB homologs received from contaminated fish consumption are enzyme inducers and/or tumor promoters (Table 5). Polychlorinated biphenyls have been shown to produce hetatocellular carcinomas, neoplastic nodules and adenofibrosis in rats and adenofibrosis and hepatomas in mice (13, 14). In these reviews Kimbrough noted an apparent association between degree of chlorination of PCB mixtures and the strength of their ability to produce tumors, induce enzymes or act as tumor promoters. This is consistent with the toxicity determined for some of the PCB congeners found in exposed humans (20, 21). Whether or not humans exposed to PCB's and other compounds at the concentrations found in the food they eat will result in latent disease such as cancer remains an open question. The persistence of these compounds provides the continous internal exposure of target organs necessary for this process if it is to occur and the mix of other aquatic contaminants in fish may provide the basis for a tumor induction interaction with the stored PCB. The role of aquatic chemical contaminants as etiologic agents in the high incidence of tumors and cancers in fish is under investigation by several investigators at a number of sites in the country (4, 5, 18). Whether or not the manifestations observed in fish exposed to aquatic chemical mixtures represents a possible outcome in humans who receive these mixtures from eating contaminated fish remains to be seen.

It is believed that the cohorts of humans identified and characterized in Michigan provide an opportunity to determine the long term outcome of exposure to halogenated biphenyls themselves (PCB silo farmers) or in combination with other aquatic contaminants (Greatt Lakes fisheaters). In both cases exposure assessment indicates that the human is a final biological receptor for these environmental chemical contaminants.

REFERENCES

1. Report to the Great Lakes Water Quality Board, *An Inventory of Chemical Substances Identified in the Great Lakes Ecosystem*. International Joint Commission, Vol 1–6, 1983
2. Committee on the Assessment of Human Health Effects of Great Lakes Water Quality, *Annual Report*. Internation Joint Commission, 142 pp, 1981
3. Aust SD, Dannan GA, Sleight SD, Fraker PJ, Ringer RK, Polin D: Toxicology of Polybrominated Biphenyls. In *Toxicology of Halogenated Hydrocarbons*, Pergamon Press, 73, 1981
4. Baumann PC: Cancer in Wild Freshwater Fish Populations with Emphasis on the Great Lakes. *J Great Lakes Res* 10:251, 1984
5. Black JJ, Evans ED, Harshbarger JC, Zeigel RF: Epizootic Neoplasms in Fishes from a Lake Polluted by Cooper Mining Wastes. *J Natl Cancer Inst* 69:915, 1982
6. Connor MS: Comparison of the Carcinogenic Risks from fish vs Groundwater Contamination by Organic Compounds. *Env Sci Technol* 18:628, 1984
7. Eyster JT, Humphrey HEB, Kimbrough RD: Partitioning of polybrominated Biphenyls in Serum, Adipose Tissue, Breast Milk, Placenta, Cord Blood, Biliary Fluid and Feces. *Arch Env Hlth* 38(1):47, 1983
8. Humphrey HEB: *Evaluation of Changes of the Level of Polychlorinated Biphenyls in Human Tissues*. Final Report to the FDA, contract no. 223-73-2209, 86 pp, 1976
9. Humphrey HEB: *Evaluation of Humans Exposed to Water*

Borne Chemicals in the Great Lakes. Final Report to the Environmental Protection Agency, Cooperative Agreement CR-807192, 198 pp. plus appendices, 1983a

10. Humphrey HEB: Population Studies of PCB's in Mihigan Residents. In: *PCB's Human and Environmental Hazards*, Ann Arbor Science, 299, 1983b

11. Humphrey HEB: The Human Population – An Ultimate Receptor for Aquatic Contaminants. *Hydrobiologia* 149:75, 1987

12. IARC Monograph, Evaluation of the carcinogenic Risk of Chemicals to Humans: Polychlorinated Biphenyls and polybrominated biphenyls 18:83, 1978

13. Kimbrough RD: The Carcinogenic and Other Chronic Effects of Persistent Halogenated Compounds. *Ann N Y Acad Sci* 320:415, 1979

14. Kimbrough RD: Halogenated Biphenyls, Terphenyls Naphthalenes, Dibenzodioxins, and Related Products. Elsevier, Holland, 136, 1980

15. Kreiss K, Roberts C, Humphrey HEB: Serial PBB Levels, PCB Levels and Clinical Chemistries in Michigan's PBB Cohort. *Arch. Env. Hlth.* 37(3):141, 1982

16. Kreiss K: Studies on Populations Exposed to Polychlorinated Biphenyls. *Env Hlth Persp* 60:193, 1985

17. Landrigan PJ, Wilcox KR, Silva J, Humphrey HEB, Kauffman C, Heath CW: Cohort Study of Michigan Residents Exposed to Polybrominated Biphenyls: Epidemiologic and Immunological Findings. *Ann. N.Y. Acad. Sci.* 320:284, 1979

18. Malins DC, Krahn MM, Brown DW, Rhodes LD, Myers MS, McCain BB, Chan SL: Toxic Chemicals in Marine Sediment and Biota From Mukilteo Washington: Relationship with Hepatic Neoplasms and Other Hepatic Lesions in English Sole. *J Natl Cancer Inst* 74:487, 1985

19. Needham LL, Barse VW, Price HA: Temperature – Programmed Gas Chromatographic Determination of Polychlorinated and Polybrominated Biphenyls in Serum. *J Assoc Off Anal Chem* 64(5):1131, 1981

20. Safe S: Polychlorinated Biphenyls (PCB's) and Polybrominated Biphenyls (PBB's): Biochemistry, Toxicology and Mechanism of Action. *Critical Reviews in Toxicology* 13(4):319, 1984

21. Safe S et al: PCB's: Structure-Function Relationships and Mechanisms of Action. *Env Hlth Persp* 60:47, 1985

22. Urabe H, Koda H, Asaha M: Present State of Yusho Patients. *Ann N Y Acad Sci* 320:273, 1979

23. Webb RG, McCall AC: Identities of Polychlorinated Biphenyl Isomers in Aroclor. *J Assoc Off Anal Chem* 55:746, 1972

24. Webb RG, McCall AC: Quantitative PCB Standards for Electron Capture Gas Chromatography. *J Chromatogr Sci* 11:366, 1973

25. Wolff MS, Thornton J, Fischbein A, Lillis R, Selikoff IJ: Disposition of Polychlorinated Biphenyl Congeners in Occupationally Exposed Persons. *Tox Appl Pharm* 62:294, 1982

CHEMICAL CARCINOGENS IN PLANTS AND INTERACTION
WITH VIRUSES AND CANCER CAUSATION

THOMAS W. BEDNAR and ELFRIEDE M. LINSMAIER-BEDNAR

INTRODUCTION

The concern during the past several decades about hazards to humans from environmental chemicals has also initiated new interest in understanding the significance of xenobiotic carcinogens in the phytosphere (86, 100). Increasing numbers of carcinogens and promoters of carcinogenesis are being found and natural plant products as well (4, 28). Although the numbers of known xenobiotic carcinogens are increasing, little systematic work has been done to explore the uptake, metabolism and the consequences of the presence of carcinogens in plants. The questions, to what extent specific plant species produce, or incorporate and sequester foreign carcinogenic chemicals, contribute such compounds to the food chain, metabolically alter, or foster their detoxification, etc. are largely unanswered. Obtaining knowledge of these events can, however, aid in understanding the environmental carcinogenic burden of human populations.

In addition to these environmental roles, eukaryotic plants, tissues and cells, being less complicated than their mammalian counterparts, can be used experimentally to study neoplastic transformation and the control of growth at the cellular, biochemical and molecular levels. The value of plant cells for studying the mechanisms involved in the complex process of initiation and development of neoplastic growth has been recognized early in this century by Smith (87) and subsequently advocated by Black (17) and Braun (24). However, plant cell systems still remain a relatively little used approach for studying the basic mechanisms of tumorigenesis. Yet, the limited number of studies conducted to date have established an important generalization. The same kinds of conditions or agents that can cause cancer in animals can also induce neoplastic growth in plant cells, namely, genetic disposition (1, 88), foreign DNA (56, 85, 101), foreign RNA (16, 74), ionizing radiation (76), direct-acting chemical carcinogens (68), and carcinogens requiring metabolic activation (8, 9, 10, 65).

Inorganic Carcinogens in Plants

Either epidemiological evidence or laboratory animal studies have implicated arsenic, cadmium, chromium, nickel, beryllium, cobalt, iron-dextran, lead, titanium, and zinc as potential carcinogens in animals and man (48, 92). In the experimental animal studies, the route of administration has largely been by injection or inhalation. Almost all studies involving oral administration via food or water have been negative. Lead has been reported to be the only inorganic carcinogen that induced malignant neoplasms following dietary administration (91).

Cadmium has been one of the most extensively studied elements with regard to its uptake and storage in plants and will serve as an example for this group of carcinogens (99). The availability of inorganic carcinogens for uptake by plants when present in the soil is governed by a significant number of physical and chemical variables in the environment. Soil pH, temperature, salinity, cation exchange capacity, water and nitrogen content, inorganic cations and anions have all been found to affect the uptake and toxicity of cadmium in higher plants (6).

Cadmium is passively taken up by the plant and translocated to the leafy vegetative portions of the plant (34, 59). Oat and barley grains have been shown to accumulate less than 25 micrograms of cadmium per kilogram dry weight tissue, while spinach and lettuce leaves acquire 3.9 to 5.2 milligrams per unit dry mass (96). It has been estimated that the average dietary intake of cadmium by adults in the United States is between 200 and 400 μg per week (26). This could be considerably higher if the diet is high in leafy vegetables grown on cadmium rich soils. The health effects of such intake are not known.

A number of these inorganic carcinogens serve as essential micronutrients for plant growth, but information about any role initiating or promoting neoplastic growth in plant cells is lacking.

Organic Carcinogens in Plants

A review of approximately 159 compounds including those found carcinogenic in the National Toxicology Program's testing protocols (37, 48, 73), together with a literature search for their uptake and metabolism, indicate that information on the fate of environmental carcinogens in plants is extremely limited. Uptake and accumulation data are largely restricted to pesticides and growth substances, only some of which are carcinogenic (38, 63).

In the limited number of studies available, conflicting evidence for uptake of various inorganic and organic carcinogens by intact plants (e.g. roots, leaves) has been reported. For example, benzo(a)pyrene was found to be taken up by a variety of plant species from sterile nutrient solution (40), while Ellwardt (43) found no uptake of polycyclic aromatic hydrocarbons including benzo(a)pyrene by pota-

H. E. Kaiser (ed.), Comparative aspects of tumor development.

toes, oats and rye grown in soil. Anthracene was reported to be taken up from the atmosphere, soil and hydroculture by soybeans (41). It appears from the reports surveyed that the differences in experimental design and the lack of standardized methodologies make comparisons between different studies difficult.

However, plant cell culture has considerable advantages in studies of uptake and metabolism of carcinogenic xenobiotics. Namely, investigations of cellular uptake and metabolism can be conducted under chemically defined and precisely controlled experimental environments. While not mimicking the natural environmental settings, such studies can define the basic physiological and biochemical potential of the plant cell in incorporating and metabolizing xenobiotic carcinogens. A recent study employing soybean and parsley cells cultured with benzo(a)pyrene produced quinones, dihydrodiols and other soluble and insoluble derivatives (82). A microsomal fraction prepared from cultured soybean cells formed quinones rather than the dihydrodiols and epoxides usually found in similar animal cell derived reaction mixtures (97). The quinones were incorporated into lignin (98). If this is a general property of plant cells when they are synthesizing lignin it would indicate the presence of an important detoxification mechanism. On the other hand, DDT (1,1,1-trichloro-2,2,-bis-[p-chlorophenyl]-ethane) can be converted to small amounts of carcinogenic DDE (1,1-dichloro-2,2-bis-[p-chlorophenyl]-ethylene) upon incubation with parsley and soybean suspension cultures. Further metabolism, however, appears to lead to detoxified polar conjugates (84). In a manner similar to mammalian cells (108), a number of oxidative enzymes in plant cells can convert some foreign compounds into highly reactive electrophilic derivatives that react with cellular macromolecules and are capable of initiating the tumorigenic process. However, as indicated earlier for uptake and accumulation, the literature on the metabolism of foreign compounds in plants is very limited and largely restricted to determining the fate of pesticides in crop species (2, 29, 38). Two key oxidative enzyme systems involved in xenobiotic metabolism in plants appear to be the P-450 enzymes and peroxidases.

A number of plant cytochrome P-450 monooxygenases have the ability to hydroxylate plant metabolites and xenobiotics (46, 50, 55). The production of plant microsomal P-450 enzymes can be increased by manganese, ethanol, phenobarbital, herbicides (81), wounding and light (12, 13) making it an effective system for both detoxification and activation of carcinogens. A number of herbicides, some of them carcinogenic, have been activated into mutagens by aqueous extracts from homogenates of *Zea mays* seedlings (79). The filamentous fungus *Cunninghamella elegans* has been shown to oxidize benzo(a)pyrene (30) as did microsomes from Jerusalem artichoke and tulip bulbs (53, 54).

Plants contain considerable amounts of peroxidases. A horseradish peroxidase-H_2O_2 reaction system effectively activated the carcinogen N-OH-acetylaminofluorene (N-OH-AAF) to a highly reactive electrophile capable of forming adducts with nucleic acid (7). Activation of N-OH-AAF and nucleic acid conjugation were demonstrated with cell-free preparations from cultured tobacco cells and the reaction increased significantly upon addition of H_2O_2 (11, 64). Thus, it was not unexpected that cultured tobacco cells were found capable of activating 2-aminofluorene into a mutagen in the Ames test (78).

Natural Carcinogens in Plants

Plants may not only act as accumulators and conduits for environmental carcinogens in the food chain, but can contribute carcinogenic natural products to the human diet as well (28, 57, 70). The common commercial mushroom *Agaricus bisporus* contains agaritine and related hydrazines which are potent stomach and lung carcinogens in mice (4). Black pepper (*Piper nigrum*) contains safrole and several related compounds containing the methylenedioxy-phenyl structure which is required for the known carcinogenic and mutagenic activity of safrole (32). Pyrrolizidine alkaloids found in many species of plants belonging to the Compositae are potent hepato-carcinogens. In some parts of the world, herbal teas, honey and remedies are prepared from plants that contain more than 1% by weight of these compounds (4, 49). Among the most toxic of plant-associated carcinogens are the aflatoxins produced by the fungus *Aspergillus flavus* when it contaminates improperly stored cereal grains (27).

In addition to producing chemicals that are complete carcinogens, many plant species produce compounds that facilitate tumor development by promoting the growth of neoplastically initiated cells. The best-known tumor promoters are the phorbol esters isolated from *Croton tiglium* (51). TPA (12-O-tetradecanoylphorbol-13-acetate), and related compounds are produced by many species of the Euphorbiaceae and Thymelaeaceae. TPA initiates its promoting effect by physically binding to the lipophilic areas of mammalian cell membranes. This association results in an inflammatory response and many diverse biochemical events. Both these effects are reversible when treatment is stopped (36). The theory (20, 21) that promoters are effective in furthering carcinogenic development by derepressing key regulator genes is becoming more widely accepted as new data about genetic controls become available from research with microbial systems and promoter-virus interactions. Thus, promotion may be the result of derepression of the regulator genes which may facilitate the expression of critical constitutive genes altered by the carcinogenic agent.

Plants can also produce numerous anticarcinogenic compounds (44, 104, 105). Some of these inhibit the metabolic activation of carcinogens from their precursor compounds. Ellagic acid, a common plant phenol derived from tannin, can inhibit the metabolic activation of polycyclic aromatic hydrocarbons such as benzo(a)pyrene, thereby preventing binding to DNA and mutagenicity (35, 109). Other compounds block the reaction of the carcinogen with the cellular target or inhibit the promotional steps of cancer development (104, 106).

Interaction of Plant-Derived Compounds and Viruses

From the previous discussion it is reasonable to assume that compounds present in plants must be included among the environmental factors that can initiate and, in addition, positively or negatively influence the carcinogenic process. A number of studies have shown that exogenous chemical agents or physical stimuli can affect the expression of oncogenic viral genes present in susceptible cells (19, 80). Table 1 lists some plant-derived compounds that initiate the ex-

Table 1. Plant-derived carcinogen and promoter-induced viral expression in host cells.

Compound	Source/Property	Virus	Effect	Reference
Mitomycin-C	*Streptomyces* sp. Carcinogen	Avian RNA Tumor Virus	Induction of Virus	(107)
TPA[1]	*Croton tiglium* Tumor Promoter	Adenovirus	Transformation of Infected Cells	(45)
TPA	Preparation from Euphorbiaceae and Thymelaeaceae species with partial chemical synthesis Tumor Promoter	Epstein-Barr Virus	Induction of Viral Antigen	(114)
Phorbol-12, 13-didecanoate	Preparation from Euphorbiaceae and Thymelaeaceae species with partial chemical synthesis Tumor Promoter	Epstein-Barr Virus	Induction of Viral Antigen	(114)
12-Deoxyphorbol-13-decanoate	Preparation from Euphorbiaceae and Thymelaeaceae species with partial chemical synthesis Tumor Promoter	Epstein-Barr Virus	Induction of Viral Antigen	(114)
3-0-Hexadecanoyl-ingenol	Preparation from Euphorbiaceae and Thymelaeaceae species with partial chemical synthesis Tumor Promoter	Epstein-Barr Virus	Induction of Viral Antigen	(114)
Mancinella Factor	Preparation from Euphorbiaceae and Thymelaeaceae species with partial chemical synthesis Tumor Promoter	Epstein-Barr Virus	Induction of Viral Antigen	(114)
Pimelea Factors P_1, P_2	Preparation from Euphorbiaceae and Thymelaeaceae species with partial chemical synthesis Tumor Promoter	Epstein-Barr Virus	Induction of Viral Antigen	(114)
TPA	*Croton tiglium* Tumor Promoter	Epstein-Barr Virus	Transformation of Human Leucocytes	(111)
Teleocidin	Indole alkaloid from *Streptomyces mediocidicus* Tumor Promoter	Epstein-Barr Virus	Introgen of Viral Antigen	(112)
Lyngbyatoxin A	Indole alkaloid from Blue-Green Alga, *Lyngbya majuscula* Tumor Promoter	Epstein-Barr Virus	Induction of Viral Antigen	(42)
Aplysiatoxin and Debromoaplysiatoxin	Polyacetates from *Lyngbya majuscula* Tumor Promoter	Epstein-Barr Virus	Induction of Viral Antigen	(42)
Aflatoxin B_1, G_1	*Aspergillus flavus,* Carcinogens	SV40	Induction of Virus	(33)
Sterigmatocystin	*Aspergillus versicolor* Carcinogen	SV40	Induction of Virus	(33)
Diterpene Esters	*Sapium sebiferum* Tumor Promoters	Epstein-Barr Virus	Induction-Barr Virus	(75)
Jacobine	Pyrrolizidine alkaloid *Senecio jacobaea* Carcinogen	Avian Tumor Virus	Induction of Virus	(77)

[1] TPA = 12-0-Tetradecanoylphorbol-13-Acetate

pression of genes in RNA and DNA viruses. In addition to the examples listed in Table 1, 12-O-tetradecanoylphorbol-13-acetate has also been shown to activate the mouse mammary tumor virus, Friend leukemia virus, Mason-Pfizer monkey virus and the endogenous murine xenotropic virus (110). In this manner, silent oncogenic viruses can be activated, produce the critical gene products, which, in turn, can transform the host cell into the cancerous phenotype (66). The mechanisms involved in viral induction are not known but may be due to DNA strand breaks (62), to inhibition of post replication repair within the host cell (113), or to other events that can cause derepression of the viral genome. The peptide products of viral oncogenes are often found associated with the plasma membrane or the nuclear and cytoplasmic membranes, but their functions in transformation still remain to be elaborated (14, 15).

Spontaneous Carcinogenesis

The carcinogenic process often appears to begin without any obvious cause. Although, by definition, very little is known about the events that initiate spontaneous cancers, they have been attributed to alterations or mutations of DNA occurring during replication, recombination, translocation of genetic elements (67), or repair of damaged DNA (83) because of the correlations between mutagenesis and carcinogenesis. It has been proposed that some of the spontaneous cancers are the result of error-prone DNA repair. In these cases, the initial damage to DNA need not be oncogenic. Support for this hypothesis has been obtained from bacteria, fungi and mammalian cells (89). DNA alterations from damage that ultimately results in a spontaneous cancer arise from background radiation, unrecognized exposure to mutagenic chemical agents, viruses, or persistent or transient metabolic imbalances within the affected cell that yield endogenous mutagenic compounds. These imbalances may be triggered by one or more co-carcinogenic events such as physical or chemical wounding that decompartmentalize the cell and start the subsequent metabolic activity and gene activation observed in the wound-healing process (60). Decompartmentalization could permit endogenous carcinogens to become metabolically activated and possibly facilitate their access to cellular DNA.

For a spontaneous cancer to develop, the events must lead to the autonomous growth of the affected cells. Autonomous growth may result from the persistent expression of normally repressed constitutive mitogenic growth factor genes such as those regulating the auxin/cytokinin biosynthesis in plant cells or the platelet-derived growth factor, epidermal growth factor or insulin-like growth factor in mammalian cells (52).

Plant cells have been found to have DNA repair systems. Wild carrot (*Daucus carota*) cells (58) and Tradescantia (*Tradescantia paludosa*) root tips (102) repaired gamma and X-ray-induced DNA strand breaks. A uracil-DNA glycosylase base-excision enzyme has been isolated from wheat germ (18). However, at present it is not known whether these systems have a role in the neoplastic transformation of plant cells.

Chemical Induction of Neoplastic Growth in Plant Cells

An early attempt to experimentally induce neoplasms in plant tissues with chemicals involved applying several known carcinogens, namely, coal tar, a red dye, and dibenz-(a,h)anthracene, to a number of different plant species. Levine (69) reported that such treatments produced swellings, new woody tissues and cell proliferation that was greater than that observed in normal wound-healing, but was considerably less than that in tumors initiated by the crown gall tumor bacteria. The mushrooms *Agaricus* and *Collybia* developed neoplastic growths in the pseudotissues of their caps when treated with diesel oil (94). Germinating pea seedlings (*Pisum satium*) have been reported to develop tumors at the junction of the cotyledon and epicotyl upon treatment with N-methyl-N-nitrosoaniline (47). Benzo(a)pyrene applied to the vascular cambium of Norway spruce (*Picea abies*) produced swellings with histological abnormalities (61).

Two significant advances in the study of experimental plant tumors occurred with crown gall tumors when first, Braun and White (22a) used tissue culture to examine the properties of the transformed tumor cells, and secondly, when Braun (23) demonstrated that fully transformed plant cells could grow in a chemically-defined culture medium without the addition of the auxin/cytokinin phytohormones. To these contributions can be added the more recent discovery and characterization of the Ti plasmid, the "tumor inducing principle" carried by the *Agrobacterium* bacillus (56, 101).

The hormone-autonomous nature of neoplastic plant cells has been demonstrated for cells from the genetic tumors of the *Nicotiana glauca* × *Nicotiana langsdorfii* tumor hybrids (31, 88), the sorrel (*Rumex acetosa*) root cells transformed by the wound tumor virus (17), and cells from neoplasms induced in cultured *Haworthia mirabiles* tissues by gamma radiation (76).

The induction of hormone-autonomous neoplasms in cultured cells by chemical carcinogens has been shown for both direct-acting compounds and compounds requiring metabolic activation (Table 2). N-methyl-N'-nitro-N-nitrosoguanidine, a reactive alkylating agent, transformed sycamore cells in liquid culture media (68). Arylamines and heteroaromatic amines, that require metabolic activation for their mutagenic and carcinogenic activities (5, 71), were found to induce cytokinin and auxin autonomous tobacco

Table 2. Induction of neoplastic growth by chemical carcinogens in cultured plant cells.

Carcinogen	Species	Neoplastic growth marker	Reference
N-methyl-N'-nitro-N-nitroso-guanidine	*Acer pseudoplantanus*	Cytokinin/ Auxin Autonomy	(68)
2-aminofluorene 2, 7-diaminofluorene 2-acetylaminofluorene	*Nicotiana tabacum*	Cytokinin Autonomy	(8, 9)
2-acetylaminofluorene	*Nicotiana tabacum*	Cytokinin/ Auxin Autonomy	(10)
Trp-P-2(1) Glu-P-1(2)	*Nicotiana tabacum*	Cytokinin Autonomy	(65)

(1) 3-amino-1-methyl-5-H-pyrido[4, 3–b]indole
(2) 2-amino-6-methyldipyrido[1, 2-a:3′, 2′-d]imidazole

cells in tissues cultured on agar-solidified media (8, 9, 10, 65). Although not yet shown to be carcinogenic, N,N'diphenylurea produced cytokinin autonomous cells in cultured bean (*Phaseolus lunatis*) tissues (72). The phytohormones, auxin and cytokinin, control mitosis, cytokinesis and subsequent developmental processes in plant growth. These processes, central to the problem of both neoplastic and normal growth, can therefore be studied with plant cells in a chemically-defined system that provides a unique means to explore the molecular mechanisms of chemical carcinogenesis.

Application of molecular biological techniques to characterize the tumor-inducing Ti plasmid from *Agrobacterium tumefaciens* has provided insight into the specific sites of auxin and cytokinin production in Ti-plasmid transformed plant cells. A gene located within the plasmid's Ti region codes for indole-3-acetamide hydrolase, the enzyme that produces indoleacetic acid, the natural auxin (95). Another region of the Ti-plasmid codes for the production of dimethylallyl-transferase, an enzyme required for the synthesis of the N-6 substituted adenine cytokinins (3). These two genetic sequences seem to fit the definition of oncogenes; their presence and expression upon infecting a host cell lead to the continual overproduction of auxin and cytokinin allowing the cell to become autonomous and to persistently grow without an exogenous supply of growth factors. Alternatively, the regulatory sequences carried in by the Ti-plasmid may trigger expression of both Ti-auxin/cytokinin genes as well as the host cell genes that code for these two phytohormones. The effect the plasmid may have on the host cell genes that regulate phytohormone production has not yet been estimated.

The arylamine carcinogens have the ability to be metabolically activated in tobacco cells (64) and, in the absence of a Ti-plasmid, presumably effect a somatic mutation (11) in those host cell oncogenes responsible for the endogenous production of auxin and cytokinin. In this way, the transformed cells may be liberated from the need for an exogenous supply of phytohormones for continued growth. The requirement for exogenous cytokinin was always lost first or at the same time the auxin system became activated. That is to say, cells requiring cytokinin, but no auxin have not been observed (10). Although growth factor involvement in the neoplastic growth in plant cells has been known for a considerable number of years, recent findings with mammalian cells have now shown that the growth factor autonomy of cancer cells results from the production of specific growth factors controlled by active oncogenes (39, 103). Much remains to be learned about both systems, but each appears to correspond to the autocrine concept developed for mammalian cells (90).

Summary

This brief overview of chemical carcinogens and plants illustrates that studies of the phytosphere in relation to environmental carcinogenesis are in their infancy. In contrast to animals which have the mobility to migrate from polluted areas, the sessile plants may have evolved better endogenous detoxification, or other protective means, to prevent or slow the progression of events that lead to cell death or neoplastic

growth during their life spans, thereby often showing no obvious chronic toxic effects from carcinogen uptake and accumulation. The current lack of biochemical knowledge about the fate of carcinogens upon uptake and metabolic alteration or sequestering in food and other plants prevents an evaluation as to whether or not this contributes to or substracts from, the human carcinogenic burden. Understanding the biochemical mechanisms by which the plant protects itself from the consequences of chemical carcinogen exposure may provide useful information for the prevention of chemical carcinogenesis in humans.

Since the studies of the crown gall tumor system early in this century (22b), it has been recognized, by those interested in understanding the fundamental biological mechanisms of neoplastic growth, that plant tumor systems can serve as models for carcinogenesis in higher organisms and man. Although some aspects of mammalian cancer development such as metastases are not mimicked by plant tumors, the basic biochemistry and molecular biology of cell replication are sufficiently similar to that in man so that important insights of what may be happening can be gained by investigating plant cell systems. Much of what is known about eukaryotic molecular biology today has been gained by studying simpler prokaryotes. Perhaps, by analogy, plant cells can serve in a similar manner to aid in understanding the fundamental cellular and molecular mechanisms regulating both normal and neoplastic cell growth.

REFERENCES

1. Ahuja MR: Genetic control of tumor formation in higher plants. *Quar Rev Biol* 40:329, 1965
2. Aizawa H: Metabolic maps of pesticides. *Acad Press NY* 243, 1982
3. Akiyoshi DE, Klec H, Amasino RM, Nester EW, Gordon MP: T-DNA of *Agrobacterium tumefaciens* encodes an enzyme of cytokinin biosynthesis. *Proc Natl Acad Sci USA* 81:5994, 1984
4. Ames BN: Dietary carcinogens and anticarcinogens. *Science* 221:1256, 1983
5. Ames BN, Gurney EG, Miller JA, Bartsch H: Carcinogens as franshift mutagens: metabolites and derivatives of 2-acetylaminofluorene and other aromatic amine carcinogens. *Proc Natl Acad Sci* 69:3128, 1972
6. Babich H, Stotzky G: Developing standards for environmental toxicants: The need to consider abiotic environmental factors and microbe-mediated ecologic processes. *Environ Health Perspect* 49:247, 1983
7. Bartsch H, Hecker E: On the metabolic activation of the carcinogen N-hydroxy-N-2 acetylaminofluorene III. Oxidation with horseradish peroxidase to yield 2-nitroso-fluorene and N-acetoxy-N-2 acetyl-aminofluorene. *Biochim Biophys Acta* 273:567, 1971
8. Bednar TW, Linsmaier-Bednar EM: Induction of cytokinin-independent tobacco tissues by substituted fluorenes. *Proc Natl Acad Sci USA* 68:1178, 1971a
9. Bednar TW, Linsmaier-Bednar EM: The potency of N-acetylaminofluorene in the production of cytokinin autonomous tobacco tissues. *Experientia* 27:1071, 1971b
10. Bednar TW, Linsmaier-Bednar EM: Induction of plant neoplasms *in vitro* by substituted fluorenes. *Chem-Biol Interactions* 4:233, 1971/72
11. Bednar TW, Linsmaier-Bednar EM, King CM: Investigations on the mechanisms of substituted fluorene-induced hormone autonomy. *In*: Proceedings of the 8 th Intl. Conf. on

Plant Growth Substances 1973, Tokyo, Hirokawa Pub. Co., 1136, 1974

12. Benveniste I, Salun JP, Durst F: Wounding induced cinnamic acid hydroxylase in Jerusalem artichoke tuber. *Phytochemistry* 16:69, 1977

13. Benveniste I, Salum JP, Durst F: Phytochrome-mediated regulation of a mono-oxygenase hydroxylating cinnamic acid in etiolated pea seedlings. *Phytochemistry* 17:359, 1978

14. Bishop JM, Varmus H: Functions and origins of retroviral transforming genes. *In*: Weiss R, Teich N, Varmus H, Coffin J, *eds*. The Molecular Biology of RNA Tumor Viruses. 2 nd Ed., Cold Spring Harbor Lab., New York, 999, 1982

15. Bishop JM: Viral oncogenes. *Cell* 42:23, 1985

16. Black LM: A virus tumor disease of plants. *Am J Bot* 32:408, 1945

17. Black LM: Viruses and other pathogenic agents in plant tissue cultures. *J Natl Cancer Inst* 19:663, 1957

18. Blaisdell P, Warner H: Partial purification and characterization of a uracil-DNA glycosylase from wheat germ. *JBC* 258:1603, 1983

19. Bockstahler L, Cantwell J: Photodynamic induction of an oncogenic virus *in vitro. Biophys J* 25.209, 1979

20. Boutwell RK: The function and mechanism of promoters in carcinogenesis. *CRC Crit Rev Toxicol* 2:419, 1974

21. Boutwell RK: Biochemical mechanism of tumor promotion. *In* Slaga TJ, Sivak A, Boutwell RK *eds., Carcinogenesis: Mechanisms of Tumor Promotion and Coccinogenesis*. Vol. 2, Raven Press, New York, 49 p, 1978

22a. Braun AC, White, PR: Bacteriological sterility of tissues derived from secondary crown-gall tumors. *Phytopathology* 33: 85, 1943

22b. Braun AC: A history of the crown gall problem. *In*: Kahl G, Schell JS eds. Molecular Biology of Plant Tumors, *Acad Press NY.*, 155, 1982

23. Braun AC: The activation of two growth-substance systems accompanying the conversion of normal to tumor cells in crown gall. *Cancer Res* 16:53, 1956

24. Braun AC: The relevance of plant tumor systems to an understanding of the basic cellular mechanisms underlying tumorigenesis. *Prog Exp Tumor Res* 15:165, 1972

25. Braun AC, White PR: Bacteriological sterility of tissues derived from secondary crown-gall tumors. *Phytopathology* 33:85, 1943

26. Burau RG: National and local dietary impact of cadmium in south coastal California soils. *Ecotoxicol and Environ. Safety* 7:53, 1983

27. Busby WF, Wogan GN: Aflatoxins *In* Searle CE (ed) Chemical Carcinogens 2nd Ed. ACS Monograph 182, ACS Wash. D.C., 945 p, 1984

28. Carr BI: Chemical carcinogens and inhibitors of carcinogenesis in the human diet. *Cancer* 55 (Suppl):218, 1985

29. Casida JE, Lykken L: Metabolism of organic pesticide chemicals in higher plants. *Annu Rev Plant Physiol* 20:607, 1969

30. Cerniglia CE, Gibson D: Oxidation of benzo(a)pyrene by the filamentous fungus *Cunninghamella elegans. J Biol Chem* 254:12174, 1979

31. Cheng T-Y: Induction of indoleacetic acid synthesis in tobacco pith explants. *Plant Physiol* 50:723, 1972

32. Concon JM, Newburg DS, Swerczek TW. Black pepper (*Piper nigrum*): Evidence of carcinogenicity. *Nutrition and Cancer* 1:22, 1979

33. Coohill TP, Moore SP: An SV40 mammalian inductest for putative carcinogens. *Mutation Res* 113:431, 1983

34. Cutler JM, Rains DW: Characterization of cadmium uptake by plant tissue. *Plant Physiol* 54:67, 1974

35. Del Tito BJ, Mukhtar H, Bickers DR: Inhibition of epidermal metabolism and DNA binding of benzo(a)pyrene by ellagic acid. *Biochem Biophys Res Commun* 114:388, 1983

36. Diamond L, O'Brien TG, Baird WM: Tumor promoters and the mechanism of tumor promotion. *Adv Cancer Res* 32:1, 1980

37. diCarlo FJ, Fung VA: Summary of carcinogenicity data generated by The National Cancer Institute/National toxicology Program. *Drug Metabolism Reviews* 15:1251, 1984

38. Dohn DR, Krieger RI: Oxidative metabolism of foreign compounds by higher plants. *Drug Metabolism Reviews* 12:119, 1981

39. Downward J, Yarden Y, Mayes E, Scrace G, Totty N, Stockwell P, Ullrich A, Schlessinger J, Waterfield MD: Close similarity of epidermal growth factor receptor and v-*erb* B oncogene protein sequences. *Nature* 307:521, 1984

40. Durmishidze SV, Devdariani TV, Kavtaradze LK, Kvartskhava LS. Assimilation and conversion of 3, 4 benzpyrene by plants under sterile conditions. *Proc Acad Sci USSR Biochem Sec* 218:409, 1974

41. Edwards NT, Ross-Todd BM, Garver EG: Uptake and metabolism of ^{14}C-anthracene by soybean. *Environmental and Experimental Botany* 22:349, 1982

42. Eliasson L, Kallin B, Patarroyo M, Klein G, Fujiki H, Sugimura T: Activation of the EBV-cycle and aggregation of human blood lymphocytes by the tumor promoters teleocidin, lyngbyatoxin A, aplysiatoxin and debromoaplysiatoxin. *Int J Cancer* 31:7, 1983

43. Ellwardt P: Variation in the content of polycyclic aromatic hydrocarbons in soil and plants by using municipal waste composts in agriculture. *In*: Proc. of a Symposium Soil Organic Matter Studies, Vol. II, *IAEA* Vienna:291, 1977

44. Fever G, Kellen JA, Kovacs K: Suppression of 7, 12 dimethylbenz(a) anthracene induced breast carcinoma by coumarin in the rat. *Oncology* 33:35, 1976

45. Fisher PB, Weinstein IB, Eisenberg D, Ginsberg HS: Interactions between adenovirus a tumor promoter and chemical carcinogens in transformation of rat embryo cell cultures. *Proc Natl Acad Sci USA* 75:2311, 1978

46. Frear DS, Swanson HR, Tanaka FS: N-demethylation of substituted 3-phenyl-1-methylureas: isolation and characterization of a microsomal mixed function oxidase from cotton. *Phytochemistry* 8:2157, 1969

47. Garrigues R, Buu-Hoi NP, Rame A: Production de tumeurs vegetales par action de la N-methyl-N nitroso-aniline compose cancerogene chez l'animal. *CR Acad Sci Paris* 273:1123, 1971

48. Gilman JPW, Swierenga SHH: Inorganic carcinogenesis *In*: Chemical Carcinogens 2 nd Ed. C.E. Searle (ed) ACS Monograph 182. ACS Wash. D.C., 577, 1984

49. Grasso P: Carcinogens in Food. *In*: C.E. Searle (ed). Chemical Carcinogens 2 nd Ed. ACS Monograph 182, ACS Wash. D.C., 1205, 1984

50. Harms H, Dehnen W, Moench W: Benzo(a)pyrene metabolites formed by plant cells. *Z Naturforsch* 32:321, 1977

51. Hecker E: Isolation and characterization of the carcinogenic principles from croton oil. *Method Cancer Res* 6:439, 1971

52. Heldin C-H, Westermark B: Growth factors: Mechanism of action and relation to oncogenes. *Cell* 37:9, 1984

53. Higashi K, Nakashima K, Karasaki Y, Frikunaga M, Mizuguchi Y. Activation of benzo(a)pyrene by microsomes of higher plant tissues and their mutagenicity. *Biochem Init* 2:373, 1981

54. Higashi K, Ikeuchi K, Karasaki YU: Use of metabolic activation systems of tulip bulbs in the Ames test for environmental mutagens. *Bull Environm Contam Toxicol* 29:505, 1982

55. Higashi K: Microsomal cytochrome P-450 in higher plants. *Gann Monograph on Cancer Research* 30:49, 1985

56. Holsters M Hernalsteens JP, Van Montagu M, Schell J: Ti-plasmids of *Agrobacterium tumefaciens*: the nature of the TIP. *In*: Kahl G, Schell JS *eds.*, Molecular Biology of Plant

Tumors. *Academic Press New York* 269, 1982

57. Homburger F, Boger E: The carcinogenicity of essential oils, flavors, and spices: A review. *Cancer Res* 28:2372, 1978

58. Howland GP, Hart RW, Yette ML: Repair of DNA strand breaks after gamma-irradiation of protoplasts isolated from cultured wild carrot cells. *Mutat Res* 27:81, 1975

59. Jarvis SC, Jones LH, Hopper MJ: Cadmium uptake from solution and its transport from roots to shoots. *Plant Soil* 44:179, 1976

60. Kahl G: Molecular biology of wound healing: the conditioning phenomenon. *In:* Kahl and Schell *eds.,* Molecular Biology of Plant Tumors. *Acad Press New York* 211 p, 1982

61. Kaiser HE: Reaction of plant tissues to mammalian carcinogens. *Abs* Panel 17, p 178 *XI Intl Cancer Congress,* Florence, 1974

62. Kaplan JC, Wilbert SM, Collins JJ, Rakusanova T, Zamansky GB, Black PH: Isolation of simian virus 40-transformed inbred hamster cell lines heterogeneous for virus induction by chemical or radiation. *Virology* 68:200, 1975

63. Kearney PC, Kaufman DD: Herbicides, chemistry, degradation and mode of action. Vol. 1 and 2, M. Dekker, New York, 1976

64. King CM, Bednar TW, Linsmaier-Bednar EM: Activation of the carcinogen N-hydroxy-2-fluorenylacetamide: Insensitivity to cyanide and sulfide of the peroxidase -H_2O_2 induced formation of nucleic acid adducts. *Chem-Biol. Interactions* 7:185, 1973

65. Kurosaki F, Shudo K, Okamoto T, Isogai Y: Induction of cytokinin autonomous tobacco callus. Transformation of cultured tobacco callus by mutagenic heteroaromatic amines. *Biochem Biophys Res Comm* 102:1130, 1981

66. Land H, Parada LF, Weinberg RA: Cellular oncogenes and multistep carcinogenesis. *Science* 222:771, 1983

67. Leder P, Battery J, Lenoir G, Moulding C, Murphy W, Potter H, Stewart T, Taub R: Translocation among antibody genes in human cancer. *Science* 222:765, 1983

68. Lescure AM, Peaud-Lenoël C: Production par treatment mutagene de lignées cellulaires d'Acer pseudoplantanus L. anergiees à l'auxine. *CR Acad Sci Paris* 265:1803, 1967

69. Levine MA: A preliminary report on plants treated with the carcinogenic agents of animals. *Bull Torrey Bot Club* 61:103, 1934

70. Miller JA, Miller EC: Carcinogens occurring naturally in foods. *Federation Proc* 35:1316, 1976

71. Miller JA, Miller EC: Some historical aspects of N-aryl-carcinogens and their metabolic activation. *Environ Health Perspect* 49:3, 1983

72. Mok M, Kim S-G, Armstrong DJ, Mok DWS: Induction of cytokinin autonomy by N, N′-diphenylurea in tissue cultures of *Phasiolus lunatus* L *Proc Natl Acad Sci USA* 76:3880, 1979

73. National Toxicology Program, United States Public Health Service, Second Annual Report on Carcinogens, Dept. Health Human Services, Washington D.C., 268p, 1981

74. Nuss DL: Molecular biology of wound tumor virus. *Adv in Virus Research* 29:57, 1984

75. Ohigashi H, Ohtsuka T, Hirota M, Koshimizu K, Tokuda H, Ito: Tigliane type diterpene-esters with Epstein-Barr virus inducing activity from *Sapium sebiferum., Agric Biol Chem* 47:1617, 1983

76. Pandey KN, Sabharwal PS. *In vitro* neoplastic transformation of plant callus tissue by gamma-radiation. *Mutat Res* 62:459, 1979

77. Pearson MN, Karchesy JJ, Deeney AO, Deinzer ML, Beaudreau GS: Induction of endogenous avian tumor virus gene expression by pyrrolizidine alkaloids. *Chem Biol Interac* 49:341, 1984

78. Plewa MJ, Weaver KL, Blair LC, Gentile JM: Activation of 2-aminofluorene by cultured plant cells. *Science* 219:1427, 1983

79. Plewa MJ, Wagner ED Gentile GJ, JM Gentile: An evaluation of the genotoxic properties of herbicides following plant and animal activation.*Mutat Res* 136:233, 1984

80. Rakusanova T, Smales WP, Kaplan JC, Black PH: Replication of simian virus 40 in simian virus 40-transformed hamster kidney cells induced by mitomycin C or ^{60}Co gamma irradiation. *Virology* 88:300, 1978

81. Reichhart D, Salun J-P, Benveniste I, Durst F: Induction by manganese, ethanol, phenobarbitol and herbicides of microsomal cytochrome P-450 in higher plant tissues. *Arch Biochem Biophys* 196:301, 1979

82. Sandermann H, Scheel D, Trenck, Th. VD: Use of plant cell cultures to study the metabolism of environmental chemicals. *Ecotoxicol and Environ Safety* 8:167, 1984

83. Sargentini NJ, Smith KC: Much of spontaneous mutagenesis in *Escherichia coli* is due to error-prone DNA repair: implications for spontaneous carcinogenesis. *Carcinogenesis* 2:863, 1981

84. Scheel D, Sandermann H: Metabolism of DDT and Kelthane in cell suspension cultures of parsley (*Petroselinum hortense* Hoffm.) and soybean (*Glycine max* L.). *Planta* 133:315, 1977

85. Schilperoort RA, Veldstra H, Warnaar SO, Mulder G, Cohen JA: Formation of complexes between DNA isolated from tobacco crown gall tumors and RNA complementary to *Agrobacterium tumefaciens* DNA. *Biochim Biophys Acta* 145:523, 1967

86. Sims RC, Overcash MR: Fate of polynuclear aromatic compounds PNA's in soil-plant systems. *Residue Reviews* 88:1, 1983

87. Smith EF: Studies on the crown gall of plants. Its relation to human cancer. *J Cancer Res* 1:231, 1916

88. Smith HH: Plant genetic tumors. *Prog Exp Tumor Res* 15:138, 1972

89. Smith KC, Sargentini NJ: Metabolically-produced "UV like" DNA damage and its role in spontaneous mutagenesis. *Photochemistry and Photobiology* 42:801, 1985

90. Sporn MB, Roberts AB: Autocrine growth factors and cancer. *Nature* 313:745, 1985

91. Sunderman FW: Metal carcinogenesis in experimental animals. *Fd Cosmet Toxicol* 9:105, 1971

92. Sunderman FW: Carcinogenic effects of metals. *Fed Proc* 37:40, 1978

93. Sunderman FW: Recent advances in metal carcinogenesis. *Ann Clin Lab Sci* 14:93, 1984

94. Thomas PT, Evans HJ, Hughes DT: Chemically induced neoplasms in fungi. *Nature* 178:949, 1956

95. Thomashow LS, Reeves S, Thomashow MF: Crown gall oncogenesis: Evidence that a T-DNA gene from the Agrobacterium Ti-plasmid pTiA6 encodes an enzyme that catalyzes synthesis of indoleacetic acid. *Proc Natl Acad Sci USA* 81:5071, 1984

96. Tjell JC, Christensen TH, Bro-Rasmussen F: Cadmium in soil and terrestrial biota with emphasis on the Danish situation. *Ecotoxicol Environ Safety* 7:122, 1983

97. Trenck Th. VD, Sandermann H: Oxygenation of benzo(a)pyrene by plant microsomal fractions. *FEBS Lett* 119:227, 1980

98. Trenck Th. VD, Sandermann H: Incorporation of benzo(a)pyrene quinones into lignin. *FEBS Lett* 125:72, 1981

99. Van Bruwaene R, Kirchmann R, Impens R: Cadmium contamination in agriculture and zootechnology. *Experientia* 40:43, 1984

100. Van Hook RI: Transport and transportation pathways of hazardous chemicals from solid waste disposal. *Environmental health Perspectives* Vol 27:295, 1978

101. Van Larebeke N, Englen G, Holsters M, Van den Elsacker S, Zaenen I, Schilperoort RA, Schell J: A large plasmid in *Agrobacterium tumefaciens* essential for crown gall-inducing ability. *Nature* 252:169, 1974

102. Veleminský J, Van't Hof J: Repair of X-ray-induced single-strand breaks in root tips of Tradescantia clones 02 and 4430. *Mutat Res* 131:143, 1984
103. Waterfield MD, Scrace GT, Whittle N, Saroobant P, Johnsson A, Wasteson A, Westermark B, Heldin C-H, Huang JS, Deuel TF: Platelet-derived growth factor is structurally related to the putative transforming protein p 28 515 of simian sarcoma virus. *Nature* 304:35, 1983
104. Wattenberg LW: Chemoprevention of cancer. *Cancer Res* 45:1, 1985
105. Wattenberg LW, Leong JL: Inhibition of the carcinogenic action of benzo(a)pyrene by flavones. *Cancer Res* 30:1922, 1970
106. Wattenberg LW, Loub WD: Inhibition of polycyclic hydrocarbon-induced neoplasia by naturally-occurring indoles. *Cancer Res* 34:1410, 1978
:07. Weiss RA, Friis RR, Katz E, Vogt PK: Induction of avian tumor viruses in normal cells by physical and chemical carcinogens. *Virology* 46:920, 1971
108. White RE, Coon MJ: Oxygen activation by cytochrome P-450. *Ann Rev Biochem* 49:315, 1980
109. Wood AW, Wang MT, Chang RL, Newmark HL, Lehr RE, Yagi H, Sayer JM, Jerina DM, Conney AH: Inhibiton of the mutagenicity of bay-region diol epoxides of polycyclic aromatic hydrocarbons by naturally occurring plant phenols: exceptional activity of ellagic acid. *Proc Natl Acad Sci USA* Vol 79:5513, 1982
110. Yamamoto N: Interaction of viruses with tumor promoters *Rev Physiol Biochem Pharmacol* 101:111, 1984
111. Yamamoto N, Zur Hausen H: Tumor promoter TPA enhances transformation of human leukocytes by Epstein-Barr virus. *Nature* 280:244, 1979
112. Yamamoto H, Katsuki T, Hinuma Y, Hoshino H, Miwa M, Fujiki H, T Sugimura: Induction of Epstein-Barr virus by a new tumor promoter teleocidin, compared to induction by TPA. *Int J Cancer* 28:125, 1981
113. Zamansky G, Little J, Black P, Kaplan J: Inhibition of post-replication repair and the enhancement of induction of SV40 virus from transformed hamster kidney cells. *Mutat Res* 51:109, 1978
114. zur Hausen H, Bornkamm GW, Schmidt R, Hecker E: Tumor initiators and promoters in the induction of Epstein-Barr virus. *Proc Natl Acad Sci USA* 76:782, 1979

POSTSCRIPT

Several significant reports have been published after the bulk of this chapter was written. A selected number of these are included in this abbreviated postscript.

A new era of cancer research began when the activation of specific viral and cellular genes were identified as necessary for the expression of the neoplastic phenotype (1) The products of such oncogenes, including the extensively studied *ras* (13), appear to function in the mitogenic and developmental processes regulated in normal mammalian cells by the platelet-derived growth factor, epidermal growth factor, insulin-like growth factors or their receptors (8, 19, 21). In plants, growth regulation involves the auxin and cytokinin growth factor systems (12, 22). Systematic studies by Hashimoto and associates (7) have shown that 2-amino-6-methyldipyrido (1,2-a: 3',2'-d) imidazole (Glu-P-1) can induce cytokinin-autonomous growth in cultured plant cells, while its acetoxy ester can mutate a plasmid-borne human c-Ha-*ras* proto-oncogene into a functional oncogene able to transform mouse fibroplasts. Evidence for a *ras* gene in *Allium cepa* has been reported more recently (2), but its

role in higher plants remains to be explored.

Tumor-inducing (Ti) plamid-infected plant cells become auxin and cytokinin autonomous. Two genes have been localized in the Ti-plasmid that code for the production of indole-3-acetamide hydrolase and tryptophane-2-monooxygenase, enzymes yielding indole-3-acetic acid, the natural 'auxin' plant growth factor (14). Another region within the Ti-plasmid codes for the enzyme dimethylallyl-transferase required for the syntheses of the N-6 substituted adenine cytokinins (15). Cultured dicotyledonous plant cells, not infected with the Ti-plasmid, can also be transformed to cytokinin autonomy with a variety of chemicals (8, 72), including N-phenyl-N'-1,2,3-thiadiazol-5-ylurea (23), none as yet shown to be carcinogenic in mammalian cells.

A key carcinogenic event is believed to occur when proto-oncogenes are mutated into stable active oncogenic forms by chemical carcinogens (5, 17, 26). Recent studies indicate that many proto-oncogenes undergo base-specific genetic modifications that effect the persistent production of an altered gene product (2, 13). Both cyclic adenosine monophosphate and inositol phosphate second messenger systems appear to be involved with oncogene products (3, 4, 10, 25).

In addition to chemical carcinogens, plant-derived tumor promoting phorbol esters not only affect expression of viral genomes in host cells, but can also trigger inactive cellular genes to transcribe their gene products (6). They act by attaching to an outer cell membrane receptor, thereby setting in motion a series of events, via the second messengers, that activate quiescent cellular genes (18) in a manner similar to that affected by exogenous growth factors (11).

A significant number of xenobiotics, many of which are agricultural chemicals, have now been examined for their ability to be metabolically activated by plant cells or plant cell preparations into mutagenic compounds as evidenced by genetic alterations in the plant cells themselves (24) or with assays such as the Ames test (16). As in animal systems, the microsomal P-450 enzymes play an important role in such activation (9). Sandermann (20) has succinctly summarized the biochemical pathways for activation by the microsomal enzymes, peroxidases and active oxygen species.

Clearly, our knowledge on the significance of the phytosphere in relation to xenobiotic environmental hazards to man is in its infancy. Therefore, we must learn more about how plants can affect man's present and future burden from environmental chemicals.

POSTSCRIPT REFERENCES

1. Baltimore D: The beginning of the molecular description of a cancer. Cell Biophys. 9:17–31, 1986
2. Barbacid M. *Ras* genes. Ann. Rev. Biochem. 56:779–827, 1987
3. Berridge MJ: Growth factors, oncogenes and inositol lipids. Cancer Surveys 5:413–430, 1986
4. Berridge MJ: Inositol triphosphate and diacylglycerol, two interacting second messengers. Ann. Rev. Biochem. 56:159–193, 1987
5. Bizub D, Wood AW and Skalka AM: Mutagenesis of the Ha-*ras* oncogene in mouse skin tumors induced by polycyclic aromatic hydrocarbons. Proc. Natl. Acad. Sci. USA 83:6048–6052, 1986
6. Colamonici OR, Trepal JB, Vidal CA, Neckers LM: Phorbol ester induces c-*sis* gene transcription in stem cell line K-562.

Mol. Cell Biol. 6:1847–1850, 1986

7. Hashimoto Y, Kawachi E, Shudo K, Sekiya T: Activation of c-Ha-*ras* proto-oncogene by *in-vitro* chemical modification with 2-amino-6-methyldipyrido (1,2-a: 3′,2′-d) imidazole (Glu-1-P) and nitroquinoline-N-oxide (4-NQO). Nucleic Acids Symp. Ser. 17:135–138, 1986

8. Heldin CH, Betsholtz C, Claessen-Welsh L, Westermark B: Subversion of growth regulator pathways in malignant transformation. Biochim. Biophys. Acta 907(3):219–244, 1987

9. Higashi, K: Metabolic activation of environmental chemicals by microsomal enzymes of higher plants. Mutat. Res. 197:273–288, 1988

10. Hiwasa T, Sakiyama S, Noguchi S, Ha J–M, Miyazawa T, Yokoyama S: Degradation of c-*amp* binding protein is inhibited by c-Ha-*ras* gene products. Biochem. Biophys. Res. Comm. 146:731–738, 1987

11. Kamata T, Kathuria S, Fujita-Yamaguchi Y: Insulin stimulates the phosphorilation level of v-Ha-*ras* protein in membrane fraction. Biochem. Res. Comm. 144:19–25, 1987

12. Letham DS, Palni LMS: The biosynthesis and metabolism of cytokinins. Ann. Rev. Plant Physiol, 34:163–197, 1983

13. Levinson AD: Normal and activated *ras* oncogenes and their encoded products. Trends Genet. 2:81–85, 1986

14. Morris RO: Genes specifying auxin and cytokinin biosynthesis in phytopathogens. Ann. Rev. Plt. Physiol. 37:509–538, 1986

15. Morris RO, Powell GK: Genes specifying cytokinin biosynthesis in prokaryotes. Bio. Essays 6:23–28, 1987

16. Plewa MJ, Wagner ED, Gentile JM: The plant cell/microbe coincubation assay for the analysis of plant-activated mutagens. Mutat. Res. 197:207–219, 1988

17. Quintanilla M, Brown K, Ramsden M, Balmin A: Carcinogen specific mutation and amplification of Ha-*ras* during mouse skin carcinogenesis. Nature 322:78–80, 1986

18. Rabin MS, Doherty PJ, Gottesman MM: The tumor promoter phorbol-12-myristate-13-acetate induces a program of altered gene expression similar to that induced by platelet-derived growth factor and transforming oncogenes. Proc. Natl. Acad. Sci. USA 83:357–360, 1986

19. Roberts AB, Sporn MB: Growth factors and transformation: Cancer Surveys 5:405–412, 1986

20. Sandermann H: Mutagenic activation of xenobiotics by plant enzymes. Mutat. Res. 197:183–194, 1988

21. Sporn MB, Roberts AB: Peptide growth factors are multifunctional. Nature 332:217–219, 1988

22. Theologis A: Rapid gene regulation by auxin. Ann. Rev. Plt. Physiol. 37:407–438, 1986

23. Thomas JC, Katterman RR: Cytokinin activity induced by thidiazuron. Plt. Physiol. 81:681–683, 1986

24. Veleminský J, Gichner T: Mutagenic activity of promutagens in plants: indirect evidence of their activation. Mutat. Res. 197:221–242, 1988

25. Wakelam MJO, Davies SA, Houslay MD, McKay I, Marshall CJ, Hall A. Normal p21[N-*ras*] couples bombesin and other growth factors to inositol phosphate production. Nature 323:173–176, 1986

26. Wiseman RW, Stowers SJ, Miller EC, Anderson MW, Miller JA: Activating mutagens of the c-Ha-*ras* proto-oncogene in chemically induced hepatomas of the male B6C3F mouse. Proc. Natl. Acad. Sci. USA 83:5825–5829, 1986

INDEX